Natural Health
ENCYCLOPEDIA
OF
HOMEOPATHY

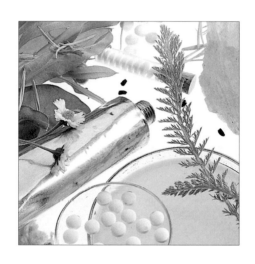

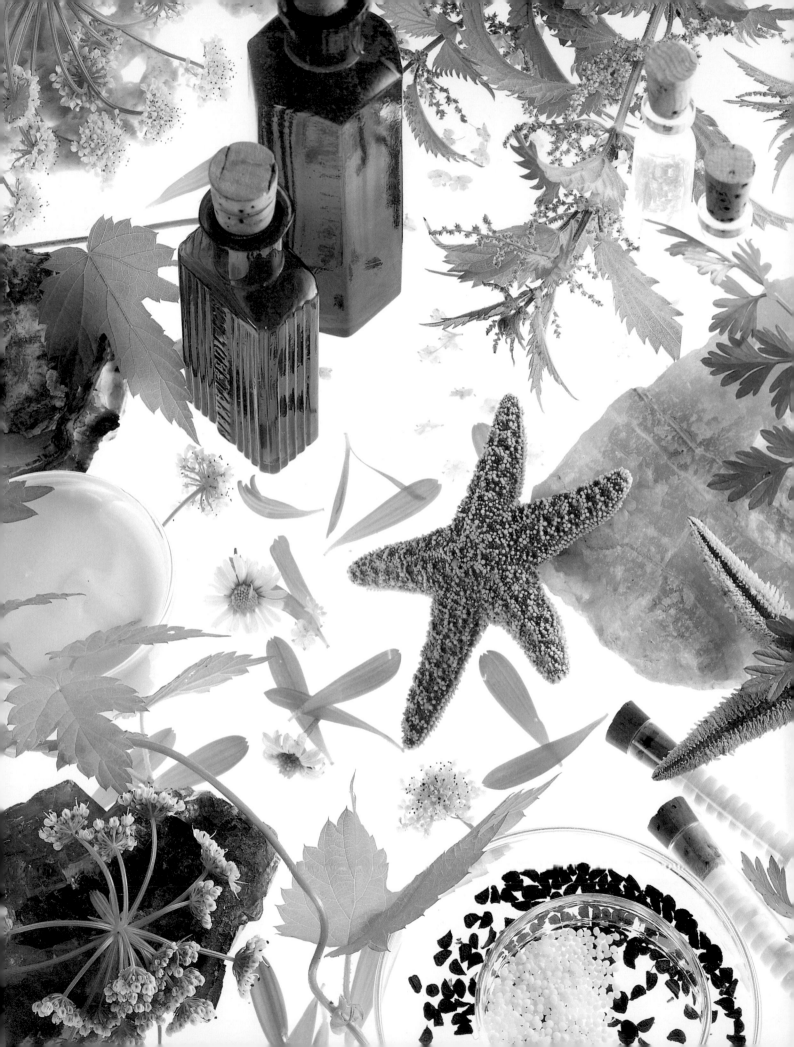

Natural Health
ENCYCLOPEDIA
OF
HOMEOPATHY

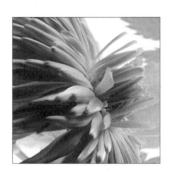
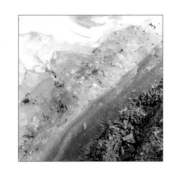
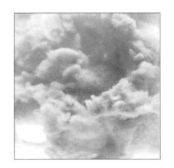

DR. ANDREW LOCKIE

A Dorling Kindersley Book

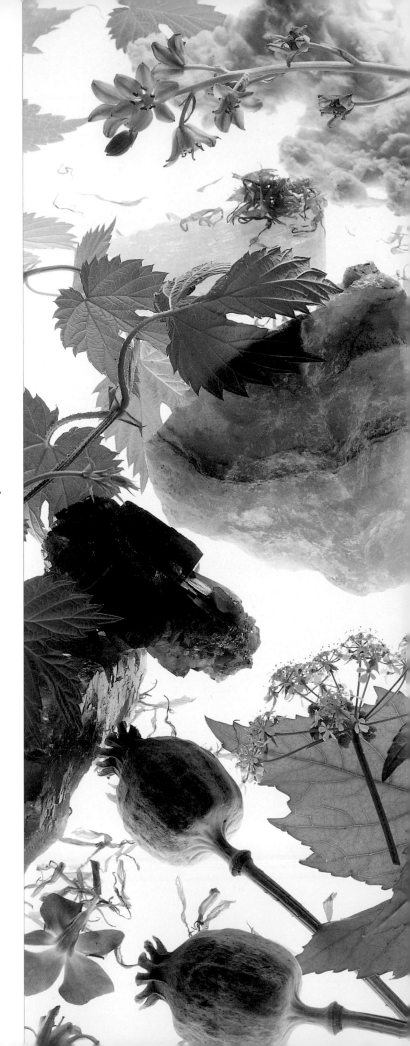

Dorling 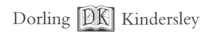 Kindersley

LONDON, NEW YORK, SYDNEY, DELHI, PARIS,
MUNICH and JOHANNESBURG

Natural Health magazine is the leading publication in the field of
natural self-care. For subscription information call 800-526-8440
or visit www.naturalhealthmag.com. Natural Health® is a
registered trademark of Weider Publications, Inc.

Senior Editor Stephanie Farrow
Project Editor (Ailments sections) Jude Garlick
Editor Joy McKnight
Senior Art Editor Hilary Krag
Designer Claudia Norris
Senior Managing Editor Krystyna Mayer
Deputy Art Director Carole Ash
DTP Designer Bridget Roseberry
Senior Production Controller Sarah Coltman
US Consultant David Riley, M.D.

IMPORTANT NOTICE

Do not try self-diagnosis of or attempt self-treatment for serious
or long-term problems without consulting a medical professional
or qualified practitioner. Do not undertake any self-treatment
while you are undergoing a prescribed course of medical
treatment without first seeking professional advice. Always seek
medical advice if symptoms persist. Do not exceed any dosages
recommended without professional guidance. Before taking
any remedy or supplement, refer to CONSULTING A PRACTITIONER,
page 176, and CHOOSING A REMEDY, page 216.

AUTHOR'S NOTE

Homeopathic remedy names are usually used in abbreviated form.
Commonly accepted abbreviations are used throughout the book.
Remedies are listed in the materia medica by Latin name.

To M, who showed me where my reset button is

First American Edition, 2000
2 4 6 8 10 9 7 5 3 1
Published in the United States by
Dorling Kindersley Publishing, Inc., 95 Madison Avenue
New York, NY 10016

Library of Congress Cataloging-in-Publication Data

Lockie, Andrew.
    Encyclopedia of homeopathy / by Andrew Lockie.
        p. cm.
    Includes index.
    ISBN 0–7894–5953–1
    1. Homeopathy—Encyclopedias. 2. Homeopathy—Popular
works. I. Title.

RX41 .L625 2000
615.5'32'03—dc21
                                                        99–049505

Reproduced in Italy by GRB Editrice, Verona
Printed and bound in China by L. Rex Printing Co. Ltd

see our complete catalog at
www.dk.com

CONTENTS

INTRODUCTION

Homeopathy is a holistic form of complementary medicine, aiming to treat the whole person rather than just the physical symptoms. It works on the principle that the mind and body are so strongly linked that physical conditions cannot be successfully treated without an understanding of the person's constitution and character.

While in conventional medicine people diagnosed with the same condition will generally be given the same medicine; in homeopathy the remedy given to a patient may well depend on a whole host of other factors, such as temperament, state of mind, and lifestyle. The key to the practice of homeopathy is the ability to understand and interpret the patient's symptoms – the outward signs of internal disorder – both before and after a remedy is given. This continuing relationship helps to make homeopaths particularly effective at discovering the underlying causes of frequently recurring ailments.

Homeopathy's safe, gentle approach complies with one of the most important rules of medical intervention – namely, that it should do no harm. Many common, everyday ailments may be treated safely and effectively at home using homeopathic remedies; should the common ailment develop into something worse, however – a cold into a chest infection, for instance – then a conventional doctor must be consulted. In general a conventional doctor should be consulted for any ailment that can be quickly and effectively treated by conventional medicine, or for any condition that requires conventional investigation. Certain serious ailments may also be alleviated using homeopathic remedies, but in the treatment of these conditions the experience of a qualified homeopathic practitioner is essential from the outset.

My aim in this book has been to give a wide-ranging and comprehensive account of homeopathy that is easy for the layman to understand and use. With several hundred homeopathic remedies available, choosing the right ones is obviously a complex matter. I have included more than 320 remedies and a great many ailments.

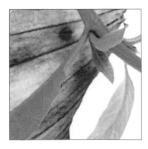 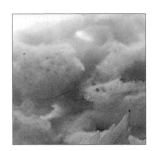 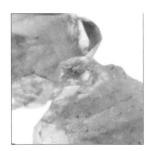

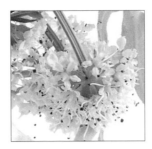
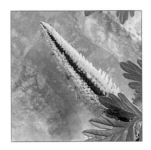
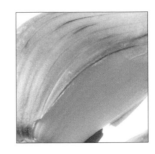

Those in the serious ailments section should under no circumstances be considered for self-treatment but always referred to a homeopathic practitioner. With their accompanying case histories, the inclusion of these serious conditions is intended to give the reader a greater insight into the way a homeopathic practitioner might approach particular problems and how consultations can help unlock a case and provide an understanding of how the illness has developed.

For this book a great deal of research has been carried out into the scientific classifications of the substances from which remedies are made, in order to correct the various errors and confusions that have crept in over the past 200 years. Thus, this book is currently the most scientifically accurate and up-to-date publication available on homeopathy. I have used current biological, zoological, and mineralogical classifications where possible, which has meant that some Latin names in this book differ from those to be found in earlier homeopathic textbooks. The remedies are listed in alphabetical order according to these Latin names in the materia medica.

It is a truism that no one system of medicine can cure every illness every time in every patient. However, an integrated approach to medicine can provide a flexible and pragmatic approach to health care, and homeopathy has an important role to play in this process. In many countries conventionally trained doctors are already turning increasingly to complementary therapies such as homeopathy to widen the range of treatments available to them.

To some extent, this is a response by the medical profession to the wishes of a growing number of patients who would like to take more responsibility for their own health. More and more people want to understand what they can do themselves to prevent illness and, if they do become ill, to understand the causes of their illness and determine how they can help themselves recover. Homeopathy offers a simple, effective, relatively inexpensive, and extremely safe way of accomplishing this, provided it is practiced with common sense.

Andrew H. Lockie

HOW TO USE THIS BOOK

THIS ENCYCLOPEDIA IS ORGANIZED into distinct sections. The first section places the therapy in its historical and contemporary context, and outlines the key principles and theories on which it is based. The second section contains an extensive materia medica, while the final sections deal respectively with serious ailments and those for which some degree of self-help may be appropriate. Guidelines for using these sections are outlined below. An appendix contains information on finding a practitioner (*see page 277*).

MATERIA MEDICA

More than 320 remedies are outlined here. The most important ones are organized in three sections according to their plant, mineral, or animal origin, while the fourth section comprises an overview of minor remedies. The remedies are listed by their Latin names. For easy reference, in the main index on page 278 the common remedy names appear in bold type.

1 **LATIN NAME** Botanical, minerological, or zoological name of the plant, mineral, or animal from which the remedy is made.

2 **REMEDY NAME** Commonly used name for the homeopathic remedy.

3 **COMMON NAMES** Commonly used name or names of the remedy source.

4 **INTRODUCTION** General information and history of the remedy source.

5 **ORIGIN** Habitat or source of the remedy substance.

6 **BACKGROUND** Historical, medicinal, or general context of the substance.

7 **PREPARATION** How the remedy is made from its primary source.

8 **REMEDY PROFILE** Outline of the principal physical, psychological, and

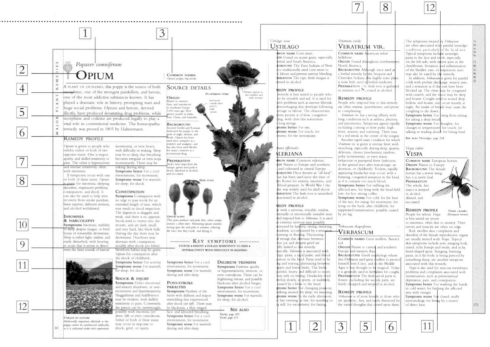

emotional symptoms associated with the remedy and the conditions treated.

9 **KEY SYMPTOMS** Primary symptoms associated with the remedy.

10 **AILMENTS** Key symptoms treated.

11 **SYMPTOMS BETTER/WORSE** Factors that improve or exacerbate symptoms.

12 **SEE ALSO** Cross-references to examples of the remedy's usage in the serious ailments and self-help sections.

SERIOUS AILMENTS

This section features certain common chronic conditions that may benefit from professional homeopathic consultation and treatment. They are not suitable for self-help. The conditions are primarily physical ailments, although some mental and emotional problems are included. They are organized into subsections according to the body system affected by each particular group of ailments. At the beginning of each subsection there is a clear, illustrated explanation of how the relevant body system works.

1 **AILMENT TITLE** Common name of the condition.

2 **INTRODUCTION** General description of the ailment and those affected by it.

3 **SYMPTOMS** Key symptoms associated with the condition.

4 **CAUSES** Principal reasons for the development of the condition.

5 **CONVENTIONAL CARE** Diagnosis and typical treatment using conventional medicine.

6 **HOMEOPATHIC MEDICINE** Typical homeopathic approach to treatment.

7 **LIFESTYLE** Recommendations concerning diet, exercise, and general lifestyle that may affect the condition and its treatment.

8 **CAUTION** Developments in the condition to watch out for, and general cautionary measures.

9 **CASE HISTORY** Details of an actual patient's experience of the condition, an outline of the homeopathic treatment prescribed, and update on subsequent progress.

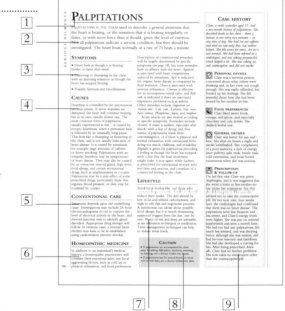

HOMEOPATHIC SELF-HELP

Arranged in chart form, this section covers a wide range of minor and acute physical, mental, and emotional ailments that may respond well to self-help measures. General conditions are organized by body system. Sections on specific ailments that are prevalent at particular stages of life follow, along with a first-aid section.

1 **SECTION TITLE** Body system or life stage to which ailments typically belong.

2 **INTRODUCTION** Body system or life stage context for the ailments in the section, and the potential of homeopathy for treating them.

3 **DISORDER** Symptoms of the ailment, along with causes, contributory factors, and possible wider implications for health. Additional self-help measures are also listed, as well as cautionary advice.

4 **SPECIFIC AILMENT** Brief description of a particular key symptom that may be associated with the disorder.

5 **PHYSICAL SYMPTOMS** Details of the particular profile of physical symptoms associated with the specific ailment.

6 **PSYCHOLOGICAL SYMPTOMS** Details of the particular psychological symptoms associated with the specific ailment.

7 **SYMPTOMS BETTER/WORSE** External or internal factors that may cause the particular combination of symptoms to improve or deteriorate.

8 **REMEDY & DOSAGE** The appropriate remedy for the set of symptoms, along with the recommended dosage and the duration of treatment.

SAFETY ISSUES

In addition to the specific cautions listed in the ailments sections, you should check the general cautions below and the warning symptoms (*see right*) before trying to treat yourself homeopathically. Unless otherwise stated, treatments recommended are for homeopathic remedies *only*; they do not advocate ingestion or application of the actual plants, minerals, or animals from which the remedy is made.

GENERAL CAUTIONS

◆ Consult a conventional doctor immediately if you have any warning symptoms (*see right*).

◆ See a conventional doctor if there is no improvement within two to three weeks (48 hours in children under five) or if symptoms get worse.

◆ Do not stop taking any prescribed conventional medication without consulting a conventional doctor first.

◆ Tell your homeopath about any prescribed conventional medication you are taking, and any other complementary treatments you are receiving.

◆ Tell a conventional doctor about any homeopathic remedies you are taking.

◆ Always check with a conventional doctor before embarking on any course of complementary treatment if you have any existing, chronic medical conditions or symptoms of illness.

◆ Do not embark on any program of vigorous exercise without consulting a conventional doctor first if you have any serious medical condition, such as high blood pressure or a heart condition, or if you are pregnant.

◆ Do not begin a course of homeopathic treatment without consulting a conventional doctor first if you are trying to conceive or are already pregnant.

◆ Do not use any herbal or aromatherapy products during pregnancy or if breast-feeding unless you are supervised by an herbal practitioner.

◆ If in any doubt about administering homeopathic treatments to children under 12 who have a chronic medical condition, or who are taking conventional drugs, consult a doctor or a medically qualified homeopathic practitioner.

◆ Do not exceed the recommended dosage of any nutritional supplements without professional supervision.

WARNING SYMPTOMS

Consult a conventional doctor immediately for:

◆ Chest pain or breathing difficulties; if there is acute pain in the chest, arms, jaw, or throat, call an ambulance.

◆ Unexplained dizziness.

◆ Persistent hoarseness, cough, or sore throat.

◆ Difficulty in swallowing.

◆ Persistent abdominal pain or indigestion.

◆ Coughing up of blood.

◆ Persistent, unexplained weight loss or fatigue.

◆ A mole that changes shape, size, or color, or itches or bleeds.

◆ Change in bowel or bladder habits.

◆ Passing of blood in the stools.

◆ Vaginal bleeding between menstrual periods, after sexual intercourse, or after menopause, or unusual vaginal discharge.

◆ Thickening of a breast, formation of a lump in a breast, or change in the shape or size of a breast; discharge or bleeding from a nipple.

◆ A lump in a testicle, or change in size or shape of a testicle; persistent failure to get an erection.

◆ Severe headaches; persistent one-sided headaches; visual disturbances.

◆ A sore or swelling that does not heal.

◆ Frequent and persistent back pain.

◆ Unexplained leg pain and swelling.

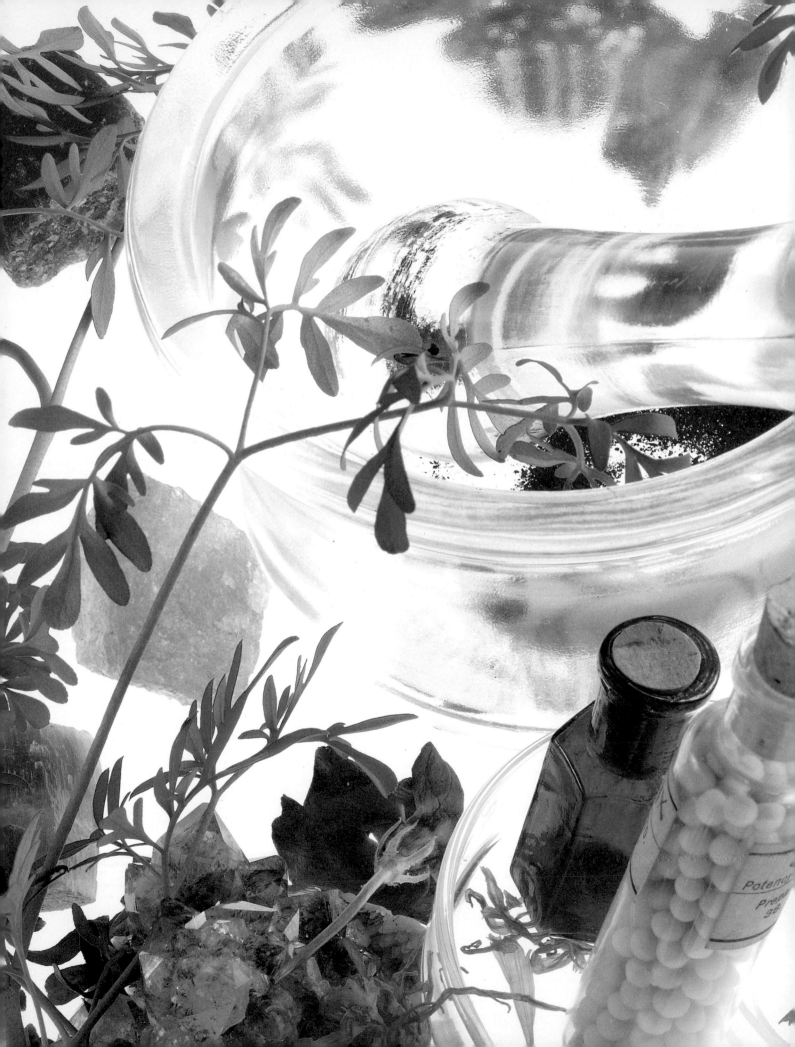

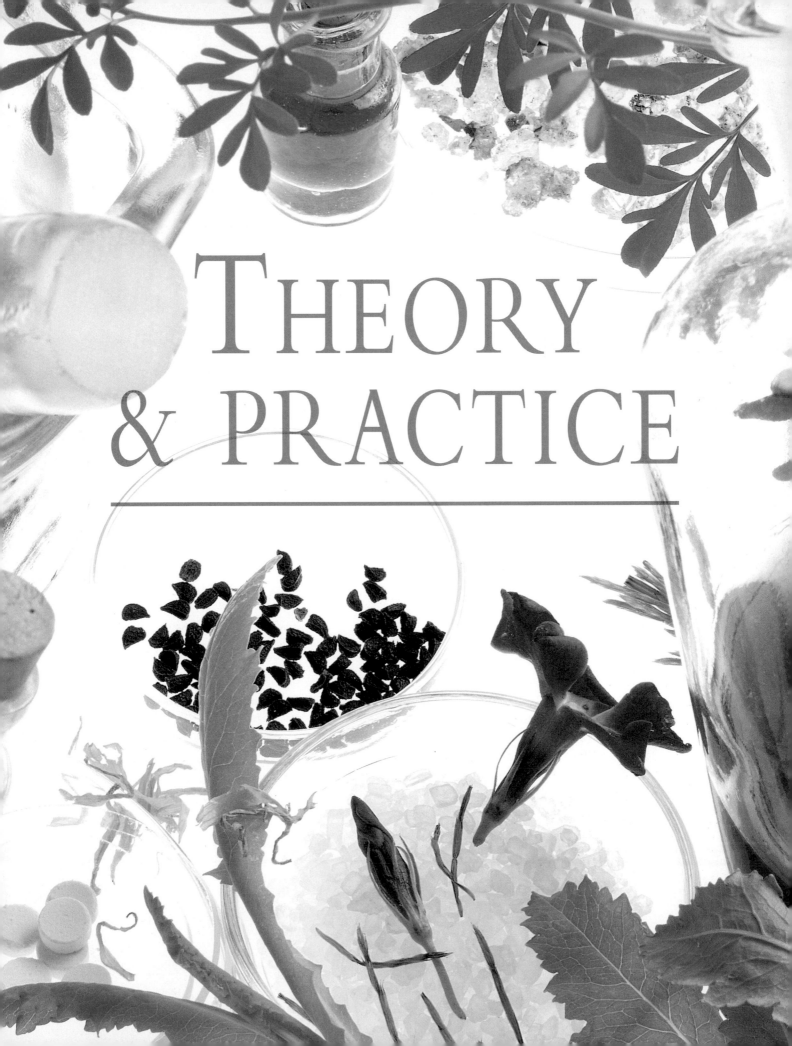

THEORY
& PRACTICE

HISTORY OF HOMEOPATHY

THE THEORIES AND PRINCIPLES OF HOMEOPATHY HAVE THEIR ORIGINS IN MEDICINAL TRADITIONS ESTABLISHED THOUSANDS OF YEARS AGO IN ANCIENT GREECE AND ROME.

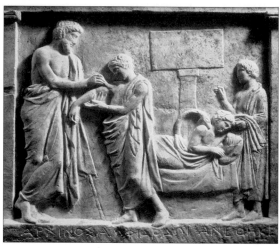

In the 5th century BCE the Greek physician Hippocrates (?460–?377 BCE) clearly established the idea that disease was the result of natural forces rather than divine intervention, and that patients' own powers of healing should be encouraged (*see page 19*). Contemporary medical theories were based upon the Law of Contraries, which advocated treating an illness by prescribing a substance that produced opposite or contrary symptoms to it. Diarrhea, for example, could be treated by a substance that caused constipation, such as aluminum hydroxide.

CLASSICAL ORIGINS OF HOMEOPATHY
This Greek votive relief, dating to the early 4th century BCE, illustrates the medicinal traditions of ancient Greece, on which both homeopathy and conventional Western medicine are based.

In contrast, Hippocrates developed the use of the Law of Similars, based on the principle that "like cures like" (*see page 18*). This theory proposed that substances capable of causing symptoms of illness in healthy people could also be used to treat similar symptoms during illness. For example, *Veratrum album* (white hellebore), which was considered effective against cholera, caused violent purging that led to severe dehydration if administered in large doses – symptoms exactly like those of cholera itself. Between the 1st and 5th centuries CE the Romans made further developments in medicine. They introduced more herbs into the pharmacopeias, improved public hygiene, and observed the structure and function of the human body. This was limited, however, by social taboo, which prevented the dissection of bodies. Existing medical knowledge was codified and rationalized by Galen (?130–?200 CE), a Roman physician, anatomist, and physiologist. He adopted many ancient Greek principles, including the Aristotelian theory of the "four humors," which claimed that the human body was made up of four humors – blood, choler (yellow bile), melancholy (black bile), and phlegm – that must be kept in balance to ensure vitality and health.

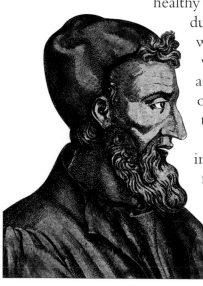

CLAUDIUS GALENUS
The Roman physician Galen added much to further understanding of the structure and function of the human body. He also established the theory of the "four humors," which influenced medicine for the next 1,400 years.

After the decline of the Roman Empire, little progress was made for centuries in the field of European medicine. A combination of herbal folklore, religious influences, and Galenic theory provided the basis for understanding and treating illness right through the 16th century. Only when the Swiss physician and alchemist Paracelsus (1493–1541) began to develop his theories did the study of medicine start to evolve again. Paracelsus revived the ancient Greek theory of the Doctrine of Signatures, which was based on the premise that the external appearance of a plant – God's "signature" – indicated the nature of its healing properties. For example, *Chelidonium majus* (greater celandine) was used to treat conditions affecting the liver and gallbladder because the yellow juice of the plant resembled bile.

Paracelsus argued that disease was linked to external factors such as contaminated food and water rather than to mystical forces, and he challenged his contemporaries to recognize the body's natural ability to heal itself, claiming that the practice of medicine should be based on detailed observation and "profound knowledge of nature and her works." According to his theories, all plants and metals contained active ingredients that could be prescribed to match specific illnesses. Concentrating on practical experiments rather than on alchemy, he laid the foundations for the early stages of chemistry and subsequent development of pharmaceutical medicine, introducing new medicines such as opium, sulfur, iron, and arsenic into the contemporary repertory. His exploration of the chemical and medicinal properties of many substances, and his advocacy of the Hippocratic concept of "like cures like," also made Paracelsus a key figure in the development of homeopathy. According to the British homeopath James Compton Burnett (1840–1901), the author of several important works on homeopathy that are still in use today, "Paracelsus planted the acorn from which the mighty oak of homeopathy has grown."

PHILIPPUS AUREOLUS PARACELSUS
One of the greatest scientists of the 16th century, Paracelsus was considered responsible for the transition from alchemy to modern chemistry. Known as the "father of chemistry," he believed in exact dosage, and stated that "it depends only on the dose whether a poison is a poison or not."

MEDICAL PRACTICES BY THE 19TH CENTURY

The period between the 16th and 19th centuries saw continued advancement in medical knowledge. The development of the printing press, and the publication of herbals in languages other than Latin, brought herbal knowledge into homes on a wide scale and decreased the monopoly of doctors and apothecaries on the treatment of illness. Hugely influential English-language herbals, such as the *Herball* of John Gerard (1545–1612) and *The English Physitian* by Nicholas Culpeper (1616–54), were published during this period.

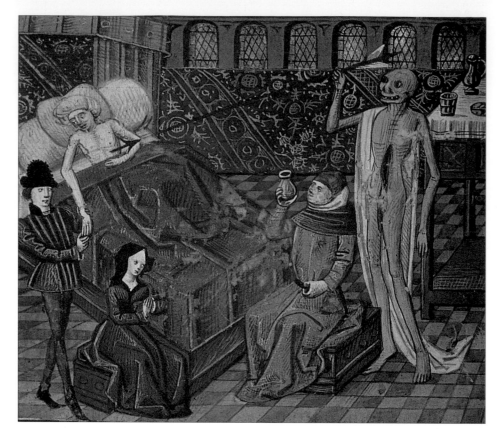

ALLEGORY OF DEATH
Between the Middle Ages and the Enlightenment there was little faith in medical practice: In this 15th-century French book illumination, doctors examine a patient's pulse and urine, while death waits in the wings.

Despite medical advances and greater dispersal of herbal lore, however, the general health of the population remained poor in many Western countries. Industrialization was accompanied by population transition from rural areas to polluted, overcrowded cities, and working conditions that were frequently unsafe. Standards of public hygiene and medical care were often low, and the mentally ill were treated in asylums. Violent medical practices, including bloodletting, leeching, and purging, became increasingly widespread and were often detrimental to people's health. Toxic substances such as lead, mercury, and arsenic were in common usage medicinally, and the cure often proved to be more harmful to patients than the illness, with some patients dying and many more suffering serious long-term side effects as a result of the drastic or extreme treatments they had received.

THE ORIGINS OF HOMEOPATHY

This was the cultural and scientific milieu in which the German doctor Samuel Christian Hahnemann (1755–1843) began practicing in 1780. He continued in practice for nine years, during which time he became increasingly disillusioned with the harsh medical methods of the day. In articles written to supplement his income, Hahnemann attacked the extreme medical practices of the day, advocating instead good public hygiene, improved housing conditions, better nutrition, fresh air, and exercise. Eventually his convictions led him to cease work as a doctor. He wrote later that it had been agony to work "always in darkness," with no secure principles in place regarding health and disease.

At this time a period of great social and political change evolved in Europe. The Industrial Revolution and the Enlightenment were accompanied by great technological and scientific advances, and increasing freedom of thought and expression. This intellectual climate encouraged important developments in the study of medicine, including the isolation of active ingredients from herbs – for example, the extraction of morphine from the opium poppy in 1803. In 1790, while translating *A Treatise on Materia Medica* by Scottish teacher, physician, and chemist Dr. William Cullen, Hahnemann began an investigation that was to prove paramount to the subsequent development of homeopathy. In his treatise Cullen argued that quinine, when isolated from *Cinchona officinalis* (*see page 49*), was a good treatment for malaria because it was an astringent. Hahnemann knew that other, more powerful astringents had no such effect on malaria. He dosed himself with quinine, recording the results and effectively beginning the first "proving" (*see page 23*). Although he did not have malaria, he found that he began to develop symptoms of the disease one after the other. With each dose of quinine the symptoms recurred and lasted for several hours, but if he stopped taking quinine his symptoms began to disappear. Hahnemann went on to test quinine on other people, noting their reactions in great detail. The test subjects were not allowed to eat heavily spiced foods or to drink alcohol or coffee, which he felt might distort the results. He repeated the proving process on other substances that were in use as medicines, such as arsenic and belladonna, and used the results to build up a "symptom picture" of each remedy's effects (*see page 23*).

SAMUEL CHRISTIAN HAHNEMANN
Born in 1755 in Meissen, Germany, Hahnemann studied at the universities of Leipzig, Erlangen, and Vienna before qualifying in medicine and chemistry in 1779. Abhorrence of the medical practices of the time led him to devise a new system of medicine, which he called homeopathy.

After conducting provings for six years, Hahnemann extended his research to the sick. Prior to prescription, he gave his patients a thorough physical examination and noted any existing symptoms. He questioned them closely regarding their lifestyle, general health, outlook on life, and other factors that made them feel better or worse. Following the principle of like cures like, Hahnemann then matched individual symptoms as closely as possible to the symptom picture of a remedy, and prescribed accordingly.

DEVELOPMENT & DEFINITION

Hahnemann's work gradually brought about the establishment of a new type of medicine. In 1796 he published his first book on the subject, entitled *A New Principle for Ascertaining the Curative Powers of Drugs and Some Examinations of Previous Principles*. He called his new system "homeopathy," from the Greek *homeo,* meaning "similar," and *pathos,* meaning "suffering." In 1810 he set out its principles in *The Organon of Rationale Medicine*, and two years later began teaching homeopathy at the University of Leipzig. During the course of his lifetime Hahnemann proved about 100 remedies, and also continued to develop and refine the theory and practice of the system (*see page 18*).

The medical establishment remained generally very skeptical of Hahnemann's theories, and he in turn continued to be intensely critical of conventional medical practice. He became known as the "raging hurricane" due to his furious tirades and sarcastic critiques during lectures at Leipzig. He also antagonized contemporary pharmacists by giving only one medicine at a time, which was contrary to their (highly lucrative) practice of generally prescribing expensive mixtures of several remedies. During the 19th century homeopathy spread rapidly across Europe to Asia and the Americas. In the US Dr. Constantine Hering (1800–80) and Dr. James Tyler Kent (1849–1916) were responsible for popularizing the therapy and introducing new ideas and practices (*see page 19*). By the time of Hahnemann's death in 1843, homeopathy was firmly established in many parts of the world, although there remained antagonism and distrust between the advocates of conventional medicine and those of homeopathy. Between 1860 and 1890 homeopathy flourished; many homeopathic hospitals and schools were opened, and many new remedies were proved, considerably enlarging the materia medica. Hahnemann's followers were often doctors who defected from conventional medicine after personally experiencing treatment. They included an English doctor, Frederick Quin (1799–1878), who was cured of cholera by the *Camphora* remedy. Quin first visited Hahnemann in Germany in 1826, and went on to introduce homeopathy to the UK, founding the first homeopathic hospital in London in 1849. During a cholera outbreak in 1854 the mortality rate at his hospital was less than half that of conventional hospitals. This information was suppressed by the national Board of Health on the grounds that "the figures would give sanction to a practice opposed to the maintenance of truth and the progress of science," illustrating the stranglehold the medical establishment had achieved within social institutions.

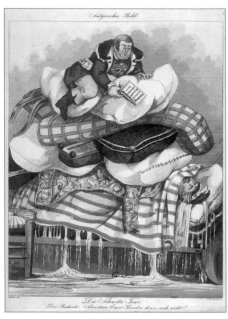

DUBIOUS MEDICAL PRACTICES
Hahnemann believed passionately that many contemporary medical practices were harmful, exploiting the infirm or gullible, and he was not alone in his criticism. Medicine was often the subject of satire for its "quackish" treatments, as shown in this 19th-century cartoon illustrating the "Sweat Cure," with the servant enquiring, "Is Your Lordship Still Not Sweating?"

DECLINE & RESURRECTION

The American Institute of Homeopathy was established in 1846, two years before the American Medical Association. By the late 19th century it was a significant part of American medical practice, with about 15 percent of doctors being practicing homeopaths. During the early 20th century, however, homeopathy became largely overshadowed by conventional medicine, principally due to the rise of the AMA.

The British Medical Association played a similar role in the UK, and divisions within homeopathy began to weaken the force of its message still further. Strict followers of Hahnemann and Kent's original theories followed "classical" or "Kentian" constitutional prescribing, believing that a person's emotional characteristics and physical symptoms should be taken into account and favoring high potencies (*see page 19*). Led by the British homeopath Dr. Richard Hughes (1836–1902), one strand of practitioners had, however, begun to prescribe based on pathological symptoms alone, favoring low doses. This unfortunate division in homeopathic practice enabled the conventional medical establishment to gain the upper hand, and by the 1920s homeopathy had been largely suppressed in the UK.

During the late 20th century there has been a resurgence in the popularity of homeopathy, possibly due to disenchantment with aspects of conventional medicine. In many countries, particularly in central Europe, its popularity never waned to the same extent as in the US and UK, although differences in practice have evolved. Single-remedy classical prescribing is prevalent worldwide, although in Germany and France complex homeopathy or polypharmacy (the use of combination remedies or several remedies) is also popular (*see page 21*). In Australia there is a strong link with naturopathy, with homeopathic remedies often incorporated into naturopathic practice. In India homeopaths have long worked successfully alongside traditional Ayurvedic medicine and conventional medicine. In the 1990s, courses in Eastern Europe pioneered by British teachers revitalized interest in homeopathy, and in Russia it continues to be implemented and developed. In South America homeopathy is widely taught in medical schools, while in the US it is undergoing a major resurgence of popularity. Figures suggest that more than 2.5 million Americans used homeopathic remedies in 1990, with upward of 800,000 people consulting homeopaths.

LONDON HOMEOPATHIC HOSPITAL
The astoundingly low mortality rate at this hospital during the 1854 cholera outbreak in London prompted a government inspector to note, "if it should please the Lord to visit me with cholera I would wish to fall into the hands of a homeopathic physician."

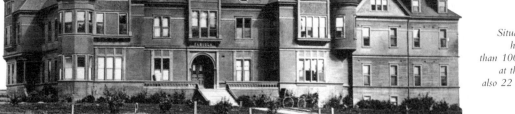

FABIOLA HOSPITAL
Situated in northern California, the Fabiola homeopathic hospital was one of more than 100 homeopathic hospitals operating in the US at the turn of the 20th century. There were also 22 homeopathic medical schools and more than 1,000 homeopathic pharmacies.

KEY PRINCIPLES & THEORIES

HOMEOPATHS BELIEVE THAT GOOD HEALTH DERIVES FROM AN EQUILIBRIUM BETWEEN THE MIND AND BODY, WHICH IS MAINTAINED BY A "VITAL FORCE" THAT REGULATES THE BODY'S SELF-HEALING CAPABILITIES.

The vitalistic concept of science had existed for many years by the time Hahnemann was developing his theories. It claims that all living things possess a subtle energy beyond their physical and chemical states, and that even inanimate matter may contain vitality. Hahnemann applied this view to both the human body and to seemingly inert substances from all the kingdoms of matter. Thus the vital force of any plant, mineral, or animal could be harnessed to produce a powerful medicine when "potentized" (*see right*). Hahnemann viewed illness as the result of an internal imbalance affecting the body's vital force and disrupting its equilibrium. If this vital force is put under strain or weakened by this imbalance, illness may develop. In stimulating the body's self-healing abilities to fight any imbalance, the vital force produces symptoms. These may manifest externally, producing such symptoms as fever or a skin rash, or may emerge as emotional or psychological states, such as weepiness or great irritability. An effective medicine must help the vital force redress the internal imbalance, enabling the symptoms produced by that imbalance to disappear, and this is what homeopaths seek to achieve. Hahnemann adopted the principle of *similia similibus curentur*, or "like cures like" (*see box*), first established in the 5th century BCE by Hippocrates. His "provings" of remedies (*see page 23*) aimed to establish the particular set of symptoms, or "symptom picture," produced by taking a substance. When the symptom picture matched the particular set of symptoms produced by an illness or imbalance in a patient, that remedy was indicated as the most effective at stimulating the vital force to treat the disorder. The key was – and in classical homeopathy still is – to establish which remedy most exactly matches a patient's symptom picture.

HIPPOCRATES
This Greek physician became known as the "father of medicine" for his work in moving healing away from mysticism and religion. He laid the foundations for the science of medicine as it is known today, and established key principles, among them the theory of "like cures like" (see box, opposite).

LIKE CURES LIKE

According to the concept of like cures like, also known as the Law of Similars, substances that are capable of provoking certain symptoms in an otherwise healthy body can also act curatively on similar symptoms in a sick person. For instance, belladonna would be used to treat scarlet fever, since the symptoms of belladonna poisoning closely resemble those of scarlet fever.

Many of the substances from which remedies are made are highly potent or possibly even poisonous. Hahnemann used only small doses of substances in his medicines, but to his consternation his patients still tended to suffer side effects, or "aggravations," as he called them. He developed a technique called "potentization" (*see page 28*), which involved diluting and shaking the medicine vigorously or banging it on a hard surface during preparation. This turbulent motion, which Hahnemann called "succussion," apparently released more potency into the medicine, even at lower dilutions. To Hahnemann's surprise, his research showed that microdilutions prepared with the additional turbulent energy provided by potentization seemed to have a much stronger effect than standard dilutions, providing a rapid and gentle effect that was long lasting. Homeopaths therefore need to give only this minimum, completely safe dosage. Hahnemann's original theories were expanded by the American homeopaths Dr. Constantine Hering and Dr. James Tyler Kent (*see page 16*). Dr. Hering developed three basic Laws of Cure to explain how illness is cured in homeopathy (*see box*), while Dr. Kent established a clear framework by which a course of treatment could be understood. Among the possible scenarios, the patient gets better; the patient gets worse; the patient's condition remains unchanged; the patient initially gets worse but then gets better. Dr. Kent laid down 12 different possible outcome scenarios, including the above, which enabled homeopaths to determine how treatment should be continued and assess whether a particular remedy had been successful or not. Since the 1970s the Greek homeopath George Vithoulkas has done a great deal of research to update the scenarios and refine the theory and practice of homeopathy.

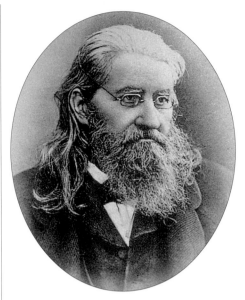

DR. CONSTANTINE HERING
This 19th-century American homeopath formulated three "Laws of Cure" that provide a useful guide for interpreting a patient's development.

LAWS OF CURE

◆ As a patient progresses toward cure, symptoms move from the inner organs of the body (those most vital to life) to the outer, less vital tissues and organs.

◆ Cure usually takes place from the top of the body to the bottom; so, for example, head symptoms clear first, gradually followed by any symptoms on the extremities.

◆ Old symptoms often resurface during the curative process, usually in reverse order of their first appearance. Immunologists claim that the body has the capacity to "remember" every "assault" on the system that it has ever reacted to, and this process confirms that capacity.

CONSTITUTION & SUSCEPTIBILITY

In homeopathic terms, a person's "constitution" describes his or her state of health, including temperament and any inherited and acquired characteristics. Homeopaths believe that healthy people resist developing sickness, despite being constantly exposed to an enormous variety of potentially harmful viruses and bacteria, since their vital force is strong and their susceptibility is therefore low. Their degree of susceptibility to illness may change, however, from hour to hour and day to day. It depends on a particular catalyst that triggers an imbalance in the vital

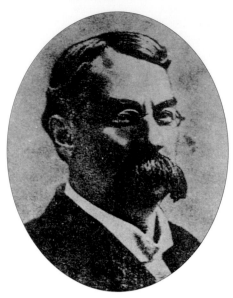

DR. JAMES TYLER KENT
This hugely influential US homeopath was responsible for establishing a clear framework on which to judge the efficacy of prescribed treatment (see page 19), and also carried out a great deal of research into new substances to enlarge the materia medica of homeopathic medicines.

force, such as exposure to the cold or heat, stress or emotional distress, overworking, exposure to pollutants, or intake of drugs (*see page 177*). Underlying "miasmatic" factors may also affect the ability of the vital force to withstand any onslaught (*see below*). Some homeopaths place great importance on the patient's "constitutional type" when they are prescribing treatment, choosing remedies whose "symptom picture" (*see page 23*) exactly match the individual's psychological and physical makeup when healthy. These remedies are taken when healthy to strengthen the patient's vital force and to build up resistance to symptoms that may develop in the future. Health problems generally fall into two categories: acute or short-term illness, arising rapidly and potentially clearing up quickly (such as a cold or minor digestive problem); and chronic, long-term ill health (such as rheumatoid arthritis or diabetes), which has a tendency to be recurrent, deep-seated, or progressively degenerative.

Homeopathic remedies work to support the self-healing powers of the vital force in its response to illness, speeding recovery from acute illness and making the duration of the illness less debilitating, aiding recovery from recurrent illness or preventing its recurrence altogether. Remedies must be carefully chosen, however, if they are to work at optimum efficiency, and chronic conditions are best treated by qualified homeopaths rather than left to self-diagnosis.

MIASMS & PREDISPOSITION

After many years of developing his ideas, Hahnemann noticed that some patients still did not seem to respond to the remedies prescribed for them, or that they relapsed after a short time. He studied these cases all together as a group, and concluded that general, inherent, higher-level themes of ill health were to blame. These he called "miasms." They can be described as the chronic effect of an underlying disease or disease susceptibility present in an individual or in previous generations of that person's family. Three particular miasms were identified by Hahnemann – *Psora* (which relates to scabies), *Sycosis* (which is linked with gonorrhea), and *Syphilis* (which is based on syphilis). Cancer and tuberculosis are regarded by some as further potential miasms. He developed remedies called "nosodes," made from the diseases themselves, to combat these miasms. Since all infected material went through the potentizing process of dilution and succussion, it became sterile and completely safe to use.

NOSODES

Hahnemann developed nosode remedies to counteract the miasms he believed to be responsible for sometimes "blocking" treatment. They were made from infected tissue or bacteria, but were perfectly safe, since the substances were sterilized and potentized. *Psorinum*, for instance, is made from scabies-infected tissue, while *Carcinosin* is derived from cancerous tissue.

The concept of a miasm proposes a model of health that has layers of predisposition or imbalance. In some cases more layers need to be peeled away than in others to reach lasting good health. At a certain stage in the treatment process, an underlying miasm may become clearly active. Treatment can then be tailored to overcome it. However, it should be emphasized that this does not mean that a person actually *has* the diseases that are implied by the names of the miasms. Rather the names describe the inheritance of a predisposition to a specific pattern of possible symptoms or a tendency to fall ill in a particular way – the person's susceptibility. For instance, *Psora* relates to slow development and poor nutrition; whereas *Sycosis* is associated with a frantic pace of life and overactivity of both mental and physical processes; and *Syphilis* describes a pattern of breakdown, decay, deterioration, and eating away.

TYPES OF HOMEOPATHIC PRACTICE

Various prescribing habits have developed in different countries or at different times. A clear conceptual division has emerged between two main schools of practice, classical and complex. Classical homeopaths generally treat with a single remedy that exactly matches the patient's inherent constitutional type and symptom picture. There are occasions, however, particularly in the case of acute illness or injury, where the physical symptoms far outweigh the emotional and other symptoms. In cases such as these a more pragmatic approach may be taken, using combinations of remedies in low potencies. Thus, for instance, five or six remedies known to be helpful for the flu might be combined in a single tablet. This is the complex approach, based on the theories of British homeopath Dr. Richard Hughes (*see page 17*), and also known sometimes as combination homeopathy or polypharmacy. In some situations, generally of an acute nature, it may be adopted by classical homeopaths, but in certain countries it is actually the standard method of prescribing. In 1948 it was officially sanctioned by the American Institute of Homeopathy, and in many European countries, such as France and Germany, polypharmacy is more common than classical homeopathy.

Further variations on the homeopathic principle include isopathy, in which a potentized microdilution of the substance causing the disorder is actually used to treat the symptoms: For example, *Apis* (which is made from the stinger of a bee) might be given to someone to treat a bee sting. A classical homeopath will generally expect a success rate of only 20 to 30 percent using this method, since it does not take into account the unique constitution of each patient. A refinement of this concept is tautopathy, in which the *exact* substance triggering the symptoms is used to make a remedy for treating those symptoms. In theory this means that the remedy for a bee sting would be prepared from the *actual bee* that had inflicted the sting. In practice the concept is most commonly used for allergic reactions, such as treating a child with a remedy made from a vaccination to which the child has reacted.

BUILDING A MATERIA MEDICA

MORE THAN 4,000 SUBSTANCES FROM THE PLANT, ANIMAL, AND MINERAL KINGDOMS HAVE BEEN TESTED SINCE HAHNEMANN FIRST DEVELOPED HIS THEORIES, RESULTING IN A MATERIA MEDICA THAT CONTAINS OVER 2,000 REMEDIES.

The reasons why particular substances were selected as homeopathic remedies are complex and varied. Many were familiar from traditional Western folk- or herbal lore. Some, such as mercury, were used in contemporary conventional medicine. Others included minerals or elements that had been used as nutritional supplements, such as zinc. Out of curiosity, or because they had a long herbal tradition or were known to have a strong, even toxic effect, different substances were tried and the information cataloged. The greatest influence came initially from herbalists in Europe but, as knowledge grew of the medicinal traditions of other cultures, more substances were tested for their homeopathic potential. European explorers and settlers filtered back information amassed on their travels. Dr. Constantine Hering (*see page 16*), for instance, visited South America and discovered the healing properties of the bushmaster snake (*see page 109*).

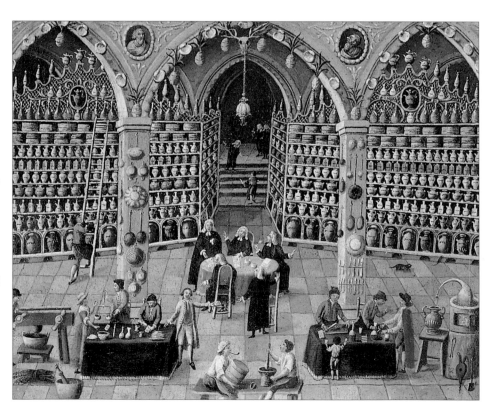

THE WORLD OF THE APOTHECARY
The eclectic assortment of plants and minerals mixed and dispensed in a standard 18th-century apothecary are illustrated in this painting of the period by an anonymous artist. Many of these medicines were tested by Hahnemann and others for their curative potential as homeopathic remedies.

Hahnemann set down strict guidelines for testing, or "proving," potential remedies. This term developed from *Prüfung*, the German word for a trial. A set of volunteers, or "provers," take a trial substance in different strengths, or potencies (*see page 19*), and make a detailed, daily record of their moods, sensations, and any symptoms that develop. Symptoms are categorized as general, relating to a temperamental picture, or specific, affecting a particular part of the body. Surrounding or provoking circumstances, and triggers that make symptoms better or worse, are all noted. Certain general, physical, and psychological affinities appear more evident than others, and some symptoms will be very common among the provers; for example, indifference to loved ones or a headache first thing in the morning that gets better after eating. These are "first-line" symptoms. Other symptoms may be experienced by only a few provers, or even one. These are known respectively as "second-line" and "third-line" symptoms. Any symptom that can be shown to be unlike the person's usual state of health will be recorded. This information is then compiled to produce a "symptom picture" that takes into account the potential variations produced by different provers' constitutional types. Often this will then be compared with information about the substance and its characteristics, possibly from its prior use within herbal or folk medicine, or from knowledge of its toxicology, to deepen understanding of the remedy.

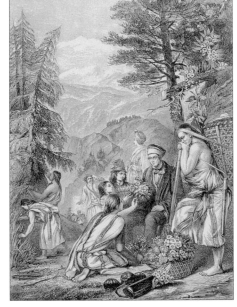

ENLARGING THE MATERIA MEDICA
Explorers to new worlds, such as the Victorian naturalist depicted in this engraving, published in 1868, collected samples and information on a wide range of plants and animals, some of which were then added to the materia medica of homeopathic remedies.

As understanding of each remedy's "symptom picture" grows, an archetypal "character" emerges. Essential or "keynote" characteristics, both mental and physical, can be established to give a thumbnail summary, enabling homeopaths to recognize cases in which a particular remedy is appropriate. Dr. James Tyler Kent (*see page 19*) carried out a great deal of research to enlarge knowledge of the remedies in the materia medica, and his work has been built on and augmented by many other practitioners.

Beyond the individual remedies, it is possible to make connections between remedies and to establish group relationships. Studying the group of remedies based on potassium or calcium compounds, for example, reveals themes such as physical weakness with all *Kalium* remedies, or sensitivity and shyness with all *Calcium* remedies. This thematic analysis is most obvious in clear categories like families of the Periodic Table, which have recently been researched by the British homeopath Jeremy Sherr. Relationships between plants within the same botanical family, or between animals with common links, can also be found. For example, all snake-based remedies tend to affect the blood and nervous system, and are for highly oversensitive individuals. The breadth of information available from some of the old provings is not complete, while other provings are very well documented. New provings tend to be carefully managed and usually give a full picture.

DEVELOPMENT OF HOMEOPATHY

HAHNEMANN'S FIRST EXPERIMENTS ON HIMSELF ARGUABLY CONSTITUTED SOME OF THE EARLIEST MEDICAL TRIALS. MEDICAL RESEARCH HAS BECOME FAR MORE SOPHISTICATED SINCE THEN, YET STRICT CLINICAL TRIALS INTO THE EFFICACY OF HOMEOPATHY WERE RARE UNTIL AS LATE AS THE 1980s.

While funding existed for major drug research due to investment by drug companies, such funding has been harder to find for homeopathic trials. Nor do homeopathic trials have the same kind of access to the research facilities of universities, hospitals, and researchers. Trials into homeopathy are further disadvantaged by the fact that so much depends on the skill and judgment of the practitioner in assessing the appropriate remedy for the patient. One of the most important issues to be addressed in trials is the influence of the placebo effect (*see box*). Clinical trials conducted by Dr. D. Taylor-Reilly in 1986 in Glasgow, Scotland, demonstrated a clear, statistically significant improvement in patients treated homeopathically that could not be attributed purely to a placebo response. He concluded that either homeopathy does work or that clinical trials do not. There have also been metanalyses, in which a large group of similar trials are analyzed as if they were one huge study, often yielding more significant results than small-scale trials might do individually. Three of the most important metanalyses to date are that led by Prof. J. Kleijnen, published in the *British Medical Journal* in 1991; that led by Dr. J. P. Boissel, which was carried out for the European Commission and published in Brussels in 1996; and that by Dr. K. Linde and others, published in *The Lancet* in 1997. All three metanalyses were done by skeptical, independent researchers, none of whom were practicing homeopaths, and all three concluded that, despite their best efforts to show otherwise, homeopathy has an action above and beyond that of merely a placebo. Valuable trials of homeopathy in veterinary medicine, undertaken by the British homeopathic veterinarian Mr. C. Day in 1984, suggest that homeopathy's action cannot be attributed purely to a placebo effect if it works on animals, since animals are not susceptible to such influences.

PLACEBO RESPONSE

In clinical drug trials, some of the test subjects are given a genuine, active medication, while others are given a placebo – an inactive medication, often a sugar pill, which is given in place of genuine treatment. Test subjects do not know whether they are receiving the active drug or the placebo. Research into the immune system has revealed that the expectations of patients can actually influence their healing processes. Thus, since they expect their medication to work, the placebo may have a therapeutic effect. Clinical trials test active drugs against a control group receiving a placebo to ensure that any positive effects take into account this placebo response. The experimental group must perform significantly better than those taking the placebo for the test drug to be deemed effective.

Various individual trials have demonstrated a degree of success for homeopathic treatment of specific ailments, such as a 1980 study by Dr. R. G. Gibson in Glasgow of homeopathic treatment for rheumatoid arthritis, and a 1994 trial of homeopathy for diarrhea in Nicaragua by American pediatrician Dr. J. Jacobs. Positive trials also exist on the efficacy of homeopathy for toothaches and teething, including a 1985 French study in Lyon by Dr. P. Berthier, and a German study published in 1994 by Dr. A. Vestweber in *Erfahrungsheilkunde*.

On the theoretical side there is ongoing research into finding a scientific explanation for how a homeopathic remedy can be effective when it has been diluted so much that not a single molecule of the remedy's base ingredient is left in the water. However, exciting research suggests several ways that water may "remember" a substance, or leave a "molecular fingerprint" of what was once there.

AN EFFECTIVE ALTERNATIVE

Formal outcome studies evaluating the effectiveness of homeopathy in the treatment of ear complaints and other conditions commonly seen in primary care have done as well as or better than traditional western medicine for those same conditions. This International Integrative Primary Care Outcomes Study (IIPCOS-1) was an international multicenter prospective outcomes study involving 29 practitioners in four countries and was coordinated by the Integrative Medical Institute. Homeopathy was as effective as conventional medicine and had a much lower incidence of side effects. Alongside clinical trials there have been a number of outcome studies that, while not being double-blind and controlled, ask patients about the outcome of their treatment. Clinical audits at the Glasgow Homoeopathic Hospital in Scotland, on patients who had already had unsuccessful conventional treatment for a range of illnesses that included depression, multiple sclerosis, and cancer, reported a significant decrease in their use of conventional medicine. A 1998 report by the Faculty of Homoeopathy in the UK argues that clinical trials consistently demonstrate the benefits of homeopathy in terms of patient care and cost-effectiveness.

In many Western countries there is a public trend away from some aspects of conventional, drug-based medicine, and sympathy with the idea of a more "holistic" way of treating the "whole person." There is growing interest from the medical establishment in exploring the possibility of integrating some complementary therapies, including homeopathy, into their treatment approaches. This is in part due to rising health-care costs, the alarming side effects of some medical treatments, and the lack of success in conventionally treating some conditions, such as cancer. If integration is to become a reality, however, high standards of education, practice, and research within homeopathy are needed. Ultimately the aim is to ensure that homeopathy is being delivered to the public by suitably qualified and regulated practitioners operating according to a strong code of ethics to protect the patient.

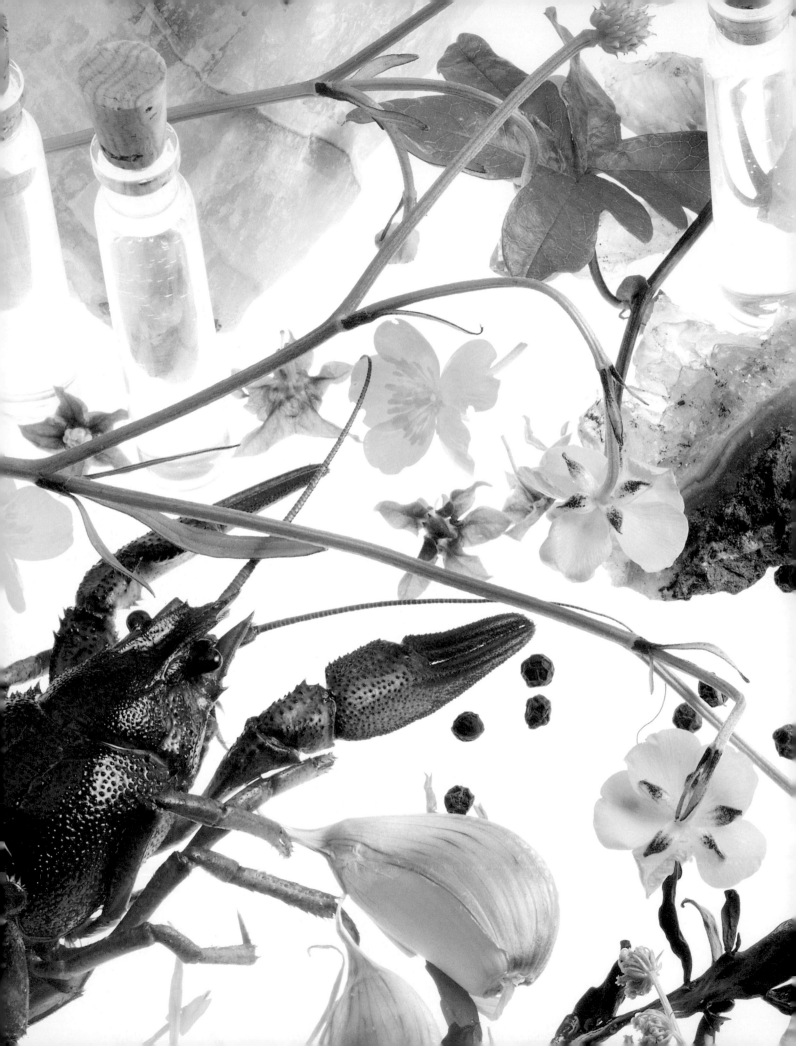

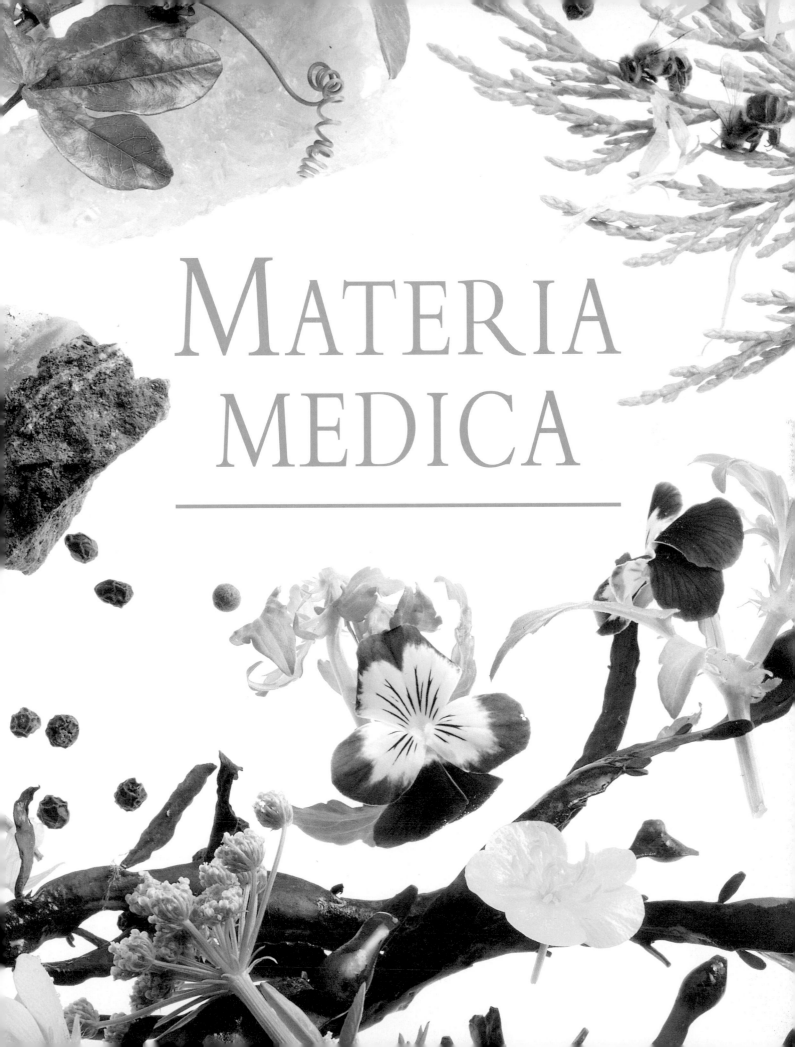

MATERIA
MEDICA

HOW REMEDIES ARE MADE

STRICTLY SPEAKING, remedies are not in themselves homeopathic. They become homeopathic only when they are prescribed according to the principle of "like cures like" (*see page 18*). When the remedy given accurately and effectively "mirrors" the patient's symptoms (*see page 177*), it can then be considered to be acting homeopathically. The experience, judgment, and skill of the practitioner are responsible for selecting the appropriate remedy. Remedies are prepared to exact guidelines but may vary in strength.

REMEDY POTENCIES

Hahnemann laid down precise guidelines for the preparation of a homeopathic remedy (*see opposite*). Measurements and methods were all strictly and scientifically controlled. He also developed a unique process called "potentization," which allowed the full strength, or potency, of the substance to be released into the remedy mixture (*see page 19*).

THE THEORY OF DILUTION

Many remedies are based on highly active or even poisonous substances. Hahnemann established that remedies needed to be diluted to a very great degree to keep patients from suffering side effects. To his surprise he discovered that, paradoxically, the more dilute the remedy, the longer its action, the deeper its effect, and the fewer doses needed. Because the remedies are diluted to such a great degree, it is highly unlikely that even a single molecule of the original substance remains. This means that although remedies may be based on highly poisonous substances, they are completely safe to use, even on children. However, this is also the main reason why homeopathy is still viewed with such skepticism by many orthodox doctors and scientists (*see page 24*).

The potency prescribed is gauged by the homeopath according to factors such as the condition to be treated, the strength of the patient, and the circumstances. Not only must the remedy given be suitable, but the potency chosen must also be appropriate for the individual patient.

SCALES OF DILUTION

Homeopathic remedies are generally prepared according to one of two scales: the decimal (*x*) and the centesimal (*c*). In the decimal scale the dilution factor is 1:10, and in the centesimal scale it is 1:100. Remedies usually have a number, such as *6c* or *12x*, after the name. This number indicates how many times it has been diluted and succussed, and on which scale; for example, the remedy *Allium cepa 6c* has been diluted and succussed six times on the centesimal scale.

More rarely, however, scales such as millesimal (*m*) and quinquagintamillesimal (*lm*) are prepared. According to these scales, remedies are diluted by factors of 1:1,000 and 1:50,000 respectively. The former is used mainly when a single, high-potency dose of a remedy is considered appropriate by the practitioner, while the latter is occasionally given for stubborn, chronic cases that seem to require the prescription of a "megadose" of a particular remedy.

DILUTING & SUCCUSSING

PREPARING A POTENCY

The mother tincture (see step 4, opposite) is usually diluted in a mixture of pure alcohol and distilled water according to one of several scales (see above, right). The ratio of alcohol to water varies depending on the base substance of the mother tincture. To produce a 1c potency, one drop of the mother tincture is added to 99 drops of an alcohol-and-water mixture and succussed. To produce a 2c potency, one drop of the 1c mixture is added to 99 drops of an alcohol-and-water mixture and succussed. To manufacture the 6c potency shown below, this process is repeated four more times.

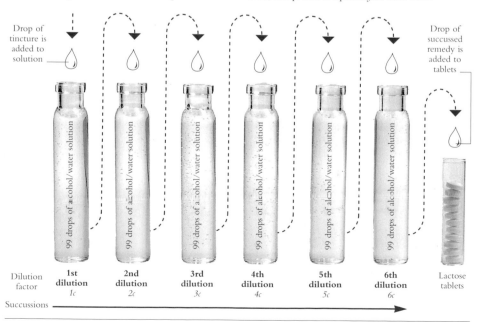

Drop of tincture is added to solution

Drop of succussed remedy is added to tablets

	1st dilution *1c*	2nd dilution *2c*	3rd dilution *3c*	4th dilution *4c*	5th dilution *5c*	6th dilution *6c*	Lactose tablets
Dilution factor	99 drops of alcohol/water solution	99 drops of alcohol/water solution	99 drops of alcohol/water solution	99 drops of alcohol/water solution	99 drops of alcohol/water solution	99 drops of alcohol/water solution	

Succussions

REMEDY STRENGTHS

According to Hahnemann's theories, the more dilute a remedy, the stronger it is and the higher the number, or "potency." A less dilute remedy is not as strong and has a lower number, or potency.

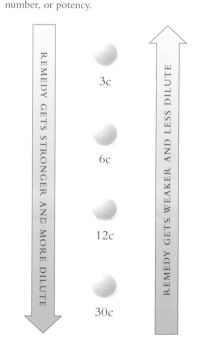

REMEDY GETS STRONGER AND MORE DILUTE

REMEDY GETS WEAKER AND LESS DILUTE

3c

6c

12c

30c

PREPARATION OF HOMEOPATHIC REMEDIES

Homeopathic remedies are made from substances derived from plant, mineral, and animal sources. Depending on their natural state, they may be prepared in a variety of different ways. Plant and animal material may be used whole or chopped, depending on its size and density. Metals that are insoluble in their natural states are combined with lactose sugar crystals and ground repeatedly to form a powder fine enough to be soluble in water, a process called trituration. Crystalline substances, seeds, and beans may also be ground up if they are hard, large, or insoluble in water.

Unlike herbal remedies, homeopathic medicines are never made in the home, but always prepared under strict conditions by a commercial manufacturer.

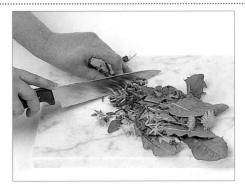

1 Plant material such as leaves, roots, and flower heads (*above*), and some animal material, such as starfish, is chopped finely, while other substances are dissolved in water or ground to prepare them for use.

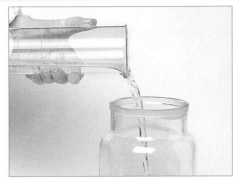

2 The substance is put in a large glass jar, into which is poured a solution of alcohol and distilled water (often 90 per-cent alcohol to 10 percent water, but this ratio varies depending on the substance).

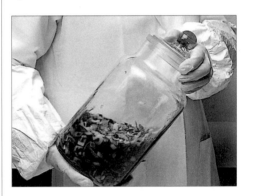

3 The mixture is left to stand for a varying length of time; mixtures that are macerated for longer periods may be shaken at intervals. Plant material may be steeped for several days or weeks, while mineral-based mixtures may be processed on to the next stage almost immediately.

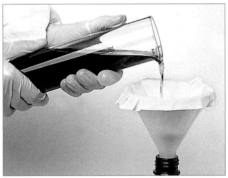

4 After being macerated for the required period of time, the mixture is poured through a filter to strain it or expressed through a press to extract the liquid. This resulting liquid becomes the "mother tincture" for the remedy, and is stored in a dark glass jar.

5 One drop of the mother tincture is diluted in a mixture of pure alcohol and distilled water according to one of several scales (*see opposite*), although the two most commonly used scales are the decimal and the centesimal.

6 This mixture is shaken vigorously (*see right*) or banged down firmly on a hard surface, a process devised by Hahnemann. He called it "succussion" and believed that the action enabled the liquid to be "potentized" (*see page 19*).

7 After the mixture has been succussed, steps 5 and 6 are repeated over and over again, as many times as necessary. Each time the resulting mixture is diluted afresh in a mixture of pure alcohol and distilled water until, finally, the required level of dilution, and therefore the required potency for the homeopathic remedy, is obtained (*see left*).

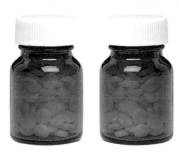

8 Once the mixture has reached the required strength and potency, a few drops of it are added to lactose tablets, pilules, granules, or powder (*see page 216*), to impregnate them with the remedy. These are then stored in dark glass bottles.

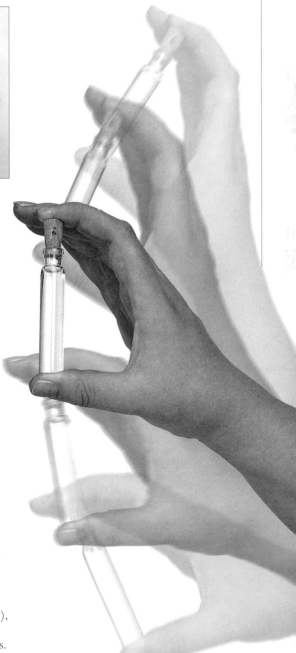

CAUTION

This information is not intended as a guide to making remedies. Homeopathic remedies should always be obtained from a reputable supplier.

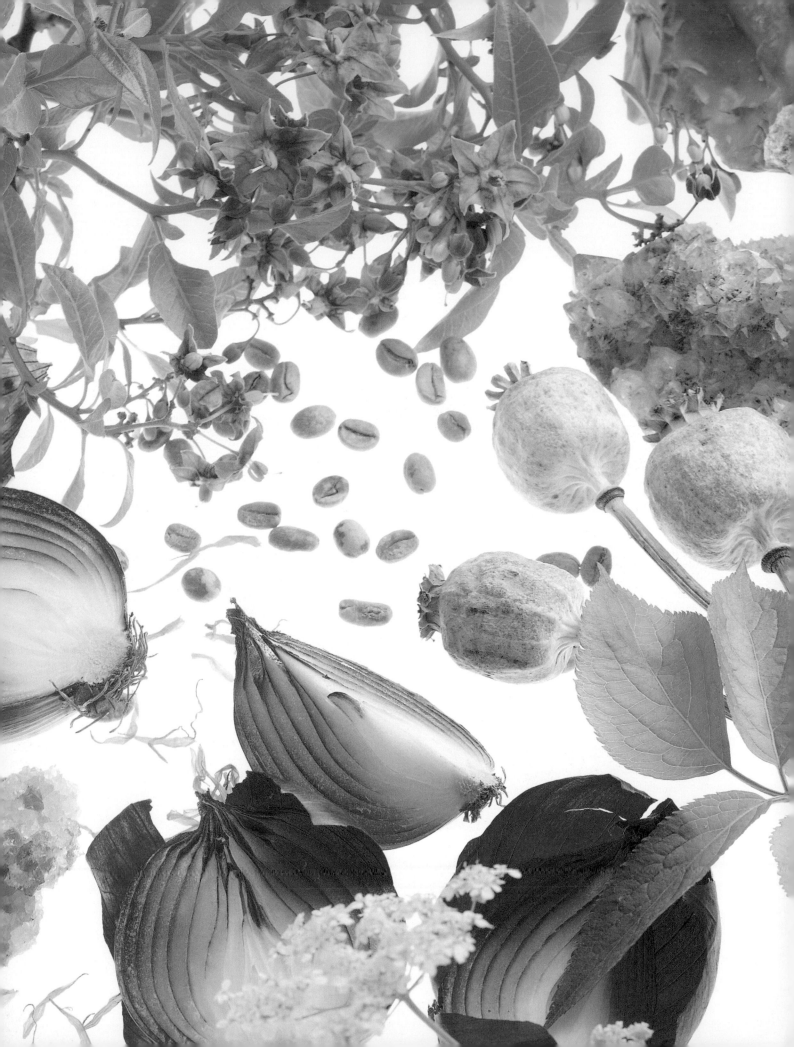

MAJOR PLANT REMEDIES

PLANTS HAVE BEEN USED FOR MEDICINAL PURPOSES

FOR THOUSANDS OF YEARS, AND THE PLANT

KINGDOM ALSO PROVIDES THE SOURCE FOR THE

MAJORITY OF HOMEOPATHIC REMEDIES. IN THIS

SECTION SOME OF THE MOST IMPORTANT PLANT-

BASED REMEDIES ARE LOOKED AT IN DETAIL.

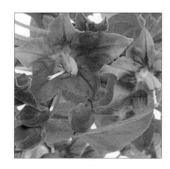 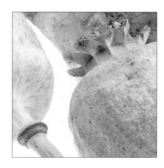 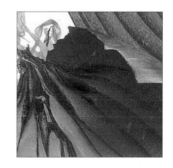

Aconitum napellus
ACONITE

COMMON NAMES
Aconite, monk's hood, wolf's bane, blue rocket, friar's cap

Historically the deadly juices derived from this plant were used as an arrow poison, hence the name aconite, from the Greek *acon,* or "dart." Until the homeopathic remedy was proved by Hahnemann in 1805, aconite was used only externally in medicine. *Aconite* became a popular alternative to the practice of bloodletting for the treatment of acute fevers and inflammations.

SOURCE DETAILS

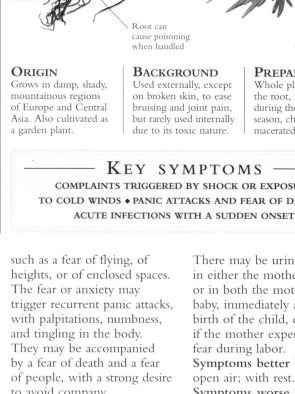

FLOWERING STEM

ACONITE
This plant is known for its poisonous alkaloids, which are found at their highest concentrations in the root.

ROOT

Hooded, blue-violet flowers appear in midsummer

Root can cause poisoning when handled

REMEDY PROFILE

Homeopaths consider using *Aconite* for people who are generally healthy and strong but develop illness rapidly and exhibit a marked sinking of strength. Physical and mental symptoms are like a great storm, arising suddenly but also subsiding quickly. Patterns of behavior are characterized by intense fear, anxiety, and restlessness, with susceptibility to extreme phobias, panic attacks, and a fear of death.

Physical symptoms often develop as a result of shock, fear, or exposure to cold, dry winds or, occasionally, intensely hot weather. Acute infections, such as colds and coughs, can be treated with the remedy, particularly at their onset. *Aconite* may also be prescribed for states of anxiety, and for mothers and infants during or immediately after childbirth.

ACUTE RESPIRATORY INFECTIONS
Symptoms Cold or flu symptoms that set in fiercely and rapidly, especially after exposure to cold, dry winds. There may be phlegm and a sore throat, possibly with a fever that makes the skin hot and dry. Croup and other acute chest infections may give rise to breathlessness, burning heat in the chest, and a hoarse, dry, barking cough.

Sleep is frequently restless and agitated; at such times, the face may be hot, flushed, and

swollen, although on rising it may become very pale. Severe headaches may develop, accompanied by raging thirst, often for cold drinks. The mouth may taste bitter, so that everything except water tastes bad. The skin is hypersensitive, causing a marked aversion to being touched.
Symptoms better With warmth; lying down.
Symptoms worse With heat; in stuffy rooms; lying on the affected area; from walking; at night; from music.

EYE & EAR INFECTIONS
Symptoms Inflamed eyes with aching, burning pain, typically due to injury or conjunctivitis. The eyes may be oversensitive to light. Ear infections develop rapidly, causing intense pain, bright red ears, and hypersensitivity to noise. Symptoms may be accompanied by a high fever and restless, fearful agitation.
Symptoms better With quiet.
Symptoms worse In light; near noise.

FEAR, SHOCK & ANXIETY
Symptoms Acute fear and anxiety accompanied by great restlessness and shocked, staring eyes with dilated pupils. Symptoms may be due to shock after witnessing a violent or frightening event, or may be triggered by phobias,

ORIGIN
Grows in damp, shady, mountainous regions of Europe and Central Asia. Also cultivated as a garden plant.

BACKGROUND
Used externally, except on broken skin, to ease bruising and joint pain, but rarely used internally due to its toxic nature.

PREPARATION
Whole plant, including the root, is unearthed during the flowering season, chopped, and macerated in alcohol.

KEY SYMPTOMS
COMPLAINTS TRIGGERED BY SHOCK OR EXPOSURE TO COLD WINDS ◆ PANIC ATTACKS AND FEAR OF DEATH ◆ ACUTE INFECTIONS WITH A SUDDEN ONSET

---

such as a fear of flying, of heights, or of enclosed spaces. The fear or anxiety may trigger recurrent panic attacks, with palpitations, numbness, and tingling in the body. They may be accompanied by a fear of death and a fear of people, with a strong desire to avoid company.
Symptoms better In the open air; with rest.
Symptoms worse In stuffy rooms; from crowds; at night.

PROBLEMS IN LABOR
Symptoms Strong fear of impending death experienced by a mother during labor.

There may be urine retention in either the mother or baby, or in both the mother and baby, immediately after the birth of the child, especially if the mother experienced fear during labor.
Symptoms better In the open air; with rest.
Symptoms worse From feeling overheated; feeling chilled; violent emotions.

SEE ALSO
Emotional problems, *page 210*; Headache, *page 218*; Respiration, *pages 226, 228*; Children's health, *page 246*

Agaricus muscarius syn. *Amanita muscaria*

AGARICUS

THIS TOXIC TOADSTOOL'S common name, fly agaric, is derived from its traditional use as a fly poison. Fly agaric contains hallucinogens that were used by Siberian shamans to induce visionary states, and it may have formed the basis of the ancient Hindu *soma* drink and the Zoroastrian *haoma* drink, due to its ability to increase strength and stamina. The fungus has sedative properties in small doses but is highly toxic: a severe overdose can be fatal, while a mild overdose can cause nausea, vomiting, diarrhea, breathing problems, and confusion, although recovery usually takes place within 24 hours. The homeopathic remedy was proved in 1828 by Dr. Stapf, and it remains the only medicinal use of fly agaric.

REMEDY PROFILE

Those in need of *Agaricus* may be anxious, insecure, or fearful, and have morbid thoughts about death. Anxiety about health may lead to an obsessive fear of having conditions such as cancer. Symptoms typically include great lethargy and an aversion to conversation, or delirium and loquacity to the point of ecstasy, elation, or hypomania.

People for whom *Agaricus* is most suitable are particularly sensitive to the cold when ill. Some symptoms are worse prior to thunderstorms and after sexual intercourse.

Agaricus is taken as a remedy for disorders of the nervous system that cause trembling, itching, and twitching and jerking of the limbs. Such conditions include epilepsy, chorea, and multiple sclerosis. *Agaricus* can be prescribed for the treatment of the delirium tremens associated with alcoholism, and for the effects of senile dementia. It is also used to treat chilblains.

NERVOUS SYSTEM DISORDERS

Symptoms Twitching and spasms in almost any muscle group in the body, caused by degenerative neurological disorders such as senile dementia or multiple sclerosis. Symptoms tend to manifest themselves diagonally from one side of the body to the other, and may be accompanied by pain that is out of proportion to the clinical condition. There may also be sharp, shooting pains, with possible convulsions and spasms. Movements may be very shaky, with clumsiness, awkwardness, and a staggering gait. Further symptoms may include facial tics or Bell's palsy, fainting, chorea, neuralgia, and sciatica.
Symptoms better With slow movement; with sleep.
Symptoms worse In cold air; before thunderstorms; after sexual intercourse.

CHOREA

Symptoms Twitching, erratic, unpredictable limb movements and a sensation that the limbs are detached from the body.
Symptoms better With slow movement; with sleep.
Symptoms worse In cold air; before thunderstorms; after sexual intercourse.

PARKINSON'S DISEASE

Symptoms General weakness with trembling and twitching limbs that exhibit the typical nervous symptoms (*see left*). The spine may be particularly

SOURCE DETAILS

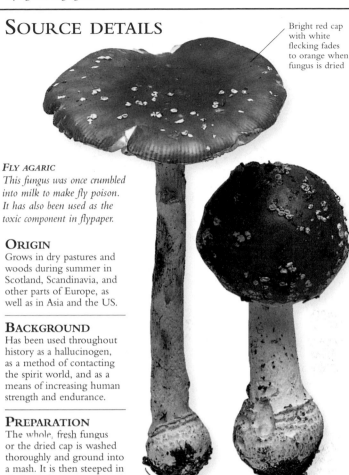

Bright red cap with white flecking fades to orange when fungus is dried

FLY AGARIC
This fungus was once crumbled into milk to make fly poison. It has also been used as the toxic component in flypaper.

ORIGIN
Grows in dry pastures and woods during summer in Scotland, Scandinavia, and other parts of Europe, as well as in Asia and the US.

BACKGROUND
Has been used throughout history as a hallucinogen, as a method of contacting the spirit world, and as a means of increasing human strength and endurance.

PREPARATION
The whole, fresh fungus or the dried cap is washed thoroughly and ground into a mash. It is then steeped in alcohol before being strained, diluted, and succussed.

KEY SYMPTOMS
TWITCHING AND SPASMS ◆ CHILBLAINS ◆ DEPRESSION OR OVEREXCITEMENT ◆ FEAR OF CANCER ◆ COMPLAINTS THAT ARE WORSE AFTER SEXUAL INTERCOURSE

---

sensitive to touch. Further symptoms may include a mental decline into great anxiety, despair, fear, and hypochondria.
Symptoms better With slow movement; with sleep.
Symptoms worse Before thunderstorms; after sexual intercourse.

CHILBLAINS

Symptoms Chilblains with burning and itching. The skin shows signs of redness and swelling.
Symptoms better With heat.
Symptoms worse In cold air; from cold compresses.

ALCOHOLISM

Symptoms Delirium tremens with marked giddiness and an impulse to fall backward. The face is puffy and red, but not hot. There may be a marked increase in appetite.
Symptoms better With slow movement.
Symptoms worse In cold air; before thunderstorms; after sexual intercourse; after eating.

SEE ALSO
Multiple sclerosis, *page 179*; Palpitations, *page 186*; Twitching eyelids, *page 220*; Chilblains, *page 230*

Allium cepa

ALLIUM CEPA

IN ANCIENT GREECE the onion was esteemed and eaten in vast quantities. One of the oldest cultivated plants, its decongestant, diuretic, and other medicinal properties have been utilized by many cultures over the centuries. In the Middle Ages its strong smell was thought to prevent infection, and it was hung outside houses to ward off the plague. Onion causes the eyes and nose to water, and is used homeopathically to treat conditions that cause the same reaction in the body, such as colds and the flu. The remedy *Allium cepa* was proved in 1847 by Dr. Constantine Hering.

REMEDY PROFILE

Melancholy, anxiety, and fear of pain are not uncommon in individuals who respond well to *Allium cepa*, but there are no marked emotional symptoms indicative of the remedy.

    Allium cepa is used primarily for the treatment of coughs and colds characterized by profuse, watery mucus that leaves the skin irritated and sore. Symptoms usually develop following exposure to cold weather and damp winds. They may be associated with hay fever, especially if accompanied by sensitivity to the scent of flowers. *Allium cepa* is also used to treat burning neuralgic pain that alternates from one side of the body to the other.

PHLEGM (MUCUS)
Symptoms Profuse, watery mucus that burns the skin of the nose and upper lip, causing it to become raw, red, and painful. The nose may seem to "drip like a faucet." Constant, violent sneezing is common, as is congestion that alternates between nostrils or affects only one nostril. *Allium cepa* is used for these symptoms in the flu, colds, and hay fever. Further remedies are needed to treat any susceptibility to hay fever itself.
Symptoms better From being in the open air.
Symptoms worse In warm rooms; in the evening.

EYE IRRITATION
Symptoms An irritating discharge that causes an urge to rub the eyes. The eyes are red, swollen, and itchy, and possibly extremely sensitive to light.
Symptoms better From being in the open air.
Symptoms worse In warm rooms; in the evening; from rubbing the eyes; coughing.

THROAT & CHEST INFECTIONS
Symptoms Laryngitis with hoarseness and a sore throat, or a cough characterized by a splitting, tearing sensation in the throat. There may be an urge to repress the cough, as it constantly irritates the throat.

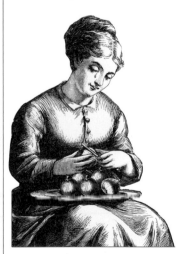

ONION EYES
Chopping onions releases a volatile oil that causes the eyes and nose to water. Shakespeare called those whose eyes were full of tears "onion-eyed."

SOURCE DETAILS

ONION
The antibiotic, anti-inflammatory, and expectorant properties of this plant are used worldwide to treat colds, coughs, and the flu.

ONION BULB

CROSS-SECTION

Layers of papery skin enclose volatile oil that stimulates tears

ORIGIN
Native to the northern hemisphere and cultivated for centuries in the Middle East. Now grown worldwide as a vegetable.

BACKGROUND
Widely used in traditional medicine: as a poultice for chilblains, infections, and arthritis; internally for gastric and bronchial infections; and to thin and purify the blood.

PREPARATION
The whole, mature bulb is gathered in summer and chopped finely. It is steeped in alcohol for ten days and shaken repeatedly, before being filtered, diluted, and succussed.

KEY SYMPTOMS
BURNING MUCUS ◆ BLAND DISCHARGE FROM THE EYES ◆ SPLITTING SENSATION IN THE THROAT ◆ PHANTOM PAINS ◆ FEELS WORSE IN WARM ROOMS

Pain may extend to the ear. Symptoms may develop rapidly on exposure to cold air, or after a cold accompanied by labored, wheezy breathing.
Symptoms better From being in the open air.
Symptoms worse In warm rooms; in the evening.

NEURALGIC PAINS
Symptoms Sharp, burning pain on alternating sides of the body, mainly in the face, head, neck, and chest. It may be due to earaches, headaches behind the brow, or a molar toothache. *Allium cepa* is also used for phantom limb pains after amputation.
Symptoms better In open air.
Symptoms worse From being in a warm room.

SEE ALSO
Allergies, *page 206*; Hay fever & allergic rhinitis, *page 224*

Aloe ferox 'Miller'
ALOE

COMMON NAMES
Aloe, Cape aloe

THE MEDICINAL PROPERTIES of the various species of aloe have been exploited for centuries. The ancient Greeks and Romans considered aloe to be a valuable tonic and purgative. The purgative quality of dried aloe gel is still valued today in herbal medicine, but the plant is probably more familiar now as the source of a soothing and effective skin lotion. The *Aloe* remedy was proved by the homeopath Dr. Helbig in 1833, and is used today mainly for digestive complaints, particularly diarrhea.

SOURCE DETAILS

Lance-shaped leaves contain a thick, clear gel

ALOE
The gel of this plant has a long history of medicinal use as a skin lotion.

Spiny leaves form in rosette shape

ORIGIN
Native to southern Africa, particularly the northern, eastern, and western capes, but now cultivated throughout the world. Found in fertile, well-drained areas with sandy soil and direct sunlight.

BACKGROUND
Traditionally, aloe gel has been used as a laxative and purgative. Various research trials conducted between 1979 and 1995 found that extracts from the plant boost immune-system functioning and may even help to treat cancer.

PREPARATION
The juice is extracted from the plant and dried to make a hard resin, which is then powdered and steeped in alcohol. The mixture is left to macerate for at least five days, after which it is filtered, and then repeatedly diluted and succussed.

REMEDY PROFILE

Homeopaths consider *Aloe* when the psychological traits exhibited include weariness, a reluctance to work, and great irritability, especially in cloudy weather. Dissatisfaction and anger are commonly directed internally, possibly producing constipation. Moreover, the person may dream about stools or involuntary soiling. Beer is a typical craving, despite the fact that it usually exacerbates any physical symptoms.

Aloe is most frequently prescribed for disorders of the large intestine. It may be taken for congestion in the pelvic organs and the head, and is also thought to counter fatigue, hemorrhoids, and the possible consequences of a sedentary lifestyle, particularly in the elderly.

DIARRHEA
Symptoms A sudden urge to pass stools, which is at its strongest particularly early in the morning, possibly forcing an early rise from bed at around 5 A.M. Accompanied by hot, explosive wind, the stools may contain mucus or jelly-like lumps. They may be passed involuntarily, giving rise to a feeling of insecurity in the rectum (this may also be an indication of colitis). Diarrhea may alternate with constipation. It is marked by incomplete, unsatisfactory stools and heavy pressure in the lower abdominal area. Symptoms generally tend to be worse prior to menstruation, or may primarily affect the elderly or those with sedentary habits.
Symptoms better From passing gas.
Symptoms worse First thing in the morning; from walking; immediately after eating; from oysters; from beer.

HEMORRHOIDS
Symptoms Hemorrhoids that resemble small bunches of grapes and protrude from the anus. They are typically accompanied by soreness and tenderness. There may be a painful, burning sensation in the rectum and anus, and flatulent diarrhea.
Symptoms better From bathing in cold water.
Symptoms worse With heat; with jarring movement; on sitting down; after eating or drinking.

HEPATITIS
Symptoms A sensation of congestion and heat in the liver. There may be rumbling and distention in the abdomen, causing it to feel full, heavy, bloated, and hot. An accumulation of gas may accompany this feeling of distention, as well as strain and tension that is felt in the area between the pubic bone and the coccyx.
Symptoms better In cold; in the open air.
Symptoms worse With heat; after eating or drinking.

HEADACHES
Symptoms Severe, painful headaches that seem to trigger a sensation of congestion in the face and in the head. These headaches frequently appear to alternate with the occurrence of hemorrhoids or diarrhea, or may be associated with pain in the lower back.
Symptoms better In the open air; from cold compresses on the head.
Symptoms worse With heat.

KEY SYMPTOMS
INVOLUNTARY STOOLS ♦ DIARRHEA WITH SUDDEN URGING, ESPECIALLY AT 5 A.M. ♦ INSECURE FEELING IN THE RECTUM ♦ HEADACHES THAT ARE BETTER FROM COLD COMPRESSES

SEE ALSO
Diarrhea, *page 238*

Anacardium orientale syn. *Semecarpus anacardium*

ANACARDIUM OR.

THE LATIN NAME of this shrub derives from the ancient Greek *kardia*, or "heart," inspired by the plant's heart-shaped, shiny, black nut. The nut yields a milky juice that turns black after it is exposed to air. In southeastern Asia this juice is combined with chalk to make an ink for marking patterns on fabric, hence the plant's common name, the marking-nut tree. The homeopathic remedy *Anacardium or.* was proved by Hahnemann in 1835. It is prescribed for both psychological and physical disorders.

REMEDY PROFILE

Anacardium or. is traditionally used for memory disturbance and a disturbed psychological state. It is considered especially apt for those who feel they are experiencing a conflict of will or are trapped between extremes of good and evil, sometimes described as "a demon sitting on one shoulder, an angel on the other." These individuals are typically prone to low self-esteem, or may exhibit hard, angry, cruel behavior. They may suspect that they are being pursued, or experience dreamlike states.

Typical physical symptoms include a feeling of constricted pain, as if bands are wrapped tightly around the body, or as if the gut or anus is plugged. In this connection, the remedy is used for certain conditions of the digestive tract. It is also used for skin irritations marked by severe itching and burning, and for minor chest pain.

PSYCHOLOGICAL PROBLEMS
Symptoms A state of inner conflict expressed in contrary and changeable behavior. This conflict may provoke behavior that is cold-hearted, violent, and cruel, with a compulsive urge to curse. Exaggerated affection toward a person or pet may be followed by cruelty or violence. An inferiority complex may be evident (*see above, right*). There may be an extremely poor memory, a

lack of concentration, and general absent-mindedness, especially at times of stress, for example, when studying for examinations. In extreme cases symptoms may be linked to a mental illness, such as depression, manic depression, or schizophrenia.
Symptoms better Lying in the sun; from hot baths; in the late morning; from eating.
Symptoms worse From mental exertion; anger; fright; under stress; from studying.

LOW SELF-ESTEEM
Symptoms Great feelings of unworthiness, irresolution, and low self-confidence, possibly with an inferiority complex, due to an inner conflict of will. Depending on the severity of the mental state, there may even be infrequent or ongoing self-abuse. Behavior patterns may be associated with prior subjection to abuse, violence, humiliation, or oppression.
Symptoms better Lying in the sun; from hot baths; in the late morning; from eating.
Symptoms worse From mental exertion; from fright; under stress; from humiliation.

DIGESTIVE DISORDERS
Symptoms Hemorrhoids, indigestion, and constipation with a painful constricted feeling, as if the gut or anus were plugged and the body wrapped by tight bands. The

SOURCE DETAILS

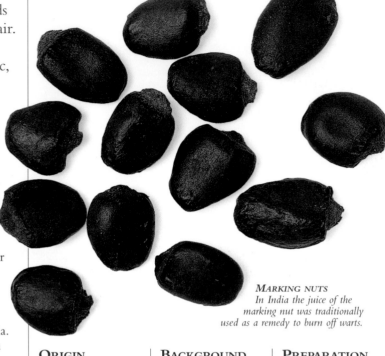

MARKING NUTS
In India the juice of the marking nut was traditionally used as a remedy to burn off warts.

ORIGIN
Native to Malaysia, Indonesia, and the Indian subcontinent, and found growing in dry, mountainous forest areas.

BACKGROUND
Arabian physicians traditionally used the juice of the marking nut to treat mental illness, memory loss, paralysis, and spasms.

PREPARATION
The ripe, dried fruit is macerated in alcohol for at least five days, before being filtered and then repeatedly diluted and succussed.

KEY SYMPTOMS

LACK OF SELF-CONFIDENCE ◆ CONFLICT OF WILLS ◆ SENSATION OF HAVING A PLUG IN THE ANUS, GUT, OR CHEST ◆ POOR MEMORY ◆ ITCHING, BURNING SKIN ERUPTIONS

---

pain may stop after eating but resumes a few hours later.
Symptoms better Immediately after eating.
Symptoms worse From a hot bath or compress; at midnight; a few hours after eating.

SKIN CONDITIONS
Symptoms Eczema and possibly patches of blistered skin, often on the forearms, causing intense itching and burning. The skin is highly sensitive. Warts are also treated with the remedy.
Symptoms better From the application of very hot water.
Symptoms worse From scratching the affected skin.

CHEST PAIN
Symptoms Sharp or pricking pain in the heart, possibly with a sense of pressure in the chest, as if it is bound by tight bands or weighed down by a small plug. An uneasy sensation may develop in the chest, possibly involving palpitations.
Symptoms better From inhaling fresh air outdoors.
Symptoms worse A few hours after eating.

SEE ALSO
Indigestion, *page 234*;
Hemorrhoids, *page 238*;
Constipation, *page 238*;
Eczema, *page 240*

Arnica montana

ARNICA

COMMON NAMES
Arnica, leopard's bane, sneezewort, mountain tobacco, mountain daisy

T HE HEALING PROPERTIES of this aromatic perennial have been recognized for over 400 years. Arnica is anti-inflammatory and promotes tissue repair. It has been used extensively in European folk medicine as an external remedy for muscle pain, and was once also prescribed as an internal treatment for dysentery and gout. Potentially toxic, its internal use is now largely limited to homeopathy. Proved by Hahnemann and published in his *Materia Medica Pura* (1821–34), *Arnica* is used to promote healing and help control bleeding. It is used mostly for shock, injury, and pain.

REMEDY PROFILE

People who respond best to this remedy may actually deny that they are ill, ignoring the severity of their condition. They generally prefer to be left alone and tend to be agitated, restless, and morose. Poor concentration and forgetfulness are typical, as are nightmares and a morbid imagination.

Arnica is usually given as a first-aid remedy following an accident, surgery, bereavement, childbirth, or dental treatment. It is also used for joint pain, fever, and some skin problems.

SHOCK, INJURY & POSTOPERATIVE CARE
Symptoms Acute and chronic consequences of shock, injury, or surgery, particularly bleeding, bruising, swelling, and aching pains. The body may feel battered and highly sensitive to discomfort, to the point where even a bed seems too hard. *Arnica* may also be prescribed to treat injuries such as a black eye or a foreign object in an eye, concussion, and nosebleeds.

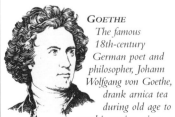

GOETHE
The famous 18th-century German poet and philosopher, Johann Wolfgang von Goethe, drank arnica tea during old age to ease his angina, since the herb was believed to stimulate a weak heart and circulation.

Symptoms better Lying down; lying with the head lower than the feet.
Symptoms worse In cold; in damp; if touched; with rest; with movement; from wine.

POSTPARTUM PAIN
Symptoms Bruised, aching pain in the vagina that may be especially distressing at night.
Symptoms better Lying down with the head lower than the feet.
Symptoms worse In cold; if touched; with movement.

TOOTH & GUM PAIN
Symptoms Pain in the teeth or sore, bruised, and bleeding gums following injury or dental work may be treated with *Arnica*.
Symptoms better Lying down.
Symptoms worse With the slightest touch; with movement.

JOINT & MUSCLE PAIN
Symptoms Arthritic pain, sprains, or strains to the joints, which feel bruised, sore, and sensitive. *Arnica* is also taken to ease swelling, bruising, and pain after a ligament tear or bone injury. Alternatively, it is used for aches in the muscles due to cramps, unaccustomed exercise, or overexertion.
Symptoms better Lying down.
Symptoms worse With the slightest touch; with movement.

SOURCE DETAILS

ORIGIN
Grows in alpine pastures and woodlands of the Pyrenees, Siberia, and central Europe, especially Switzerland and Germany.

BACKGROUND
Traditionally used externally as an ointment to improve local blood supply and speed healing in the treatment of bruises, sprains, and muscle pain.

PREPARATION
The whole flowering plant, including the root, is steeped in alcohol, filtered, diluted, and succussed.

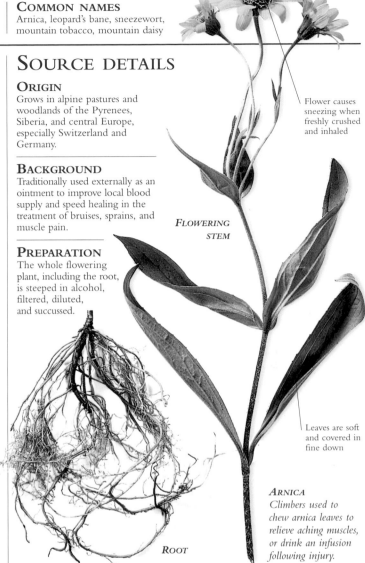

Flower causes sneezing when freshly crushed and inhaled

FLOWERING STEM

Leaves are soft and covered in fine down

ARNICA
Climbers used to chew arnica leaves to relieve aching muscles, or drink an infusion following injury.

ROOT

KEY SYMPTOMS
TRAUMA ◆ BRUISING ◆ POSTOPERATIVE CARE ◆
TENDENCY TO DENY ILLNESS ◆ BRUISED, SORE FEELING ◆
BED SEEMS TOO HARD

FEVER
Symptoms A hot head, cold body, and exhaustion. Stools, flatulence, and perspiration tend to have a characteristic odor of rotten eggs, and there may be incontinence of stools and urine. *Arnica* is also prescribed for recurring fevers such as typhoid or malarial fever.
Symptoms better Lying down; lying with the head lower than the feet.
Symptoms worse In cold surroundings; in damp; with the slightest touch.

SKIN CONDITONS
Symptoms Hard, dry, swollen skin due to insect bites, bed sores, small, painful boils, red, blistering skin eruptions, or varicose ulcers.
Symptoms better Lying down.
Symptoms worse In cold; in damp; if touched.

SEE ALSO
Circulation, *pages 184, 230*; Breast problems, *page 201*; Grief, *page 213*; Men's health, *page 264*; Dizziness, *page 266*

Artemisia cina syn. *A. maritima* 'Linn'

CINA

COMMON NAMES
Levant wormseed, European wormseed,
Tartarian southernwood

PURPORTEDLY NAMED after Artemisia, the queen of Persia in the 4th century BCE who was renowned for her botanical skills, this family of plants has been valued by many medicinal traditions, from ancient Roman to Chinese. *Artemisia cina* was identified as a remedy for intestinal worms by the ancient Greeks, and its active constituent, santonin, is still used in worm medicines. In 1829 *Cina* was proved by Hahnemann, who felt that the plant's "valuable curative properties" went well beyond its traditional role in herbalism.

REMEDY PROFILE

Cina is typically perceived as a children's remedy and is given for intestinal worms or muscle twitches, associated with great irritability when scolded or in discomfort. Those affected cannot bear to be touched, held, or even observed – they often consider themselves ugly. Restlessness, a frantic state of mind, picking the nose, and grinding the teeth are typical symptoms in those for whom *Cina* is appropriate. Sleep is often fitful and plagued by night terrors. All symptoms may be worse at night.

These people may have an "anxiety of conscience," a groundless feeling of having done something wrong, which manifests itself as touchiness and obstinacy. They may be survivors of childhood abuse.

In addition to its primary use for worms, *Cina* has also been given to treat convulsions and seizures in children. Today it is still given as a treatment for worms, as well as for temper tantrums, violent coughing, muscle twitches, and sleep problems in children.

INTESTINAL WORMS
Symptoms Worms evident in whitish-colored stools. Cutting, pinching pain is felt in the belly, which may be bloated. There is an urge to grind the teeth at night, and to pick the nose and scratch the rectum, both of which are itchy. The appetite may be

nonexistent, enormous, or changeable, with potential cravings for sweet foods. There is often intense irritability and great restlessness.
Symptoms better With movement; bending down.
Symptoms worse In summer heat; at night; if touched.

TEMPER TANTRUMS
Symptoms Extreme irritability in children, especially chubby ones with variable appetites. Tantrums may be due to being scolded or to worms (*see left*). Typical *Cina* symptoms such as teeth-grinding may be present.
Symptoms better Lying on the abdomen; from being carried.
Symptoms worse If touched; from being stared at.

COUGHS & COLDS
Symptoms Whooping cough or severe, gagging cough, with limb spasms before a coughing fit. The chest feels constricted, making breathing difficult. Speaking or sudden movement may trigger coughing. In children the body tends to stiffen prior to a coughing fit. Violent sneezing may cause pressure buildup in the head, and the nose may be alternately blocked and runny. There may be an urge to pick the nose, and nosebleeds often result. Intense ill-humor and irritability are often evident.
Symptoms better From being still; in the daytime.

SOURCE DETAILS

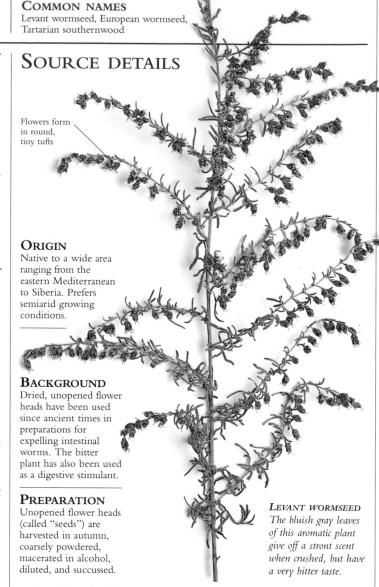

Flowers form in round, tiny tufts

ORIGIN
Native to a wide area ranging from the eastern Mediterranean to Siberia. Prefers semiarid growing conditions.

BACKGROUND
Dried, unopened flower heads have been used since ancient times in preparations for expelling intestinal worms. The bitter plant has also been used as a digestive stimulant.

PREPARATION
Unopened flower heads (called "seeds") are harvested in autumn, coarsely powdered, macerated in alcohol, diluted, and succussed.

LEVANT WORMSEED
The bluish gray leaves of this aromatic plant give off a stront scent when crushed, but have a very bitter taste.

KEY SYMPTOMS
TEETH-GRINDING ◆ IRRITABILITY AND TOUCHINESS ◆ TEMPER TANTRUMS ◆ RAVENOUS APPETITE ◆ DESIRE TO LIE ON THE HANDS AND KNEES ◆ ITCHY NOSE THAT IS CONSTANTLY RUBBED

Symptoms worse On getting up; from walking outside; during sleep; at night.

TWITCHING MUSCLES
Symptoms Jerking muscles and spasms, especially in the hands and feet, associated with irritability. *Cina* is often used if twitching or convulsions are triggered by touch or by being scolded.
Symptoms better From bending down.
Symptoms worse If touched; at night; in summer heat.

SLEEP PROBLEMS
Symptoms Difficulty in falling asleep, or restless sleep with twitching, jerking limbs.
Symptoms better From being rocked violently; lying on the hands and knees.
Symptoms worse From night terrors; being turned over.

SEE ALSO
Temper tantrums, *page 246*

Atropa belladonna

BELLADONNA

COMMON NAMES
Deadly nightshade, belladonna, dwale, devil's cherries, sorcerer's cherry, witches' berry

T HIS DEADLY GENUS is named after the Greek Fate Atropos, who held the power of life and death over mortals. In the 16th century Italian ladies used deadly nightshade to make their eyes sparkle, hence *bella donna*, which is Italian for "beautiful woman." *Belladonna* was one of the first homeopathic remedies, developed in 1799 by Hahnemann for scarlet fever, after he observed that symptoms of deadly nightshade poisoning closely matched those of scarlet fever.

SOURCE DETAILS

DEADLY NIGHTSHADE
Despite this plant's poisonous nature, it has been used as an antispasmodic, relaxant, and sedative in herbalism, and for acute inflammation, pain, and fever in homeopathy.

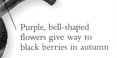

Purple, bell-shaped flowers give way to black berries in autumn

REMEDY PROFILE

Belladonna is a major remedy for acute illnesses of sudden, violent onset. It is usually given to people who are generally fit and energetic, but restless and agitated when ill. They are prone to sudden, explosive anger, marked by the desire to strike out or even to bite.

Typical symptoms linked with *Belladonna* include high fever, dilated pupils, flushed skin, and throbbing pain, particularly in the head, due to rapid blood circulation. There is often hypersensitivity to light, noise, and touch, and also to rapid temperature changes.

Belladonna is typically given for acute pain, inflammation, or infection, chiefly of the upper respiratory tract. It may also be used to treat menstrual pain, sunstroke, febrile convulsions, cystitis, nephritis (inflamed kidneys), teething pain, and mastitis during breast-feeding.

ACUTE FEVER & PAIN
Symptoms Sudden onset of high fever and hypersensitivity in all the senses. The face may be hot, flushed, and dry, with bright eyes and dilated pupils. Although the lips and mouth remain pale, the tongue is often bright red. Any inflammation is red, radiates heat, and throbs painfully. Fever is commonly followed by perspiration, and may develop into delirium. There is little thirst, or just a craving for sour drinks.

Other symptoms include throbbing pain in the eyes, which are swollen, red, and sensitive to light; a tearing, pounding pain deep in the ear; and a pulsating headache (*see below, right*).
Symptoms better In warm rooms; from sitting or standing erect.
Symptoms worse Near noise; if touched; with movement; lying down; in drafts.

SORE THROAT & DRY COUGH
Symptoms Constricted, dry, burning throat, a tender neck, and red, swollen tonsils, notably on the right side. There may be a painful, racking cough and fever (*see above*).
Symptoms better In warm rooms; with rest.

ORIGIN
Native to Europe, western Asia, north Africa, and North America, but now cultivated worldwide. Thrives in chalky soil, woods, and wasteland.

BACKGROUND
Used traditionally for swelling and inflammations, colic, and ulcers. It formed part of a sleeping potion in Chaucer's time, and six centuries later, provides an anesthetic still used in conventional medicine.

Leaves have weaker effect than root, and for this reason are preferred for herbal medicines

PREPARATION
As it comes into flower, the whole fresh plant, including the root, is dug up. It is chopped and pounded to a pulp, then the juice is expressed. This juice is steeped in alcohol before being filtered, diluted, and succussed.

KEY SYMPTOMS
HOT, FLUSHED, RED FACE ♦ HIGH FEVER ♦
DELIRIUM ♦ DESIRE FOR SOUR THINGS ♦
SENSITIVITY TO LIGHT, NOISE, AND MOVEMENT

Symptoms worse In cold drafts; around 3 P.M.; from swallowing foods or drinks.

HEADACHE & MIGRAINE
Symptoms Violent, throbbing pain. During a migraine, pain starts in the back of the head, radiates to the right brow area, and settles behind the eye.
Symptoms better From pressure on the head; lying in the dark; cold compresses.
Symptoms worse In light; near noise; with movement; from menstruating.

MENSTRUAL PAIN
Symptoms Menstrual flow is extremely heavy and painful. The blood is hot and may be bright red or clotted.
Symptoms better From standing or sitting erect.
Symptoms worse With the slightest movement.

SEE ALSO
Rosacea, *page 193*; The flu, *page 224*; Children's health, *page 246*; Breast-feeding problems, *page 262*

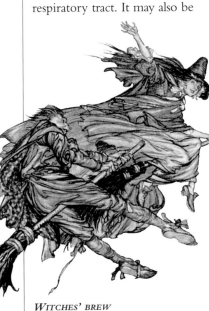

WITCHES' BREW
In medieval Europe deadly nightshade became linked with witchcraft and was thought to help witches to fly.

Baptisia tinctoria

BAPTISIA

COMMON NAMES
Wild indigo, indigo weed,
horsefly weed, rattleweed

THE FAMOUS INDIGO DYE obtained from this plant is reflected in its name, *tinctoria*, from the Latin *tingere*, "to dye." Wild indigo was used medicinally by Native Americans and by New World settlers, primarily as an antiseptic wash for wounds. Modern herbalists use it internally and externally as an antiseptic and immune-system stimulant. The homeopathic remedy was proved in a small-scale trial in the 1850s by Drs. Douglas, Hadley, Burt, and others, and introduced into the repertory by Dr. Thompson in 1857.

SOURCE DETAILS

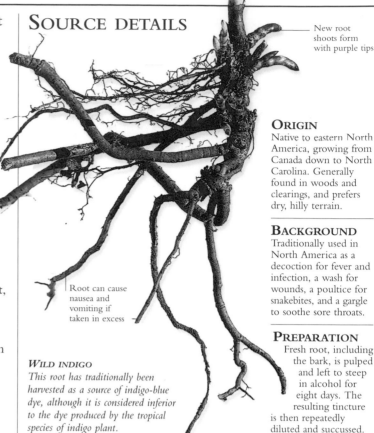

New root shoots form with purple tips

ORIGIN
Native to eastern North America, growing from Canada down to North Carolina. Generally found in woods and clearings, and prefers dry, hilly terrain.

BACKGROUND
Traditionally used in North America as a decoction for fever and infection, a wash for wounds, a poultice for snakebites, and a gargle to soothe sore throats.

PREPARATION
Fresh root, including the bark, is pulped and left to steep in alcohol for eight days. The resulting tincture is then repeatedly diluted and succussed.

Root can cause nausea and vomiting if taken in excess

WILD INDIGO
This root has traditionally been harvested as a source of indigo-blue dye, although it is considered inferior to the dye produced by the tropical species of indigo plant.

REMEDY PROFILE

Baptisia is prescribed almost exclusively for acute feverish illness with a characteristic set of symptoms. These include confusion or even stupor, as though drunk. The lethargy or exhaustion brought on by illness is so profound that the person even falls asleep during conversations. Nightmares and delirium are common, notably a sensation that the body is scattered in pieces. This feeling can lead to difficulty in falling asleep, as can sensations of suffocation or breathlessness.

Typical physical symptoms include foul breath, a yellowish brown tongue, and a bitter-tasting mouth. The face may be swollen and flushed dark red, with drooping eyelids.

First developed for typhoid fever, *Baptisia* is now used mostly for acute fever, severe flu, and gastrointestinal infections, as well as for sore throats and septic infections.

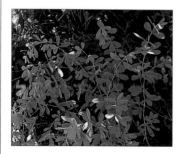

WOUND HEALER
The herb's wound-healing properties were first recognized by the Native Americans of the Northeast, such as the Mohicans.

ACUTE FEVER
Symptoms A high fever or the flu, often of sudden onset, alternating with severe chills. The face may be darkly flushed; the tongue tends to be deep red or even brown in color, and is possibly coated and dry down the center. Lethargy may accompany these symptoms, with the body feeling tender and bruised and the muscles sore, stiff, and heavy. The bed may feel too hard, resulting in bouts of restlessness and curling up tightly in order to try and ease discomfort.
Symptoms better From being indoors.
Symptoms worse From being in the open air; in cold, wind, fog, and humid heat; on waking; from walking.

INTESTINAL INFECTIONS
Symptoms Exhausting attacks of diarrhea, with acute fever (*see above*) and possibly even delirium. The tongue may have a yellowish coating and there may be a bitter taste in the mouth. Stools are particularly foul-smelling and cause painful irritation around the anus. There may also be blood in the stools and a pink rash on the abdomen, possibly indicating typhoid fever.
Symptoms better From being indoors; with rest.
Symptoms worse From walking in the open air.

KEY SYMPTOMS
SEVERE INFECTION ◆ CONFUSION AND STUPOR ◆ SENSATION THAT THE BODY IS SCATTERED IN PIECES ◆ AVERSION TO OPEN AIR ◆ OFFENSIVE-SMELLING DISCHARGES

THROAT INFECTIONS
Symptoms Stupor, flushing, and fever (*see above, left*). The throat is sore, and the tonsils may be dark red and swollen. The gums and throat may be affected by ulcers, which are not necessarily painful. The lips may be blue, cracked, or bleeding. Swallowing solid food without gagging may be impossible, but drinking small quantities of liquid is bearable. A marked thirst and copious drinking may be followed by the scant passage of urine. A related ear infection may be quick to set in, especially in the right ear.
Symptoms better From being indoors; with rest.
Symptoms worse From walking in the open air.

SEPTIC CONDITIONS
Symptoms Foul-smelling canker sores in the mouth and throat, with a foul-smelling discharge. The breath, sweat, and urine may have an offensive odor. The symptoms set in rapidly, with stupor and fatigue, and may be due to an incomplete miscarriage, or to septicemia or other septic states marked by acute fever.
Symptoms better From being indoors; with rest.
Symptoms worse From walking in the open air.

SEE ALSO
The flu, *page 224*; Sore throat, *page 226*; Canker sores, *page 232*; Diarrhea, *page 238*

Berberis vulgaris
BERBERIS

T HIS STRONGLY ASTRINGENT and healing plant was used by ancient Greek and Arabian physicians to cool the blood during fevers and to treat jaundice and gastrointestinal disorders, while Native Americans used it for peptic ulcers. Western herbalists give barberry for liver problems caused by drug or alcohol abuse, and Ayurvedic doctors advocate it as a detoxicant and liver tonic. In traditional Chinese medicine it is taken for diarrhea. Barberry contains alkaloids that are thought to inhibit cancer. The homeopathic remedy was proved by Dr. Hesse in 1835, and is taken largely for urinary and digestive disorders with sharp or colicky pain.

SOURCE DETAILS

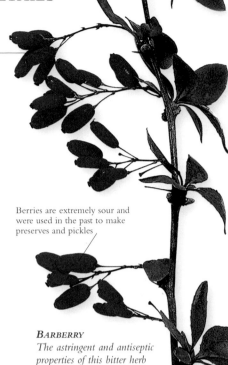

All parts of barberry plant are harmful if eaten, except red berries

ORIGIN
Native to Europe and naturalized in North America. Grows wild in woods and hedges, and on bushy chalk hills, and is commonly cultivated as a garden plant or herb.

BACKGROUND
Traditionally used in many cultures to treat digestive and gallbladder complaints, and also thought to lower fever, control bleeding, and reduce inflammation.

PREPARATION
The bark of the small or medium-sized root branches is dried and chopped, then steeped in alcohol, filtered, diluted, and succussed.

Berries are extremely sour and were used in the past to make preserves and pickles

BARBERRY
The astringent and antiseptic properties of this bitter herb make it an effective digestive tonic for gastrointestinal infections and peptic ulcers.

REMEDY PROFILE

People who respond well to *Berberis* are prone to lethargy, inertia, and listlessness. They can find it difficult to sustain any mental effort or to think straight. They can be especially anxious at twilight, when objects may appear larger than life and distorted so that they may be mistaken for monsters.

Typical physical symptoms for those who need *Berberis* include pallor, hollow eyes and cheeks, and dry mucous membranes. *Berberis* is given for a particular type of pain, typically described as deep, sharp, neuralgic or colicky pain radiating outward, and often shifting from one part of the body to another. This type of sudden pain is often linked with kidney infection, arthritis, or gout. *Berberis* has a strong affinity with the urinary and digestive systems, and is used mainly in the treatment of kidney disorders.

KIDNEY DISORDERS
Symptoms Kidney infection with tenderness and pain in the kidney area, as if water is trying to bubble through the skin. Urine is dark yellow or green with a reddish, branlike sediment. *Berberis* may help kidney stones with severe, sharp, neuralgic or colicky pain radiating from the kidneys to the bladder and down the legs.
Symptoms better With rest; lying on the painful side.
Symptoms worse From standing; with movement; with sudden jarring or jolts.

CYSTITIS
Symptoms Burning or sharp, cutting pains from the bladder to the urethra, with green or dark yellow urine that contains a reddish, branlike sediment. Pain from the spermatic cord to the testes may make sexual intercourse painful.
Symptoms better After urinating.
Symptoms worse From urinating; from standing.

GALLBLADDER PROBLEMS
Symptoms Sharp, radiating, tearing pain in the area of the gallbladder, extending toward the stomach. Colic may cause a stabbing, stitchlike pain that radiates from the liver area. There may be an inflamed gallbladder or gallstones with associated biliary colic (pain in the upper abdomen), which may sometimes develop into jaundice with pale stools.
Symptoms better With rest.
Symptoms worse From pressure on the abdomen; from standing; with movement.

LOWER-BACK PAIN
Symptoms Pain in the lower back that radiates outward or down the thigh, accompanied by stiffness and possibly by a stitch in the abdomen or the side of the body.
Symptoms better With rest.
Symptoms worse Lying; from sitting; from standing; with movement; from treading heavily down stairs.

JOINT PAIN
Symptoms General joint and muscle aches in the arms and legs, with sharp pains radiating outward and down the limbs. Gout and arthritic pain may also respond to *Berberis*.
Symptoms better In the afternoon.
Symptoms worse With movement; from treading heavily down stairs.

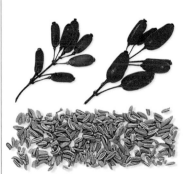

FEVER TONIC
In ancient Egypt, the red berries of the barberry plant were macerated with fennel seeds to make a drink for fevers.

KEY SYMPTOMS
COLICKY KIDNEY PAINS ◆ RADIATING PAINS ◆ LETHARGY AND LISTLESSNESS ◆ COLICKY PAINS IN THE REGION OF THE GALLBLADDER

SEE ALSO
Gastroenteritis, *page 236*; Cystitis, *page 260*

Bryonia alba

BRYONIA

DIOSCORIDES, the famous Greek physician of the 1st century CE, advocated bryony for gangrenous wounds, and the ancient Greeks and Romans also used it for epilepsy, vertigo, paralysis, gout, and coughs. In 17th-century England the herbalist Culpeper found bryony useful for phlegm, coughs, and shortness of breath. In 1834 Hahnemann proved the homeopathic remedy, which is used mostly for slow-starting ailments accompanied by pain on the slightest movement.

REMEDY PROFILE

Bryonia is mainly used for people who are highly irritable when ill. Often clean-living, meticulous individuals, they can be contrary and capricious if ill, wanting things that, when given, are promptly rejected. They may feel tired, taciturn, languid, and angry if disturbed. Anxiety is common, especially about financial security.

The chief physical symptom treated by *Bryonia* is pain felt on the slightest movement. It is often accompanied by infrequent spells of great thirst, and dry lips, mouth, and eyes. Illness sets in slowly, typically after overexposure to heat or cold. *Bryonia* is useful for chest inflammation, pneumonia, bad headaches, and rheumatic pains. It may also be taken for some forms of constipation and breast pain.

DRY COUGHS

Symptoms Great dryness in the mouth, throat, chest, and mucous membranes, with a tickly cough and sharp chest pains. Pressing the chest during a coughing fit may alleviate pain in the head, chest, or ribcage, as may lying still and breathing gently. Coughs may be linked to colds, pleurisy, or bronchitis.
Symptoms better With rest; lying still; from pressure on the chest.
Symptoms worse In warm rooms; in the morning; from deep breathing; with movement; from eating.

COLDS & THE FLU

Symptoms Red, sore, swollen nose, a hoarse, constricted throat, and a dry cough (*see below, left*). The lips are often cracked and itchy, and the mouth is dry, with a white-coated tongue. Sharp, shooting ear pains may develop, as may sore eyes with sensitivity to movement and heavy eyelids. There may be an intense, aching headache (*see below*), raging thirst, and copious perspiration.
Symptoms better With rest.
Symptoms worse Bending forward; with movement.

HEADACHES

Symptoms Bursting, splitting, headache over the forehead or left eye, so that even moving the eyeball hurts. Pain extends to the back of the head, then the whole head, often lasting all day. The mouth may be dry, and there may be great thirst.
Symptoms better From cold compresses; from pressure on the head; closing the eyes.
Symptoms worse With eye or body movement; from drinking while hot; overeating.

JOINT PAIN

Symptoms Joints and muscles are hot, swollen, stiff, and prone to stabbing pain, usually due to gout, tenosynovitis, or arthritis, or after an injury.

SOURCE DETAILS

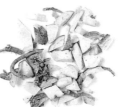

WHOLE ROOT

BRYONY
The root of this plant has a bitter taste and unpleasant smell. In excessive amounts, it can cause death within hours, usually from inflammation of the digestive tract.

Fresh root can cause severe skin irritation

CHOPPED ROOT

PULPED ROOT

ORIGIN
Grows mainly in hedges and woodlands of southern England, and in central and southern Europe.

BACKGROUND
Used traditionally for shortness of breath, coughing, and the clearing of phlegm from the chest.

PREPARATION
The fresh root is unearthed before the plant flowers, chopped, pulped, macerated in alcohol for ten days, diluted, and succussed.

KEY SYMPTOMS

PAIN UPON THE SLIGHTEST MOVEMENT ◆
DRY MUCOUS MEMBRANES ◆ GREAT THIRST ◆ ANXIETY ABOUT
FINANCIAL SECURITY ◆ IRRITABILITY

Symptoms better From pressure on the affected area.
Symptoms worse From cold compresses; with the slightest movement; with jarring.

CONSTIPATION

Symptoms Large, hard stools that look black or burned. The rectum may be particularly dry, with burning pain after passing a stool. Rumbly, colicky pains in the abdomen are common.
Symptoms better With rest.
Symptoms worse In hot weather; in the morning; with movement; from cold drinks.

BREAST PROBLEMS

Symptoms Breasts are pale, hard, and hot, with sharp pains, particularly in women who are pregnant or breast-feeding. Milk supply may be excessive.
Symptoms better With heat; with rest.
Symptoms worse With movement.

SEE ALSO
Breast problems, *page 201*; Bronchitis, *page 228*; Coughs, *page 228*; Constipation, *page 238*; Breast pain, *page 258*

Cannabis sativa 'Indica'

CANNABIS IND.

COMMON NAMES
Cannabis, marijuana, hashish,
Indian hemp, bhang bhanga

FIRST MENTIONED in a Chinese herbal dating to 2700 BCE, cannabis has long been an important medicine in the herbal repertories of many cultures. By the 19th century cannabis had become a standard painkiller in Europe. More recently, it has been prescribed as a conventional medicine in some countries to relieve nausea caused by chemotherapy and spasms due to multiple sclerosis. The plant is also an illegal recreational drug, and its prohibition extends to medicinal uses in many countries. The homeopathic remedy *Cannabis ind.* was proved by the American Provers' Union in 1839 and introduced by Dr. Trinks in 1841.

SOURCE DETAILS

CANNABIS
The active ingredient in this plant, tetrahydrocannabinol, causes mild euphoric effects when ingested or smoked.

Leaves are long and deeply serrated

REMEDY PROFILE

The behavior of those who benefit most from *Cannabis ind.* alternates between sweet and gentle, and desperate or even paranoid. Typical physical symptoms include a marked increase in appetite and thirst, especially for sweet foods and cold drinks.

Cannabis ind. is prescribed primarily to treat abnormal psychological states, such as confusion, disorientation, loss of memory, overexcitement, unwarranted fears, or paranoia. The remedy is also given for physical conditions such as headaches, urinary-tract infections, and pain in the legs.

In the paranoid state there is generally fear and anxiety, particularly a fear of losing control and becoming insane. There may be disorientation, memory loss, and confusion, even when in well-known environments. Travel or relocation may cause distress. Hallucinations that distort time, space, and distance are not uncommon.
Symptoms better In open air; with rest; from walking.
Symptoms worse In the dark; from tobacco; coffee.

DISORDERED MENTAL STATES
Symptoms Marked swings in thought and mood between a gentle state and paranoia. The gentle state is marked by mild euphoria, an overactive brain, and headstrong views, particularly about esoteric subjects such as astrology and Unidentified Flying Objects. Wonderful and enlightening ideas occur in rapid succession, but they are equally quickly forgotten. The slightest thing may trigger hysterical giggling. Prophetic dreams, out-of-body experiences, or an apparent ability to predict the future may also be experienced.

HEADACHES
Symptoms An opening and closing sensation at the top of the head, as if shock waves are passing through the brain. The head may shake involuntarily and feel as if it is separate from the body. A stooping posture may be adopted due to a sensation of heavy pressure on the brain or to a migraine.
Symptoms better With rest; from deep breathing.
Symptoms worse From exertion; from tobacco; from alcohol; from coffee.

URINARY-TRACT INFECTIONS
Symptoms A dull, burning, aching, or stitchlike pain in the right kidney. Urine may

ORIGIN
Native to China and central western Asia, but now grown worldwide, although usually subject to legal restrictions.

BACKGROUND
Important in cultures such as ancient Egypt, China, and India, as a strong analgesic, sedative, and anti-inflammatory.

PREPARATION
The flowering tops and seeds are finely chopped, macerated in alcohol for ten days, then filtered, diluted, and succussed.

KEY SYMPTOMS
MOODS SWING BETWEEN OVEREXCITEMENT AND PARANOIA ◆ OUT-OF-BODY EXPERIENCES ◆ BURNING PAIN IN THE URETHRA ◆ "OPENING AND SHUTTING" SENSATIONS IN THE HEAD

---

be profuse and colorless, with erratic flow due to obstructed urination. There may be urethritis (inflammation of the urethra) with mucus discharge and burning, stinging pain.
Symptoms better With rest; from deep breathing.
Symptoms worse In the morning; from tobacco; from alcohol; from coffee.

PAIN OR PARALYSIS IN THE LEGS
Symptoms Shooting pains that rise up the legs when walking. Exhaustion may

follow even a very short walk. Alternatively, there may be a sensation of paralysis in the lower limbs. These symptoms are frequently accompanied by a backache.
Symptoms better With rest; from deep breathing.
Symptoms worse From walking; during menstruation.

SEE ALSO
Confusion, *page 266*

Carbo vegetabilis

CARBO VEG.

CHARCOAL'S HARDNESS and durability have in the past made it a popular material for staking out land boundaries. Its ability to absorb gases and toxins in the body gained charcoal a reputation as a "purifier," and in the 18th and 19th centuries it was used in dressings for skin ulcers and in mouthwashes. Hahnemann proved and published the homeopathic remedy in his *Chronic Diseases* (1821–34). It became known as the "corpse reviver" for its ability to restore severe collapse.

REMEDY PROFILE

People who need *Carbo veg.* may be in a state of physical and mental collapse. It is used for debilitated states ranging from a simple faint or fatigue to exhaustion or more serious collapse. Those affected may never have fully recovered from a previous illness. Symptoms include extreme weariness on making the least effort, a patchy memory, and anxiety at night, along with a fear of the supernatural.

Typical physical symptoms include a cold, clammy body, a sallow face, weakness, and numbness or burning pain in the limbs. A tendency to suffer from trapped gas is common.

Despite usually feeling cold, people who respond to *Carbo veg.* like fresh air, especially if it is fanned over their faces. They may crave junk foods, coffee, candy, and salt, and long for alcohol although it makes them feel sick. In common with herbalists, homeopaths often give the remedy for flatulence and weak digestive functioning. *Carbo veg.* may also be taken for respiratory problems, or for a poor, sluggish constitution, particularly in the elderly.

FATIGUE
Symptoms Weakness, severe exhaustion, or low vitality. The skin is cold and pale, but the body feels hot inside, and there is a bitter taste in the mouth. *Carbo veg.* can be used for loss of vitality, fatigue, or shock during convalescence.
Symptoms better From burping; from being fanned.
Symptoms worse In warm, wet weather; in the evening; lying down; from rich, fatty foods; from wine; coffee.

CHRONIC FATIGUE SYNDROME
Aching, burning pains all over the body, and swollen, tender glands. Confusion, difficulty in concentrating, and anxiety may be evident, along with other symptoms of fatigue (*see above*).
Symptoms better In the afternoon; lying down.
Symptoms worse In cold, damp weather; at night; from exertion; from talking.

INDIGESTION & FLATULENCE
Symptoms Indigestion and flatulence that occur regardless of diet. Regurgitation of food

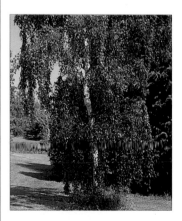

SILVER BIRCH
Wood from silver birch, beech, or poplar trees is commonly burned to make the type of charcoal used in homeopathy.

SOURCE DETAILS

ORIGIN
Made from silver birch, beech, or poplar trees, which grow on moors, heaths, woodland, and mountains throughout the northern hemisphere.

BACKGROUND
Used in traditional and conventional medicine for ulceration, septic diseases, flatulence, and indigestion. Also known for its deodorant and disinfectant properties.

PREPARATION
Fist-sized bits of wood are cut, heated until red hot, and sealed in an airtight earthenware jar. The resulting ash is then triturated, diluted, and succussed.

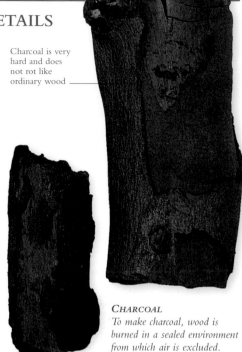

Charcoal is very hard and does not rot like ordinary wood

CHARCOAL
To make charcoal, wood is burned in a sealed environment from which air is excluded.

KEY SYMPTOMS
LISTLESS BEHAVIOR ♦ CONFUSION ♦ COLDNESS ♦ COLLAPSE ♦
PERSON FEELS BETTER FROM FANNED AIR ♦ FLATULENCE ♦
DESIRE FOR SWEETS, COFFEE, SALT, AND ALCOHOL

---

may be accompanied by sour burps, smelly gas, diarrhea, and bloating so that the skin of the stomach is stretched taut. Overeating may trigger nausea, dizziness, fainting, and morning headaches where the head feels heavy and hot.
Symptoms better In cold, fresh air; from passing wind; from burping.
Symptoms worse In the morning; lying down; from rich, fatty foods; from milk, coffee, or wine.

BREATHING PROBLEMS
Symptoms Spasmodic cough, whooping cough, asthma, and bronchitis in the elderly. There may be cold perspiration and weakness, choking, gagging, and vomiting of mucus. A desire for fresh air is common, as is a feeling of suffocation.
Symptoms better From fresh air; from being fanned; from sitting up.

Symptoms worse In warm, wet weather; from overheating; at night; from rich foods.

POOR CIRCULATION
Symptoms Reduced energy and lack of coordination due to poor circulation of oxygen around the body. The skin on the face, hands, and feet may be cold and blue. Hoarseness and a cold tongue and breath are common, and there may also be cold, puffy legs with a tendency for bleeding varicose veins to form.
Symptoms better In cold, fresh air; from burping.
Symptoms worse Lying down; in the evening; from milk, coffee, or fatty foods.

SEE ALSO
Chronic fatigue syndrome, *page 205*; Indigestion, *page 234*; Bloating & flatulence, *page 236*

Cephaelis ipecacuanha

IPECAC.

A PORTUGUESE FRIAR living in Brazil in the early 17th century first recorded the medicinal properties of ipecacuanha, a traditional remedy used by Brazilian Indians. Its name is from the Portuguese for "sick-making plant," since in large doses it causes nausea, vomiting, and even cardiac failure. In conventional medicine, drugs derived from the root are used to loosen phlegm in the respiratory tract and to induce vomiting. *Ipecac.* was proved by Hahnemann in 1805 and is used especially to relieve persistent nausea.

REMEDY PROFILE

Irritability is common in those who respond best to *Ipecac.*, and children suited to the remedy may scream and howl. When ill these people can be capricious and hard to please, asking for things and then changing their minds. Illness can prompt them to become morose, depressed, impatient, and contemptuous of those around them.

Physical symptoms generally linked with *Ipecac.* are persistent nausea, with or without vomiting, and a tendency to hemorrhage. Despite any vomiting, the tongue is clean and unfurred. There is often oversensitivity to movement and a constant feeling of being hot on the inside and cold on the outside. These symptoms appear rapidly, are generally intermittent, and may also include coughing fits and breathing difficulties. *Ipecac.* is also used for headaches, migraines, and gynecological problems linked to the general tendency to bleed very easily.

NAUSEA & VOMITING
Symptoms Persistent nausea that is not necessarily relieved by vomiting is a key symptom associated with *Ipecac.* There is a bloated, swollen feeling in the abdomen, and cramping, colicky pain that may be most severe around the navel, while the stomach may seem to "flop" inside the abdomen. Vomit consists mostly of undigested food or bile. Belching and excess saliva production are common, the mouth remains moist, and there is little thirst. The tongue tends to be clean and unfurred.

If gastroenteritis is the cause, there may be copious, watery, greenish-colored diarrhea that contains undigested food. If the skin is itchy, with sweat forming on the brow, then the symptom picture may indicate gallbladder problems. The nausea is very enervating, and may be accompanied by a weak pulse and fainting.
Symptoms better In fresh air.
Symptoms worse With warmth; lying down; with movement; from opiate drugs or tobacco; from eating.

COUGHS & WHEEZING
Symptoms An irritating, dry, rattling, loose cough, usually triggered by warm, humid weather. Breathing may be wheezy and asthmatic, and the chest may feel constricted. Although little phlegm may be produced, coughing may be violent and accompanied by nosebleeds, retching, nausea, vomiting, or coughing up of blood. These symptoms may be indicative of conditions such as bronchitis, whooping cough, and childhood asthma.
Symptoms better In fresh air; from sitting up.
Symptoms worse With heat and warmth; in the winter; lying down; with movement.

SOURCE DETAILS

Root is strongly emetic and used to induce vomiting

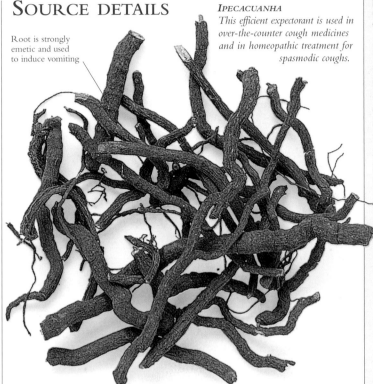

IPECACUANHA
This efficient expectorant is used in over-the-counter cough medicines and in homeopathic treatment for spasmodic coughs.

ORIGIN
Native to Central and South America and cultivated particularly in Brazil; this plant's preferred habitat is tropical rainforest.

BACKGROUND
A traditional Brazilian cure for dysentery that was taken to Europe in 1672, it is still used today by herbalists for amebic dysentery.

PREPARATION
The root is dug up and the firmest dark rootlets dried, powdered, and macerated in alcohol. They are then filtered, diluted, and succussed.

KEY SYMPTOMS
PERSISTENT NAUSEA AND VOMITING ◆ CLEAN, UNFURRED TONGUE ◆ BRIGHT RED BLEEDING ◆ EXCESSIVE MUCUS PRODUCTION AND A COUGH ◆ IRRITABILITY

MIGRAINE
Symptoms Migraine pain in the whole head, with severe nausea and vomiting. The pain extends to the face, teeth, and tongue. The face is pallid, or blue around the lips and eyes.
Symptoms better For fresh air.
Symptoms worse For warmth; for lying down; for movement; for stress; for embarrassment.

GYNAECOLOGICAL PROBLEMS
Symptoms Extremely heavy menstrual flow, possibly with nausea and fainting. Between menstrual periods there may be irregular spotting or a sudden, gushing flow of bright red blood from the uterus that proves slow to clot. *Ipecac.* may also be prescribed for morning sickness, for hemorrhaging in connection with a displaced placenta, and for bleeding and nausea in the aftermath of a miscarriage.
Symptoms better In fresh air.
Symptoms worse During and after labor; with movement.

SEE ALSO
Asthma, *page 181*; Nausea & vomiting, *page 236*; Morning sickness, *page 262*

Chamomilla recutita syn. *Matricaria chamomilla*

CHAMOMILLA

THE NAME OF THIS PLANT derives from the Greek *chamaimelon*, or "earth apple," so called because of the applelike scent of its blossoms. Culpeper, the 17th-century English herbalist, advocated chamomile for strengthening the uterus, especially after an arduous labor. Herbalists recommend it for external use as a poultice or cream for treating skin complaints such as eczema or burns. *Chamomilla*, proved by Hahnemann and published in his *Materia Medica Pura* (1821–34), is used for ailments with extreme sensitivity to pain, especially in children.

REMEDY PROFILE

Chamomilla works best for those exhibiting an extremely low pain threshold, as well as anger, marked irritability, and hostility. Often hypersensitive, they are bad-tempered, easily offended, and impossible to please. They flush easily when angry, and hate being touched. Bad temper, anger, or stress exacerbate physical symptoms.

Chamomilla is often given to children who are snappy, wail when ill, and are pacified only if being carried and cuddled by someone walking around.

Typical *Chamomilla* symptoms are great irritability and pain that seems unbearable. The remedy is given for teething pain, fever, stomach pain with diarrhea, menstrual or labor pains, and sore, inflamed nipples during breast-feeding.

IRRITABILITY
Symptoms Hypersensitivity to pain, and hostility and anger that triggers physical problems. Things may be demanded then promptly thrown away.
Symptoms better From being carried; from perspiring.
Symptoms worse From being touched; being put down.

TOOTHACHES, TEETHING & EARACHES
Symptoms Excruciating pain in the teeth or ears, with fever (*see below*). Toothaches flare up after a hot drink or if a tooth is pressed. Swollen glands may cause face and neck pain, and the ears, nose, and throat may feel blocked and numb. Babies teething may scream angrily, insist on being carried, and have greenish diarrhea.
Symptoms better In cold; from being carried.
Symptoms worse With heat; from warm foods and drinks.

FEVER
Symptoms A hot, flushed state, often with one cheek red and the other pale. There may be irritability, shivering, and a tendency to sweat easily.
Symptoms better In cold.
Symptoms worse With heat; from warm foods and drinks.

COLIC & DIARRHEA
Symptoms Colicky pain in the abdomen, possibly with pale green diarrhea that smells like rotten eggs. Colic in children may cause restlessness and arching of the back.
Symptoms better From warm compresses on the abdomen; from fasting.
Symptoms worse With heat; from fresh air; from anger.

MENSTRUAL & LABOR PAIN
Symptoms Menstrual cramps or labor pains, possibly severe enough to cause sweats, anger, or fainting. Anger may trigger nonmenstrual bleeding.
Symptoms better From being driven in a car.
Symptoms worse With heat; in drafts; in wind; in damp; from anger; if touched.

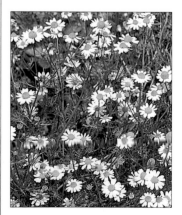

HEALING HERB
This herb is called "the plant's physician" since, when grown alongside sickly garden plants, it is reputed to aid their recovery.

SOURCE DETAILS

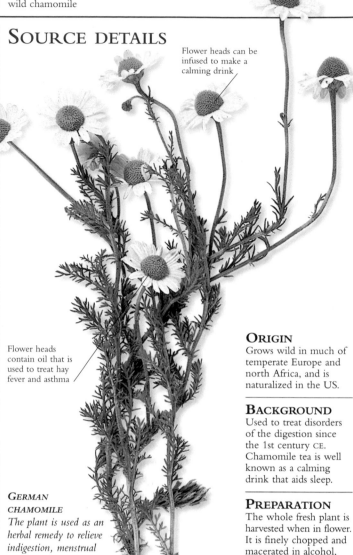

Flower heads can be infused to make a calming drink

Flower heads contain oil that is used to treat hay fever and asthma

GERMAN CHAMOMILE
The plant is used as an herbal remedy to relieve indigestion, menstrual pain, migraines, gout, and rheumatic pains.

ORIGIN
Grows wild in much of temperate Europe and north Africa, and is naturalized in the US.

BACKGROUND
Used to treat disorders of the digestion since the 1st century CE. Chamomile tea is well known as a calming drink that aids sleep.

PREPARATION
The whole fresh plant is harvested when in flower. It is finely chopped and macerated in alcohol, before being filtered, diluted, and succussed.

KEY SYMPTOMS
IRRITABILITY ◆ HYPERSENSITIVITY TO PAIN ◆ CHILDREN WANT TO BE CARRIED ◆ TEETHING PROBLEMS ◆ ONE CHEEK RED AND THE OTHER PALE ◆ GREENISH DIARRHEA

SEE ALSO
Toothache, *page 232*; Teething, *page 246*; Temper tantrums, *page 246*; Sleeplessness, *page 248*; Breast-feeding problems, *page 262*

Chelidonium majus
CHELIDONIUM

BECAUSE THIS PLANT FLOWERS as the swallows are migrating, Dioscorides, the famous Greek physician of the 1st century CE, named it after the Greek *khelidon*, or "swallow." In traditional medicine its juice was used for skin, liver, and gallbladder disorders. The homeopathic remedy was proved by Hahnemann and published in his *Materia Medica Pura* (1821–34).

REMEDY PROFILE

An aggressive, domineering personality is typically linked with *Chelidonium*. Those who respond well to the remedy tend also to be practical rather than intellectual people who do not like to "waste time" analyzing their emotions.

Typical physical symptoms include cravings for hot drinks and cheese. There is a feeling of heaviness, with symptoms tending to be right-sided.

Chelidonium is used mainly for liver conditions, or spleen, kidney, gallbladder, intestinal, and lung complaints. It may also be given prior to surgery linked to hepatitis or gallstones.

HEPATITIS
Symptoms An enlarged liver, with pain extending to the back and right shoulder blade, and jaundiced, yellow skin.

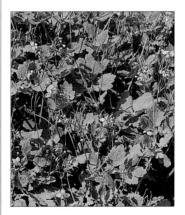

EYE TONIC
Dioscorides, believing that swallows used the plant's sap to sharpen their eyesight, advocated it for similar uses in humans.

The abdomen feels distended and tight, as if bound. There may be a strong craving for, or aversion to, cheese.
Symptoms better From a hot bath; from passing stools; from pressure on the affected area; from hot foods and drinks, such as hot milk.
Symptoms worse Lying on the right side; around 4 A.M. or 4 P.M.

GALLSTONES
Symptoms A sharp, constant pain on the upper right side of the abdomen, behind the ribs, possibly due to a gallstone trapped in a bile duct. The pain may resemble that of hepatitis (*see above*). It is often exacerbated by fatty foods, and may extend to the back and right shoulder blade (*see right*). There may be nausea and vomiting, and inflammation of the bile duct that may lead to jaundice or inflammation of the gallbladder.
Symptoms better From a hot bath; from passing stools; from pressure on the affected area; from hot foods and drinks, such as hot milk.
Symptoms worse Lying on the right side; around 4 A.M. and 4 P.M; from fatty foods.

HEADACHES
Symptoms A sensation of heaviness on the right side of the head. There may also be facial numbness and neuralgia (especially above the eye), and

SOURCE DETAILS

Yellow flowers resemble poppies, which belong to same plant family

GREATER CELANDINE
The freshly crushed plant exudes a sticky, orange sap, which herbalists use to treat warts and corns.

ORIGIN
Native to Europe, north Africa, and western Asia, and now naturalized in North America. Grows in banks and hedges.

BACKGROUND
Used in Western and Chinese herbalism as a muscle relaxant and antispasmodic, and to clear cataracts.

PREPARATION
The whole flowering plant, or the root, is chopped, pulped, and macerated in alcohol for at least ten days.

KEY SYMPTOMS

RIGHT-SIDED COMPLAINTS ◆ PRACTICAL, DOMINANT NATURE ◆ LIVER AND GALLBLADDER PROBLEMS ◆ PAIN IN THE RIGHT SHOULDER BLADE ◆ PERSON FEELS BETTER WITH HOT DRINKS

a yellow-coated tongue that retains teethmarks. These symptoms may be linked to an existing liver disorder (*see left*).
Symptoms better From a hot bath; from bending backward; from pressure on the affected area; hot foods and drinks.
Symptoms worse Lying on the right side; with movement; around 4 A.M. and 4 P.M.

SHOULDER PAIN
Symptoms Shoulder pain with icy coldness in the fingertips and muscles that feel sore to the touch. There may be associated nausea and perspiration.
Symptoms better From having a hot bath; from pressure on the affected area; from bending backward.
Symptoms worse Lying on

the right side; with movement; from coughing; around 4 A.M. and 4 P.M.

PNEUMONIA
Symptoms Breathlessness and pain on coughing or breathing deeply, with pneumonia that chiefly affects the right lung and, possibly, liver problems.
Symptoms better From hot foods and drinks.
Symptoms worse With warmth; lying on the right side; with movement; from coughing.

SEE ALSO
Cancer, *page 208*

Cimicifuga racemosa
CIMICIFUGA

THIS NORTH AMERICAN PLANT'S genus name is derived from the Latin words *cimex,* "bug," and *fugere,* "to flee," a reference to its properties as an insect repellent. Native Americans used the root to treat gynecological problems, and its beneficial effect on conditions arising during menopause was confirmed in German studies published in 1995. *Cimicifuga* was proved in 1852 by Drs. Hempel, Wells, Paine, and Mears, a team of US homeopaths.

REMEDY PROFILE

Primarily a women's remedy, *Cimicifuga* is particularly suited to those whose emotions swing between overexcitement and depression. They tend to have very intense emotional lives, possibly marked by fears of death and insanity. Emotional symptoms often alternate with physical ones, such as chilliness and sharp pains, especially on the left side of the body. Symptoms may intensify during menstruation.

Cimicifuga acts upon the nerves and uterine muscles. It is prescribed mostly for gynecological problems; for head, neck, and back pain; and for emotional symptoms.

MENOPAUSE

Symptoms Severe hot flashes, fainting spells, and other typical menopausal symptoms, but in an extreme form. Depression and irrational fears are common (*see right*).
Symptoms better In the open air; from bending over; with gentle movement.
Symptoms worse In cold; from sitting; emotional stress.

MENSTRUAL PROBLEMS

Symptoms Heavy menstrual flow, with dark-red, clotted blood, shooting, cramping pains radiating across the pelvis into the thighs, and bearing-down pains in the lower back. Menstruation is often too frequent, too early, or absent. Before menstruation there may be burning breast pain and congestion in the head. Premenstrual syndrome, depression (*see below, right*), and irrational fears are commonly associated with the remedy.
Symptoms better In the open air; from bending over; with gentle movement.
Symptoms worse In cold; from sitting; under stress.

PREGNANCY

Symptoms Vomiting, nausea, and lack of sleep. Lower back pain and a bruised feeling all over the body are common, with abdominal pains shooting from side to side. There may be depression and irrational fears (*see below, right*). *Cimicifuga* may also be prescribed for protracted labor and recovery from an early miscarriage.
Symptoms better In the open air; from bending over; with gentle movement.
Symptoms worse In cold; from sitting; emotional stress.

HEAD & NECK PAIN

Symptoms Headaches in the top or side of the head, which may dull thought, or pain or

RATTLEROOT
The seed pods of this plant make a rattling noise in the wind that is similar to that of the rattlesnake.

SOURCE DETAILS

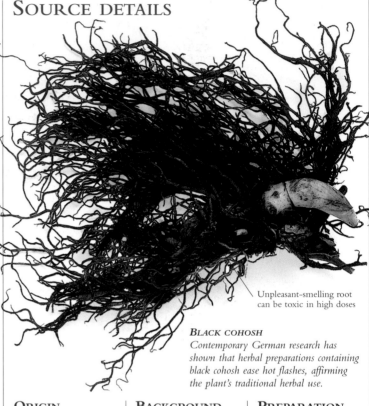

Unpleasant-smelling root can be toxic in high doses

BLACK COHOSH
Contemporary German research has shown that herbal preparations containing black cohosh ease hot flashes, affirming the plant's traditional herbal use.

ORIGIN
Indigenous to Canada and eastern parts of the US, but now also grown in Europe. Prefers moist, shady conditions, such as those to be found in woods and hedges.

BACKGROUND
Traditionally used by Native Americans for health problems in women. Used in contemporary herbal medicine as a sedative and antidepressant.

PREPARATION
Fresh root and rhizome are harvested in autumn. They are pounded to a pulp, then mixed with alcohol and left to stand before being strained, filtered, and succussed.

KEY SYMPTOMS
DEPRESSION ◆ NECK AND BACK PAIN ◆ FEAR OF DEATH ◆
GREAT EXCITABILITY ◆ MENSTRUAL IRREGULARITIES

---

stiffness in the neck or nape of the neck, which may radiate to the upper back or shoulders.
Symptoms better In the open air; from wrapping up; lying flat; from pressure on the neck and head.
Symptoms worse In cold, wind, drafts, and dampness; from weather changes; from physical strain; menstruating; from menopause; at night.

DEPRESSION

Symptoms Black moods and heavy sighing, alternating with euphoria, loquaciousness, and a tendency to jump from topic to topic. Possible fears of insanity and death worsen with the onset of the menopause. *Cimicifuga* may also be given for postpartum depression, especially when accompanied by feelings of imprisonment.
Symptoms better In open air; with gentle movement.
Symptoms worse From menstruating; from pregnancy; after giving birth; from menopause.

SEE ALSO

Depression, *page 212*; Headache, *page 218*; Painful periods, *page 256*; Heavy periods, *page 258*

Cinchona officinalis
CHINA

THE SOURCE OF THIS REMEDY is Peruvian bark, which was taken from South America to Europe by Jesuits in the 17th century. This bark is of particular historical significance for homeopaths, since quinine extracted from it became the subject of Hahnemann's first homeopathic proving. In 1790 he tested quinine on himself, and noticed that it caused symptoms similar to the malaria for which it was prescribed as a cure (*see page 15*). He developed the remedy *China*, which has become a key treatment for malarial symptoms and exhaustion due to fluid loss or long-term illness.

REMEDY PROFILE

China is thought to work best for idealistic, artistic people. Despite problems articulating their feelings, they prefer meaningful talk to trivial chat, but their own intensity often tires them, causing irritability, laziness, depression, violence, or intolerance. Easily offended, they may feel paranoid and mistreated, or that they have been born unfortunate, as if the world is hostile to them. A highly active imagination can lead to a preoccupation with future plans and to egocentric, heroic fantasies that later cause embarrassment.

Physical symptoms may be linked to weaknesses in the liver and digestive system and generally include a dislike of butter and other fatty foods, and cravings for alcohol and foods that are sweet or spicy.

The remedy is used for exhaustion following illness or extreme fluid loss. It is also given for fever, insomnia, gastric upsets, and headaches.

EXHAUSTION

Symptoms Extreme lethargy, with weak, jumpy muscles, and oversensitivity to noises, smells, and touch. Fatigue can be due to extensive fluid loss caused by diarrhea, severe vomiting, or possibly breast-feeding. It can also be a result of anemia, possibly linked to blood loss or heavy menstrual flow, or to debilitating illness, such as chronic fatigue syndrome (CFS).
Symptoms better Lying down.
Symptoms worse If touched; near noise; from walking.

FEVER

Symptoms Intermittent high temperature with shivering chills and profuse sweats. Thirst may be absent during sweats, but is marked with the chills. The skin may be sallow or flushed, and sensitive to the slightest touch.
Symptoms better With warmth; with sleep; from firm pressure on the affected area.
Symptoms worse In cold; in drafts; at night; in autumn.

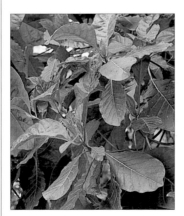

SOURCE OF QUININE
Since its introduction into Europe in the 17th century, cultivation of this bitter-tasting evergreen shrub has attained worldwide significance. It is now grown commercially in many tropical regions.

SOURCE DETAILS

ORIGIN
Native to the tropical forests of South America, but now grown in southeast Asia, India, Sri Lanka, and East Africa.

BACKGROUND
In the 17th century Jesuits used quinine, extracted from Peruvian bark, as a cure for malaria. It was widely adopted in Europe as a treatment for fevers.

PREPARATION
The bark is macerated in alcohol for at least five days, before being filtered, diluted, and then succussed.

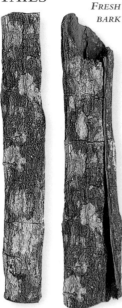

FRESH BARK

DRIED BARK

PERUVIAN BARK
The bark of this tropical tree yields quinine, which causes symptoms similar to those of malaria if taken in large doses.

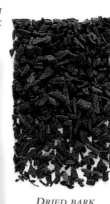

KEY SYMPTOMS
EXHAUSTION AFTER FLUID LOSS ◆ GREAT IMAGINATION ◆ DESIRE FOR ALCOHOL AND FOR SWEET OR SPICY FOODS

INSOMNIA
Symptoms Sleeplessness due to excited thoughts and heroic fantasies. Even the slightest noise disrupts sleep. The mind tends to be very clear in the evening and at night.
Symptoms better For warmth.
Symptoms worse For cold; for draughts.

DIGESTIVE DISORDERS
Symptoms Indigestion accompanied by ineffectual burping and a sensation that food is stuck behind the breastbone. The abdomen may feel bloated. Wind that is difficult to expel may cause pain or, alternatively, pain may remain even after expulsion of wind. There may be attacks of profuse, watery, painless diarrhoea. The appetite may be disturbed, causing either great hunger at night or a complete loss of appetite that, however, returns after the first mouthful of a meal. A bitter taste in the mouth may arise from an unsettled stomach.

In addition, *China* may be prescribed to treat digestive symptoms arising as a result of gastroenteritis and disorders of the gallbladder.
Symptoms better With warmth; with rest; from firm pressure on the affected area.
Symptoms worse At night; after eating; from sour foods; from drinking, especially tea.

HEADACHES
Symptoms Throbbing pain in the head, possibly linked to facial neuralgia, nosebleeds, tinnitus, or liver disorders.
Symptoms better With warmth; from firm pressure on the painful area; with sleep.
Symptoms worse In cold; in drafts; at night; in the autumn; if lightly touched, such as combing the hair.

SEE ALSO
Chronic fatigue syndrome, page 205

Coffea cruda syn. *C. arabica*

COFFEA

COMMON NAMES
Coffee, Arabian coffee

NATIVE TO ETHIOPIA, COFFEE was reportedly first drunk in the Middle East, introduced to Europe in the 17th century, then taken by Europeans to the East and to South America. It has been incorporated into Ayurvedic medicine, which uses unripe beans to treat headaches and ripe, roasted beans for diarrhea. Coffee's main active constituent, caffeine, has been used medicinally as an analgesic, a diuretic, a digestive tonic, and a stimulant to the nervous system. Modern medicine combines caffeine with conventional analgesics such as aspirin to make over-the-counter painkillers. However, coffee has long had a reputation for being simultaneously helpful and harmful: excessive consumption upsets the digestion, drains the body of calcium, and can cause nervousness. Dr. Stapf proved the homeopathic remedy in 1823.

REMEDY PROFILE

Drinking too much coffee produces symptoms that are very similar to those treated by *Coffea*. Homeopaths often prescribe it for those with overactive minds and thoughts that race uncontrollably. This is generally accompanied by restlessness and nervousness.

Coffea is also useful for those who experience overly excited or ecstatic states, perhaps precipitated by narcotics, a series of events, or a sudden shock, such as very good or very bad news. Such states can frequently trigger excessive exhilaration or despair, with an inability to calm down and insomnia or headaches. The nerves are taut, and the senses may be so acute that fresh air, noises, smells, and tastes seem unbearable. Hypersensitivity to pain, to the point where pain causes intense despair, is not unusual. *Coffea* may also help insomnia, palpitations, overexcitement, and hot flashes during menopause.

INSOMNIA
Symptoms Excess mental activity, making the mind race with thoughts and ideas. Sleep may be impossible for long periods, despite tiredness, due to a frustrating inability to switch off the mind. Any sleep obtained is interrupted by the slightest noise, since the nerves are stretched taut. Symptoms may often be due to pressure or stress involving work deadlines or exam revision.
Symptoms better With warmth; with rest.
Symptoms worse In cold, windy weather; near noise, odors, and if touched.

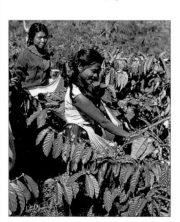

*AN IMPORTANT COMMERCIAL CROP
In Brazil and the West Indies the entire production of this important export crop is said to originate from a single plant that was introduced to the Americas in 1822.*

SOURCE DETAILS

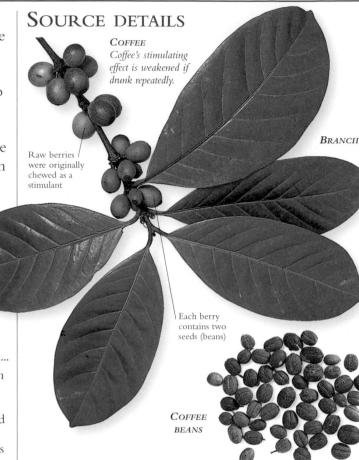

COFFEE
Coffee's stimulating effect is weakened if drunk repeatedly.

Raw berries were originally chewed as a stimulant

BRANCH

Each berry contains two seeds (beans)

COFFEE BEANS

ORIGIN
Native to Ethiopia, but now grown in tropical areas worldwide. South America and African countries such as Kenya and Tanzania supply the bulk of the world's crop.

BACKGROUND
Originally an African stimulant and drink that spread to Arabia and was used by Muslims to stay awake in all-night prayer. In England, the Church linked it with the devil.

PREPARATION
Ripe, unroasted coffee beans are macerated in alcohol for at least five days before being filtered. The resulting liquid is then repeatedly diluted and succussed.

KEY SYMPTOMS
OVERSTIMULATION LEADING TO SLEEP PROBLEMS ◆ EXTREME SENSITIVITY TO PAIN ◆ RESTLESSNESS AND NERVOUSNESS

HEADACHES
Symptoms One-sided pain in the head, which feels as if a nail is being driven into it. Pain sets in on waking, and can seem unbearable. It can extend to the ears and teeth (*see right*), with possible facial neuralgia. Common triggers are tension, stress, or an overactive mind.
Symptoms better From cold compresses; lying or sitting still in darkness.
Symptoms worse In fresh air; near noise; from tea or coffee.

TOOTHACHE
Symptoms Pain that shoots downward from the teeth to the tips of the fingers.
Symptoms better From ice or cold water on the affected area
Symptoms worse With heat; from menstruation; hot foods.

SEE ALSO
Toothache, page 232; Insomnia, page 244

Conium maculatum

CONIUM

COMMON NAMES
Hemlock, spotted hemlock

GENERATIONS OF STORYTELLERS have woven the poison hemlock into their tales. The Greek physician Dioscorides and the Roman natural historian Pliny used it in the 1st century CE to calm sexual urges, as a painkiller, and for skin complaints, nervous disorders, and breast tumors. Hahnemann proved and published the homeopathic remedy in his *Chronic Diseases* (1821–34).

REMEDY PROFILE

Conium is prescribed for people whose minds are dulled by illness, so that they seem mentally paralyzed, tired, and depressed, with "fixed" ideas and an aversion to company. These people tend to be very materialistic when young, but ultimately lose interest in possessions.

The remedy is prescribed for cysts or tumors in the reproductive organs. It is used if physical symptoms, such as gradual stiffening of the legs, "mirror" the mental paralysis. *Conium* may help if illness is due to mental strain, grief, or old age. In the elderly, it is thought to restore vitality and counter premature aging. It is also used for giddiness, as well as for emotional and physical problems due to sexual excess or suppression of the sex drive.

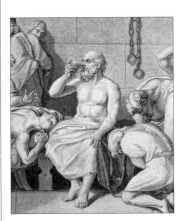

SOCRATES
The famous philosopher was condemned to die by drinking hemlock in 399 BCE, when it was used in ancient Greece as a "state poison" for capital punishment.

CYSTS, TUMORS & CANCER
Symptoms Hard lumps in the prostate, testicles, breasts, ovaries, or uterus, with sharp local pain and a possible feeling of internal itchiness. Breast tumors may be accompanied by secondary lumps in the armpits.
Symptoms better From local pressure; with movement.
Symptoms worse From injury; exertion; at night; from the pressure of tight clothing.

SWOLLEN BREASTS
Symptoms Enlarged, tender, hard breasts prior to menstrual periods, with heaviness in the legs and a reduced sex drive.
Symptoms better From pressure on the breasts; letting the arms hang down; from fasting; expressing emotion.
Symptoms worse In cold; lying down; from turning over in bed; with movement.

ENLARGED PROSTATE
Symptoms A sensation of heaviness in the prostate and frequent interruption of urine flow, possibly with a discharge from the penis and impotency.
Symptoms better From firm local pressure; from walking.
Symptoms worse From injury; from exertion; lying down; from tight clothing.

NERVOUS DISORDERS
Symptoms Cold, trembly, weak legs, with giddiness and sensitivity to light. Weakness

SOURCE DETAILS

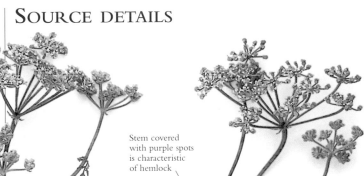

Stem covered with purple spots is characteristic of hemlock

HEMLOCK
The toxins in this plant cause paralysis, primarily of the respiratory nerves, which leads to death by suffocation if taken in excess.

ORIGIN
Common in hedges, damp meadows, along riverbanks, and on waste ground throughout much of Europe, Asia, and North America.

BACKGROUND
Used in ancient Rome for epilepsy, mania, chorea, swellings, and tumors. In 19th-century Europe hemlock was given as a painkiller.

PREPARATION
The fresh flowering plant, including the root, is macerated in alcohol and then diluted and succussed.

KEY SYMPTOMS

MATERIALISTIC NATURE WITH FIXED IDEAS ◆ COMPLAINTS THAT ARE TRIGGERED BY SUPPRESSION OF SEXUAL FEELINGS ◆ TENDENCY TO DEVELOP TUMORS

---

may eventually extend to the entire body. These symptoms are common in advancing age.
Symptoms better With warmth; with movement; letting the limbs hang down.
Symptoms worse From injury; from exertion; with jarring; from eating.

SEXUAL PROBLEMS
Symptoms Extreme sexual excitement with premature ejaculation or impotence in men, and vaginal discharge

and irregular menstruation in women. Suppression of sexual activity may cause anxiety, depression, and forgetfulness.
Symptoms better From pressure on the genitals.
Symptoms worse From sexual excess or celibacy.

SEE ALSO

Breast problems, *page 201*; Prostate problems, *page 202*; Cancer, *page 208*; Breast pain, *page 258*

Cucumis colocynthis syn. *Citrullus colocynthis*

COLOCYNTHIS

COMMON NAMES
Colocynth, bitter apple, bitter cucumber

IN THE OLD TESTAMENT it is related that the prophet Elisha turned this bitter, toxic gourd into an edible fruit during famine, but colocynth was generally used as a drastic purgative, and also to induce abortion. Ingesting the pulp causes inflammation of the bowels and severe cramps. The homeopathic remedy, which was proved by Hahnemann in 1821, is used to treat these same symptoms, as well as colicky pains, neuralgia, and cramps in the pelvis.

REMEDY PROFILE

Colocynthis works best on those whose symptoms are brought on by suppressed anger. These people tend to be generally restless, anxious, and reserved, but easily irritated or angered. They have a strong sense of right and wrong, and can feel humiliated if their opinion is contradicted; the humiliation then gives way to indignation. *Colocynthis* is prescribed if the physical complaint, such as neuralgia or a digestive disorder, is brought on by, or exacerbated by, repressed anger.

The remedy is used chiefly for acute pain, specifically colicky abdominal pain; cramping in the hips, kidneys, and ovaries; headaches; or shooting nerve pain in the face, neck, and limbs. It may also be prescribed for gout and rheumatic pain in the neck.

COLIC & DIARRHEA

Symptoms Intense, twisting, spasmodic pains just below the navel. Often of sudden onset, the pain is generally linked to repressed anger but may also have a physical cause, such as gallstones. Other symptoms include nausea, vomiting, and diarrhea with copious, thin, green or yellowish stools. The abdomen may feel bloated, and pressing on the site or passing gas may bring relief.

Colocynthis may be prescribed for infantile colic if a baby screams, gets red in the face, and draws the legs up to abdomen. The pain is usually most intense in the evening, lasting from a few minutes to several hours.
Symptoms better With warmth; bending over; from passing gas or stools; coffee.
Symptoms worse With anger; before diarrhea or passing stools; from drinking; from eating, particularly fruits.

FACIAL NEURALGIA

Symptoms Searing pain on the right side of the face, maybe extending to the ear. The burning, lacerating pain often comes in acute waves. There may also be a headache with right-sided facial neuralgia.
Symptoms better From firm pressure on the affected area; with sleep; from coffee.
Symptoms worse With anger; if touched; with movement.

MENSTRUAL PROBLEMS

Symptoms Cramping pain in the uterus or ovaries during menstruation. Alternatively, menstrual periods may cease entirely following bouts of extreme anger.
Symptoms better In heat; from the application of firm

SOURCE DETAILS

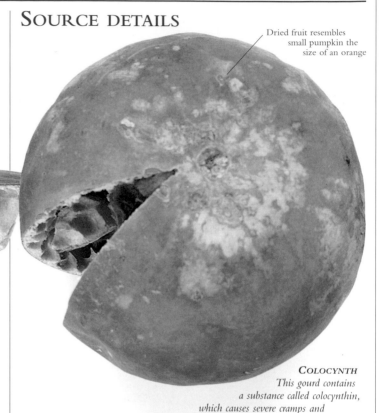

Dried fruit resembles small pumpkin the size of an orange

COLOCYNTH
This gourd contains a substance called colocynthin, which causes severe cramps and gastrointestinal inflammation if ingested.

Seeds are considered nutritious but are not used in homeopathy

ORIGIN
Native to Turkey, but can now be found growing in many hot, dry, sandy regions throughout the world.

BACKGROUND
Used in ancient Greece as a strong purgative and for complaints ranging from mania to lethargy, edema, and dropsy.

PREPARATION
The dried, deseeded fruit is powdered and macerated in alcohol, before being diluted and succussed.

KEY SYMPTOMS

CONDITIONS THAT ARE TRIGGERED BY REPRESSED ANGER ◆ COLICKY PAINS THAT ARE RELIEVED BY PRESSURE ◆ INDIGNATION ◆ NEURALGIC PAINS THAT ARE BETTER WITH WARMTH

---

pressure to the affected area.
Symptoms worse In cold; from anger; emotional stress.

NEURALGIC PAINS

Symptoms Sharp pains down the outer side (usually the right side) of the thigh, leg, and foot. These severe, tearing pains are often accompanied by backache, followed by numbness and weakness in the limbs. Sciatica and sharp, cramping pain in the kidneys, hips, or pelvis may also be helped by this remedy.

Symptoms better With warmth; bending over; lying on the painful side; from firm pressure on the affected area.
Symptoms worse In cold; in drafts; with anger; with the slightest movement, even breathing deeply, lying on the nonpainful side.

SEE ALSO

Irritable bowel syndrome, *page 189*; Ulcerative colitis, *page 190*; Sciatica, *page 218*; Gastroenteritis, *page 236*; Colic, *page 246*

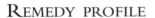

Datura stramonium
STRAMONIUM

COMMON NAMES
Thorn apple, devil's apple, stinkweed, false castor oil

ASTRONG hallucinogen, thorn apple was used in the salves of medieval folk healers and in Native American shamanistic rites. It relaxes the muscles of the bronchial tubes and digestive and urinary tracts, and reduces mucus secretions. *Stramonium*, proved by Hahnemann and published in his *Materia Medica Pura* (1821–34), is used for violent brain activity, often due to nervous disorders.

REMEDY PROFILE

People who respond best to *Stramonium* may experience rage and violence, particularly sudden outbursts accompanied by strong fears. The anger may be rooted in profound fear, following abuse or an accident. The fear may take the form of terror of the dark or of water. Those affected may also manifest hyperactive or overt sexuality. They are prone to stammering, and may have religious delusions, praying and proselytizing incessantly. Sleep may exacerbate symptoms.

Stramonium is prescribed for fevers and chest complaints accompanied by the typical rages and terrors. It is also used, if the characteristic traits are evident, for delirium, tics, convulsions, Parkinson's disease, epilepsy, and other nervous-system disorders.

The remedy is sometimes prescribed to treat chorea and for some serious psychological problems, such as mania, manic depression, and schizophrenia, particularly if they are accompanied by hallucinations or violence.

FEVER
Symptoms High fever with a burning thirst. There may be night terrors, fear of the dark, hallucinations, delirium, or febrile convulsions. The limbs may twitch involuntarily, and the heart and pulse may be "in turmoil."
Symptoms better With warmth; in light.
Symptoms worse In cloudy weather; with sleep; in darkness; from being left alone; looking at shiny, reflective surfaces; from swallowing.

VIOLENCE & MANIA
Symptoms Excitability with disorientation, confusion, a tendency to violence, and fear of the dark. Writhing, bouts of garrulousness, and incoherent muttering are common, and there may be hallucinations, visions, and imaginary voices. Symptoms may be triggered by the trauma of childbirth, by alcoholism or drug addiction, or by more serious conditions such as schizophrenia.
Symptoms better With warmth; in light.
Symptoms worse If touched; in darkness; from looking at shiny, reflective objects; from looking at dark water.

CHOREA
Symptoms Involuntary, jerky, twitches of the face, limbs, or trunk, often with stammering. Symptoms may be caused by extreme fright, a head injury, a bad reaction to vaccination, or meningitis. In extreme cases there may be facial grimacing, convulsions, or epilepsy.
Symptoms better With warmth; in light.
Symptoms worse In windy weather; if touched; from looking at shiny, reflective objects; looking at dark water.

SOURCE DETAILS

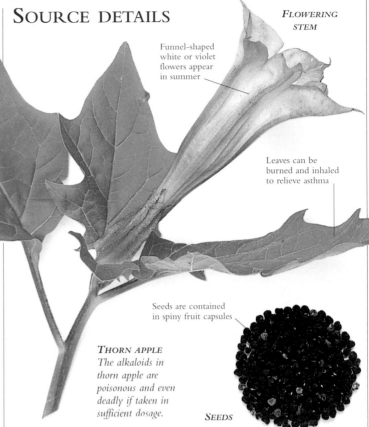

FLOWERING STEM

Funnel-shaped white or violet flowers appear in summer

Leaves can be burned and inhaled to relieve asthma

Seeds are contained in spiny fruit capsules

THORN APPLE
The alkaloids in thorn apple are poisonous and even deadly if taken in sufficient dosage.

SEEDS

ORIGIN
Thought to be native to both South America and western Asia, but now found growing in many temperate areas, often on wasteland.

BACKGROUND
Introduced to Europe in the 16th century and traditionally used as a narcotic, a painkiller, an anti-inflammatory, and to treat convulsions.

PREPARATION
The fresh leaves and flowers, or the seeds, are chopped and macerated in alcohol, before being filtered, diluted, and succussed.

KEY SYMPTOMS
ANGER ACCOMPANIED BY FEAR ♦ FEAR OF THE DARK ♦ FEAR OF WATER ♦ STAMMERING ♦ TREMBLING AND CONVULSIONS

ASTHMA
Symptoms Breathlessness, tightness in the chest, or a dry, wheezy cough. Attacks occur with, or after, fits of intense rage or fear.
Symptoms better With warmth; in light.
Symptoms worse In darkness; in the morning; in the evening; from looking at dark water.

BRONCHITIS
Symptoms Wheezing that is associated with shortness of breath, or a cough that generates yellow or green phlegm. Strong fear or anger may trigger or exacerbate the symptoms.
Symptoms better With warmth; in light.
Symptoms worse In darkness; in the morning; in the evening; from looking at dark water.

SEE ALSO
Irritable bowel syndrome, *page 189*; Phobias, *page 211*

Delphinium staphisagria

STAPHYSAGRIA

As LONG AGO AS THE 5th century BCE, ancient Greek physicians were using this plant to purge the bowels and to induce vomiting. Applied externally, it was given as an antidote to stings and bites. Its common name, stavesacre, comes from the ancient Greek *staphis,* "raisin" and *agria,* "wild." The plant's seeds are a powerful poison. The homeopathic remedy, proved by Hahnemann in 1819, is typically used to treat people who tend to suppress their emotions, especially anger.

REMEDY PROFILE

Staphysagria is most appropriate for people who bottle up their emotions, especially rage. They tend to be extremely sensitive, particularly to criticism or rudeness. Irritation and anger can bubble away inside them, although they appear mild-natured and yielding on the surface, avoiding confrontation. When their emotions finally erupt, they often overreact and tremble with anger.

Common physical symptoms include perspiration, gas, and stools that smell of rotten eggs. Cravings for alcohol and sweet foods are typical. Suppressing emotions may cause headaches, depression, or an increased sex drive. Despite shyness, the libido is often high and there is a tendency to masturbate.

Staphysagria is most commonly prescribed for cystitis and other urogenital disorders, and for joint pains and neuralgia, skin conditions, insomnia, and toothaches.

UROGENITAL PROBLEMS
Symptoms Cystitis in either sex after sexual intercourse, especially on the first occasion, or on the first occasion with a new partner. In men there may be urine retention, linked to an enlarged prostate, and the testicles may wither or develop lumps. There may also be other urinary problems, such as urethritis, bed-wetting, and symptoms that develop following urogenital surgery and catheterization.

Symptoms better With warmth; after meals.
Symptoms worse From the slightest touch or pressure; from suppressing emotions.

JOINT PAIN
Symptoms Bruised, sore, weak, or immobile limbs. The right shoulder may be painful, and there may be neuralgia. Joints may have bony nodules.
Symptoms better In warmth.
Symptoms worse If touched; with movement.

SKIN CONDITIONS
Symptoms Easily infected, unhealthy-looking skin that is slow to heal if cut. Stinging pains persist in slow-healing wounds or scars. The remedy may help speed wound-healing after surgery, particularly if the temperament matches the remedy profile. There may be skin eruptions such as eczema and psoriasis with dry, thick crusts and itching, or weepy, scaly skin that burns before and after being scratched. After being scratched an itch may occur elsewhere on the body.
Symptoms better In warmth.
Symptoms worse If touched; from suppressing emotions.

HEADACHES
Symptoms Compressing pain as though a weight is boring through the forehead, or a numb sensation in the head, with dizzy spells that intensify on sitting or lying down.
Symptoms better In warmth;

SOURCE DETAILS

STAVESACRE
This plant has been used herbally for centuries as an emetic and a treatment for head lice, warts, and itching.

ORIGIN
Native to Europe and now grown in Asia and southern Europe. Prefers chalky, loamy soil in areas of waste ground and cornfields.

BACKGROUND
In Western herbal medicine the seeds of the plant can be used to make an ointment for treating head lice and other parasites.

PREPARATION
The seeds of the plant are gathered once it has finished flowering. They are then dried, triturated, and succussed.

SEEDS

FLOWERING STEM

Delicate, pale-blue or purple flowers appear in summer

KEY SYMPTOMS
CONDITIONS GENERATED AS SIDE EFFECTS OF SURGERY, PARTICULARLY UROGENITAL SURGERY ◆ SUPPRESSED EMOTIONS ◆ INCREASED SEX DRIVE AND MASTURBATION

---

from yawning.
Symptoms worse From mental exertion; in the early morning; from anger.

INSOMNIA
Symptoms Exhaustion and frequent yawning. Despite the fatigue, there is difficulty in falling into a deep sleep, and even after sleeping there may be bad temper, irritability, and continued exhaustion.
Symptoms better In warmth.
Symptoms worse From an afternoon nap; from emotional stress; from sexual excess.

TOOTHACHE
Symptoms Decay associated with black, loose teeth, causing pain in the affected area that is worse from being touched.
Symptoms better In warmth; with rest.
Symptoms worse From biting and chewing; touching the affected area.

SEE ALSO
Palpitations, *page 186*; Psoriasis, *page 195*; Infertility, *page 203*; Grief, *page 213*; Sties, *page 220*; Cystitis, *page 260*

Helleborus niger

HELLEBORUS

COMMON NAMES
Black hellebore, Christmas rose

As early as 1400 BCE the Roman natural historian Pliny wrote of using black hellebore for mental conditions. Ancient Greek and Roman philosophers would drink an infusion of the plant to increase their concentration before prolonged debates. The herb is extremely toxic and is now used only in homeopathy, since herbalists believe that it is too strong to be used safely. *Helleborus* was proved by Hahnemann and published in his *Materia Medica Pura* (1821–34).

SOURCE DETAILS

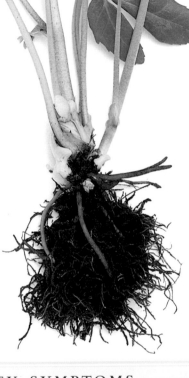

BLACK HELLEBORE
This plant is poisonous if ingested in all but the smallest doses. It was used in medieval medicine to expel an excess of "black bile," a bodily "humor" (see page 12) linked with insanity.

ORIGIN
Grows naturally on rocky or mountainous sites in southern Europe. Flowers from winter to spring and is widely cultivated as a popular garden plant.

BACKGROUND
Used in the past by herbalists as a treatment for lice, and as a local anesthetic, purgative, heart tonic, and means of inducing an abortion. The leaves were used as a heart stimulant for the elderly.

PREPARATION
The tincture is prepared from the fresh root of the plant. This is dug up in the winter, chopped, and macerated, then filtered and succussed.

REMEDY PROFILE

The people who benefit most from taking this remedy are characteristically dull and sluggish. It is best suited to those who feel stupefied and have slow mental processes. They commonly experience anguish, irritability, apathy, and depression. These people frequently feel as though their brains are in turmoil, and do not understand what is going on around them. Although they may beg for help, they are generally inconsolable.

Physical symptoms generally worsen between 4 P.M. and 8 P.M., and improve in warmth and when lying covered up.

Helleborus is prescribed for mental states that feature sluggishness and stupefaction. Acute inflammatory nervous conditions may be helped, as may headaches, digestive problems, and depression. Symptoms may follow as a result of a concussion, brain surgery, or a bout of meningitis or encephalitis.

NERVOUS SYSTEM DISORDERS
Symptoms Stupefaction and dullness, possibly even giving an impression of stupidity or mental disorder. Questions are answered slowly and with great effort. The body feels numb and the brain loses control over the muscles, so that objects drop easily from the hands. Forgetfulness and poor concentration, with the memory becoming totally blank, are common. In extreme cases symptoms may be associated with Alzheimer's disease, including memory loss, anxiety, and disorientation.
Symptoms better From being wrapped up; lying quietly at rest and undisturbed.
Symptoms worse In cold air; from being uncovered; from exertion; during the night; between 4 P.M. and 8 P.M.

BRAIN INFLAMMATION
Symptoms Swelling of the brain tissue, possibly caused by encephalitis or meningitis. Symptoms typically include convulsions, and the head tends to feel very hot while the body feels very cold. There is a feeling of stupor and sluggishness.
Symptoms better From being wrapped up; lying quietly at rest and undisturbed.
Symptoms worse In cold air; from being uncovered; from exertion; during the night; between 4 P.M. and 8 P.M.

HEADACHES
Symptoms A headache or a migraine with mental dullness, possibly after injury or surgery. The headache often begins in the back of the head or in the neck, and there may be a need to pull the head down toward the body. Dizziness and vertigo causing vomiting may accompany the pain.
Symptoms better With warmth; with rest.
Symptoms worse From being uncovered; from exertion; from stooping; between 4 P.M. and 8 P.M.

DIGESTIVE DISORDERS
Symptoms Painful bowel urges with watery diarrhea and mucus. Bowel movements are so disoriented and sluggish that constipation may also occur. There is often a lack of thirst and a dry mouth.
Symptoms better With warmth and warm coverings.
Symptoms worse In cold; from being uncovered; at night; between 4 P.M. and 8 P.M.

DEPRESSION
Symptoms Blank stares, involuntary sighs, and black moods, especially between 4 P.M. and 8 P.M. The lips and clothes may be picked at.
Symptoms better From being wrapped up warmly.
Symptoms worse During the night; from exertion.

KEY SYMPTOMS

MENTAL DULLNESS AND SLUGGISHNESS ◆
CHILLINESS ◆ TENDENCY TO DROP THINGS ◆ PERSON
FEELS WORSE BETWEEN 4 P.M. AND 8 P.M.

SEE ALSO
Depression, *page 212*; Headache & migraine, *page 218*; Digestion, *page 234*; Irritability, *page 244*

Hyoscyamus niger
HYOSCYAMUS

COMMON NAMES
Henbane, common henbane, black henbane, hairy henbane, stinking nightshade, stinking Roger, hog's bean, cassilata

HENBANE WAS ADVOCATED by the Greek physician Dioscorides in the 1st century CE as a painkiller and soporific. The Latin name comes from the Greek *hys*, "pig," and *kyamos*, "bean" – perhaps because pigs are not poisoned by eating it, while humans are. It was the method by which Shakespeare had Hamlet's father murdered, and the famous Dr. Crippen used henbane to murder his wife. *Hyoscyamus*, proved by Hahnemann in 1805, is used for emotional disorders and coughs.

REMEDY PROFILE

Hyoscyamus is the best remedy for those with paranoid traits and behavioral problems. The typical *Hyoscyamus* pattern is incoherent, excited behavior, muttering, and obscene sexual exhibitionism. Laughter at inappropriate times is common, as is a sense of being ostracized in a private world.

In addition, *Hyoscyamus* is used for physical conditions associated with involuntary twitching, such as delirium, and for fits of dry coughing. Homeopaths may prescribe it for certain types of convulsion, such as petit mal, epilepsy, and, in children, febrile convulsions with a rapid rise in temperature. In some cases, the remedy may be given for schizophrenia and Parkinson's disease, if accompanied by marked withdrawal, obscenity, and inappropriate laughter.

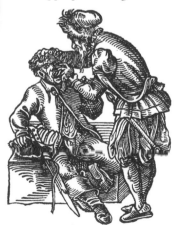

PAINKILLER FOR TOOTHACHES
In the Middle Ages, the Latin name for henbane was Dentaria, signifying its use as an herbal remedy for toothaches.

BEHAVIORAL PROBLEMS
Symptoms Violent outbursts and a desire to shock, with behavior ranging from simple foolishness to shameless sexual exhibitionism. Characteristic impulses are to appear naked, masturbate, and handle the genitals. Lewdness, promiscuity, or an erotic obsession may develop. Jealousy is common, and in children is often due to a new baby in the family.
Symptoms better In warmth.
Symptoms worse From fright; from emotional stress.

DELIRIUM
Symptoms
Twitching, starts, and facial grimaces, with the typical *Hyoscyamus* mental state (*see left*). Mania is possible, triggered by fever, addiction, brain injury, or the trauma of childbirth. Despite a meager flow, there may be a frequent desire to urinate. Constant fumbling with the hands or clothing is common. There may be convulsions, possibly with involuntary urination.
Symptoms better From sitting up; from walking around; with movement.
Symptoms worse If touched, lying down; from emotional stress or trauma.

PARANOIA
Symptoms Severe paranoia and jealousy, with intense suspicion of being watched, deceived, or even poisoned.

SOURCE DETAILS

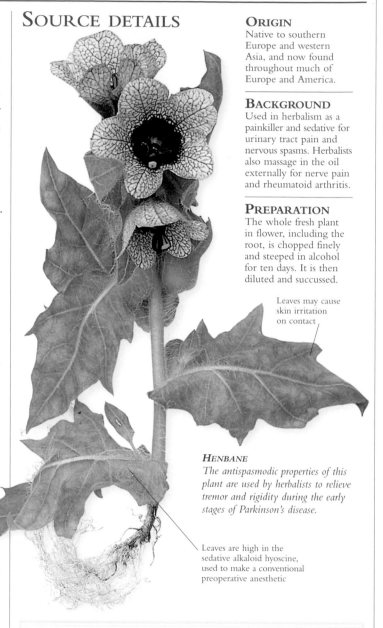

HENBANE
The antispasmodic properties of this plant are used by herbalists to relieve tremor and rigidity during the early stages of Parkinson's disease.

Leaves may cause skin irritation on contact

Leaves are high in the sedative alkaloid hyoscine, used to make a conventional preoperative anesthetic

ORIGIN
Native to southern Europe and western Asia, and now found throughout much of Europe and America.

BACKGROUND
Used in herbalism as a painkiller and sedative for urinary tract pain and nervous spasms. Herbalists also massage in the oil externally for nerve pain and rheumatoid arthritis.

PREPARATION
The whole fresh plant in flower, including the root, is chopped finely and steeped in alcohol for ten days. It is then diluted and succussed.

KEY SYMPTOMS
BEHAVIORAL PROBLEMS WITH EROTIC TENDENCIES ◆
DELIRIUM AND PARANOIA ◆ SPASMODIC COUGH ◆
LAUGHTER AT INAPPROPRIATE TIMES

Symptoms better In warmth.
Symptoms worse Around the time of menstruation; from emotional stress.

COUGH
Symptoms Dry, spasmodic, tickly cough. Suffocating fits of coughing trigger spasms severe enough to cause doubling up and coughing blood.

Symptoms better From sitting up.
Symptoms worse Lying down.

SEE ALSO
Stroke, *page 187*

Ignatia amara syn. *Strychnos ignatia*

IGNATIA

ST. IGNATIUS' BEAN SEEDS were traditionally worn by natives of the Philippine Islands as amulets to prevent and cure all manner of diseases. The Spanish Jesuits introduced the seeds into Europe from the Far East in the 17th century. They contain strychnine, a powerful poison that acts on the nervous system when ingested. The homeopathic remedy *Ignatia* was proved and published by Hahnemann in his *Materia Medica Pura* (1821–34).

REMEDY PROFILE

Ignatia is best suited to people, especially women, who are experiencing strong emotional problems, such as a broken relationship or acute grief after a death. They are frequently emotionally fragile, artistic, and hypersensitive. Prone to mood swings and feelings of self-pity, they may have a rather brittle air, often laughing and crying at the same time. Suppressing their emotions can lead to hysteria. High expectations of those close to them are typical, and they find it hard to break the bond with their partner if disillusioned in love.

Contradictory physical symptoms are typically treated with *Ignatia*, such as indigestion that is relieved by eating, or a sore throat that is better from swallowing solid food. There is often great sensitivity to pain, with a tendency to yawn and sigh frequently. There is also a dislike of crowds, and a fear of birds, especially chickens.

Ignatia is used to treat illness that develops from emotional stress. Such conditions include headaches, nervous tics and twitches, digestive disorders such as nausea and vomiting, and a sore throat.

GRIEF & DISTRESS
Symptoms Fainting, crying and laughing simultaneously, or hysterical behavior due to an inability to express emotions. There may also be insomnia.
Symptoms better From breathing deeply; from eating.
Symptoms worse From anxiety; from emotional stress; from coffee; from tobacco.

HEADACHES
Symptoms Sharp, spasmodic pain, as if a nail is sticking into the side of the head, with a hot, heavy sensation in the head and possible dizziness, especially after emotional stress.
Symptoms better Lying on the affected side; from resting the head on a surface.
Symptoms worse From loud talking; from stooping; from being in a smoky room.

NERVOUS DISORDERS
Symptoms Twitches, nervous tics, or numbness in the face or limbs, possibly escalating to hysterical paralysis, convulsions, or chorea (random, jerky twitches of the face or limbs). *Ignatia* is used if symptoms are

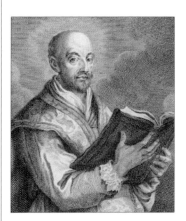

ST. IGNATIUS LOYOLA
This 16th-century Catholic priest from Spain founded the Jesuit order and gave his name to the Ignatia amara *tree.*

SOURCE DETAILS

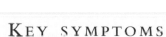

ST. IGNATIUS' BEAN
The seeds are very bitter, due to the poisonous strychnine they contain.

Pebblelike, heavy seed pods are embedded in bitter pulp of fruit

ORIGIN
Native to the East Indies, China, and the Philippine Islands. This large tree bears a bitter fruit that contains the seeds within its pulp.

BACKGROUND
In the late 17th century the Dutch used the seeds of St. Ignatius' bean to treat conditions such as gout, cholera, asthma, and epilepsy.

PREPARATION
The dried seeds are powdered before being steeped in alcohol for at least five days. This is followed by filtration, dilution, and succussion.

KEY SYMPTOMS
AILMENTS TRIGGERED BY GRIEF ◆ TENDENCY TO BOTTLE
UP EMOTIONS ◆ FEAR OF BIRDS ◆ SENSATION AS IF
THERE IS A LUMP IN THE THROAT

---

triggered by shock, grief (*see left*), or other strong emotions.
Symptoms better With warmth; from changing position; from firm pressure on the affected area; after eating.
Symptoms worse In cold air; if touched; from emotional stress; from strong smells.

DIGESTIVE DISORDERS
Symptoms Nausea and vomiting that is alleviated by eating, typically with burping, hiccuping, and profuse, bitter-tasting saliva in the mouth. There may be hunger unsated by eating. A prolapsed rectum with sharp, upward-shooting pain may be helped by *Ignatia*, as may diarrhea, constipation, or hemorrhoids that have been triggered by emotional stress.
Symptoms better Lying or pressing on the affected area;

from changing position; from urinating; from eating.
Symptoms worse In cold air; if touched; from strong smells; from coffee; from tobacco.

SORE THROAT
Symptoms A constantly sore, tickly throat that feels as if there is a lump in it, yet seems better from eating solids. There may also be a racking cough.
Symptoms better With warmth; from changing position; from eating.
Symptoms worse If touched; in cold air; from emotional stress; from coffee; tobacco.

SEE ALSO
Grief, *page 213*; Hiccups, *page 234*; Insomnia, *page 244*; Absent periods, *page 256*

Lilium lancifolium syn. *L. tigrinum*

LILIUM

COMMON NAME
Tiger lily

THE LILIUM GENUS comprises around 100 species of bulbous plant, including the tiger lily. This was introduced to the West from China, Korea, and Japan where it was cultivated as a food plant for centuries. The tiger lily has not generally been adopted into the Western herbal repertory, but it forms the basis of an important homeopathic remedy for uterine pain and emotional problems. *Lilium* was proved in 1867 by Dr. E. W. Payne of Maine.

SOURCE DETAILS

Bright petals curl up to reveal distinctive spots

TIGER LILY
The bright-orange flowers of this lily appear in late summer and early autumn.

REMEDY PROFILE

Lilium is traditionally linked with people who are hurried and impatient, and generally trying to do too many things at once. They often feel wild and out of control, and may even fear that they are going insane. They like to be the center of attention and can be quick to anger if they are not. Alternatively, they may be filled with feelings of remorse, especially of a religious nature, and torment themselves endlessly about their behavior.

A conflict between very high moral standards and intense sexual urges is characteristic in these people. The suppression of their sexual desire generally aggravates frustration and anger. They are often sensitive to criticism, easily offended, irritated, even by kindness, and hurried beyond reason. People who respond well to this remedy typically have a burning sensation in their hands, and prefer cool weather.

Lilium is prescribed chiefly for female reproductive-system disorders. It is also given for states of despair and depression, and for urinary complaints, angina, and poor circulation.

WOMEN'S HEALTH
Symptoms Disorders of the female reproductive organs, such as uterine prolapse, vulval itching, and a bearing-down pain in the pelvis. In addition, the ovaries may be swollen and menstruation is often painful. Fibroids may also be treated with the remedy.
Symptoms better In cool, fresh air; lying on the left side.
Symptoms worse With warmth; with jarring; after a miscarriage.

DEPRESSION
Symptoms A sense of despair and need for religious salvation is characteristic in people who need *Lilium*. They are easily offended and feel that people are deliberately annoying them. They may have a fear of developing an incurable disease and look for a reason to grieve.
Symptoms better From being occupied; in company.
Symptoms worse From sympathy; after a miscarriage or menstruation.

URINARY DISORDERS
Symptoms Cystitis with burning, stinging pain during and after urination. There is often a constant urge to pass urine, although only a small amount is passed at a time. Irritation in the genital area is experienced during both day and night. The symptoms usually affect women.
Symptoms better In cool, fresh air; lying on the left side.
Symptoms worse With warmth; at night; with jarring; after a miscarriage.

ORIGIN
Native to China and Japan, but now grown worldwide, almost always for ornamental purposes. Prefers moist, acid soil in full sun, but with its base in shade.

BACKGROUND
Introduced to Europe and the Western world from China and Japan, and has since become a popular ornamental flower for cultivation in gardens.

PREPARATION
The stalk, leaves, and flowers of the fresh plant are finely chopped and soaked in alcohol for at least ten days. The mixture is then filtered, diluted, and succussed.

KEY SYMPTOMS

HURRY AND IMPATIENCE ◆ INTENSE SEXUAL URGES ◆ PREFERENCE FOR COOL, FRESH AIR ◆ SENSATION AS THOUGH THE HEART IS BEING GRIPPED

HEART DISORDERS
Symptoms Angina with numbness in the right arm and pain in the heart, as if it is being gripped. The heart may feel as if it is going to burst, as though it is hanging by a thread, or as though it is being alternately grasped and released. A rapid or irregular pulse is common. Palpitations may occur, especially during pregnancy.
Symptoms better In cool, fresh air; lying on the left side; from rubbing or pressing the area around the heart.
Symptoms worse Lying down at night.

SEE ALSO
Angina, *page 185*

Lycopodium clavatum

LYCOPODIUM

THIS PLANT'S ROOT was said to bear a resemblance to a wolf's foot, hence its folk name "wolf's claw," and Latin name, from the Greek *lykos*, or "wolf" and *podos*, or "foot." The plant has been used medicinally since the Middle Ages. Since the 17th century, the spores alone were given for gout and urine retention. Modern herbalists use the spores externally for wounds and eczema. Proved by Hahnemann in 1828, the remedy is used for digestive disorders and anxiety.

SOURCE DETAILS

SPRIG

Scaly spikes shoot up in summer, developing tips of yellow spore cases

Straggly stem is covered with shiny, scaly leaves

CLUB MOSS
This plant has water-repellent spores that stop pills from sticking together.

SPORES

REMEDY PROFILE

Lycopodium is prescribed when anticipatory anxiety features strongly in the psychological symptoms. Lack of confidence is often hidden by a veneer of arrogance or sarcasm. There is a dislike of close company but also of being left alone.

Physical symptoms usually focus on digestive problems, with excessive bloating and gas. Complaints are often right-sided, or move from the right to the left of the body. Another typical physical trait, poor physical stamina, is often worse in the afternoons. Desire for sweet foods is common. *Lycopodium* is also used for kidney and prostate problems, headaches, and chest infections.

ANXIETY
Symptoms Fear of inferiority and of failing, despite an air of quiet self-possession. Such fears may lead to exaggeration of the truth to bolster self-esteem. Insomnia, talking and laughing while asleep, and night fears are typical, as is apprehension on waking. Anticipatory anxiety,

such as fear of public speaking, exams, or stage fright, often leads to digestive disorders (*see below*). Low self-esteem may result from poor memory or dyslexia. An aversion to change is often due to the challenges it brings. The demands of emotional commitment may be avoided, possibly resulting in sexual problems such as promiscuity, frigidity, or erectile dysfunction.
Symptoms better From being active; from gentle exercise in fresh air; from warm foods and drinks.
Symptoms worse In extreme heat or cold; in stuffy rooms; from being inactive; between 4 P.M. and 8 P.M.

DIGESTIVE DISORDERS
Symptoms Indigestion caused by anticipatory anxiety (*see left*), eating late at night, or eating foods that can cause gas, such as onions, cabbage, and beans. There may be a rumbling, bloated abdomen due to acrid, sour gas, insatiable hunger with discomfort after eating even small amounts of food, nausea, vomiting, constipation, and bleeding hemorrhoids.
Symptoms better In cool air; at night; from loose clothes; with movement; from warm foods and drinks.
Symptoms worse From tight clothes; between 4 A.M. and

ORIGIN
Native to temperate areas throughout the northern hemisphere, and commonly found growing on moorland and in mountainous areas and forests.

BACKGROUND
Traditionally used for its antibacterial and sedative action, it has also been given by herbalists as a digestive, a diuretic, to treat kidney stones, and to lower fever.

PREPARATION
The spikes are cut in summer and their spores are collected. These are then steeped in alcohol for at least five days, before being filtered, diluted, and succussed.

KEY SYMPTOMS
ANTICIPATORY ANXIETY ◆ LACK OF SELF-ESTEEM ◆ FLATULENCE AND CONSTIPATION ◆ DESIRE FOR SWEET FOODS ◆ PERSON FEELS WORSE BETWEEN 4 P.M. AND 8 P.M.

---

8 A.M. and 4 P.M. and 8 P.M.; from overeating; from cold foods and drinks.

UROGENITAL PROBLEMS
Symptoms Urine with a sandy sediment due to kidney stones, or genital herpes. An enlarged prostate in men may be helped by the remedy.
Symptoms better At night; in cool, fresh air; being active; from warm foods and drinks.
Symptoms worse With heat; between 4 P.M. and 8 P.M.

CHEST INFECTIONS
Symptoms Dry, sore, tickling cough, burning chest pain, and fast, labored breathing, which

may be worse when lying on the back. The throat is swollen and sore, notably on the right side. Thick, yellow phlegm may cause severe congestion.
Symptoms better From loose clothes; in cool air; at night; from warm foods and drinks.
Symptoms worse In stuffy rooms; from tight clothes; between 4 P.M. and 8 P.M.; from fasting or overeating; from cold drinks.

SEE ALSO
Prostate problems, *page 202*;
Bloating & flatulence, *page 236*;
Erectile dysfunction, *page 264*

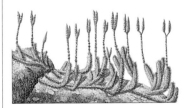

FIERY SPORES
The spores of this small, straggly moss are flammable and ignite explosively; in the past, they were used to make fireworks.

Papaver somniferum

OPIUM

COMMON NAMES
Opium poppy

A PLANT OF EXTREMES, this poppy is the source of both morphine, one of the strongest painkillers, and heroin, one of the most addictive substances known. It has played a dramatic role in history, prompting wars and huge social problems. Opium and heroin, derived illicitly, have produced devastating drug problems, while morphine and codeine are produced legally to play a vital role in conventional medicine. The homeopathic remedy was proved in 1805 by Hahnemann.

REMEDY PROFILE

Opium is given to people who exhibit either or both of two opposite states. One is stupor, apathy, and dulled sensitivity to pain. The other is hyperactivity and intense sensitivity, often with insomnia.

If symptoms occur with one or both of these states, *Opium* is given for insomnia, sleeping disorders, respiratory problems, constipation, and shock. It can also be used to help treat recovery from stroke paralysis, brain injuries, delirium tremens, and alcohol withdrawal.

INSOMNIA & NARCOLEPSY

Symptoms Insomnia, inability to sleep despite fatigue, or brief bouts of irresistible drowsiness. Sleep is either light, restless, and easily disturbed, with hearing so acute that it seems to detect even the faint sounds of insects'

movements, or very heavy, with difficulty in waking. Sleep may be so deep that breathing becomes irregular or even stops momentarily. There may be talking during sleep.
Symptoms better In a cool environment; with movement.
Symptoms worse With warmth; with sleep; shock.

CONSTIPATION

Symptoms Constipation with no urge to pass stools for an extended length of time, which may result in fecal impaction. The digestion is sluggish and weak, and there is no appetite. Stools tend to retreat into the rectum, and are dark, small, and very hard, like black balls. During the day there may be drowsiness. Diarrhea may alternate with constipation, notably after shock (*see below*). Newborn babies may be given *Opium* for constipation after the shock of childbirth.
Symptoms better With activity.
Symptoms worse With warmth; from shock.

SHOCK & INJURY

Symptoms Either emotional and sensory shutdown, or over-excitement and hypersensitivity. Sluggishness and indifference may be evident, with dulled sensitivity to pain. Conversely, the person can be overwrought, possibly with insomnia (*see above, left*) or even convulsions. Either or both of these states may occur in response to shock, grief, or injury.

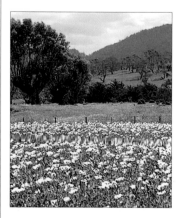

UNIQUE IN NATURE
Medicinally important alkaloids in this poppy cannot be synthesized artificially, so it is cultivated under strict supervision.

SOURCE DETAILS

ORIGIN
Native to western Asia, and introduced to southeast Europe 3,000 years ago. Now grown mostly in India, Iran, China, and Australia.

BACKGROUND
Dedicated by the ancient Greeks and Romans to the gods of night, dreams, and death. Opium has been used since antiquity as a sedative and analgesic, and has also been used illicitly for many centuries as a recreational drug.

PREPARATION
Sticky latex (sap) from the unripe, green seed pods is dried, dissolved in alcohol, and succussed.

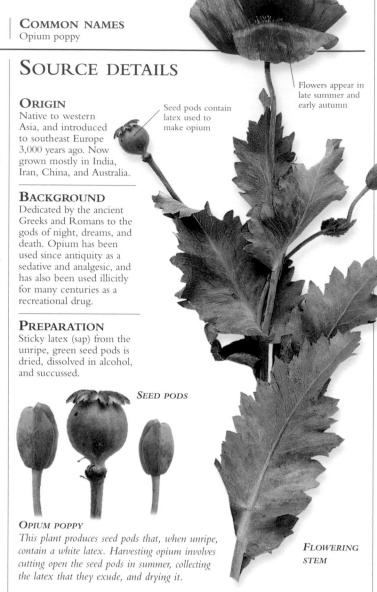

Flowers appear in late summer and early autumn

Seed pods contain latex used to make opium

SEED PODS

FLOWERING STEM

OPIUM POPPY
This plant produces seed pods that, when unripe, contain a white latex. Harvesting opium involves cutting open the seed pods in summer, collecting the latex that they exude, and drying it.

KEY SYMPTOMS
STUPOR ◆ APATHY ◆ DULLED SENSITIVITY TO PAIN ◆ HYPERACTIVITY WITH DIFFICULTY IN SLEEPING

Symptoms better In a cool environment; with movement.
Symptoms worse With warmth; with sleep.

POSTSTROKE PARALYSIS

Symptoms Paralysis of the limbs with dullness and stupor resembling that experienced after shock (*see left*). There may be blackouts, a blue-tinged face, and labored breathing.
Symptoms better In a cool environment; with movement.
Symptoms worse With warmth; with sleep.

DELIRIUM TREMENS

Symptoms Extreme apathy or hypersensitivity, tremors, or even convulsions. There can be frightening visions, and possibly blackouts after alcohol binges.
Symptoms better In a cool environment; with movement.
Symptoms worse With warmth; from alcohol.

SEE ALSO
Stroke, *page 187*; Grief, *page 213*

Pulsatilla pratensis subsp. *nigricans*

PULSATILLA

COMMON NAMES
Small pasqueflower,
meadow anemone

SMALL PASQUEFLOWER has been used medicinally since the age of classical Greece. The name derives from the archaic term for Easter, *Pasch*, since the plant flowers around the time that the festival occurs. Roman legend says that this plant sprang from the tears of the goddess Venus, and was hence used to treat weepiness. *Pulsatilla* was proved by Hahnemann in 1805 and is used for a variety of disorders, ranging from colds and coughs to digestive and gynecological conditions.

REMEDY PROFILE

People who respond best to *Pulsatilla* are sweet-natured, gentle, and compliant. They will avoid confrontation, but their moods change frequently and rapidly, and they can be stubborn in their demands for attention and sympathy. Their physical symptoms can be equally changeable. Easily moved to laughter or tears, they are highly prone to weepiness when ill but are soon consoled by hugs. Other common traits are a dislike of stuffy rooms or fatty foods, a lack of thirst, and a preference for fresh air.

Pulsatilla is given for labor, menstruation, menopause, and pregnancy problems. It is used for respiratory illness marked by yellowish green phlegm, eye complaints, and indigestion with variable symptoms.

WOMEN'S HEALTH
Symptoms Short, variable, late, or absent menstrual flow with severe pain. There may be delayed onset of menstruation in puberty. Severe premenstrual syndrome may respond to the remedy, particularly if it is accompanied by indigestion, weepiness, and mood swings. In pregnancy, if the general symptom picture fits, *Pulsatilla* is given for stress incontinence, fatigue, indigestion, and morning sickness (especially if this is brought on by fatty foods). It may also act on the uterine muscles to help turn a malpresented or breech baby in the uterus during labor.

Symptoms better From fresh air; with gentle exercise; from crying; from sympathy.
Symptoms worse With heat; lying on the left side; in the evening; from rich, fatty foods.

COLDS & COUGHS
Symptoms An alternately runny or blocked nose, with smelly, thick, yellowish green phlegm, and a reduced sense of taste and smell. There may be wet, spasmodic coughing, with yellowish green mucus and shortness of breath, which is worse when lying on the left side. Violent coughing fits tend to occur in the evening and at night; they may be triggered by lying down and frequently cause sleep to be disturbed. *Pulsatilla* may be prescribed for the flu when there is fever with alternate hot and cold flashes, a lack of thirst, and possibly an earache.
Symptoms better In fresh air; with gentle exercise; from crying; from sympathy.
Symptoms worse In stuffy environments; lying down.

SINUSITIS
Symptoms Yellowish phlegm, weepiness, and headaches. The sinuses are tender to the touch. Sharp pains may begin on the right side of the face, but tend to move around.
Symptoms better In fresh air; with gentle exercise.
Symptoms worse In stuffy environments; in cold; in the evening.

SOURCE DETAILS

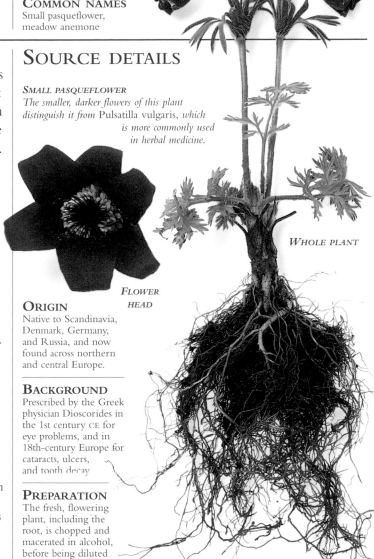

SMALL PASQUEFLOWER
The smaller, darker flowers of this plant distinguish it from Pulsatilla vulgaris, *which is more commonly used in herbal medicine.*

FLOWER HEAD

WHOLE PLANT

ORIGIN
Native to Scandinavia, Denmark, Germany, and Russia, and now found across northern and central Europe.

BACKGROUND
Prescribed by the Greek physician Dioscorides in the 1st century CE for eye problems, and in 18th-century Europe for cataracts, ulcers, and tooth decay.

PREPARATION
The fresh, flowering plant, including the root, is chopped and macerated in alcohol, before being diluted and succussed.

KEY SYMPTOMS
WEEPINESS ◆ CONDITIONS THAT IMPROVE WITH SYMPATHY ◆ DESIRE FOR OPEN AIR ◆ THICK, YELLOWISH GREEN PHLEGM

EYE INFECTIONS
Symptoms Profuse, yellowish green, foul-smelling discharge from the eye, with sensitivity to light and possible indigestion (*see below*). *Pulsatilla* may help conjunctivitis and itchy styes.
Symptoms better In fresh air; from bathing the eyes in cold water.
Symptoms worse In warm rooms; in the evening.

DIGESTIVE DISORDERS
Symptoms Variable, including indigestion, nausea, vomiting, diarrhea, and painful, itchy hemorrhoids. No two stools are alike. The mouth is dry, but there is no thirst and a craving for, or aversion to, rich foods that exacerbate the symptoms.
Symptoms better In fresh air; with gentle exercise.
Symptoms worse With heat; lying on the left side; in the evening; from rich, fatty foods.

SEE ALSO
Respiration, *pages 180, 224*; Digestion, *pages 189, 234*; Sties, *page 220*; Women's health, *page 256*

Solanum dulcamara

DULCAMARA

COMMON NAMES
Bittersweet, woody nightshade,
bitter nightshade, felonwort

SINCE THE TIME OF ANCIENT ROME, bittersweet has been used to treat a wide range of ailments. One such ailment, abscesses called "felons" on the fingertips, inspired one of the plant's common names, felonwort. The 18th-century Swedish naturalist Carolus Linnaeus prescribed the plant to treat fever and inflammatory infections. The homeopathic remedy, proved in 1811 by Hahnemann, is traditionally associated with people who are highly susceptible to dampness and chills.

REMEDY PROFILE

Dulcamara is typically given to people who are sensitive to cold and dampness, with symptoms caused by rapid temperature changes or cold, wet weather.

In the symptom picture for *Dulcamara*, these physical factors outweigh psychological traits, but some confusion, irritability, impatience, and restlessness may be evident, possibly with a domineering attitude, notably toward family members.

Susceptibility to respiratory infections causing thick, yellow mucus is typical. Hay fever and other allergic reactions are also common, as are head and joint pain, eczema, and diarrhea.

COLDS & COUGHS
Symptoms Sore throat, with a thick, yellow discharge from the nose and the eyes. Thick mucus may be due to sinusitis,

as may painful pressure and congestion in the head. A stiff neck is common, perhaps with back and limb pain. There may also be conjunctivitis, a rattling cough, bronchitis, or even pneumonia. **Symptoms better** With warmth; in dry, settled weather; with movement. **Symptoms worse** In cold, damp weather; at night.

HAY FEVER & ASTHMA
Symptoms Nasal congestion, with profuse, watery discharge from the eyes and constricted breathing. Exposure to animal fur, grass pollen, dust mites, and other allergens may aggravate the severity of symptoms. **Symptoms better** With warmth; in dry, settled weather; with movement. **Symptoms worse** In cold, damp weather; at night.

HEAD & FACIAL PAIN
Symptoms Pain in a specific part of the head, or with a sensation of heaviness, nausea, or confusion. Neuralgic face pain, perhaps caused by Bell's palsy, may be treated, or pain due to sinusitis (*see above, left*). **Symptoms better** In dry, fine weather, from keeping still; from expelling phlegm. **Symptoms worse** In cold, damp weather; in winter.

SKIN CONDITIONS
Symptoms Thickened, crusty, itchy skin, notably on the scalp, which bleeds when scratched.

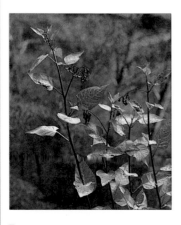

BOTANICAL RELATIONS
This plant belongs to a diverse botanical family of plants that also includes tobacco, the potato, and deadly nightshade, which it closely — and confusingly — resembles.

SOURCE DETAILS

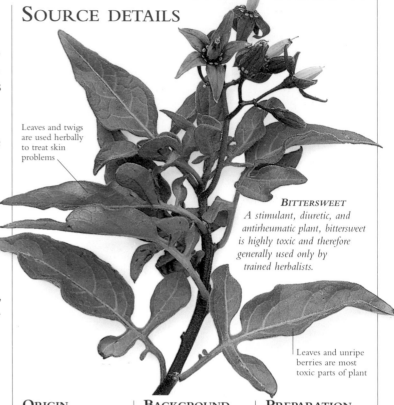

Leaves and twigs are used herbally to treat skin problems

BITTERSWEET
A stimulant, diuretic, and antirheumatic plant, bittersweet is highly toxic and therefore generally used only by trained herbalists.

Leaves and unripe berries are most toxic parts of plant

ORIGIN
Native to north Africa, Europe, and northern Asia, and naturalized in North America. Grows in moist, shady soil.

BACKGROUND
Has a long history of use as an anti-inflammatory and a liver tonic. Stem extracts have been used for warts and eczema.

PREPARATION
Fresh green stems and leaves are picked just before the plant flowers, then finely chopped and macerated in alcohol.

KEY SYMPTOMS
CONDITIONS THAT ARE AFFECTED BY WEATHER CHANGES FROM HOT TO COLD ◆ DOMINEERING NATURE ◆ SENSITIVITY TO COLD AND DAMPNESS ◆ ASTHMA ◆ HIVES IN HUMID CONDITIONS

Dulcamara is also used to treat hives (urticaria) brought on by sweating in humid conditions; large, flat, smooth warts, especially on the palms of the hands; and ringworm, often found on the scalps of children. **Symptoms better** With warmth; in dry weather. **Symptoms worse** In cold, damp weather; before menstruation.

DIARRHEA
Symptoms Slimy, yellow or green stools, maybe with traces of blood. There may be nausea, and pain before passing stools. In children, symptoms may be triggered during teething.

Symptoms better With warmth; with movement. **Symptoms worse** In cold; in dampness; with rest.

JOINT PAIN
Symptoms Stiffness and pain, aggravated by dampness. **Symptoms better** With warmth; with movement. **Symptoms worse** In cold; in damp; from extremes of temperature; from inactivity.

SEE ALSO
Severe eczema, *page 194*; Sore throat, *page 226*

Strychnos nux-vomica

NUX VOMICA

COMMON NAMES
Poison-nut tree, Quaker buttons (seeds), nux vomica, vomit weed

THE POISON-NUT TREE was taken to Europe from southeast Asia in the 15th century. Strychnine, the toxic alkaloid from its seeds, was famous as a poison before 17th-century physicians discovered its stimulating effect on the digestive and nervous systems. Small doses can be diuretic, stimulate the appetite, and aid digestion, but excessive amounts can be fatal. *Nux vomica* was proved by Hahnemann in 1805.

REMEDY PROFILE

Nux vomica is chiefly linked to workaholic personalities who drive themselves to stress and excess. Ambitious and pushy, they thrive on challenges, and often work in entrepreneurial or managerial jobs. The typical pattern is of someone who is oversensitive and intolerant of criticism, yet perfectionist and often very critical of others. Such highly driven people tend to overload their bodies at play as well as at work. They tend to have high sex drives, consume too much rich food, coffee, and alcohol, and abuse drugs. This indulgence can create tension and sleeplessness, and often leads to digestive disorders (most seriously, peptic ulcers, irritable bowel syndrome, or liver problems when the body can no longer keep up with the lifestyle).

If the profile matches, *Nux vomica* is given for irritability, insomnia, digestive symptoms, colds and the flu, asthma, cystitis, and menstrual or pregnancy problems. Typically symptoms are worse from cold, noise, light, and odors.

IRRITABILITY & INSOMNIA
Symptoms Hangover-type symptoms, with disrupted sleep and great irascibility, due to an excessive lifestyle with too much alcohol, coffee, or other stimulants. A headache that feels as if a nail has been driven into the forehead is typical, as is waking at around 4 A.M.

feeling very irritable and unable to sleep again until morning.
Symptoms better With warmth; with rest; from hot drinks.
Symptoms worse In cold; in open air; near noise; in light; from strong odors.

DIGESTIVE DISORDERS
Symptoms Indigestion, and vomiting with painful retching. Diarrhea is accompanied by abdominal cramps, and nausea by colicky pain. Constipation may make it difficult to empty the bowel fully. Hemorrhoids and constipation may be due to rectal spasms. The abdomen is often bloated and flatulent. There may be cravings for stimulants or spicy, fatty, or rich foods, even though these only aggravate symptoms.
Symptoms better With warmth; from resting; with sleep; from firm pressure on the abdomen; in the evening.
Symptoms worse In cold; if touched; near noise; from mental overexertion; repressing emotions; between 3 A.M. and 4 A.M.; from stimulants; from eating spicy foods.

COLDS & THE FLU
Symptoms Runny phlegm by day, especially in warm rooms, but a blocked nose at night. There may be sneezing, a sore throat and dry, tickly cough, headaches, and watery, sensitive eyes, or the flu with aching muscles and a shivery fever.

SOURCE DETAILS

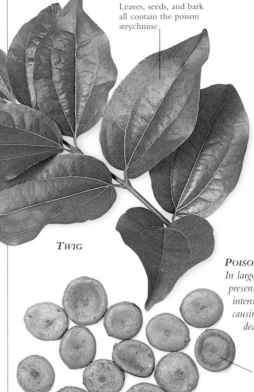

Leaves, seeds, and bark all contain the poison strychnine

TWIG

POISON-NUT TREE
In large doses, the strychnine present in this plant induces intense spasms of the diaphragm, causing respiration to cease and death by suffocation.

Buttonlike seeds are obtained from fruit of tree

SEEDS

ORIGIN
Native to southeast Asia, the tree grows in sandy soil in dry forests of India, Burma, Thailand, China, and Australia.

BACKGROUND
A rat poison in medieval Europe, and also used to treat the plague. Indian herbalists use the bark to treat cholera, and in Nepal it is prescribed for menstrual problems, rabies, and paralysis.

PREPARATION
The dried, ripe seeds are steeped in alcohol for at least five days, before being filtered, diluted, and successed.

KEY SYMPTOMS
IRRITABILITY ◆ OVERLY CRITICAL NATURE ◆ TENDENCY TO BE HIGHLY DRIVEN AND AMBITIOUS ◆ CHILLINESS ◆ DESIRE FOR RICH FOODS AND STIMULANTS ◆ INDIGESTION AND CONSTIPATION ◆ SLEEPLESSNESS

Symptoms better With warmth; from sleep; being left alone; in the evening.
Symptoms worse In cold, dry weather; if touched; near noise; with overexertion; between 3 A.M. and 4 A.M.

WOMEN'S HEALTH
Symptoms Cystitis with spasmodic pain in the bladder, and a frequent but ineffectual urge to urinate. Early, irregular, or heavy menstruation with cramping pains is treated with the remedy, as is menstruation preceded by faintness, and premenstrual syndrome with a violent temper. In pregnancy *Nux vomica* may be used to

help ease fatigue, frequent urination, numbness in the arms, leg cramps, constipation, and morning sickness.
Symptoms better With warmth; with sleep; in the evening; from firm pressure on the affected area; from being left alone.
Symptoms worse From mental overexertion; if touched; near noise; from stimulants; from spicy foods.

SEE ALSO
Headache, *page 218*; Indigestion, *page 234*; Irritability, *page 244*; Cystitis, *page 260*; Morning sickness, *page 262*

Thuja occidentalis
THUJA

ARBOR VITAE WAS USED by Native Americans as a source of hard-wearing wood and of herbal medicine for fever, coughs, menstrual problems, headaches, and muscle and joint pain. European settlers later incorporated it into their herbal lore, and it has also become a popular ornamental tree in European gardens. The remedy *Thuja* was proved by Hahnemann and published in his *Materia Medica Pura* (1821–34).

REMEDY PROFILE

Serious, sensitive people who are easily upset and feel that they are unloveable respond best to *Thuja*. They may try to present a pleasing image to the world but, if reactions are negative, they neglect their appearance, becoming secretive and depressed. Delusions about the body may be evident, as may fanatical ideas or paranoia, with a feeling that others are trying to manipulate them. They tend to sleep badly.

Thuja is used for skin and urogenital disorders, headaches, and respiratory or menstrual problems. Typically there is localized pain, exhaustion, and rapid weight loss. Symptoms may be due to health changes following a vaccination, or date back to a bout of gonorrhea.

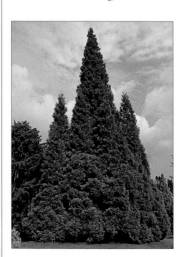

DURABLE HARDWOOD
The wood of this tree is very resistant to decay, and was traditionally used by Native Americans to make canoes, bows, and roofing material.

SKIN CONDITIONS
Symptoms Large, "cauliflower" warts, and warts that weep, sting, or are on stalks. There may be scaly patches on covered body areas, itchy skin complaints, brown "age spots," and ridged, weak, or deformed nails. *Thuja* is widely used as an ointment for warts.
Symptoms better From free flow of discharges and phlegm.
Symptoms worse In cold and dampness; after gonorrhea; after a vaccination.

UROGENITAL PROBLEMS
Symptoms Swollen, inflamed urethra, with urine stream split and weak, and frequent strong urges to urinate, perhaps with trickling incontinence. In men urethral infection is common, usually with a discharge and possibly affecting the prostate gland. In women there may be vaginal infection, often with profuse discharge. Inflammation may spread through the pelvic area. Genital warts and herpes may develop, as may ulcers and uterine polyps. *Thuja* may also be given to treat suppressed gonorrhea.
Symptoms better In warm air; from drawing up the limbs.
Symptoms worse In cold and damp; with movement; from urinating; from gonorrhea.

HEADACHES
Symptoms Piercing neuralgic pain due to stress, exhaustion, or overexcitement, or related to inflamed gums, tooth decay, or infected sinuses.
Symptoms better From tilting the head backward.
Symptoms worse From sexual excess; from tea.

CATARRH & SINUSITIS
Symptoms Chronic sinus or respiratory problems, usually with foul-smelling, green or yellow-green phlegm. Asthma may respond to *Thuja*, as may nasal polyps with thick, green, bloody mucus containing pus.
Symptoms better In warm air; from expelling phlegm.
Symptoms worse In cold and dampness; during menstruation; from tobacco.

SOURCE DETAILS

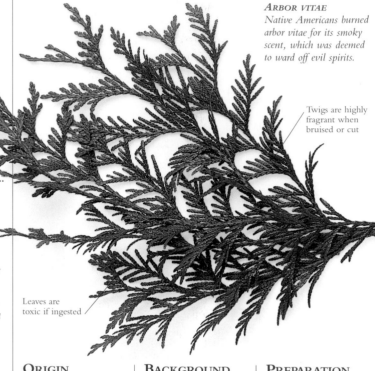

ARBOR VITAE
Native Americans burned arbor vitae for its smoky scent, which was deemed to ward off evil spirits.

Twigs are highly fragrant when bruised or cut

Leaves are toxic if ingested

ORIGIN
Native to Canada and eastern US, but now also widely cultivated as an ornamental tree. Prefers swamps and other wetlands.

BACKGROUND
Featured in the *US Pharmacopoeia* until 1894. Used in modern herbalism to treat warts, cancer, phlegm, and other conditions.

PREPARATION
The fresh leaves and twigs of the one-year-old plant are chopped finely and macerated in alcohol, then filtered, diluted, and succussed.

KEY SYMPTOMS

WARTS AND POLYPS ♦ FEELING OF BEING UNLOVEABLE ♦ COMPLAINTS THAT DEVELOP AFTER VACCINATION OR GONORRHEA ♦ DELUSIONS ♦ NAIL PROBLEMS ♦ PHLEGM

MENSTRUAL PROBLEMS
Symptoms Early or scant menstrual periods. There may be menstrual pain that is localized over the left ovary. Ovarian cysts may also respond to *Thuja*.
Symptoms better Drawing up the limbs; lying on the affected side or on the back.
Symptoms worse On the left side; during menstruation; after gonorrhea.

SEE ALSO
Prostate problems, *page 202*; Depression, *page 212*; Warts, *page 242*

Veratrum album

VERATRUM ALB. | COMMON NAMES
White hellebore, false hellebore

EXTREMELY TOXIC in all its parts, white hellebore was reputedly used in ancient Rome on the tips of weapons. Its toxicity has limited white hellebore's role in herbal medicine, although the plant has been used in insecticides and veterinary medicine. The remedy was proved by Hahnemann between 1826 and 1830. Along with *Camphor*, it was successfully used to treat victims of the 19th-century cholera epidemic in Europe, helping to make Hahnemann's reputation.

REMEDY PROFILE

Veratrum alb. is thought to work best on those who appear restless, self-righteous, overly critical, haughty, melancholy, and solitary, or who loathe being alone. A hyperactive or manic state, possibly with repetitive behavior, may be evident in people who are best suited to this remedy.

Typical physical symptoms include a poor immune system; extremely cold skin and perspiration, with chilliness possibly extending to the breath and tongue; a blue pallor; a rapid pulse; weakness; anemia; extreme thirst; or cravings for fruit or ice cream. Symptoms tend to become worse in damp cold, at night, following a bowel movement, and after eating fruit.

The remedy is usually given for debilitating gastrointestinal problems with severe vomiting and diarrhea. It is also used to treat collapse and some psychological problems.

DIARRHEA

Symptoms Severe diarrhea, possibly with vomiting (*see below, right*), due to cholera, dysentery, gastroenteritis, or other digestive disorders. Stools are watery, green, or colorless. Painful cramps may accompany attacks, and exhaustion may follow (*see below*), caused by dehydration and exhaustion. There may be a great thirst for cold water and a ravenous appetite, as well as cravings for sour foods, ice, and salt.
Symptoms better Lying down; from hot drinks, warm foods, and milk.
Symptoms worse If touched; with movement, from cold drinks.

COLLAPSE

Symptoms Weakness with a clammy, sweaty forehead, blue-tinged skin, dehydration, and possible fainting. This may be due to cramps, violent vomiting, and diarrhea (*see above*), especially during pregnancy. Other potential causes include acute fright, menstrual pain, or heatstroke.
Symptoms better From being covered; lying down.
Symptoms worse If touched; at night; from bowel movements; from cold drinks.

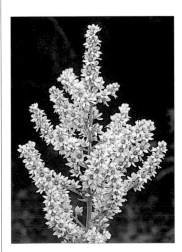

A STRONG IRRITANT
This hardy perennial produces greenish white flower heads from early to late summer and can grow up to 5 ft (1.5 m) high. It is a strong irritant to the skin.

SOURCE DETAILS

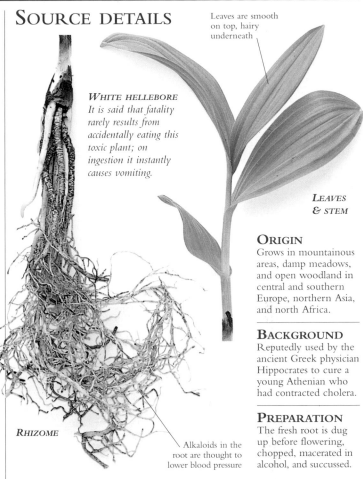

Leaves are smooth on top, hairy underneath

WHITE HELLEBORE
It is said that fatality rarely results from accidentally eating this toxic plant; on ingestion it instantly causes vomiting.

LEAVES & STEM

RHIZOME

Alkaloids in the root are thought to lower blood pressure

ORIGIN
Grows in mountainous areas, damp meadows, and open woodland in central and southern Europe, northern Asia, and north Africa.

BACKGROUND
Reputedly used by the ancient Greek physician Hippocrates to cure a young Athenian who had contracted cholera.

PREPARATION
The fresh root is dug up before flowering, chopped, macerated in alcohol, and succussed.

KEY SYMPTOMS
PROFUSE DIARRHEA ◆ VOMITING WITH EXHAUSTION ◆ COLD PERSPIRATION ◆ BLUE-TINGED SKIN ◆ FAINTING ◆ HYPERACTIVITY OR MELANCHOLY

EMOTIONAL PROBLEMS

Symptoms Behavioral disorders such as hyperactivity in some children or emotional disturbances due to the trauma of childbirth. Behavior may be sullen and indifferent. There may be adult insecurity about social position or a lack of one, alternating with ruthless ambition and delusions of grandeur or of becoming the victim of some tragedy.
Symptoms better Lying down; in children who are carried quickly.
Symptoms worse At night; from fright; before and during menstruation; from injured pride.

VOMITING & NAUSEA

Symptoms Violent vomiting with nausea, a cold feeling in the abdomen, clammy sweat, salty saliva, and possibly also diarrhea and collapse (*see left*).
Symptoms better Lying down; from being covered; from hot drinks, warm foods, and milk.
Symptoms worse If touched; with the slightest movement; at night; from cold drinks.

SEE ALSO
Nausea & vomiting, *page 236*; Diarrhea, *page 238*

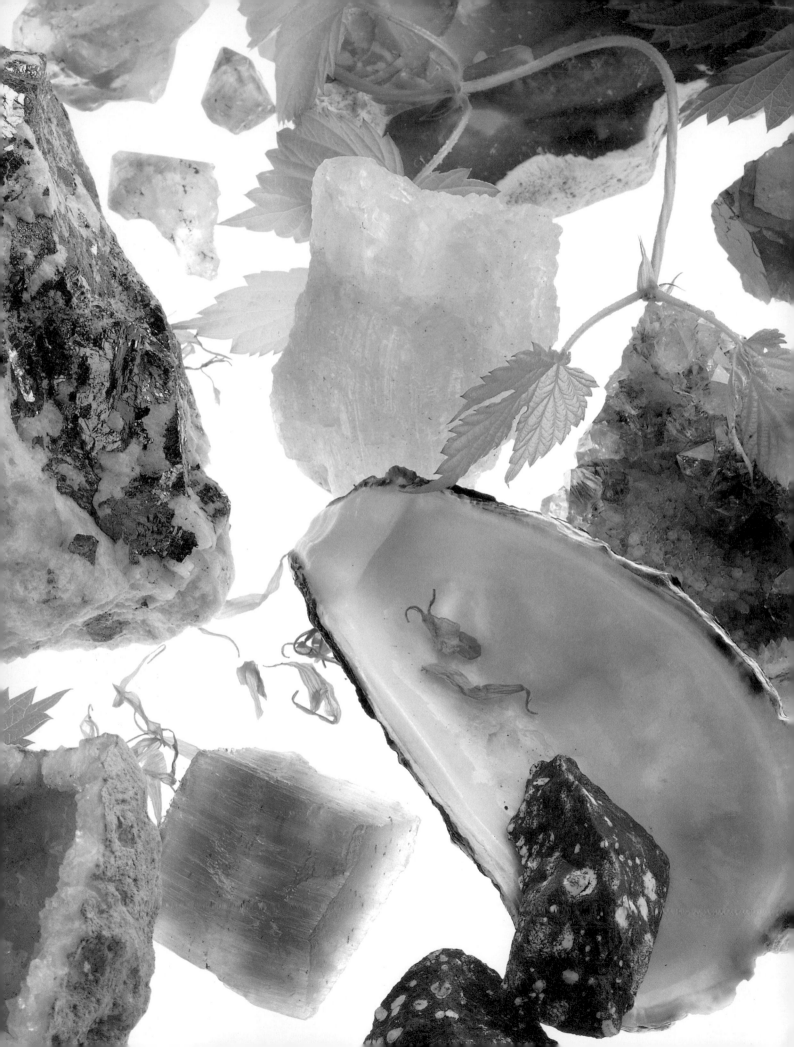

MAJOR MINERAL REMEDIES

ALTHOUGH NOT USED AS COMMONLY FOR HEALING

PURPOSES AS PLANTS, NATURALLY OCCURING

MINERALS AND MANUFACTURED MINERAL AND

CHEMICAL COMPOUNDS DO HAVE A LONG MEDICINAL

TRADITION. THIS SECTION OUTLINES THE MAJOR

MINERAL-BASED HOMEOPATHIC REMEDIES.

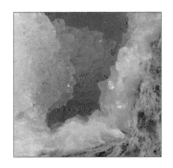 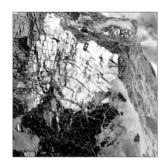 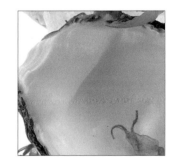

Acidum arsenicosum syn. *Arsenicum album*

ARSEN. ALB.

ARSENIC IS WELL KNOWN as a deadly poison. In the past it was used to make flypaper and wallpaper, sometimes leading to accidental poisonings: Napoleon's death has recently been attributed to arsenic used to color his wallpaper, which may have formed a deadly gas in damp, moldy conditions. *Arsen. alb.*, proved by Hahnemann and published in his *Materia Medica Pura* (1821–34), is given chiefly to treat the mucous membranes of the digestive and respiratory tracts.

REMEDY PROFILE

Those most suited to *Arsen. alb.* are affectionate, sensitive, and stable in good health, but may be prone to restlessness, stress, and anxiety about their health, with a deep need for reassurance. Illness brings rapid physical and mental exhaustion and chaos, which heightens their fears and vulnerability, and can cause severe anxiety or pessimism. Perfectionists by nature, they are intolerant of disorder, and when under stress or ill may develop phobias or obsessions, for example, about cleanliness. They like alcohol, warm drinks, and warm, sour, sweet, and fatty foods.

Arsen. alb. is a key remedy for asthma and breathlessness. It is also prescribed for violent digestive upsets with diarrhea and vomiting, headaches, burning eye inflammation, and itchy, weepy skin complaints.

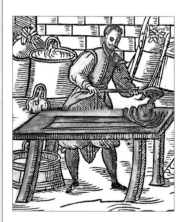

ARSENIC & ALCHEMY
Alchemists derived the name arsenic from the Greek arsen, *or "male," due to their belief that all elements had specific genders.*

RESPIRATORY ILLNESS
Symptoms Asthma or severe breathlessness, possibly brought on by stress or anxiety. There is typically susceptibility to colds, violent sneezing, and hay fever. Burning, watery phlegm causes the nostrils and lips to become dry, cracked, and sensitive. Weakness and extreme fatigue are common.
Symptoms better With warmth; with movement; from sitting upright.
Symptoms worse In cold, dry, windy weather; between midnight and 2 A.M.; under stress; on the right side of the body; from cold food.

DIGESTIVE DISORDERS
Symptoms Indigestion and colitis, aggravated by stress and anxiety. Watery, offensive-smelling stools cause soreness around the anus and burning pain in the rectum. There may be vomiting or diarrhea followed by exhaustion and dehydration. Excessive consumption of alcohol, ripe fruit and vegetables, and iced foods may cause gastroenteritis. If there is any fever, the body feels hot to the touch while chilled inside, or cold to the touch but burning inside.
Symptoms better With warmth; with movement; lying with the head propped up; from sips of water.
Symptoms worse From exposure to the cold; between midnight and 2 A.M.; under stress; from cold foods.

SOURCE DETAILS

ARSENIC
In the past doctors used arsenic to treat eczema, but it is now considered too toxic.

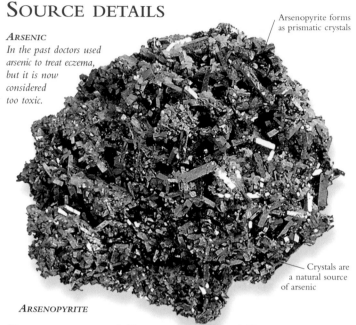

Arsenopyrite forms as prismatic crystals

Crystals are a natural source of arsenic

ARSENOPYRITE

ORIGIN
Extracted from the mineral arsenopyrite, which is found in Norway, Sweden, Germany, England, and Canada.

BACKGROUND
Has long been used in the US and Europe as a preservative for tanning animal hides, and is also traditionally used to make rat poison.

PREPARATION
Arsenic is triturated by being ground repeatedly with lactose sugar until it is soluble in water. It is then further diluted and succussed.

KEY SYMPTOMS

ANXIETY ABOUT HEALTH ◆ RESTLESSNESS AND EXHAUSTION ◆ CHILLINESS ◆ THIRST FOR SMALL SIPS OF WATER ◆ BURNING PAINS THAT ARE BETTER WITH WARMTH

FOOD POISONING
Symptoms Burning, stinging vomiting, with exhaustion and dehydration, and nausea on the sight or smell of food.
Symptoms better For warmth; for movement; for sips of water.
Symptoms worse For cold; between midnight and 2 A.M.

HEADACHES
Symptoms Pain beginning at the bridge of the nose and extending over the entire head, with dizziness, vomiting, and nausea. Excitement, stress, and anxiety may aggravate the pain.
Symptoms better From cold air; from cold compresses.
Symptoms worse From stress or excitement; from over-heating; from tobacco smoke; from the smell of food.

EYE INFLAMMATION
Symptoms Inflamed, stinging eyes with burning pains and sensitivity to bright light.
Symptoms better From warm compresses.
Symptoms worse In cold air; from tobacco smoke.

ECZEMA
Symptoms Itching, burning, cracked skin. Scratching causes weeping, bleeding, raw skin.
Symptoms better From warm compresses.
Symptoms worse From anxiety; at night.

SEE ALSO
Respiration, *page 180*; Digestion, pages *188, 234*; Skin, pages *192, 240*; Depression, *page 212*; Anxiety, *page 244*

Acidum hydrofluoricum
FLUORIC AC.

COMMON NAME
Hydrofluoric acid

FLUORINE, A COMPONENT of hydrofluoric acid, is found chiefly in the mineral fluorite (fluorspar). It is essential for healthy teeth and gums, and a compound of it, fluoride, is often added to toothpastes and the water supplies in some countries to help prevent tooth decay. Some homeopaths believe that fluorine intake from these sources can be excessive and can, in certain people, cause health problems that may be treated with this remedy. *Fluoric ac.* was proved by Dr. Constantine Hering and published in his *Guiding Symptoms of Our Materia Medica* (1879–91).

REMEDY PROFILE

Fluoric ac. suits people who are energetic, lively, and bustling in the early stages of illness, but rapidly become exhausted and forgetful as it progresses.

Spiritually and emotionally these people have a tendency to be extremely limited, and they are highly materialistic. As a result, they generally neglect their relationships, showing indifference to family and loved ones. Often, they cut themselves off from others. Their shallow relationships indicate an inability to connect deeply with others. Prone to self-satisfaction and egotism, they dislike any responsibility or commitment in their relationships. They tend to be dominant in relationships, and may become obsessed with sexual intercourse. An excessive sexual drive may lead to amoral and promiscuous behavior.

Fluoric ac. is used to treat fibrous tissue disorders, usually affecting the bones, teeth, nails, hair, and veins. It is prescribed for certain sexual problems, varicose veins, hair loss and baldness related to prolonged illness, and ear and nasal discharges. It may also help osteomyelitis (bone infection).

SEXUAL PROBLEMS
Symptoms In men, especially in old age, increased sexual desire and erections at night, perhaps preventing sleep. The scrotum may swell, and varicoceles (testicular varicose veins) may develop. There may be nymphomania.
Symptoms better From a cold shower; after a short sleep.
Symptoms worse With heat; at night; from alcohol.

TOOTH DECAY
Symptoms Teeth decay easily, perhaps becoming discolored, mottled, and brittle.
Symptoms better No specific factors.
Symptoms worse No specific factors.

NAIL CONDITIONS
Symptoms Weak, distorted, and crumbling nails that tend to grow too quickly, becoming too thick in some places or corrugated in others.
Symptoms better No specific factors.
Symptoms worse From alcohol.

VARICOSE VEINS
Symptoms Prominent, painful, enlarged veins in the backs of the calves and insides of the legs. The affected area may ache, and the pain may be aggravated by standing for prolonged periods of time.
Symptoms better In fresh air; from cold compresses.
Symptoms worse With heat; at night; from alcohol.

SOURCE DETAILS

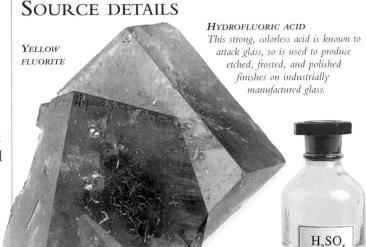

YELLOW FLUORITE

HYDROFLUORIC ACID
This strong, colorless acid is known to attack glass, so is used to produce etched, frosted, and polished finishes on industrially manufactured glass.

H₂SO₄

Yellow fluorite is one of several different-colored forms of the crystalline mineral

SULFURIC ACID

ORIGIN
Prepared by distilling fluorite (fluorspar) with sulfuric acid to create hydrogen fluoride gas, which is then dissolved in water to produce hydrofluoric acid.

BACKGROUND
Prescribed in traditional Chinese medicine for the treatment of anxiety, insomnia, and coughs. Used industrially in the manufacture of enamel, glass, and jewelry.

PREPARATION
Hydrofluoric acid is first dissolved in alcohol, before being repeatedly diluted further in alcohol and succussed between each dilution.

KEY SYMPTOMS
MATERIALISTIC AND UNSPIRITUAL NATURE ◆ INDIFFERENCE TO LOVED ONES ◆ PREOCCUPATION WITH SEXUAL INTERCOURSE ◆ WEAKNESS IN THE BONES, NAILS, AND HAIR

ALOPECIA
Symptoms Patchy baldness in both sexes, perhaps after prolonged illness. Hair tends to fall out easily, and new growth is typically dry and brittle.
Symptoms better In fresh air; from cold compresses.
Symptoms worse With heat; from alcohol.

DISCHARGES FROM THE EARS & NOSE
Symptoms Ear infection with profuse discharge after a period of stress, prolonged illness, or depression. Copious mucus may "drip like a faucet" from the nose, and may be associated with hay fever.
Symptoms better From being in open air; in a cool room; after a short sleep.
Symptoms worse With heat; at night; from alcohol.

BONE CONDITIONS
Symptoms Painful, inflamed, tender bones following injury or a bone infection such as osteomyelitis, with swelling around the infected bone.
Symptoms better In a cool room; from bathing in cold water; after a short sleep.
Symptoms worse With heat; at night; from alcohol.

SEE ALSO
Cancer, *page 208*

Acidum nitricum

NITRIC AC.

NITRIC ACID WAS FIRST developed by Arabian chemists in the 11th century. By the 18th century it was in use medicinally for burning off warts, and for treating skin complaints, syphilis, chest infections, and fevers. It has many modern commercial applications, being used in the manufacture of fertilizers, varnishes, nylon, lacquers, chemicals, and explosives. *Nitric ac.* was proved by Hahnemann and published in his *Chronic Diseases* (1821–34). He used it chiefly for painful skin conditions, and for miasms such as *Sycosis* (*see page 20*).

SOURCE DETAILS

NITRIC ACID
Produced commercially from ammonia, this acid is highly corrosive and gives off fumes that are extremely irritant and toxic if inhaled.

ORIGIN
Chemically prepared from sodium nitrate (a white, soluble mineral) and sulfuric acid (a corrosive liquid produced from sulfur).

BACKGROUND
Used in 18th-century Europe to burn off warts and as a treatment for chest and bladder complaints, kidney stones, and fever.

PREPARATION
Made by diluting one part nitric acid in nine parts pure alcohol. This mixture is then diluted and succussed.

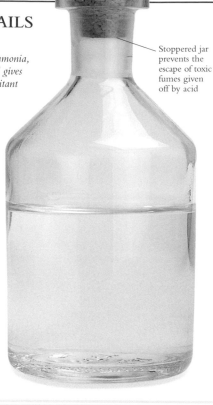

Stoppered jar prevents the escape of toxic fumes given off by acid

REMEDY PROFILE

An underlying discontent is evident in those who respond best to *Nitric ac.* This may be due to the extreme discomfort of their physical symptoms. Their behavior is often bitter and unforgiving, and they tend to dwell in the past. They are typically selfish, bad-tempered, explosively angry, and critical. Hypersensitivity may cause these people to worry that they are offending others, to be easily offended themselves, or to feel that others are trying to deceive them.

Prolonged emotional and mental suffering often leads to ill-health in these individuals. They fear death and worry incessantly about their health, often believing that their own suffering is much worse than others' and must therefore be treated immediately. Discharges such as urine and perspiration are typically offensive-smelling. A tendency to feel the cold is common, as are cravings for fat and salt. Any jarring motion, such as that of a moving car or train, usually makes them feel worse, as does drinking milk.

Nitric ac. is used mainly for painful skin ailments, especially where the mucous membranes meet the skin of the mouth, nose, or anus. The conditions treated by this remedy often manifest in the skin before going on to affect the internal organs. It is also used for warts, hemorrhoids, anal fissures, canker sores, and phlegm.

SKIN CONDITIONS
Symptoms Cracked, broken skin, and fissures that bleed slightly but easily. The nipples may be sore and cracked. Severe acne may develop, as may boils, facial blackheads, pimples, and skin ulcers. The skin is prone to profuse, foul-smelling sweat. Skin complaints are accompanied by splinter-like, cutting pains that appear and disappear suddenly.
Symptoms better With warmth; from warm compresses; from steady, even pressure on the affected area.
Symptoms worse In cold; if touched.

WARTS
Symptoms Big, jagged, moist warts on the hands, with sharp pain and possible bleeding. There may be anal warts with splinterlike pain, notably after passing stools (*see below*). Stools and urine often smell foul.
Symptoms better From warm coverings.
Symptoms worse If touched; from washing.

HEMORRHOIDS
Symptoms Extremely painful hemorrhoids, possibly with bleeding and splinterlike pain, a burning sensation, and rectal ulcers. Passing stools may involve great strain and effort but little result. Agonizing pain may follow straining or passing a stool, possibly lasting for hours. Hemorrhoids may be accompanied by nausea, vomiting, constipation, and foul-smelling anal discharges.
Symptoms better From warm compresses; from pressure on the hemorrhoids.
Symptoms worse If touched; with the slightest jar.

ANAL FISSURES
Symptoms A cracked, sore rectum with splinterlike pains and bleeding, due to tearing on passing a stool. Agonizing pain when passing stools may lead to constipation.
Symptoms better From warm coverings.
Symptoms worse If touched; with jarring movement.

CANKER SORES
Symptoms Sharp, splinter-like pain with sores on the tongue, or in the mouth or throat. There may be halitosis with bleeding gums. The gums may feel soft and spongy and the teeth may be loose.
Symptoms better From hot compresses.
Symptoms worse If touched; from swallowing; after eating.

PHLEGM
Symptoms Profuse, yellow burning phlegm, raw nostrils with splinterlike pain, and green crusts on the nostrils on waking. Nosebleeds may occur.
Symptoms better In mild weather.
Symptoms worse In winter; in cold, damp air; at night; from fatty foods; from milk.

KEY SYMPTOMS

ANXIETY ABOUT HEALTH ◆ SPLINTERLIKE PAINS ◆ CRACKS IN MUCOUS MEMBRANES AT ORIFICES ◆ OFFENSIVE-SMELLING DISCHARGES ◆ IRRITABILITY ◆ OVERSENSITIVITY ◆ CHILLINESS

SEE ALSO
Candidiasis, *page 200*; Cancer, *page 208*

Acidum phosphoricum
PHOSPHORIC AC.

COMMON NAMES
Phosphoric acid, glacial phosphoric acid, orthophosphoric acid

PHOSPHORIC ACID is widely used in the drinks industry to give soft drinks a fruity, acidic flavor. It is also used industrially to rustproof metals, and in the manufacture of sugar, fertilizers, detergents, waxes, polishes, and pharmaceutical products. *Phosphoric ac.*, proved by Hahnemann and published in his *Materia Medica Pura* (1821–34), is prescribed primarily for profound exhaustion, and is also a useful addition to the traveler's first-aid kit for treating mild diarrhea.

REMEDY PROFILE

Phosphoric ac. is especially suited to mild, calm, gentle people who tend to be sensitive and emotionally dependent on others. When in good health they are usually strong, but their constitutions are easily undermined by debilitating illness, emotional trauma, or repeated drug abuse, leading to severe exhaustion.

Profuse perspiration and chilliness are typical symptoms, as are loss of appetite and a craving for refreshing drinks and juicy fruits. The remedy is used for acute grief or stress, severe exhaustion, diarrhea, and headaches. It is also given for childhood growing pains and insomnia or exam nerves.

GRIEF OR SHOCK
Symptoms Apathy, lethargy, and total indifference, brought on by emotional trauma, such as shock or acute grief, possibly due to a broken love affair or the death of a loved one. The memory may become poor, and there may be premature graying of the hair or hair loss.
Symptoms better In warmth.
Symptoms worse Near noise; from emotional stress.

EXHAUSTION
Symptoms Extreme physical fatigue and mental sluggishness, leading to listlessness and apathy. Possible causes include mental or emotional strain such as overwork, exam nerves (*see right*), grief, or shock (*see above*). Drug abuse or severe loss of fluids may also trigger this form of exhaustion. Hair loss or premature graying of the hair may be associated symptoms if acute shock, grief, or stress is the cause. Headaches (*see below*), lack of concentration, poor memory, and insomnia may also occur.
Symptoms better With sleep; from short naps.
Symptoms worse From physical exertion; from emotional stress; on waking.

DIARRHEA
Symptoms Profuse, watery, thin stools, especially during hot weather. Stools are often passed involuntarily, and are accompanied by flatulence and a distended, bloated feeling in the abdomen, possibly with cramping pain. The diarrhea does not in itself cause fatigue, although exhaustion follows after eating or due to loss of fluids (*see left*).
Symptoms better With warmth; from short naps; from passing stools.
Symptoms worse In cold; in drafts; from emotional stress; from standing; from eating dry foods.

HEADACHES
Symptoms Pain that is like a crushing weight on the temples or the top of the head, possibly with dizziness and eye strain. These headaches particularly affect schoolchildren, especially girls, who are overstudying for exams (*see right*), and those

SOURCE DETAILS

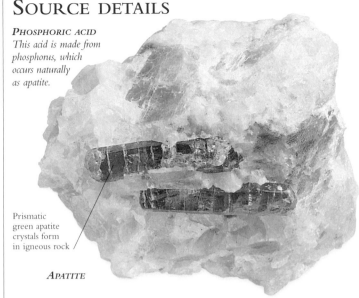

PHOSPHORIC ACID
This acid is made from phosphorus, which occurs naturally as apatite.

Prismatic green apatite crystals form in igneous rock

APATITE

ORIGIN
Produced by grinding a phosphate rock such as apatite into a powder and then mixing it with sulphuric acid.

BACKGROUND
Once used by doctors in Europe and the US to stimulate the digestion; now taken to lower high blood-calcium levels.

PREPARATION
Phosphoric acid is dissolved in alcohol in a ratio of 1:9. It is then repeatedly diluted and succussed.

KEY SYMPTOMS
AILMENTS THAT ARE TRIGGERED BY GRIEF ◆ FATIGUE ◆ APATHY ◆ CHILLINESS ◆ CRAVINGS FOR FRUITS AND JUICY FOODS

---

stressed at work. They may also be caused by exhaustion, grief (*see left*), or prolonged periods of standing or walking.
Symptoms better With warmth; with movement; from short naps; from pressure on the affected area.
Symptoms worse In cold; from emotional stress; from overstudying; from loss of fluids; near noise; from music; from talking; in the evening.

GROWING PAINS
Symptoms Rapid growth and development of a gangly frame, causing growing pains in the limbs in children. An over-active libido may develop, characterized by frequent masturbation accompanied by feelings of guilt that may ultimately cause emotional strain and exhaustion (*see left*).
Symptoms better With warmth; from short naps; from pressure on the affected area.
Symptoms worse With fatigue; from emotional stress.

EXAM NERVES
Symptoms Headaches (*see left*), with possible eye strain due to overstudying. Dizziness and even complete exhaustion (*see left*) may accompany the headaches. Girls are especially prone to this type of stress.
Symptoms better With warmth; with movement.
Symptoms worse In cold; from emotional stress; from overstudying; near noise; from music; from talking.

SEE ALSO
Diabetes, *page 191*; Chronic fatigue syndrome, *page 205*; Grief, *page 213*

Aluminum oxydatum
ALUMINA

SIGNIFICANT AMOUNTS of aluminum absorbed into the body are thought by some to cause the mental processes to slow down. Some evidence suggests that it may aid the development of Alzheimer's disease. Sources of ingested aluminum in humans may include drinking water, baking powder, food additives, and indigestion remedies. *Alumina*, proved by Hahnemann and published in his *Materia Medica Pura* (1821–34), is given chiefly for sluggish states and dementia.

REMEDY PROFILE

Alumina is best suited to those who are generally sluggish. They may be in a state of deep despair, and fear that something awful is about to happen. Fear of insanity is not uncommon, especially on sighting sharp objects and knives, which may even trigger suicidal thoughts. Reactions to external stimuli and questions are slow, yet despite this, these people often feel a sense of haste, hurry, and confusion.

Typical physical symptoms include dry, gray skin and dry, sore mucous membranes. In addition, there may be a lack of coordination, weakness, and fatigue, possibly associated with chronic illness.

Alumina is typically used for elderly people who are senile, and confused, with a poor memory. It is also suited to delicate babies. The remedy is given to treat fatigue, nervous complaints, constipation, and unusual food cravings.

FATIGUE
Symptoms Great weakness, sluggishness, and exhaustion. The skin is pallid, and the legs are heavy and tired, even when sitting. This weakness may be the result of chronic illness.
Symptoms better In damp weather; with moderate exertion; while eating.
Symptoms worse In warm rooms; on waking; lying or sitting down.

NERVOUS DISORDERS
Symptoms Numbness, "pins and needles," a sensation of muscle paralysis and fatigue, and slow, weak movements. The extremities may become uncoordinated (locomotor ataxia), and the eye muscles may be affected, causing drooping eyelids and squinting.
Symptoms better In fresh air; in the evening.
Symptoms worse In cold air; in the morning; from salty and starchy foods.

DEMENTIA
Symptoms Deterioration of mental processes leading to sluggish and absent-minded behavior. Those affected may forget who they are and feel as if they are talking, hearing, or smelling through someone else's senses. There is often a sense of being adrift from the body. Elderly people are most commonly affected. The remedy may be given to treat Alzheimer's disease.
Symptoms better In damp weather; in the evening; with moderate exertion.
Symptoms worse In warm rooms; on waking.

CONSTIPATION
Symptoms Sluggish bowels or severe constipation. The rectum characteristically feels paralyzed, and great effort is required to expel even small, soft stools. Pregnant women, newborn babies, and children are most commonly affected. *Alumina* may also help elderly or sedentary people who have severe constipation and no urge to pass stools.
Symptoms better In fresh air; in the evening; from warm foods and drinks.

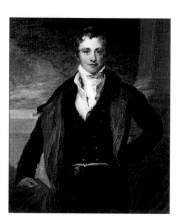

SIR HUMPHREY DAVY
This 19th-century chemist and inventor, who also invented the Davy lamp, gave aluminum its original name, alumium.

SOURCE DETAILS

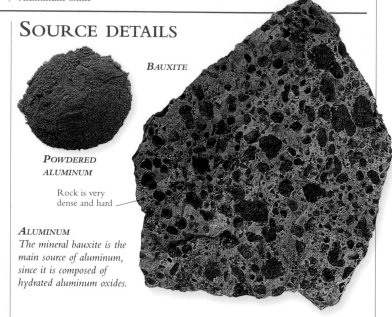

BAUXITE

POWDERED ALUMINUM

Rock is very dense and hard

ALUMINUM
The mineral bauxite is the main source of aluminum, since it is composed of hydrated aluminum oxides.

ORIGIN
Obtained from bauxite, a dense mineral that is predominantly found in Ghana, Jamaica, the US, France, Italy, Hungary, Indonesia, and Russia.

BACKGROUND
Used as an antacid in indigestion remedies, and in cooking utensils. Controversially thought by some to be a factor in triggering the onset of Alzheimer's disease.

PREPARATION
Aluminum-oxide crystals are extracted from bauxite using an industrial process. They are then triturated with lactose sugar, filtered, diluted, and succussed.

KEY SYMPTOMS
SENSE OF FEELING HURRIED AND FLUSTERED ◆
FATIGUE AND SLUGGISHNESS ◆ FAILING MEMORY ◆ DRYNESS
OF THE SKIN AND MUCOUS MEMBRANES

Symptoms worse In cold air; with heat; in the morning; from salty and starchy foods.

APPETITE DISORDERS
Symptoms A dry mouth and throat, with cravings for dry foods or inedible substances such as pencils, chalk, clay, tea leaves, and coffee grounds. The cravings appear to be for substances that actually contain aluminum.
Symptoms better In fresh air; in the evening; from warm foods and drinks.
Symptoms worse From starchy, salty, processed foods.

SEE ALSO
Constipation, *page 238*

Ammonium carbonicum
AMMONIUM CARB.

COMMON NAMES
Ammonium carbonate, sal volatile

For MANY CENTURIES ammonium carbonate was used in the West to treat "blood poisoning" arising from scarlet fever infection. From the 19th century, however, its main medicinal use was in smelling salts (also called sal volatile or salts of ammonia), which were used to revive and stimulate those who had fainted. Hahnemann proved and published the remedy in his *Materia Medica Pura* (1821–34). It is considered particularly useful for states of collapse.

REMEDY PROFILE

This remedy is best suited to people who polarize between a fast, excitable, idealistic state and one that is absent-minded, confused, and chaotic. Their initial idealism may lead them to misjudge their own abilities, resulting in disappointment, resentment, or a feeling that they will never succeed.

These people typically search for values and beliefs as a means of establishing a structure and overview for their lives. If these structures begin to drop away, perhaps due to stress or illness, for example, they typically try to "battle on," exhausted and muddled. They are sensitive to other people and to any distress they may be experiencing, but are also inclined to be challenging and disobedient. They have a tendency to be forgetful, gloomy, weepy, and bad-tempered, especially during cloudy weather.

Physical symptoms typically treated with *Ammonium carb.* include severe fatigue, skin eruptions, chesty respiratory conditions such as bronchitis, and problems generated by a sluggish circulation. It may also be used for scarlet fever.

FATIGUE
Symptoms Extreme fatigue, possibly with great weakness, fainting, irritability, and depression. The temperament typically changes from idealistic and positive to gloomy, chaotic, confused, absentminded, and

hysterical. An overwhelming sensation that "things cannot go on like this" may be felt, with initial zest and sparkle giving way to a scattered, exhausted feeling. Ultimately, these symptoms may lead to feelings of depression and nervous exhaustion.
Symptoms better In warm, dry surroundings; from raising the feet.
Symptoms worse In cloudy weather; with continuous movement.

RESPIRATORY ILLNESS
Symptoms A sensation of oppression in the chest, with a recurrent, dry, tickling, rattling cough. The cough may be persistent enough to cause retching, especially at night, and severe enough to cause palpitations. The remedy is commonly used for bronchitis and other chest problems.
Symptoms better In warm, dry surroundings; from pressure on the chest; from raising the feet.
Symptoms worse In cloudy weather; with continuous movement.

POOR CIRCULATION
Symptoms Breathlessness, wheezing, palpitations, and fatigue, particularly following exertion. Symptoms are often accompanied by a flushed, puffy face, and are typically caused by inefficient circulation of blood by the heart.
Symptoms better In warm,

SOURCE DETAILS

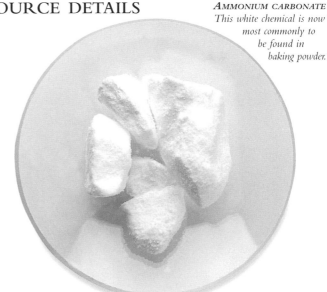

AMMONIUM CARBONATE
This white chemical is now most commonly to be found in baking powder.

ORIGIN
Chemically prepared from the crystalline compounds sodium carbonate (*see page 91*) and ammonium chloride (*see page 123*).

BACKGROUND
Traditionally mixed with alcohol and lavender to make smelling salts, a pungent concoction for reviving someone who has fainted.

PREPARATION
The crystalline solid is diluted in distilled water. The resulting solution is repeatedly diluted and succussed to potentize it.

KEY SYMPTOMS
MENTAL SLUGGISHNESS ◆ FATIGUE ◆ FAINTING AND WEAKNESS ◆
BREATHLESSNESS ◆ SENSE OF COMPRESSION IN THE CHEST ◆
PERSON FEELS WORSE FROM COLD AND DAMPNESS
---

dry surroundings; from raising the feet.
Symptoms worse In cloudy weather; with continuous movement.

SKIN CONDITIONS
Symptoms Skin eruptions such as boils, pimples, and red blotches that are often slow to clear. *Ammonium carb.* is used for rashes, hives (urticaria), and erysipelas with violent itching. The skin is generally prone to allergic reactions and sensitive, especially to water, and there is often a dislike of bathing or washing. The skin eruptions are commonly considered an indication of more serious internal problems, and are usually accompanied by a flushed and puffy face due to a weak circulation (*see left*).
Symptoms better In warm,

dry surroundings; from pressure on the skin.
Symptoms worse In cloudy weather; with continuous movement.

SCARLET FEVER
Symptoms A rash of tiny, red spots spreading rapidly over the body from the neck and the upper trunk, accompanied by a sore throat, headache, and fever.
Symptoms better From pressure on the affected area; lying on the abdomen.
Symptoms worse In cold; in damp; between 3 a.m. and 4 a.m.

SEE ALSO
Depression, *page 212*

Argentum nitricum
ARGENTUM NIT.

M EDIEVAL ALCHEMISTS called this compound lunar caustic. They used its antibacterial and caustic properties for cauterizing wounds. If ingested in large amounts, silver nitrate is highly poisonous and may turn the body blue. It is now used for manufacturing photographic film and plates, and as a backing for mirrors. *Argentum nit.* was first proved by Hahnemann, but then given a more thorough proving by Dr. J. O. Müller of Vienna in 1845.

REMEDY PROFILE

Argentum nit. is best suited to people who are extroverted, cheerful, and impressionable. Suggestible and impulsive, they may have difficulty in controlling their far-ranging minds and emotions, and readily laugh, cry, lose their tempers, or become anxious. They may be nervous, phobic, and superstitious. Motivated people who think, talk, and act rapidly, they are always in a hurry, and are frequently to be found in careers that require quick thinking and a good memory, or where the emphasis is on performance.

Typical physical symptoms include a "sensitive" digestion, a lack of physical control, with awkwardness and tremors, and a tendency to feel the heat. *Argentum nit.* is used for certain nervous, mental, and digestive problems where these key physical and mental symptoms are evident.

ANXIETY & PHOBIAS
Symptoms Anxiety, possibly accompanied by palpitations, tremors, awkwardness, sweats, insomnia, and even vomiting (*see right*). There is typically a feeling of being out of control, and the imagination may become overactive, spiraling off to exacerbate fears and heighten anxieties or phobias. Common triggers include stage fright, anticipatory anxiety, and phobias such as claustrophobia, vertigo, or fear of water or the dentist. People who respond to

this remedy usually feel very anxious about their health.
Symptoms better In fresh air; in cool surroundings; from pressure on the head, such as a tight bandage around it.
Symptoms worse With warmth; in hot weather; at night; with movement; lying on the left side; from emotional stress.

DIGESTIVE DISORDERS
Symptoms Diarrhea, loud, explosive burping, a distended abdomen, and flatulence. The stools are smelly, watery, and green. There may be vomiting exacerbated by nervousness or anticipatory anxiety (*see below, left*). If symptoms persist, colitis or irritable bowel syndrome (*see below*) may develop. The digestion is "sensitive," with possible cravings for salty or sweet foods, although the latter may trigger headaches or diarrhea.
Symptoms better In fresh air; in cool surroundings; from pressure on the abdomen.
Symptoms worse With warmth; in hot weather; lying on the left side; from emotional stress; sweet foods.

IRRITABLE BOWEL SYNDROME
Symptoms Constipation that alternates with flatulence and diarrhea. There is a fluttery, tense feeling in the stomach and pain in the upper left abdomen. The stools are usually coated with mucus.

SOURCE DETAILS

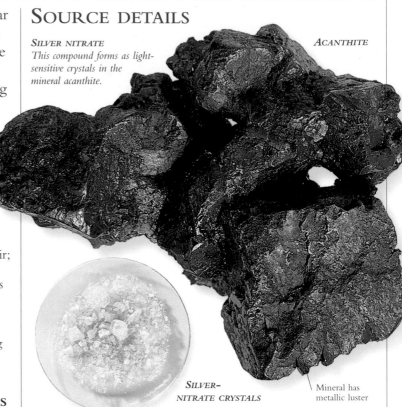

SILVER NITRATE
This compound forms as light-sensitive crystals in the mineral acanthite.

ACANTHITE

SILVER-NITRATE CRYSTALS

Mineral has metallic luster

ORIGIN
Found in acanthite, which usually occurs as crystals in hydrothermal veins in Norway, the US, and South America.

BACKGROUND
Used in 19th-century North America for eye infections and warts, and still included in some modern wart medicines.

PREPARATION
Pure crystals of silver nitrate are dissolved in alcohol before being repeatedly diluted and succussed.

KEY SYMPTOMS
ANXIETY ♦ IMPULSIVENESS ♦ PHOBIAS ♦ CRAVING FOR SWEET FOODS, WHICH AGGRAVATE SYMPTOMS ♦ DIGESTIVE PROBLEMS WITH FLATULENCE ♦ TENDENCY TO FEEL HOT

Symptoms better In fresh air; in cool surroundings; from pressure on the abdomen.
Symptoms worse With warmth; in hot weather; lying on the left side; from emotional stress.

NERVOUS DISORDERS
Symptoms The limbs feel weak, bruised, and trembling. There is often giddiness and a tendency to stagger in the dark. The remedy is also used for twitching with numbness, which may follow a stroke or brain injury, or which may be linked to epilepsy, especially if attacks occur after a fright or

during menstruation. The weakness and heaviness of the limbs may eventually lead to a feeling of paralysis. *Argentum nit.* may also be prescribed for multiple sclerosis, if the mental and physical symptoms fit the profile.
Symptoms better In fresh air; in cool surroundings.
Symptoms worse With warmth; during menstruation.

SEE ALSO
Multiple sclerosis, *page 179*;
Digestion, *pages 188, 234*;
Emotional problems, *page 210*;
Exam nerves, *page 254*

Aurum metallicum

AURUM MET.

COMMON NAME
Gold

THE ANCIENT EGYPTIANS were one of the earliest civilizations to master the art of mining and working gold. In many cultures it was ascribed great value on the basis of its rarity and splendor. As early as the 7th century BCE, gold was fashioned into coins and used as a means of exchange, paving the way for today's world economy. Gold also plays a role in conventional medicine, being used in the treatment of rheumatoid arthritis. Hahnemann proved the homeopathic remedy in 1818.

REMEDY PROFILE

Those who are most suited to *Aurum met.* often feel as if they do not accomplish as much as they should. They tend to be workaholics, always striving to attain the tough standards that they set for themselves. If they consider that they have failed in this, a feeling of emptiness and despair may follow.

There is a marked tendency toward hypersensitivity in these people, both emotionally and physically, with smell, taste, hearing, and touch all being highly acute. As a result of being emotionally overcharged, they tend to overreact to criticism or contradiction, exploding into fierce anger with trembling and flushing.

Aurum met. is prescribed for depression and grief. It is also given to treat circulatory problems such as palpitations and angina, and for headaches, disorders of the reproductive system, and bone pains.

for show but lacks substance: it glitters but is not gold. In extreme cases this may lead to severe clinical depression and suicide. There may be a longing for death, possibly provoking suicidal thoughts, although a fear of death may coexist simultaneously.

Other symptoms include irritability, feelings of guilt or of being forsaken, perhaps associated with a shock, such as the death of a loved one, or a failed romance.
Symptoms better With rest; from walking; in fresh air.
Symptoms worse With mental concentration or exertion; from emotional stress, particularly at night.

ANGINA
Symptoms Palpitations, high blood pressure, breathlessness, and chest pains behind the breastbone that extend along the arm to the fingertips. There may also be the sensation that the heart is about to stop, and that the blood vessels are hot. The heart may not feel properly lodged in the chest, and may seem to shake with every movement.
Symptoms better With warmth; with rest; in fresh air.
Symptoms worse At night; from mental or physical exertion; from emotional stress.

DEPRESSION
Symptoms Anxiety and a sense of worthlessness, disenchantment with life, and despair. There is commonly an empty feeling, as though everything is just

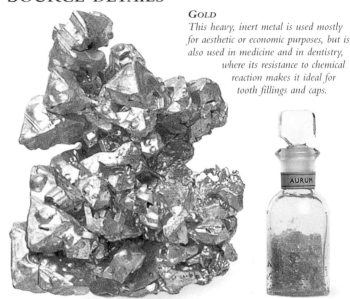

GOLD
This heavy, inert metal is used mostly for aesthetic or economic purposes, but is also used in medicine and in dentistry, where its resistance to chemical reaction makes it ideal for tooth fillings and caps.

GOLD NUGGET   *GOLD FLAKES*

SOURCE DETAILS

ORIGIN
Found in hydrothermal veins, and sometimes as nuggets or grains lying in streambeds or sand in Australia, South Africa, and North America.

BACKGROUND
Given by 12th-century Arabian physicians for heart problems, gold was also used in blood tests and for tuberculosis in the early 20th century.

PREPARATION
Gold is purified from a nugget or extracted from an ore. It is then triturated with lactose sugar, filtered, diluted, and succussed.

KEY SYMPTOMS
WORKAHOLIC NATURE ◆ DESPAIR AT ANY PERCEIVED FAILURES ◆
BOUTS OF ANGER AND VIOLENCE ◆ ANGINA ◆ PAINS IN THE
BONES ◆ PERSON FEELS WORSE AT NIGHT

REPRODUCTIVE-SYSTEM PROBLEMS
Symptoms Inflammation of the testes and undescended testicles in boys. In women, *Aurum met.* is used for painful menstruation, fibroids, a prolapsed uterus, causing a dragging feeling in the pelvis, and a sensation that the uterus is enlarged. There may be sterility, leading to depression.
Symptoms better With rest; from walking; in fresh air; from washing in cold water.
Symptoms worse In cold; at night; from emotional stress.

BONE PAIN
Symptoms Deep, gnawing, debilitating bone pains, often on the right side of the jaw bone and in the bones of the

nose. Alternatively, there may be wandering, debilitating rheumatic pains in the muscles.
Symptoms better With warmth; with rest; in fresh air.
Symptoms worse At night; from exertion; emotional stress.

HEADACHES
Symptoms Severe, pounding, unbearable pain, with blood veins pulsing in the temples.
Symptoms better With rest; in fresh air.
Symptoms worse At night; from exertion; emotional stress.

SEE ALSO
Palpitations, *page 186*; Arthritis, *page 197*; Infertility, *page 203*; Cancer, *page 208*; Emotional problems, *page 210*

GOLDEN BUDDHA
Religious icons are often made of gold in honor of the deity depicted. Gold may also be offered as a tribute.

Barium carbonicum syn. *Baryta carbonica*

BARYTA CARB.

COMMON NAME
Barium carbonate

ALCHEMISTS IN THE 17th century gave barium the name *lapis solaris*, due to its luminous qualities when heated. Its compounds are used in radiology, although as a pure element barium is very poisonous. Commercially barium carbonate is used as a pottery glaze, and to make porcelain, glassware, and optical glass. *Baryta carb.*, proved by Hahnemann and published in his *Chronic Diseases* (1821–34), is prescribed mainly for problems in childhood and old age.

REMEDY PROFILE

Physical, emotional, or mental development is usually slow in those who respond best to *Baryta carb.* They tend to be shy and introverted, often because they are insecure and feel that they are worthless. They may require excessive reassurance, and are prone to fears and anxieties. Emotional immaturity can cause them to feel inadequate in relationships and social situations.

Typical physical traits linked with *Baryta carb.* include nail-biting when anxious and a tendency to have sweaty, smelly feet. The remedy is used for slow development in children and for those with Down's syndrome, and is also given for senile dementia in the elderly. In addition, *Baryta carb.* is used to treat recurrent colds and coughs, sore throats, swollen tonsils, anxiety and phobias, and impotence.

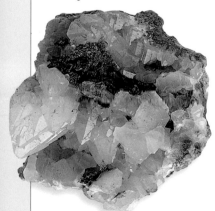

WITHERITE
Barium carbonate occurs naturally as witherite, which was discovered in 1783 by a British scientist, William Withering.

GROWTH DISORDERS IN CHILDREN
Symptoms Delayed physical development in children, such as late development of speech and walking, possibly caused by Down's syndrome. The genitals and other parts of the body may not develop properly, typically resulting in a large head and short stature.
Symptoms better No specific factors.
Symptoms worse From emotional stress.

PROBLEMS OF THE ELDERLY
Symptoms Senile dementia with childish, confused, and embarrassing behavior. The short-term memory may be impaired, and paranoia or depression may develop. There may be hair loss. A frequent desire to urinate may progress eventually to incontinence. These symptoms may be associated with a stroke.
Symptoms better From not thinking about symptoms.
Symptoms worse From emotional stress; in company.

SWOLLEN TONSILS
Symptoms A raw throat with inflamed tonsils and a burning pain on swallowing. There may be retching that is aggravated by swallowing solid foods. The neck glands may swell and harden, and there may be excess production of saliva. Symptoms may be indicative of mumps, especially in children.

SOURCE DETAILS

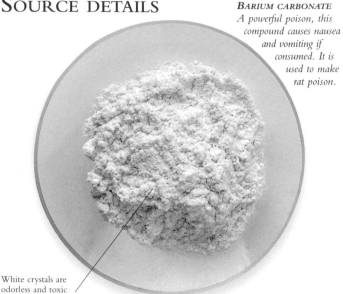

BARIUM CARBONATE
A powerful poison, this compound causes nausea and vomiting if consumed. It is used to make rat poison.

White crystals are odorless and toxic

ORIGIN
Barium chloride is precipitated with a weak solution of ammonia to form white, odorless crystals of barium carbonate.

BACKGROUND
Prescribed medicinally in Europe in the late 19th and early 20th centuries as a treatment for tuberculosis and glandular swelling.

PREPARATION
Once the crystals of barium carbonate have been chemically prepared, they are mixed with lactose sugar and triturated.

KEY SYMPTOMS
PHYSICAL, MENTAL, AND EMOTIONAL IMMATURITY ♦
LACK OF CONFIDENCE ♦ SWOLLEN TONSILS ♦
OFFENSIVE-SMELLING PERSPIRATION ON THE FEET

Symptoms better With warmth; in fresh air.
Symptoms worse In extreme heat; in cold; from having damp feet; from thinking about symptoms.

ANXIETY & PHOBIAS
Symptoms Intense, often irrational, fears and anxieties, possibly triggered by negative recollections of school days, or by memories of physical or sexual abuse. There is often a tendency to bite the nails.
Symptoms better From walking alone in open air; not thinking about symptoms.
Symptoms worse From emotional stress; in company.

RESPIRATORY ILLNESS
Symptoms Recurrent colds, coughs, and bronchitis. The nostrils may feel dry and raw.

Symptoms better With warmth; in fresh air.
Symptoms worse In extreme heat; in cold; from having damp feet; from thinking about symptoms.

IMPOTENCE
Symptoms Bouts of erectile dysfunction or low libido in men, possibly so pronounced that they actually fall asleep during sexual intercourse.
Symptoms better From not thinking about symptoms.
Symptoms worse In cold, from having damp feet; from emotional stress.

SEE ALSO
Stroke, *page 187*; Prostate problems, *page 202*; Confusion, *page 266*; Senile dementia, *page 266*

Calcium carbonicum Hahnemanni

CALC. CARB.

OYSTER SHELLS ARE THE natural source of calcium carbonate used in this remedy, but the compound also occurs naturally in marble, chalk, pearls, limestone, and coral. It is one of several calcium salts used in homeopathy. The human body needs calcium to function efficiently, since various essential compounds are produced when it combines with protein in the body. Hahnemann proved the remedy and published it in his _Chronic Diseases_ (1821–34).

REMEDY PROFILE

Calc. carb. is best suited to shy, placid, sensitive, contemplative people who may also have an agitated, excitable side, notably in the face of cruelty. Cautious and fearful worriers, they are calmed by reassurance. They are forgetful, lacking in energy, and inherently clumsy, often spraining ankles and wrists.

As children these individuals develop slowly, teething and walking later than the average age. Both adults and children may sweat heavily, mostly on the scalp, and have a sluggish circulation. There may be an aversion to meat, dairy foods, and coffee, and cravings for candy, eggs, or indigestible things such as chalk or soap. They are prone to constipation and sour-smelling sweat, and may be sensitive to the cold.

Calc. carb. is prescribed for anxiety-related conditions, and for bone, joint, and dental problems, digestive disorders, headaches, and certain ailments affecting women's health.

ANXIETY & PHOBIAS

Symptoms Worry and fears that may escalate into obsessive behavior, mainly focusing around fears that other people will "see through them" and consider them unable to cope or "fakes." Anxiety may be due to irrational fears, typically of darkness, poverty, illness, death, or failure. Worry and anxiety dreams may result in sleep being disrupted or prevented, leading to insomnia.

Symptoms better In dry weather; in the late morning; after breakfast.
Symptoms worse In cold weather; toward evening; from mental exertion.

BONE & JOINT PAIN

Symptoms Backache, bone growths, bunions, or joint pain, perhaps caused by an arthritic condition, an inflammatory joint problem such as tennis elbow, or a slow-mending sprain. Broken bones tend to be slow to heal.
Symptoms better Lying on the affected side; in the late morning; in dry weather.
Symptoms worse In cold; in damp; from sweating; physical exertion; before menstruating.

DENTAL PROBLEMS

Symptoms Painful teething in children, with sore gums, fever, and a sweaty scalp. The child is irritable and makes a chewing motion with the jaws. _Calc. carb._ is also used for slow tooth development, weak, crumbly teeth, and dental decay in children and adults
Symptoms better In warm weather; from rubbing or lying on the affected area.
Symptoms worse With heat or cold in the mouth; with a direct air current on the tooth.

DIGESTIVE DISORDERS

Symptoms Indigestion with flatulence, bloating, and sour burping, or constipation with sour-smelling, hard, pale stools.

SOURCE DETAILS

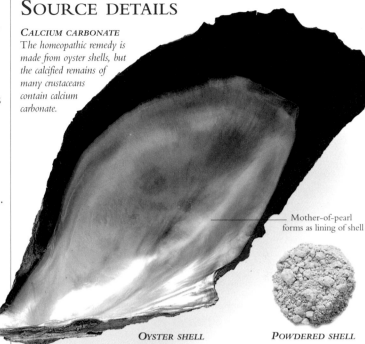

CALCIUM CARBONATE
The homeopathic remedy is made from oyster shells, but the calcified remains of many crustaceans contain calcium carbonate.

Mother-of-pearl forms as lining of shell

OYSTER SHELL

POWDERED SHELL

ORIGIN
Secreted by oysters between the inner and outer layers of their shells. In this form it is commonly called mother-of-pearl.

BACKGROUND
Previously given as an antacid, and now used in dentistry, in making furniture and jewelry, and in the building and chemical industries.

PREPARATION
The shells are cleaned and dried, and the mother-of-pearl is removed from the outer shell. It is then triturated with lactose sugar.

KEY SYMPTOMS

FEARS AND ANXIETIES ◆ DELAYED DEVELOPMENT ◆ SOUR-SMELLING DISCHARGES ◆ SENSITIVITY TO THE COLD ◆ AVERSION TO DAIRY PRODUCTS ◆ CRAVINGS FOR CANDY AND EGGS

Symptoms may improve when accompanied by constipation. They are often triggered by anxiety and agitation (_see left_).
Symptoms better In the late morning; after breakfast.
Symptoms worse In cold; in damp; on waking; from sweating; with physical exertion; before menstruating.

HEADACHES

Symptoms Sharp head pain, often right-sided, and possibly with dizziness, congestion, or phlegm. Migraines with nausea and bursting pain may develop.
Symptoms better In the late morning; in dry weather.
Symptoms worse In cold; in damp; before menstruating; in spring.

WOMEN'S HEALTH

Symptoms Burning vaginal itching, with a thick, yellow or white discharge, due to a yeast infection. There may be heavy menstrual flow or premenstrual syndrome (PMS), possibly with enlarged, painful breasts and dizziness. Menopausal symptoms may include breast pain and heavy bleeding.
Symptoms better With warmth; with rest.
Symptoms worse In cold; with exertion; emotional stress.

SEE ALSO

Respiration, _page 180_;
Palpitations, _page 186_; Skin, _pages 192, 194_; Reproduction, _page 198_; Immune system, _page 204_

Calcium phosphoricum
CALC. PHOS.

COMMON NAMES
Calcium phosphate, phosphate of lime

IN NATURE, THE MINERAL SALT calcium phosphate exists as apatite, found predominantly in north Africa. Calcium phosphate is the main constituent of bones and teeth, accounting for about 60 percent of the average human skeleton. Dr. Wilhelm Schüssler chose it in 1873 as one of the 12 mineral or tissue salts that he considered vital for a healthy body (*see page 90*). The remedy, proved by Dr. Constantine Hering in 1837, is given primarily for bone and teeth problems.

SOURCE DETAILS

CALCIUM PHOSPHATE
Although calcium phosphate exists in a natural state, it is manufactured in a laboratory for use in homeopathy.

ORIGIN
Manufactured from dilutions of phosphoric acid and calcium hydroxide (also called limewater). The two solutions react to form calcium phosphate as a cloudy, white precipitate.

BACKGROUND
Used in the manufacture of glass, in fertilizers, as a stabilizer in plastics, and as a leavening agent in baking. Additionally used by dentists as a polishing powder for teeth.

PREPARATION
The white calcium phosphate precipitate is filtered, dried, and triturated with lactose sugar.

Calcium phosphate forms as white precipitate when the two solutions are mixed

REMEDY PROFILE

Usually sociable and sensitive, people who respond best to *Calc. phos.* are prone to feelings of great insecurity with regard to their health and friends. They may get depressed, worn down, and weary, feeling poorly nourished on both a physical and emotional level. This feeling often leads them to be restless and uncertain of what they want. Constantly seeking new stimulation and contacts, they like to travel and meet people but tend to feel dissatisfied, bored, and irritable without knowing why. As children they exhibit similar discontent with no real cause.

Calc. phos. is used to treat bone conditions such as joint disorders, fractures that are slow to heal, and slow growth in children. Teething problems and weak teeth are also treated with the remedy, as are fatigue, anemia (possibly after illness), migraines, and disorders of the digestive system.

BONE & JOINT CONDITIONS
Symptoms Pain and stiffness in the neck and back. Joints may be painful, possibly due to arthritis, inflamed tendons, slow healing of fractures, or ligament sprains. There may be abnormality of the bones in a joint, causing them to fuse and become immobile, or leading to curvature of the spine.
Symptoms better In summer; in warm, dry weather.
Symptoms worse In cold, damp weather; from worry or grief; from overexertion; from lifting heavy objects.

TEETHING
Symptoms Slow or difficult teething, typically with colds, coughs, and diarrhea. Once teeth have formed, they tend to be weak and decay easily.
Symptoms better In summer; in warm, dry weather.
Symptoms worse In cold, damp weather.

FATIGUE
Symptoms General feeling of being undernourished and unwell. Weakness, exhaustion, and anemia may follow illness or emotional stress. There may also be susceptibility to the cold and to drafts.
Symptoms better In summer; after a very hot bath.
Symptoms worse In cold, damp weather; from worry or grief; from overexertion; from lifting heavy objects; from sexual excess.

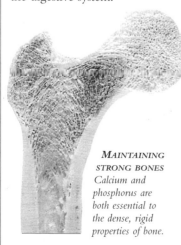

MAINTAINING STRONG BONES Calcium and phosphorus are both essential to the dense, rigid properties of bone.

GROWTH DISORDERS
Symptoms Slow growth in children and adolescents, or rapid growth during puberty, typically accompanied by numbness and a crawling sensation in the hands and feet. The fontanelle may be slow to close in babies.
Symptoms better In warm, dry weather.
Symptoms worse In cold, damp weather; from puberty; during teeth development.

HEAD PAIN
Symptoms Severe headaches with pain along the cranial sutures (the joints linking the bones of the cranium). These may intensify into migraines.
Symptoms better In summer; in warm, dry weather.
Symptoms worse In cold, damp weather; from worry or grief; from overexertion; from lifting heavy objects.

DIGESTIVE DISORDERS
Symptoms Indigestion, pain after eating, and heartburn. Adults may find it difficult to eat and be nourished by food, possibly due to cramps, nausea, vomiting, and diarrhea. There may be cravings for candy, and for salty foods such as smoked meats. Children may have chronic abdominal pain. Babies have great difficulties feeding, persistently vomiting even breast milk, and suffering from cramps and colic after feeding.
Symptoms better In summer; in warm, dry weather.
Symptoms worse In cold, damp weather; from dwelling on symptoms; drinking milk.

SEE ALSO
Rosacea, *page 193*; Rheumatoid arthritis, *page 197*; Breast problems, *page 201*; Phobias, *page 211*

Causticum Hahnemanni
CAUSTICUM

COMMON NAME
Potassium hydrate

UNIQUE TO HOMEOPATHY, this compound of potassium was specially devised and proved by Hahnemann, who published it in his *Chronic Diseases* (1821–34). Hahnemann noted that the compound caused an astringent sensation and a burning taste on the tongue. Interestingly, *Causticum* is a major homeopathic first-aid remedy for severe burns and a remedy for pain with a burning sensation. Other ailments for which it is taken include local paralysis, incontinence, sore throats, and coughs.

REMEDY PROFILE

Those for whom *Causticum* may be most helpful tend to be serious and introspective. They feel the effect of grief for prolonged periods and may become mentally weakened, absentminded, hopeless, anxious, and prey to fears or fanciful ideas. Forgetfulness and a need to check on their fears and fancies can lead to a compulsive need to check and recheck everything they do. Acutely sympathetic to the sufferings of others, they tend to react strongly to others' distress or to any perceived injustices; at best sympathetic and idealistic, they are often politically active.

These people frequently have a tendency to feel chilly and to be affected by changes in the weather, by cold, dry weather, and by getting wet. *Causticum* is most often prescribed for weakness, which may progress to paralysis, of the nerves and muscles, especially of the bladder, larynx, vocal cords, upper eyelids, and the right side of the face. Muscle weakness may show both as twitching and as stiffness that causes mobility problems.

TREMORS & PARALYSIS

Symptoms Muscle weakness with tremors and drooping of the upper eyelids. There may be a stammer, particularly at times of anger or excitement, and dizziness accompanied by a lack of coordination. Facial neuralgia or paralysis (Bell's palsy) is possible, especially on the right side, or there may be a form of slow-developing paralysis. Minor or severe seizures may occur, from petit mal fits to serious convulsions, with a susceptibility to jerking and twitching in extreme cases.
Symptoms better With warmth; from washing.
Symptoms worse In dry, cold winds; in the evening; from exertion.

URINARY DISORDERS

Symptoms Bed-wetting that may be long-term in children, and urine incontinence in the elderly. A need to urinate frequently may be experienced, or the reverse, where urine is retained due to temporary paralysis. There may be stress incontinence on jarring the body, for example, when running, or when coughing, sneezing, or laughing. This is particularly prevalent in women during pregnancy and after giving birth. Cystitis, with a strong urge to urinate accompanied by an inability to actually do so, may also be treated by *Causticum*. Both men and women who respond to this remedy may experience a loss of sexual pleasure or an aversion to sexual intercourse.
Symptoms better With warmth; from washing.
Symptoms worse In dry, cold winds; in the evening; from coffee.

SOURCE DETAILS

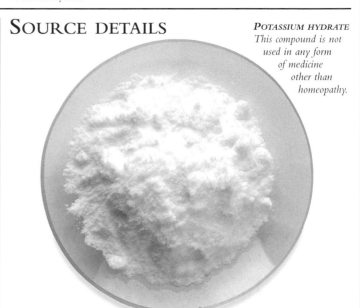

ORIGIN
Hahnemann used equal parts of slaked lime (calcium hydroxide) and sulfate of potash (potassium bisulfate) to make this remedy.

BACKGROUND
Created by Hahnemann, who wanted to produce a particularly caustic mixture, this compound was new to the medical repertory of the time.

PREPARATION
Slaked lime and sulfate of potash are combined and dissolved in purified water. This solution is then further diluted and succussed.

KEY SYMPTOMS

EXTREME SENSITIVITY ◆ INTOLERANCE OF INJUSTICE ◆ GRADUAL PARALYSIS ◆ RAW, BURNING PAIN ◆ PERSON FEELS WORSE IN COLD, DRY, WINDY WEATHER

SKIN CONDITIONS

Symptoms Large warts that may bleed easily on the hands, face, and fingertips, especially near the nails; scars that do not heal well; and slow-healing burns that blister. Boils, blisters, eczema, herpes, and acne may also be helped by the remedy.
Symptoms better With warmth; from washing.
Symptoms worse In dry, cold winds; in the evening; from exertion.

SORE THROAT

Symptoms A dry, raw, and burning throat with a constant need to swallow or to clear mucus from the throat, possibly with a choking sensation. The larynx and vocal cords may be inflamed and hoarse. Tightness and a tearing pain in the chest may be related to asthma.
Symptoms better With warmth; from washing.
Symptoms worse In dry, cold winds; in the evening; from overusing the voice.

COUGH

Symptoms A dry, deep cough that racks the chest, with a persistent tickle in the throat and difficulty coughing hard enough to expectorate mucus.
Symptoms better In warm, moist weather; with warmth in bed; from cold drinks.
Symptoms worse In dry, cold winds; in the evening; with exertion.

SEE ALSO

Multiple sclerosis, *page 179*;
Skin, *pages 192, 242*; Emotions, *page 210*; Laryngitis, *page 228*; Bed-wetting, *page 248*

Cuprum metallicum
CUPRUM MET.

COMMON NAME
Copper

COPPER'S NAME IS DERIVED from the Greek *Kupris*, or Cyprus, after the island on which the ancient Greeks found the metal. Although used by doctors as late as the 1880s in ointments for healing wounds, coppersmiths have long known of copper's toxic nature. Chronic copper poisoning produces symptoms such as coughs, colic, diarrhea, and difficulty in assimilating food. Acute copper poisoning can cause convulsions, paralysis, and even death. These factors suggested to Hahnemann, who proved *Cuprum met.* in 1834, the remedy's strong affinity with similar symptoms.

SOURCE DETAILS

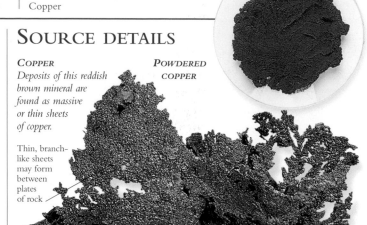

COPPER
Deposits of this reddish brown mineral are found as massive or thin sheets of copper.

Thin, branch-like sheets may form between plates of rock

POWDERED COPPER

COPPER

ORIGIN
Deposited worldwide in rocks, and mined in many countries, such as Chile. Copper has many uses and can be alloyed to form harder metals such as bronze.

BACKGROUND
The first metal to be utilized for tools, and also an essential trace element in many foods, vital for maintaining a healthy body and for good bone growth.

PREPARATION
The metal is triturated with lactose sugar, then ground repeatedly until it forms a powder fine enough to be soluble in water. It is then filtered, diluted, and succussed.

REMEDY PROFILE

Emotions tend to be both rigidly suppressed and intensely felt in those for whom *Cuprum met.* is best suited. Adolescents may suppress their sexual urges as being too strong to cope with, so that any later release of tension may appear extreme. Psychological contrasts can also be extreme, ranging from yielding to headstrong, or from closed-down mental dullness to destructive anger or even violent insanity.

Typical physical symptoms include a pale, drawn face, with blue lips and cold hands and feet. Symptoms may be violent, becoming worse if menstruation is late, or if any eruptions and bodily discharges are suppressed by medication, being chilled, or getting wet.

The remedy is associated primarily with problems of the nervous, respiratory, and digestive systems. Cramping, which may be extreme, may affect the fingers, toes, legs, and stomach. A common feature is exhaustion, perhaps following illness, lack of sleep, or exhausting mental strain.

CRAMPS, CONVULSIONS & EPILEPSY
Symptoms The muscles feel knotted up, particularly in the legs, feet, and calves. Cramps and muscle spasms appear in the limbs, especially at night. They start with twitching and jerking in the toes, and then spread further up the feet, ankles, and calves. Other symptoms are cold extremities, blue lips, and facial grimacing.

Muscle spasms may be marked in pregnancy and after childbirth. Extreme cramps or convulsions may occasionally be triggered. Young children may exhibit great anger or teething problems. Muscle spasms and convulsions linked to epilepsy may be violent, starting in the fingers and toes and spreading to the center of the body. There may be rashes and perspiration on the feet, which is worse if suppressed, by chilling the feet, for example.
Symptoms better From perspiring; from cold drinks.
Symptoms worse In hot weather; at night; if touched; from suppressing emotions; suppressing sweats and rashes.

COUGHS & ASTHMA
Symptoms Long, spasmodic, violent coughing fits, possibly associated with whooping cough. Breathing is labored, rapid, and may seem to stop during coughing fits. The face may be pale, with blue lips and a metallic taste in the mouth.
Symptoms better From perspiring; from cold drinks.
Symptoms worse In hot weather; in cold air; if touched; from vomiting; from suppressing emotions.

KEY SYMPTOMS
SPASMS AND CRAMPS ◆ SUPPRESSION OF EMOTIONS ◆ AILMENTS THAT ARE TRIGGERED BY SUPPRESSION OF RASHES AND DISCHARGES ◆ PERSON FEELS BETTER FROM COLD DRINKS

ABDOMINAL CRAMPS
Symptoms Spasmodic, often violent, colicky pain, possibly with nausea, vomiting, or diarrhea. The abdomen is hot, tender, and sore, and there is a blue line at the margin of the gums, and a metallic taste in the mouth. A gurgling sound on drinking may be due to a spasm of the esophagus. Exhaustion may follow (*see right*), with loss of appetite. *Cuprum met.* is also used for nausea associated with cholera.
Symptoms better From perspiring; from cold drinks.
Symptoms worse In hot weather; if touched; from vomiting; from suppressing emotions.

EXHAUSTION
Symptoms Fatigue following hard work, lack of sleep, or restless sleep. There may be cramps and headaches between the eyes. Exhaustion may also be the result of abdominal cramps and vomiting (*see left*).
Symptoms better From perspiring.
Symptoms worse In hot weather; from emotional stress; from suppressing sweats and rashes; during pregnancy.

SEE ALSO
Cramps, *page 230*

Ferrum metallicum
FERRUM MET.

COMMON NAME
Iron

IRON IS ESSENTIAL IN THE BODY for the formation of hemoglobin, the oxygen-carrying substance in red blood cells. A diet deficient in iron or an inability to absorb iron into the body can lead to anemia, fatigue, and breathlessness. *Ferrum met.* was probably proved and published by Hahnemann between 1821 and 1834. It is prescribed to help the body cope with anemia caused by blood loss and is thought by some to help the body absorb iron more efficiently.

REMEDY PROFILE

Emotional traits that indicate a need for *Ferrum met.* include moodiness, nervous irritability, sensitivity, and an intolerance of contradiction. A compulsion to do certain tasks may lead to feelings of failure, restlessness, and neglected duty. This sense of compulsion easily turns into its opposite: extreme fatigue, weakness, and depression.

Typical physical symptoms include pale lips and face, a tendency to flush easily, and a rosy look that suggests good health but is actually caused by poor circulation. Perspiration may be cold, clammy, and profuse. Bouts of dizziness may occur, as well as sensitivity to cold and to noise. Mental and physical activity are subject to weakness and severe fatigue. Circulatory and digestive problems frequently occur, possibly with marked appetite loss. Movement may be painful and difficult due to back, joint, and head pain.

ANEMIA
Symptoms Pale face that flushes easily, and pale lips, with great fatigue (*see above, right*).

MARS, ROMAN GOD OF WAR
Alchemists, noting how iron deficiency caused moods to be at war in people, linked iron with warlike Mars.

Ferrum met. is given for anemia from blood loss, often due to heavy periods or problems in pregnancy.
Symptoms better In summer; with gentle movement.
Symptoms worse From violent exertion; menstruation.

SEVERE FATIGUE
Symptoms Extreme physical and mental fatigue, the latter causing great sensitivity to noise. There is no desire to work but a need to lie down.
Symptoms better From walking slowly in fresh air.
Symptoms worse At night; from violent exertion; from loss of bodily fluids.

CIRCULATORY PROBLEMS
Symptoms Painful varicose veins, particularly in pregnancy. There may be hemorrhages such as nosebleeds, especially in children. Throbbing blood vessels with headaches are also possible, as are neuralgic pains (*see right*), hot flashes, fever, or palpitations, aggravated by heat.
Symptoms better With gentle movement.
Symptoms worse With heat; at night; lying down; with the loss of bodily fluids.

DIGESTIVE DISORDERS
Symptoms Nausea brought on by eating, which causes a reluctance to eat. There may be sudden vomiting, either while eating or hours later, at around midnight. Typical

SOURCE DETAILS

HEMATITE
This opaque mineral is the most important source of iron ore, containing up to 70 percent iron.

Hematite often forms as kidney ore, so called because of its shape

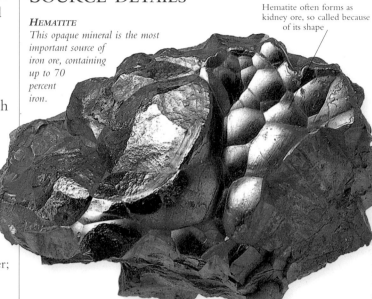

ORIGIN
From iron ores such as hematite, found in Canada, the US, and Venezuela. Iron is the second most common metal on the Earth.

BACKGROUND
So prominent in history that it gave its name to the Iron Age, and also a highly important trace element for the working of the human body.

PREPARATION
Powdered iron is ground with lactose sugar to triturate it. It is then dissolved in water, and repeatedly diluted and succussed.

KEY SYMPTOMS
CHILLINESS ◆ INTOLERANCE OF NOISE, CONTRADICTION, EGGS, AND FATTY FOODS ◆ TENDENCY TO FLUSH EASILY ◆ PERSON FEELS BETTER WITH GENTLE MOVEMENT
---

symptoms include constipation or cramping pains in the stomach or abdomen. The digestion is weak, with an intolerance of eggs and fatty foods. Teething children may develop diarrhea while eating. *Ferrum met.* can also be used to treat postoperative nausea.
Symptoms better With gentle movement.
Symptoms worse At night; from eating; from eggs; from fatty foods.

BACK & JOINT PAIN
Symptoms Stiffness of the lower back and neck, sciatica, arthritis, especially in the shoulders, and painful daytime cramps and coldness in the feet. Despite fatigue and an aversion to brisk movement, pain or restlessness causes a compulsion to keep moving.
Symptoms better With gentle movement.
Symptoms worse At night; from beginning to move.

HEADACHES
Symptoms Throbbing pains in the forehead, often lasting for several days, with possible dizziness and scalp pain.
Symptoms better Lying down; from firm pressure on the affected part of the head.
Symptoms worse From going down steps; from writing; from stooping.

SEE ALSO
Chronic fatigue syndrome, *page 204*; Headache, *page 218*; Varicose veins, *page 230*; Nausea & vomiting, *page 236*

Ferrum phosphoricum

FERRUM PHOS.

MADE FROM IRON PHOSPHATE, *Ferrum phos.* is one of Dr. Wilhelm Schüssler's "biochemic tissue salts," thought to counter deficiencies in the body (*see page 90*). This German homeopath believed that the remedy strengthened the blood vessel walls, restoring normal blood flow in cases of acute inflammation, hemorrhaging, or congestion. Dr. J. C. Morgan proved the remedy in 1876. It is given for the initial stages of infections and for inflammatory conditions.

REMEDY PROFILE

Ferrum phos. is most suited to alert, sociable, open-natured people who are sensitive and sympathetic, but who like to take action if something has upset them. Often overexcited and talkative, they may have difficulty concentrating. While their temperament is generally imaginative, cheerful and lively, it may alternate rapidly with an indifferent, depressed state.

Ferrum phos. may be given for the early stages of infection, respiratory problems, earaches, fever, and digestive, circulatory, and urogenital disorders.

FEVER
Symptoms Slow-developing fever with hot flashes, excessive perspiration, intense thirst, and areas of acute inflammation.
Symptoms better In cold; from pressure on the inflamed area; from being left alone.
Symptoms worse At night; before starting to perspire; from physical exertion.

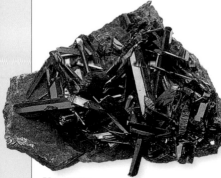

VIVIANITE
A natural source of iron phosphate, this mineral is commonly found coating the fossilized remains of fish and bones.

RESPIRATORY ILLNESS
Symptoms A slow-developing cold, possibly with a nosebleed and dry, hacking cough, often with chest pain. There may be hoarseness and a sore throat, typical of laryngitis. Other symptoms may include short, panting breaths, possibly due to pneumonia or pleurisy.
Symptoms better With gentle exercise.
Symptoms worse At night; between 4 A.M. and 6 A.M.; before starting to perspire.

EARACHE
Symptoms Pain and itching in the ear, possibly with hearing loss. Pain may be one-sided.
Symptoms better In cold; from pressure on the ear.
Symptoms worse At night; from physical exertion.

DIGESTIVE DISORDERS
Symptoms Indigestion, sour burps, and vomiting of seemingly undigested food, with poor appetite and an intense thirst. There may be diarrhea that has a tendency to recur during the summer, or that may be linked to irritable bowel syndrome. Another possible symptom for which *Ferrum phos.* may be given is constipation accompanied by hemorrhoids. Blood in the stools may indicate the initial stages of dysentery.
Symptoms better from getting gentle exercise.

SOURCE DETAILS

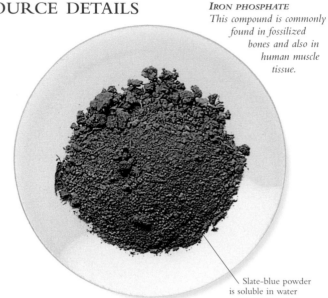

IRON PHOSPHATE
This compound is commonly found in fossilized bones and also in human muscle tissue.

Slate-blue powder is soluble in water

ORIGIN
Chemically prepared for manufacturing homeopathic remedies, although vivianite is a natural source of iron phosphate.

BACKGROUND
Used by Dr. Wilhelm Schüssler to make a "biochemic tissue salt" for treating the early stages of inflammatory conditions.

PREPARATION
Prepared chemically from iron sulfate, sodium phosphate, and sodium acetate. The powdered mineral is then triturated.

KEY SYMPTOMS
COLDS ACCOMPANIED BY TEMPORARY DEAFNESS ◆
CONDITIONS THAT APPEAR GRADUALLY ◆ HOT FLASHES ◆
PALE FACE THAT FLUSHES EASILY

Symptoms worse With heat; in sun; with jarring; with movement; at night; from cold drinks; from sour foods.

POOR CIRCULATION
Symptoms Varicose veins, hemorrhages, and nosebleeds with bright red blood, and a weak, rapid pulse. The face tends to flush easily. There may be weakness and pallor, possibly indicating anemia.
Symptoms better From cold compresses.
Symptoms worse With heat; with jarring; with movement.

RAYNAUD'S DISEASE
Symptoms Fingers and toes are white, cold, numb, tingling, and burning, due to restricted blood flow when blood vessels contract in the cold. As the blood flow is restored, the fingers turn blue, then red.
Symptoms better From pressure on the fingers; from walking at a slow pace.
Symptoms worse In cold air; from jarring the fingers.

UROGENITAL PROBLEMS
Symptoms A short menstrual cycle, or possibly a dry vagina, dragging uterine pain, and nocturnal stress incontinence in women, or a marked loss of libido in men.
Symptoms better From getting gentle exercise.
Symptoms worse During the night; if touched.

SEE ALSO
Colds, *page 224*

Graphites
GRAPHITES

COMMON NAMES
Graphite, blacklead, plumbago

GRAPHITE IS A CARBON MINERAL that contains traces of iron. The name derives from the Greek *graphein* meaning "to write." The main constituent of pencil lead, graphite is also used in the production of lubricants, polishes, batteries, and electric motors. The remedy, proved by Hahnemann and published in his *Chronic Diseases* (1821–34), is often given for skin complaints and for anxiety with lack of confidence.

REMEDY PROFILE

Those who respond best to *Graphites* tend to be more physically than intellectually oriented. These practical types prefer action to discussion, and are seen as "the ones who are going to cope." They can, however, be lethargic, notably on waking. Seemingly moody, pessimistic, and agitated, under the surface they are deeply emotional, often sad, and easily moved to tears by music.

These people are especially susceptible to certain physical symptoms affecting the skin, nails, mucous membranes, and the left side of the body. Symptoms are often linked to glandular problems. Sensitivity to the cold and headaches after skipping meals are typical.

SKIN & NAIL CONDITIONS
Symptoms Irritated, cracked, dry skin behind the ears, and on the nostrils, knees, nipples, and fingertips. Eczema or psoriasis may ooze a honey-colored discharge. Cracked skin may bleed and easily become infected. There may be old scars that ulcerate and burn, cold sores around the mouth, and herpes blisters around the genitals.

GRAPHITE IN PENCILS
Pencils have been made using graphite since 1562, when the first pencil factory opened in England.

Symptoms better With warmth; in fresh air; in the dark; with sleep; from eating.
Symptoms worse In cold; during menstruation; from sweet foods; from seafood.

ANXIETY & SHYNESS
Symptoms Self-doubt, lack of self-confidence, shyness, and indecision. There is a tendency to anticipate the worst, to be full of anxiety, and to become upset over the slightest thing, which frequently causes depression or overexcitement. Concentration may be poor, and may even develop into dementia. Fastidiousness and perfectionism are further common *Graphites* traits.
Symptoms better From walking in fresh air; from being in a moving vehicle.
Symptoms worse On waking; from hearing music.

EYE, EAR & NOSE CONDITIONS
Symptoms Swollen, red, dry eyelids due to blepharitis, and sties with a yellow discharge. There may be an ear discharge with an itchy infection of the outer ear. A cracking sound, especially while eating, may occur, as may deafness related to otosclerosis (a middle-ear disorder). Hot sweats (often due to a hormonal imbalance) may be followed by nosebleeds.
Symptoms better With warmth; from fresh air.
Symptoms worse In cold; on the left side; before and during menstruation.

SOURCE DETAILS

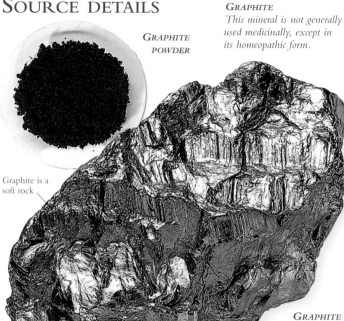

GRAPHITE POWDER

GRAPHITE
This mineral is not generally used medicinally, except in its homeopathic form.

Graphite is a soft rock

GRAPHITE ROCK

ORIGIN
Forms within other rocks, such as granite, slate, schist, and marble. Commonly found in Sri Lanka, Mexico, and North America.

BACKGROUND
Dr. S. Weinhold, a German contemporary of Hahnemann, noted that workmen in a mirror factory cured cold sores with graphite.

PREPARATION
Graphite powder is triturated with lactose sugar to make it soluble. After being dissolved in water it is repeatedly diluted and succussed.

KEY SYMPTOMS
POOR CONCENTRATION ◆ INDECISIVENESS ◆ CONDITIONS THAT MAINLY AFFECT THE LEFT SIDE ◆ WEEPING ON HEARING MUSIC ◆ CHILLINESS ◆ CRACKED SKIN WITH A HONEYLIKE DISCHARGE

DIGESTIVE DISORDERS
Symptoms Constipation, bloating, and flatulence, maybe with cramps. There may be rectal itching, hemorrhoids, anal fissures, and stomach pains with hunger or vomiting. Bland foods are preferred to meat and salty or sweet foods.
Symptoms better With warmth; in fresh air.
Symptoms worse In cold; during menstruation; from sweet foods; from seafood.

MENSTRUAL PROBLEMS
Symptoms Irregular, scant, menstruation and swollen, hard, painful breasts before and during menstruation. There may be itchy genitals and constipation (*see above*).

Symptoms better From wrapping up warmly.
Symptoms worse At night; from scratching.

ERECTILE PROBLEMS
Symptoms Impotence in men with a high libido at an early age. Priapism (persistent, sore erection) may affect men who dislike sexual intercourse.
Symptoms better From walking in fresh air.
Symptoms worse From sexual excess; masturbation.

SEE ALSO
Eczema, *pages 194, 240*;
Reproduction, *page 198*;
Emotional problems, *page 210*;
Phlegm, *page 226*

Hepar sulfuris calcareum

HEPAR SULF.

DOCTORS IN THE 18TH CENTURY used calcium sulfide externally for ailments such as acne, boils, and gout. It is still used in veterinary medicine and industrially in paint manufacture. The homeopathic remedy was first used by Hahnemann in 1794, as an antidote to the side effects of mercury, a common medicine at the time (*see page 85*). *Hepar sulf.* is now given primarily for respiratory problems such as croup and coughs, and for skin infections.

REMEDY PROFILE

People who respond best to *Hepar sulf.* are touchy, both mentally and physically. They are patient and methodical workers, but this tolerance does not extend to others, and they are often critical, irritable, and hard to please. They are also oversensitive and quick to take offense. Illness heightens their irritability and impetuosity, and anger, pain, or anguish may drive them to violent outbursts. They may have low self-esteem and feel as though they are rejected by others.

Often hypersensitive, these people tend to have a low pain threshold and to complain out of proportion to their illness. They lack internal warmth, and will feel the cold keenly, especially dry cold. Symptoms are usually worse at night, and aggravated by the least touch on the affected area. Common cravings are for fatty foods and for sour tastes such as vinegar.

Hepar sulf. is generally used where there is an infection, particularly in the respiratory system or skin. It is especially appropriate for ailments that are accompanied by swollen glands, particularly in the neck or groin, or if there is a high fever alternating with chills.

smell of old cheese. Contact with cold air triggers sneezing. The nostrils may feel sore and raw. Colds may begin with a tickly throat (*see below*). There may be sinusitis, with pain in the facial bones and the bridge of the nose. Pain is often right-sided and extends to the ear, notably on swallowing. There may be a piercing earache with a foul-smelling ear discharge.
Symptoms better With warmth; in warm, wet weather; from eating.
Symptoms worse In cold and cold drafts; if touched; from undressing.

SORE THROAT

Symptoms A hoarse voice, sore throat, and swollen tonsils, often due to a cough (*see below*) or quinsy (abscesses around the tonsils). There may be weeping abscesses on the gums or glands, with sharp, splinterlike pain, especially on swallowing, that may spread to the ear.
Symptoms better In warm, wet weather; from wrapping the throat.
Symptoms worse In cold; from touching the throat; from swallowing; cold drinks.

COUGHS & CROUP

Symptoms A dry, hacking, crowing cough, often causing a sore throat (*see above*). If the cough is loose, a coughing fit may be triggered by touching the throat, and may cause a choking feeling. Thick phlegm may be lodged in the chest.

COLDS & PHLEGM

Symptoms Cold or the flu with fever, sneezing, sweating, and need for warmth. Profuse phlegm may be watery at first, then blood-stained, thick, and yellowish in color, with a

SOURCE DETAILS

ORIGIN

A form of calcium sulfide using powdered oyster shell (*see page 77*) and flowers of sulfur (*see page 99*).

BACKGROUND

Used by 18th-century doctors for goiter, gout, rheumatic pain, and tuberculosis.

PREPARATION

Flowers of sulfur and powdered oyster shell are heated, dissolved in acid, and triturated with lactose sugar.

CALCIUM SULPHIDE
Hahnemann developed his own form of calcium sulfide using flowers of sulfur and powdered oyster shell instead of ordinary lime.

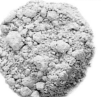

OYSTER SHELL

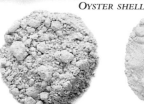

POWDERED OYSTER SHELL   *FLOWERS OF SULFUR*

KEY SYMPTOMS

VIOLENT OUTBURSTS ◆ EXTREME SENSITIVITY ◆ CHILLINESS ◆
OFFENSIVE-SMELLING DISCHARGES ◆ SPLINTERLIKE PAINS ◆
CRAVING FOR SOUR FOODS AND DRINKS

Coughs tend to be dry in the evening and loose in the morning. The symptoms of croup are similar, but with a barking cough and difficulty coughing up phlegm.
Symptoms better In warm, wet weather; from wrapping up warmly.
Symptoms worse In cold; in the morning and evening; from touching the throat.

SKIN CONDITIONS

Symptoms The skin chaps or roughens easily, and eruptions such as acne are inflamed and sore, with foul-smelling, yellow pus. Eruptions are slow to heal and prone to infection, perhaps leaving scars. Infections such as sties, boils, and cold sores may be accompanied by the typical yellow discharge. Abscesses and ulcers bleed easily.

Symptoms better With warmth; from warm compresses.
Symptoms worse In cold; from undressing; if touched.

DIGESTIVE DISORDERS

Symptoms Nausea, vomiting, or chronic diarrhea, usually accompanied by a grumbling abdomen. Stools are typically pale, soft, and have a sour odor, as does urine.
Symptoms better In warm, wet weather, with warmth; from eating.
Symptoms worse In cold; from undressing.

SEE ALSO

Eczema, *pages 194, 240*; Earache, *page 222*; Sinusitis, *page 226*; Mild acne, *page 240*; Tonsillitis, *page 250*; Croup, *page 250*

Hydrargyrum metallicum syn. *Mercurius solubilis Hahnemanni*

MERC. SOL.

COMMON NAMES
Mercury, quicksilver, black oxide of mercury, ammonionitrate of mercury

EGYPTIAN PAPYRI dating from 1600 BCE record the early medicinal use of mercury, which later spread to the Greeks, Romans, and Arabs. Its use persisted through to 1900 in the West as an aggressive treatment for syphilis and other diseases, until its toxic effects were deemed too dangerous. *Merc. sol.* was proved by Hahnemann and published in his *Materia Medica Pura* (1821–34). It is given primarily for ulcers, glandular problems, and offensive-smelling discharges.

REMEDY PROFILE

People who benefit most from *Merc. sol.* are anxious and restless. A need for stability and order gives them a conservative facade. In trying to restrain an inner sense of urgency, they become insecure, introverted, and suspicious, appearing detached and even arrogant in their dealings with people. They bottle up feelings of conflict until they explode in a blind rage. If ill, they slow down in mind and body, but never lose their inner sense of restlessness. Illness may bring on confusion, a weak memory, hesitant speech, and weepiness. Constant hunger is typical, with cravings for bread, butter, and cold drinks such as milk or beer, but aversions to other alcoholic drinks, coffee, meat, and sweet foods.

Typical physical symptoms include abscesses, ulcers, fever, swollen glands, and copious sweating. Bodily discharges, such as sweat, saliva, urine, and stools, are often foul-smelling. Symptoms are worse at night, and are aggravated by extremes of heat or cold (moderate temperatures are necessary for recovery). Excessive salivation is common, as is constant swallowing and dribbling on the pillow at night.

MOUTH & THROAT CONDITIONS

Symptoms Canker sores on the tongue, walls of the mouth, and gums. Sore, raised, cream-colored patches may form in the mouth, usually indicating oral thrush. A sore throat may become ulcerated, and tonsillitis may set in. Abscesses may form in the roots of the teeth, causing painful swelling. Gums may become painfully inflamed and prone to bleeding (gingivitis). The teeth may also ache and loosen. Pain brought on by toothache or a sore throat may extend to the ears. Other typical symptoms treated by *Merc. sol.* include a bitter taste in the mouth, halitosis, swollen glands, fever (*see below, right*), and a yellow-coated tongue that may bear tooth marks.
Symptoms better With rest; from moderate temperatures; applying warm compresses.
Symptoms worse In extreme heat or cold; from sweating; hot or cold foods and drinks.

PHLEGM & COLDS

Symptoms Watery, yellow or greenish phlegm that has a strong odor, with constant sneezing, and a raw, burning sensation in the nose. Chills, aches, fever (*see right*), and the flu are accompanied by a bitter-tasting mouth, a headache, and a sore throat (*see above*). Pain in the sinuses may extend to the teeth (*see above*) and ears (*see right*).
Symptoms better With rest; from moderate temperatures.
Symptoms worse In extreme heat or cold; from lying on the right side; from sweating.

SOURCE DETAILS

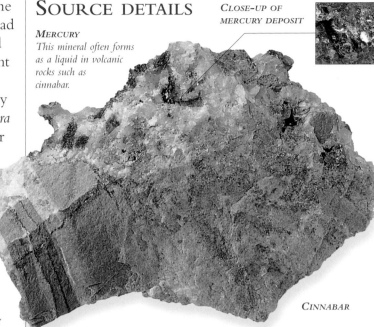

MERCURY
This mineral often forms as a liquid in volcanic rocks such as cinnabar.

CLOSE-UP OF MERCURY DEPOSIT

CINNABAR

ORIGIN
Mercury deposits are extracted from cinnabar, an ore found near hot springs and volcanic vents in Spain, Italy, the US, Peru, and China.

BACKGROUND
Advocated by Paracelsus, a 16th-century scientist, and used medicinally for centuries: Charles II and George Washington were both prescribed it.

PREPARATION
Mercury is dissolved in nitric acid, forming a gray powder precipitate. This is then filtered, dried, and triturated until soluble.

KEY SYMPTOMS

FOUL-SMELLING DISCHARGES ◆ RESERVED, SUSPICIOUS STATE OF MIND ◆ INSECURITY ◆ COPIOUS PERSPIRATION THAT DOES NOT RELIEVE CONDITIONS ◆ PERSON FEELS WORSE AT NIGHT

EYE & EAR INFECTIONS

Symptoms Light-sensitive, swollen, watery, or inflamed eyes that exude a nasty yellow, greenish, or blood-flecked discharge, which may be due to conjunctivitis. *Merc. sol.* is also used for ear pains with a thick, yellow-green, bloody, and foul-smelling discharge.
Symptoms better With rest; from moderate temperatures.
Symptoms worse In extreme heat or cold; at night; from stooping; if touched.

FEVER

Symptoms High temperature with profuse, offensive-smelling perspiration that chills the skin. The fever often occurs with swollen glands, neuralgic pain, and a vicelike headache.
Symptoms better With rest; in moderate temperatures.
Symptoms worse In changes in temperature; from intense heat; from sweating; at night; lying on the right side.

THRUSH

Symptoms Itchy, burning vaginal discharge in women, and itchy, red spots on the penis in men, with a discharge.
Symptoms better Bathing in cool water; with rest.
Symptoms worse If touched; in humidity.

SEE ALSO

Pneumonia, *page 183*;
Osteoarthritis, *page 196*; Mouth, *page 232*; Children's health, *page 246*

Iodum
IODUM

COMMON NAME
Iodine

IODINE IS ESSENTIAL FOR the proper functioning of the thyroid gland. A deficiency of iodine produces symptoms such as weak muscles, weight loss, mental sluggishness, and fatigue. The condition is rare in the West because potassium iodide, a salt of iodine, is added to table salt. The homeopathic remedy, proved in 1837 by Hahnemann (in association with Drs. Trinks, Gross, Gerdorff, and Hartlaub), is used mainly to treat the many symptoms associated with an overactive thyroid gland and the accelerated metabolism it produces.

REMEDY PROFILE

Those for whom *Iodum* is most suitable are talkative, with a marked mental restlessness and irritability due to anxiety, and sudden urges to engage in exhausting activities. Their behavior is obsessive, with a compulsion to keep frantically busy, yet in a disorganized, forgetful way. Despite causing physical and mental fatigue, this frenzy is preferable to inactivity, when frightening thoughts heighten anxiety.

Iodum is given for symptoms caused by an overactive thyroid gland (hyperthyroidism) and the accelerated metabolism it causes. Psychological symptoms may include eating disorders and anxiety that may manifest as violent rages if meals are not ready as soon as hunger is felt.

Physical symptoms include protruding eyes and eye pain linked with hyperthyroidism; nausea with a clean tongue and excess salivation, great thirst, respiratory problems, enlarged glands, and excessive sweating. These people tend to feel the heat and constantly try to keep cool, preferring cool clothing and finding warm surroundings uncomfortable.

OVERACTIVE METABOLISM
Symptoms Staring eyes (exophthalmos) and a distressed expression on the face, which may be swollen. The skin and hair are usually dry. There may be vertigo, with hot flashes, fainting, and throbbing head pain with a rush of blood to the head. Other symptoms include an increased appetite yet a noticeable weight loss (*see below*) and overheating (*see below, right*). Symptoms may be linked to hyperthyroidism.
Symptoms better In fresh air; with movement; from eating.
Symptoms worse In warm surroundings.

EATING DISORDERS
Symptoms Rapid, noticeable weight loss and emaciation despite an insatiable appetite. An excessive thirst is typical. The liver may become enlarged, with possible signs of jaundice, and the pancreas may be painful. Chronic diarrhea linked to nervousness or to particular

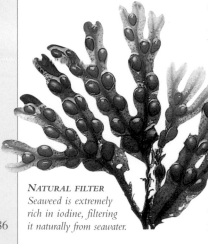

NATURAL FILTER
Seaweed is extremely rich in iodine, filtering it naturally from seawater.

SOURCE DETAILS

Granules are heavy and slightly soluble in water

IODINE
This bluish-black element is commonly used in medicine, in photography, and in dyes.

ORIGIN
Once extracted from slowly burned seaweed, but now generally prepared chemically by industrial processes.

BACKGROUND
Chinese herbalists used burned seaweed to treat thyroid problems 2,000 years ago. It is also a well-known antiseptic.

PREPARATION
The remedy is made by dissolving iodate salts in alcohol, then repeatedly diluting and succussing the mixture.

KEY SYMPTOMS
LOSS OF WEIGHT WITH INCREASED APPETITE ◆ HEAT INTOLERANCE ◆ LACK OF THIRST ◆ ENLARGED GLANDS THAT THEN WASTE AWAY ◆ ANXIETY AND RESTLESSNESS

---

foods may be present, as may constipation with pale stools.
Symptoms better In fresh air; with movement; from eating.
Symptoms worse In warm surroundings; from anxiety.

COUGH
Symptoms Dry, spasmodic, choking cough, possibly with gagging, retching, or vomiting. There may be copious mucus and a rattling sound in the chest, but no expectoration if symptoms are due to asthma or pneumonia. Children with this cough may become stiff, pale, or blue.
Symptoms better In fresh air.
Symptoms worse In warm surroundings; from overeating; from cold nights after hot days.

RESPIRATORY ILLNESS
Symptoms Profuse, watery, excoriating mucus in the nose, possibly with hay fever, or a dry, obstructed nose with enlargement of the adenoids. Asthma with hay fever may also be helped by *Iodum*.
Symptoms better In fresh air; with movement; from eating.
Symptoms worse In warm surroundings.

HEAT INTOLERANCE
Symptoms Physical distress and feverishness in warm surroundings. The slightest physical activity may cause marked sweating.
Symptoms better In fresh air; in cool surroundings; from wearing cool clothing.
Symptoms worse In warm surroundings.

SEE ALSO
Rheumatoid arthritis, *page 197*; Prostate problems, *page 202*; Blockage of the eustachian tube, *page 222*

Kalium bichromicum

KALI. BICH.

COMMON NAMES
Potassium dichromate, potassium bichromate,
bichromate of potash

Potassium dichromate, the compound used to make this remedy, is also used industrially for a variety of purposes, such as the manufacture of chrome pigments. The homeopathic remedy was proved by Dr. Drysdale and published in 1864. Like other *Kali.* remedies, it has a strong affinity with the mucous membranes; it is often used for conditions that produce profuse mucus, and for certain skin problems. Unlike other *Kali.* remedies, it may help stomach complaints.

REMEDY PROFILE

People who benefit most from *Kali. bich.* tend to have regular habits and like to go into great detail about even minor issues. They often have quite a black-and-white view of the world and a strong sense of morality.

The symptom picture may include pain in localized areas, and joint pain alternating with diarrhea in summer. There is generally a desire for beer and possibly a sensation as if there is a hair on the tongue.

Kali. bich. is considered to have a beneficial effect on the mucous membranes, and is consequently prescribed for respiratory-tract ailments marked by excessive phlegm. It is also given for indigestion and headaches, and for skin conditions with discharges, such as ulcers and acne with burning pains. *Kali. bich.* is also used to treat joint pain.

PHLEGM & SINUSITIS
Symptoms Constant yellow-green phlegm that is stringy or slimy and proves difficult to expel. At night, phlegm may accumulate in the nose or run down the back of the throat. The phlegm may sometimes become dry and hard. The sinuses are inflamed, and there is sharp pain at the bridge of the nose. Glue ear may develop, marked by earache and a thick, yellow discharge from the affected ear. Phlegm that becomes blocked in the nose may cause a headache (*see right*), possibly with vomiting.

Symptoms better With warmth; lying in a warm bed; from firm pressure on the bridge of the nose.
Symptoms worse In cold; from stooping; in the morning; in spring and fall.

SORE THROAT, COUGHS & CROUP
Symptoms The throat and tonsils are swollen. A tickle in the throat develops into a dry, hoarse cough. Stringy mucus lines the larynx and is hard to expel. Chest pains may spread to the back and shoulders. There may be a dry mouth, painful canker sores, and a yellow tongue, possibly with digestive problems (*see below*).
Symptoms better With warmth; on balmy days; lying in a warm bed; expelling mucus; at night.
Symptoms worse In cold and dampness; in the morning; in spring and fall; from breathing deeply.

INDIGESTION
Symptoms Sharp, knifelike pains that radiate to the loins, and a sore spot in the stomach as if an ulcer has developed there. There may be an impression that the digestive processes have stopped, with a heavy feeling in the abdomen immediately after eating. An aversion to meat is a common symptom, as is a craving for beer, but drinking beer often causes vomiting and diarrhea.
Symptoms better From passing gas; from burping.
Symptoms worse In cold; in spring and fall; from rich, heavy foods; from beer.

HEADACHES
Symptoms Pain at the same time each day. Localized pain may extend slowly across the whole head, possibly due to sinusitis (*see left*). The onset of a migraine is marked by dim and blurred vision. There may be nausea, and stringy mucus may be present in the throat.
Symptoms better With warmth; from firm pressure on the bridge of the nose.
Symptoms worse In cold; from bending over.

SKIN CONDITIONS
Symptoms Facial acne that causes small, solid, red bumps producing a yellow discharge. There may be itchy, blisterlike rashes, with burning pains, skin ulcers with raised edges, and blisters on the soles of the feet. Round, depressed scars develop on the area after the eruptions or ulcers have healed.
Symptoms better In cool weather.
Symptoms worse In hot weather; if touched.

JOINT PAIN
Symptoms Pain in the joints that appears and disappears suddenly. Sharp pains may move around the joint area.
Symptoms better With warmth; lying in a warm bed.
Symptoms worse In cold; from sudden or extreme heat; in the summer.

SOURCE DETAILS

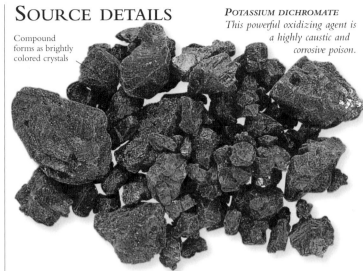

Compound forms as brightly colored crystals

POTASSIUM DICHROMATE
This powerful oxidizing agent is a highly caustic and corrosive poison.

ORIGIN
Does not occur in nature, so generally produced chemically by combining neutral yellow potassium chromate with hydrochloric acid.

BACKGROUND
Used for industrial purposes such as the dyeing of fabric and wood-staining. Also used in photography, and as a component of electric batteries.

PREPARATION
Potassium dichromate crystals are finely ground (triturated) with lactose sugar until soluble in water. They are then filtered, diluted, and succussed.

KEY SYMPTOMS

GREAT ATTENTION TO DETAIL ♦ REGULAR HABITS ♦
LOCALIZED PAIN ♦ TOUGH, STRINGY, YELLOW-GREEN PHLEGM ♦
PERSON FEELS WORSE BETWEEN 2 A.M. AND 5 A.M.

SEE ALSO
Rheumatoid arthritis, *page 197*; Sinusitis, *page 226*; Glue ear, *page 250*

Kalium carbonicum

KALI. CARB.

POTASSIUM CARBONATE is a compound of the alkali metal potassium. Used by the ancient Egyptians to make glass, the compound is still widely used in the manufacture of glass, soap, and other products. In the body potassium is present in every cell in a delicate balance with sodium. Any disturbance of this balance causes many problems, including muscle weakness and cardiac arrhythmia. Hahnemann proved the remedy and published it in his *Chronic Diseases* (1821–34).

SOURCE DETAILS

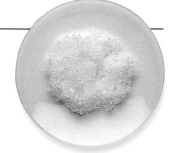

POTASSIUM CARBONATE

POTASSIUM CARBONATE
This white, odorless compound of potassium is a powerful alkali, used in industry and in the making of other potassium compounds.

Wood ash is a common source of potassium carbonate

WOOD ASH

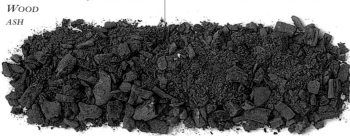

REMEDY PROFILE

People for whom *Kali. carb.* is suitable tend to be irritable, touchy, and possessive, feeling at odds with everyone, hating to be touched, yet wanting company. Conservative and "proper," they have a strong sense of duty and responsibility. Emotional upsets are felt as a strong sense of fear or anxiety, hitting them like a blow in the stomach. These people fear many things: the future, loss of self-control, death, and even the supernatural.

Among the typical physical symptoms associated with the remedy are great sensitivity to drafts and the cold. It is prescribed for recurrent fever, coughs, colds, and other respiratory problems, including asthma. There may be sharp, shooting pains in parts of the body, and swelling above the eyes. Underlying anemia may cause fatigue and weakness.

Symptoms typically tend to be worse in the early hours of the morning, and insomnia is another feature of the *Kali. carb.* profile. Those for whom the remedy is appropriate tend to be middle-aged or older, stout or obese, and have a desire for sweet foods.

COUGHS & COLDS
Symptoms Dry, hacking cough with expectoration in the morning of foul-tasting, yellowy-green mucus. The cough may be whooping or wheezy, with vomiting and a chilly feeling in the chest. *Kali.* *carb.* is also used for recurrent colds that settle in the throat, with hoarseness or voice loss due to becoming very chilly after profuse sweating.
Symptoms better With warmth; from sitting up and leaning forward.
Symptoms worse In cold air and drafts; between 2 A.M. and 4 A.M.

ASTHMA
Symptoms Particularly bad asthma that makes it impossible to lie down comfortably, perhaps with a dry cough that may disrupt sleep between 2 A.M. and 4 A.M.
Symptoms better Being propped up; from sitting up straight; from bending forward with the head on the knees.
Symptoms worse In cold air and drafts; lying down; from exertion.

JOINT PAIN
Symptoms Sharp pain in the shoulders, arms, hips, and legs that is worse on the left side. The arms may feel weak, and the legs are often restless. Arthritis in the joints may be severe enough to cause the deformities characteristic of rheumatoid arthritis. Sciatica pains may prompt a need to sit up or turn over in bed.
Symptoms better With warmth; with movement.
Symptoms worse In cold air and drafts; between 2 A.M. and 4 A.M.; lying on the affected area.

ORIGIN
Originally prepared by percolating wood ash and evaporating the resulting solution in iron pots: hence the name "potash." Now made chemically.

BACKGROUND
Rarely prescribed internally for medicinal purposes, since it is highly caustic, but traditionally used in external treatments such as skin lotions.

PREPARATION
Potassium carbonate is triturated by being ground repeatedly with lactose sugar until it is soluble in water. This solution is then diluted and succussed.

KEY SYMPTOMS
SENSITIVITY TO THE COLD ◆ SHARP, SHOOTING PAINS ◆ ANXIETY THAT IS FELT IN THE STOMACH ◆ STRONG SENSE OF DUTY ◆ PERSON FEELS WORSE BETWEEN 2 A.M. AND 4 A.M.

BACK PAIN
Symptoms Pain that begins in the small of the back, often severe enough to make it uncomfortable to stay in bed. The pain is worse on the left side, extending to the genitals, thighs, and lower limbs. It may be particularly severe during pregnancy and labor and after injury, childbirth, or pregnancy termination.
Symptoms better With warmth; in the open air.
Symptoms worse In cold air; from drafts; between 2 A.M. and 4 A.M.; for long periods of sitting; before menstruating.

KIDNEY DISORDERS
Symptoms Kidney stones or other diseases of the kidney, with shooting pains in the small of the back. Pains may be worse on the left side. The eyelids may be puffy.

Symptoms better With warmth; with movement.
Symptoms worse In cold air and drafts; between 2 A.M. and 4 A.M.

INSOMNIA
Symptoms Insomnia, with difficulty getting to sleep, or falling asleep but waking between 2 A.M. and 4 A.M. Getting back to sleep seems impossible. There may be talking during sleep.
Symptoms better With warmth; in the open air.
Symptoms worse In cold air and drafts; lying on the left side of the body; before menstruating.

SEE ALSO
Asthma, *page 181*; Palpitations, *page 186*; Osteoarthritis, *page 196*; Whooping cough, *page 250*; Incontinence, *page 268*

Kalium phosphoricum
KALI. PHOS.

COMMON NAMES
Potassium phosphate, phosphate of potash,
potassium dihydrogen orthophosphate

POTASSIUM HELPS TO STORE energy in the body's cells, maintain the rhythm of the heartbeat, and ensure the transmission of nerve impulses. A deficiency of potassium in the body is rare, since it is found in most foods. *Kali. phos.* is one of the 12 Schüssler "tissue salts," which were designed to counter any deficiency in the body (*see page 90*). Proved by Dr. H. C. Allen of Chicago in 1892, the remedy is prescribed mainly for nervous collapse and exhaustion.

REMEDY PROFILE

Extreme mental and physical exhaustion, particularly after a period of overwork or stress, is typically treated with *Kali. phos.* For this reason it may be given to students experiencing nervous collapse. Often down-to-earth individuals with a strong sense of morality, those who respond to *Kali. phos.* tend to be conservative and dogmatic in their opinions. Distressing news events, such as famine or violence, can easily upset them. Extroverted behavior is typical of them, yet when fatigued they become nervous, introverted, and over-sensitive. Illness makes them uncommunicative, withdrawn, and averse to company, even that of family members.

Typical physical symptoms include an inability to keep the feet still, drooping of the left eyelid, yellowish bodily discharges, a tendency to sweat excessively yet to be sensitive to the cold, and spinal pain. In addition to fatigue, *Kali. phos.* is given for gnawing hunger pains, headaches, and insomnia.

CHRONIC FATIGUE SYNDROME
Symptoms Physical and mental exhaustion following an acute illness or overwork. Extreme tenderness and weakness in the muscles may be accompanied by a slight fever. There is general lethargy, depression, frustration, anger, and irritability. Heightened sensitivity causes susceptibility to the cold and flinching at the slightest noise or bright light. The tongue is coated yellow.
Symptoms better With heat; with gentle movement; from sleep; from eating.
Symptoms worse In cold; from the slightest excitement; from physical exertion; from worry; near noise.

ABNORMAL DISCHARGES
Symptoms Purulent yellowy-orange discharge from the vagina, bladder, or lungs, or present in the stools.
Symptoms better With heat; from sleep; with rest.
Symptoms worse From physical and mental exertion; from drinking milk.

HUNGER PAINS
Symptoms Empty, nervous feeling in the stomach, related to stress and possibly with a headache (*see right*). Gnawing hunger pains cause waking at about 5 A.M., but food brings only temporary relief. Frequent eating between meals is typical. Sweet foods such as chocolates are often craved, and there may be a strong aversion to bread.
Symptoms better With heat; with gentle movement; eating.
Symptoms worse From mental exertion; worry; from cold drinks; drinking milk.

EXCESS PERSPIRATION
Symptoms Excessive sweating that occurs only during bouts of illness, notably with severe

SOURCE DETAILS

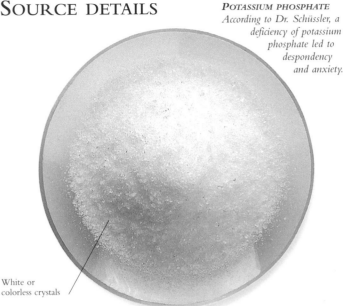

*POTASSIUM PHOSPHATE
According to Dr. Schüssler, a deficiency of potassium phosphate led to despondency and anxiety.*

White or colorless crystals

ORIGIN
A solution of potassium carbonate (*see opposite*) is combined with dilute phosphoric acid to form potassium phosphate as a precipitate.

BACKGROUND
Used in conventional medicine as one of the various compounds administered in solution to patients who are fed intravenously.

PREPARATION
The precipitated crystalline compound of potassium phosphate is dried, then triturated with lactose sugar until soluble in water.

KEY SYMPTOMS
MENTAL AND PHYSICAL EXHAUSTION ◆ YELLOWY-ORANGE DISCHARGES ◆ CHILLINESS ◆ PERSON FEELS BETTER WITH GENTLE MOVEMENT

---

fatigue (*see left*). Perspiration tends to have a characteristic smell of onions. It may appear on the head and face, especially after the slightest excitement or exertion, or after meals.
Symptoms better From sleep.
Symptoms worse From physical and mental exertion.

HEADACHES
Symptoms Head pain, generally only on one side of the head, with a nervous, empty sensation in the stomach (*see left*).
Symptoms better In fresh air; from eating.
Symptoms worse In cold.

INSOMNIA
Symptoms Sleeplessness accompanied by an empty, nervous sensation in the pit of the stomach and possible hunger pains (*see left*).
Symptoms better With heat; with gentle movement.
Symptoms worse In cold, dry air; from mental exertion; from worry.

BACK PAIN
Symptoms Sore, bruising pain down the spine. The limbs feel heavy and cold.
Symptoms better With heat; with gentle movement; sleep.
Symptoms worse From mental exertion; if touched; from going up steps or stairs.

SEE ALSO
Chronic fatigue syndrome, *page 205*; Headache, *page 218*; Insomnia, *page 244*

Magnesium phosphoricum

MAG. PHOS.

O F ALL THE MINERALS present in the human body, magnesium is exceeded in quantity only by potassium. Magnesium regulates mineral balance and a deficiency can cause neuralgic pains. *Mag. phos.* is known as the "homeopathic aspirin" because it is commonly taken for minor aches and pains. Proved by Drs. W. P. Wessehoeft and J. A. Gann, it was published in Dr. H. C. Allen's *Medical Advances* (1889) and is most often prescribed for cramping pain or neuralgia.

REMEDY PROFILE

Mag. phos. is considered most suitable for outgoing people who are prone to impulsive and restless behavior. Often sensitive, artistic, intellectual individuals, they also have a tendency to be forgetful and unable to concentrate. In addition, they may be prone to irritability, nervousness, and exhaustion. These people fear the dark, thunderstorms, and confrontation with others.

A hypochondriac streak is a common trait in these people, marked by sensitivity to the cold and regular complaints of muscle cramps. Symptoms are generally worse on the right side. There may be craving for sugar and an aversion to coffee.

Mag. phos. is usually taken for menstrual or neuralgic pains, headaches, sharp abdominal pain, toothaches, and earaches.

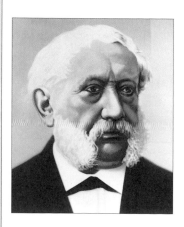

DR. WILHELM SCHÜSSLER
In 1872–73 this German homeopath claimed that deficiencies in body function could be countered using 12 "tissue salts," among them Mag. phos.

ABDOMINAL CRAMPS
Symptoms Sharp, colicky cramps such as those associated with irritable bowel syndrome. The pain is often right-sided and appears and disappears rapidly. Its intensity may cause restlessness and cries of pain. The abdomen is bloated, and there is a lot of gas that is not eased by burping. Severe cases may cause doubling up.
Symptoms better With heat; from pressure on the abdomen.
Symptoms worse In cold.

NEURALGIA
Symptoms Sharp, radiating, cramping pains that appear and disappear rapidly anywhere in the body, prompting cries of pain and restlessness. Muscles are stiff, numb, and awkward, especially after exertion.
Symptoms better With heat; from hot baths; from firm pressure on the affected area.
Symptoms worse In cold air; at night.

MENSTRUAL CRAMPS
Symptoms Sudden cramping, shooting pains in the lower abdomen during menstruation.
Symptoms better With heat; from doubling up; hot drinks.
Symptoms worse On the right side; before menstruation.

HEADACHES
Symptoms Spasmodic, shooting pains on the right side or the back of the neck, spreading over the head and settling around the right eye.

SOURCE DETAILS

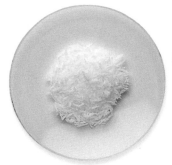

SODIUM PHOSPHATE

MAGNESIUM PHOSPHATE
This compound does not exist in nature but is prepared chemically from sodium phosphate and epsomite.

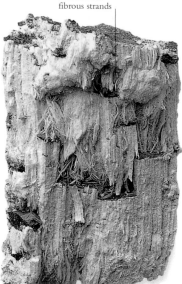

Mineral has fibrous strands

EPSOMITE (MAGNESIUM SULFATE)

ORIGIN
Sodium carbonate and phosphoric acid are used to make sodium phosphate. Magnesium sulfate forms in caves and on rock faces as epsomite.

BACKGROUND
The human body needs magnesium to break down nutrients, and this magnesium compound was chosen as a "tissue salt" by Dr. Schüssler (*see below, left*).

PREPARATION
Magnesium sulfate and sodium phosphate are mixed in water and left to crystallize. The resulting crystals are then triturated with lactose sugar.

KEY SYMPTOMS

CRAMPING PAIN ♦ SENSITIVE, ARTISTIC, INTELLECTUAL TEMPERAMENT ♦ COMPLAINTS THAT TEND TO AFFECT THE RIGHT SIDE OF THE BODY ♦ PERSON FEELS BETTER IN WARMTH

Characteristically the face is red and throbbing. Such headaches are common in teenage girls.
Symptoms better With heat; from pressure on the head.
Symptoms worse In cold.

TOOTHACHE
Symptoms Dull, throbbing pain, or sharp twinges of pain, common in teething infants.
Symptoms better With heat, from warm compresses; firm pressure on the gums or tooth.
Symptoms worse In cold drafts; if touched.

CRAMPS
Symptoms Sudden onset of stabbing cramps in the arms, fingers, wrists, and hands, which are especially common

in instrumentalists and writers.
Symptoms better With heat; from firm pressure on the affected area.
Symptoms worse In cold.

EARACHE
Symptoms Pains in the ear that are spasmodic and shooting, especially following exposure to cold wind.
Symptoms better With heat; from firm pressure on the ear.
Symptoms worse In cold; from turning the head.

SEE ALSO
Colic, page 246; Painful periods, page 256

Natrum carbonicum

NAT. CARB.

COMMON NAMES
Sodium carbonate, soda ash, washing soda

Roughly 35 million tons of sodium carbonate are produced industrially each year, particularly for use in making glass, ceramics, paper, and detergents. Traditionally its use in medicine was largely confined to external remedies; as a homeopathic remedy, it is used for digestive problems, nervous disorders, and skin complaints. *Nat. carb.* was proved by Hahnemann, with Drs. Gross, Hering, Langhammer, and others and published in Hahnemann's *Chronic Diseases* (1821–34).

SOURCE DETAILS

Crystals form when brine and seawater absorb carbon dioxide

SODIUM CARBONATE
Sodium carbonate is used worldwide in products such as household cleaners, water softeners, and soap.

ORIGIN
Once extracted from the ashes of burned seaweed, now prepared chemically using sodium chloride, ammonia, and carbon dioxide.

BACKGROUND
Traditionally used in 19th-century Western medicine as a treatment for burns, eczema, phlegm, and vaginal discharges.

PREPARATION
Sodium carbonate is mixed with lactose sugar and triturated to grind it into a powder fine enough to be soluble in water.

REMEDY PROFILE

People for whom *Nat. carb.* is most suited are very sensitive. They usually have an inability to assimilate things on both an emotional and a physical level. For example, there may be an emotional inability to tolerate noise, music, thunderstorms, hot weather, and even other people. Physically, this inability to assimilate things might, for example, manifest as digestive problems. These people tend to devote their lives to one person, sacrificing everything to this relationship. Prone to suppressing emotions, they tend to act cheerful even when sad, which compounds the mental strain, fatigue, and irritability they often feel.

People who respond to *Nat. carb.* may find that mental stress or physical exercise when tired aggravates their symptoms.

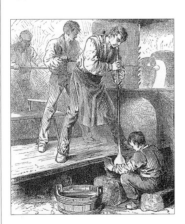

GLASSMAKING
For centuries this compound has been used as an ingredient in glass, and up to 50 percent of all sodium carbonate made today is still used for that purpose.

DIGESTIVE DISORDERS
Symptoms Indigestion with burping, sourness, and a feeling of nausea. There is a marked intolerance of milk, so that ingestion of even the smallest amount often causes diarrhea. The abdomen may feel painful when touched, and there may be thirst, especially when the stomach is upset. An empty, gnawing sensation in the stomach is common, especially around 5 A.M., and may be assuaged by getting up and eating something sweet. Constant nibbling, especially of bread and sweets, is a typical accompanying symptom.
Symptoms better From pressure on the abdomen; with movement; from eating little and often.
Symptoms worse With heat and in the sun; with sympathy and fuss; from drinking milk.

COLDS & PHLEGM
Symptoms Colds that are aggravated by sitting in a draft, with phlegm running down the back of the throat. The phlegm may smell foul.
Symptoms better From perspiring.
Symptoms worse In drafts; every second day.

HEADACHES
Symptoms Headaches that alternate with pain in the stomach, accompanied by sensitivity to noise and music. Headaches may be caused by studying or other demanding mental activity, or by over-exposure to the sun. There may be a feeling of dizziness.
Symptoms better With movement; from eating.
Symptoms worse In the sun and hot weather; in drafts; from thunderstorms; from mental exertion.

SKIN CONDITIONS
Symptoms A wide variety of skin complaints, such as warts, moles, blisters, and corns, with either very dry skin or a tendency to perspire very easily. There may be extreme sensitivity to sunlight, with the result that even the slightest exposure may cause sunburn or sunstroke.
Symptoms better From pressing on, rubbing, or scratching the affected skin.
Symptoms worse With heat.

ANKLE WEAKNESS
Symptoms Easily sprained or dislocated ankles, particularly in children.
Symptoms better Rubbing or pressing on the ankle.
Symptoms worse From over-exertion.

EXHAUSTION
Symptoms Nervous fatigue due to overexposure to the sun or overwork. The legs may feel weak and heavy.
Symptoms better Rubbing or pressing on the affected area.
Symptoms worse With heat;

KEY SYMPTOMS

DEVOTED NATURE TOWARD LOVED ONES ◆ SUPPRESSION OF EMOTIONS ◆ WEAK ANKLES ◆ SENSITIVITY TO SUNLIGHT ◆ INTOLERANCE OF MILK

SEE ALSO

Infertility, *page 203*; Allergies, *page 206*; Phobias, *page 211*; Depression, *page 212*

NAT. MUR.

Natrum chloratum syn. *N. muriaticum*

SODIUM CHLORIDE, the main ingredient of this remedy, occurs naturally as the mineral halite, or rock salt, and in saltwater. An essential part of the human diet, deficiency causes fatigue and muscle cramps, while excess intake is thought to exacerbate high blood pressure and heart disease. In conventional medicine salt is administered as saline solution, often to replace fluid loss. *Nat. mur.* was proved and published by Hahnemann in his *Chronic Diseases* (1821–34).

REMEDY PROFILE

Nat. mur. is most suitable for sensitive people who are easily wounded by criticism. They keep a tight rein on emotions, but this can lead to moodiness and self-absorption. Despite a desire for company, they feel awkward in social situations and isolate themselves to avoid being hurt, thus seeming self-reliant and stoical. Inhibition and self-awareness may restrict them: for instance, they may be unable to urinate in a public restroom. They are often conscientious, diligent, and loyal in their relationships.

Suppressing strong emotions such as depression, anxiety, or grief, is often a cause of illness. These people hate sympathy. They are prone to colds, crave salt, feel worse in stuffy heat or sunshine, and from eating, physical exertion, and sweating.

COLDS

Symptoms Profuse, runny mucus that tends to resemble uncooked egg white and may slip down the throat. There may be a dry, hacking cough.
Symptoms better In fresh air; from bathing in cool water.
Symptoms worse With heat; between 9 A.M. and 11 A.M.

HEADACHES

Symptoms A hammering, bursting headache or migraine above the eyes, possibly with vision disturbances such as zigzag lines.
Symptoms better From pressure on the eyes; lying in the dark.
Symptoms worse With heat; in light; near noise; with movement; from reading; between 10 A.M. and 3 P.M.

SKIN CONDITIONS

Symptoms Greasy skin and hair, with dandruff around the hairline. Warts, boils, psoriasis, hives (urticaria), hangnails, and cold sores on the nose and lips may be helped by the remedy.
Symptoms better In fresh air; from bathing in cool water; from perspiring; from fasting.
Symptoms worse With heat; in sunshine; in sea air; after menstruating.

MOUTH & THROAT CONDITIONS

Symptoms Cold sores, canker sores, dental abscesses, and gingivitis (bleeding gums). The lips may be cracked and dry, with a split running down the center of the lower lip. The tongue is bright red with a white coating, and has a tendency to develop blisters.

SOURCE DETAILS

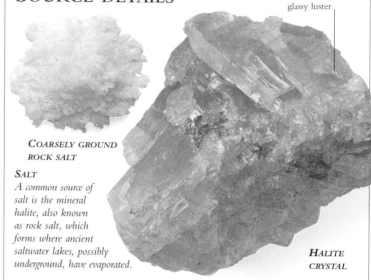

Halite has a glassy luster

COARSELY GROUND ROCK SALT

SALT
A common source of salt is the mineral halite, also known as rock salt, which forms where ancient saltwater lakes, possibly underground, have evaporated.

HALITE CRYSTAL

ORIGIN
Rock salt is obtained from underground sources in the form of halite. Salt is also produced when sea water is evaporated.

BACKGROUND
Historically of immense economic value in trade as a preservative and a condiment, but has had limited medicinal uses outside homeopathy.

PREPARATION
Rock salt is dissolved in boiling water, filtered, and evaporated to make pure sodium chloride, which is then triturated with lactose sugar.

KEY SYMPTOMS

AILMENTS THAT ARE BROUGHT ON BY SUPPRESSION OF EMOTIONS ♦ PERSON FEELS WORSE WITH CONSOLATION ♦ CRAVING FOR SALT ♦ DISCHARGES THAT RESEMBLE EGG WHITE

Extreme thirst, a bitter-tasting mouth, and halitosis are also typical symptoms. A sore throat may occur, producing white mucus and the sensation of having a lump in the throat.
Symptoms better In fresh air; from fasting.
Symptoms worse With heat; in sea air; with emotional stress.

WOMEN'S HEALTH

Symptoms Vaginal discharge that resembles uncooked egg white, usually due to candida. Fatigue may develop before and after menstrual periods. Premenstrual syndrome is marked by water retention and severe headaches (*see above, left*). Menstruation may be irregular, and shock or grief may stop it entirely. A dry, sore vagina may even lead to vaginismus (painful spasms during sexual intercourse).

Symptoms better In fresh air; lying on the right side.
Symptoms worse With heat; from emotional stress.

DIGESTIVE DISORDERS

Symptoms Constipation with hard, dry stools, colicky pains with nausea, and possibly anal fissures, rectal bleeding, and backache. There may be sour burps and a bitter taste in the mouth. Any diarrhea is evident only during the day.
Symptoms better In fresh air; from tight clothing; lying on the right side; from fasting.
Symptoms worse With heat; from emotional stress.

SEE ALSO

Skin, *page 192*; Migraine, *page 218*; Respiration, *page 224*; Gingivitis, *page 232*; Cold sores, *page 242*

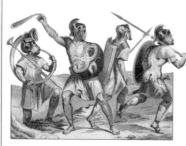

SALT MONEY
Roman soldiers were paid a salarium reserved for buying sal, or "salt." This became the origin of the word "salary."

Petroleum rectificatum syn. *Oleum petrae*

PETROLEUM

PETROLEUM (from the Latin *petra*, or "rock," and *oleum*, "oil") is formed by the decomposition of animal matter in rock sediment deposits on the seabed. Over time, heat and pressure transform this organic material into petroleum, or crude oil. It is used in the manufacture of many goods, from fertilizers to paints and plastics to explosives. Proved by Hahnemann and published in his *Chronic Diseases* (1821–34), the remedy is prescribed mainly for skin complaints and nausea.

REMEDY PROFILE

Those who are best suited to *Petroleum* can be irritable and argumentative, and may lose their tempers easily. Known for their inability to make decisions, they tend also to be forgetful, which may lead to confusion and disorientation, to the point of losing their way even in familiar streets. A strange sense of physical duality may be experienced, as if their bodies are divided, or not entirely their own.

Symptoms are usually worse during the day and in winter. These individuals generally feel chilly, and prone to offensive-smelling perspiration from the feet and armpits even in cold weather. An aversion to rich, fatty foods is also common. Inhaling petrochemical fumes may aggravate symptoms and cause weakness and irritability.

Petroleum is often given for skin problems such as eczema, psoriasis, and chilblains. It is also used for complaints such as diarrhea, nausea, travel sickness, morning sickness, halitosis, and migraine.

ECZEMA & PSORIASIS
Symptoms The skin is dry and leathery with deep cracks, especially on the palms of the hands, the tips of the fingers, and in the folds of the skin, for example behind the ears or the knees. Extreme itchiness may provoke scratching that causes bleeding and possible infection. The itching tends to be worse at night. There may

be psoriasis, with thick patches of scaly, inflamed skin causing great discomfort. In addition the skin may be prone to cold sores, boils, and chilblains (*see below*). *Petroleum* is especially appropriate if the symptoms are due to hard manual labor or regular exposure to chemicals.
Symptoms better In warm weather; after eating.
Symptoms worse From the heat of the bed; in winter.

CHILBLAINS
Symptoms Intensely itching, burning skin, especially on the hands, feet, and toes. The skin may be scratched raw, causing a weepy discharge to develop and possibly infection to set in.
Symptoms better In dry weather; from warm air.
Symptoms worse In cold, damp weather; if touched.

DIARRHEA & NAUSEA
Symptoms Diarrhea that is present only during the day. Constant, ravenous hunger may even lead to getting out of bed to eat snacks during the night. Hunger increases after a bowel movement, but there is a cutting pain in the abdomen that is worse after eating. An aversion to cabbage, peas, beans, meat, and fatty foods is characteristic. There may be nausea accompanied by vomiting, dizziness, and pressing head pain at the back of the skull (*see right*). Another associated symptom may be halitosis with a strong odor of

garlic. Symptoms may be linked to morning sickness, motion sickness (*see below*), or eating disorders such as bulimia nervosa, anorexia nervosa, or other psychological conditions that cause long-term bingeing.
Symptoms better Temporarily after eating; from passing stools; from bending double.
Symptoms worse In cold weather; with movement; in the morning; when eating.

MOTION SICKNESS
Symptoms Nausea and vomiting when traveling, often with a severe headache (*see right*). Nausea may develop on the slightest movement, with increased salivation.
Symptoms better Temporarily after eating.
Symptoms worse In cold weather; in fresh air; with movement.

MIGRAINE
Symptoms Severe headache, with a sensation of great heaviness at the back of the head. The scalp is sensitive to the cold and to touch. The head may feel sensitive, as if a cold breeze is blowing on it, or numb and wooden. A degree of temporary deafness is a possible associated symptom, and there may be an accompanying feeling of nausea (*see left*).
Symptoms better From pressure on the temples.
Symptoms worse In cold; if touched; from shaking when coughing.

SOURCE DETAILS

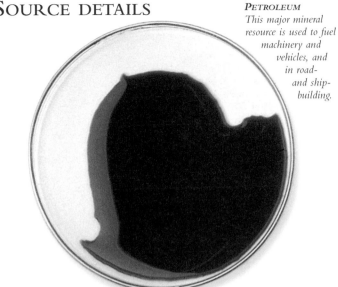

PETROLEUM
This major mineral resource is used to fuel machinery and vehicles, and in road- and ship-building.

ORIGIN
Extracted from deposits, mainly concentrated in the North Sea, the Persian Gulf, and parts of North and South America.

BACKGROUND
Used as fuel in the form of gasoline, paraffin, and diesel. Petroleum jelly is used in conventional medicine as an emollient and protective dressing.

PREPARATION
The remedy is made by distilling purified crude oil or petroleum. This solution is then diluted using sulfuric acid, and succussed.

KEY SYMPTOMS
CRACKED SKIN ◆ CHILLINESS ◆ AVERSION TO FATTY FOODS ◆ IRRITABILITY ◆ OFFENSIVE-SMELLING PERSPIRATION ◆ PERSON TENDS TO FEEL WORSE IN WINTER

SEE ALSO
Psoriasis, *page 195*

Phosphorus
PHOSPHORUS

PHOSPHORUS WAS DISCOVERED in the 17th century by the German alchemist Hennig Brand. He kept his method of extracting it from urine a secret, but it was soon discovered by the Irish chemist Robert Boyle. The name is derived from the Greek *phosphoros*, or "light-bringing," since the element glows in the dark. Unstable, highly toxic white (or yellow) phosphorus had been used to make fireworks and matches since 1669; by 1845 it had been replaced by the nontoxic red form. The remedy was proved by Hahnemann and published in his *Chronic Diseases* (1821–34).

REMEDY PROFILE

People who love being the center of attention respond best to *Phosphorus*. Like a match that sparks readily but burns out intensely, they are artistic, expressive, and affectionate, but may offer more than they can sustain. Illness or stress rapidly exhausts their energy, making them lethargic and indifferent toward loved ones, but highly responsive to any sympathy offered. They feel better after short naps. Vague anxieties crystallize into concrete fears when ill, leading to nervous fatigue and tension.

Cravings for salty, spicy, or sweet foods, and cold sodas or cold milk are typical. Warm foods or drinks may upset the stomach, as may cold drinks once they have warmed up in the stomach.

Phosphorus is prescribed for circulation problems, bleeding, digestive disorders, chest complaints, and burning pains.

LITTLE MATCH GIRL
Before 1845 those involved in the manufacture and sale of matches made with white phosphorus often developed "phossy jaw," a gangrenous condition caused by inhaling phosphorus fumes that killed off the bone in the jaw.

POOR CIRCULATION
Symptoms The extremities feel burning hot yet are cold to the touch. Erratic blood flow may cause a weak pulse, hot flashes, fainting, dizziness, or palpitations. There may be burning neuralgic pain (*see below, right*), and a sense of suffocation, possibly triggered by emotion or menopause.
Symptoms better In cold; from a massage; lying on the right side; from sleeping.
Symptoms worse Lying on the left side; from thundery weather; emotional stress.

BLEEDING
Symptoms Profuse, bright red blood flow, especially from the nose, gums, and lining of the stomach. Menstrual flow may be heavy. The skin bruises easily and anemia may set in.
Symptoms better In cold; from a massage; lying on the right side; from sleeping.
Symptoms worse Lying on the left side; from thundery weather; emotional stress.

DIGESTIVE DISORDERS
Symptoms Nausea, vomiting, and constipation, often due to food poisoning, stress, stomach ulcers, or gastroenteritis. Other symptoms include a saliva-filled mouth and burning pain in the stomach, or heartburn. Stools are long, ribbonlike, and may be blood-streaked. Ice-cold

SOURCE DETAILS

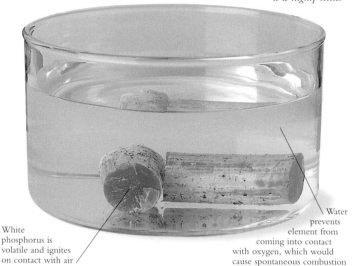

White phosphorus is volatile and ignites on contact with air

Water prevents element from coming into contact with oxygen, which would cause spontaneous combustion

ORIGIN
A pale yellow element with a distinct odor, occuring in the mineral calcium phosphate in volcanic regions. The main deposits are found in North Africa.

BACKGROUND
Used medicinally for headaches, pneumonia, measles, rheumatic pain, malaria, and epilepsy until the 19th century, when its toxic nature became widely known.

PREPARATION
White phosphorus is used for the remedy. This waxy substance is insoluble in water, so it is dissolved in alcohol, filtered, then repeatedly diluted and succussed.

KEY SYMPTOMS
AFFECTIONATE, OPEN NATURE ♦ TEARFULNESS ♦ CRAVINGS FOR COLD DRINKS & SALTY FOODS ♦ BURNING PAINS ♦ PERSON FEELS WORSE LYING ON THE LEFT SIDE OF THE BODY

---

foods and drinks are craved, but then cause vomiting once they warm up in the stomach.
Symptoms better Lying on the right side; from eating; from cold foods or drinks.
Symptoms worse Lying on the left side; in stuffy rooms; from emotional stress; from warm foods or salt.

RESPIRATORY ILLNESS
Symptoms A sore throat and dry, tickly cough, possibly causing retching and vomiting. Phlegm is streaked with dark-red blood. Chest tightness may be due to asthma, bronchitis, or pneumonia. Colds tend to go straight to the chest.
Symptoms better From sitting up; lying on the right side of the body; from sleep; from cold foods or drinks.
Symptoms worse Lying on the left side; from laughing; from warm foods or drinks.

BURNING PAINS
Symptoms Burning neuralgic pains in the limbs, spine, or stomach, possibly with pins and needles and numbness, especially in the limbs, spine, or shoulder blades.
Symptoms better From cold compresses; from a massage.
Symptoms worse In windy weather; from emotional stress.

SEE ALSO
Respiration, *pages 180, 224*; Palpitations, *page 186*; Digestion, *pages 188, 234*; Reproduction, *page 198*

Platinum metallicum
PLATINA

COMMON NAME
Platinum

THE CHIBCHA INDIANS of Columbia were the first people recorded as using platinum, back in 1735. Its name derives from the Latin *platina*, meaning "little silver." Today it is considered more valuable than gold or silver, and plays a key role in modern technology. A costly, malleable metal, platinum is fashioned into coinage, jewelry, surgical instruments, and dental alloys. It is used industrially to refine oil and reduce pollution from exhaust fumes. The homeopathic remedy was proved by Drs. Staph and Gross, two pupils of Hahnemann, and published in the latter's *Chronic Diseases* (1821–34).

SOURCE DETAILS

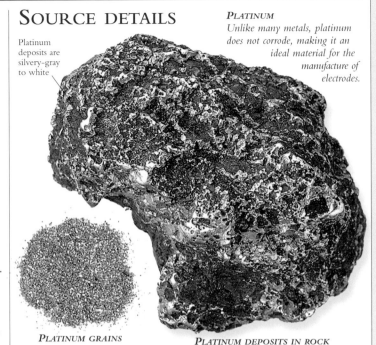

Platinum deposits are silvery-gray to white

PLATINUM
Unlike many metals, platinum does not corrode, making it an ideal material for the manufacture of electrodes.

PLATINUM GRAINS

PLATINUM DEPOSITS IN ROCK

ORIGIN
Usually forms as grains in or by nickel deposits. Found mainly in South America but also in Canada and Russia.

BACKGROUND
Given as a remedy for treating syphilis in the 19th century, but not otherwise widely used until the 20th century.

PREPARATION
Grains of platinum are boiled in acid, washed, and dried. They are then triturated with lactose sugar.

REMEDY PROFILE

Chiefly a remedy for women, *Platina* is best suited to those who tend to be haughty and passionate. High expectations set for themselves and their partners are frequently not met, causing disappointment. They often dwell on the past, and may feel that others have deserted them. A sense of isolation may lead them to become independent and introspective. Narcissistic tendencies are accompanied by a feeling that they deserve the very best of everything. If this is denied them, they may become rather arrogant and depressed. Weeping may bring relief. Curiously, objects often appear to these people to be smaller than they actually are.

Platina suits those with alternating emotional and physical symptoms. Any pain increases and decreases slowly. Secretions such as menstrual blood and tears tend to be sticky. The libido is often high. *Platina* is used for sexual and menstrual problems in women and nervous system disorders in both men and women.

MENSTRUAL PROBLEMS
Symptoms Heavy, brief, or absent menstruation. Heavy menstrual flow may contain blood clots. There may be painful uterine cramps that are worse as menstruation begins, with a sense of constriction and numbness in the lower abdomen. Pain may also be felt around the ovaries.
Symptoms better From walking in the open air; in sunshine; from stretching.
Symptoms worse If touched; in the evening; from emotional stress; from nervous fatigue.

OVERSENSITIVITY OF THE FEMALE GENITALIA
Symptoms Hypersensitive vulva and vagina during and between menstrual periods that may cause rapid stimulation during sexual intercourse, or else extreme pain and even fainting. The vaginal muscles may spasm involuntarily (vaginismus). There may be genital itching, a high libido, and a tendency to masturbate. The pain is intermittent, not necessarily occurring every time sexual intercourse takes place, but tends to be worse as menstruation begins. It can make vaginal examination and wearing a sanitary napkin or tampon highly uncomfortable.
Symptoms better From walking in the open air; in sunshine; from stretching.
Symptoms worse If touched; in the evening; from emotional stress; from nervous fatigue.

NUMBNESS & CRAMPS
Symptoms Cold, numb skin, cramps in the calves, and a constricted feeling in the limbs, especially the thighs, as if the limbs are tightly bandaged.
Symptoms better From walking in the open air; in sunshine; from stretching.
Symptoms worse If touched; in the evening; from emotional stress; from nervous fatigue.

HEAD & FACIAL PAIN
Symptoms Pain and a sense of constriction in the head that builds up and disappears slowly. There may be neuralgic pains in the face that alternate with numbness, or painless paralysis of the face due to Bell's palsy.
Symptoms better Walking in the open air; with movement.
Symptoms worse If touched; from bending backward.

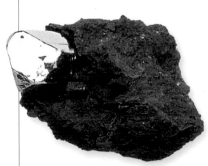

SPERRYLITE CRYSTAL
Sperrylite is one of several minerals in which platinum is deposited. This is the largest known platinum ingot, found in Transvaal, South Africa, in the 1920s.

KEY SYMPTOMS
HIGH EXPECTATIONS ◆ HYPERSEXUALITY ◆ NUMBNESS ◆ SENSE OF CONSTRICTION, AS IF BANDAGED ◆ PERSON FEELS BETTER IN THE OPEN AIR

SEE ALSO
Depression, *page 212*

Plumbum metallicum

PLUMBUM MET.

COMMON NAME
Lead

ALTHOUGH LEAD HAS BEEN widely used since Roman times, its toxicity was not recognized until the 20th century. It is now banned from paints to prevent children from being poisoned by chewing lead-based toy or crib paint, and it is being phased out of gasoline because of fears that it may impair mental development in children. Physical symptoms of lead poisoning include wrist drop and colicky abdominal pains. *Plumbum met.* was proved by Drs. Hering, Hartlaub, Trinks, and Menning and published in Allen's *Encyclopedia of Pure Materia Medica* (1874–79).

REMEDY PROFILE

While the profile for *Plumbum met.* is associated mainly with physical symptoms, irritability, timidity, restlessness, apathy, anxiety, and depression are all psychological factors that may be linked to *Plumbum met.* The emotional traits may begin in childhood: children suited to the remedy are restless, with a weak memory and emotional instability. Adults who respond best to *Plumbum met.* have a tendency to be self-centered, with self-destructive impulses.

There may be difficulties in perception, a reduced ability to express thoughts, and memory loss. These symptoms show a lack of emotional pliability that may be echoed by a loss of physical flexibility. Thus the remedy is given for sclerotic (tissue-hardening) conditions such as arteriosclerosis, which thickens and hardens arteries, and Dupuytren's contracture, a disorder affecting one or both of the hands, in which one or more fingers become fixed in a bent position.

A POISONOUS COSMETIC
To maintain a lily-white complexion, fashionable Elizabethan women used to apply lead to their faces to strip off the surface layers of skin and reveal the white skin beneath.

NEUROLOGICAL CONDITIONS

Symptoms Spasms, trembling, and muscle weakness (*see below*). The joints may be rigid and, between spasms, movement is slow. If the sensory nervous system is affected, there may be vision disturbances and a loss of feeling, so that external sources of pain, such as the heat of an oven or pin-pricks, are not felt. These symptoms may indicate a progressive neurological disorder such as multiple sclerosis or Parkinson's disease. Symptoms may also occur after a stroke (often due to arterio-sclerosis blocking the blood supply to the brain – another example of the thickening and hardening traits linked to the remedy), possibly with pain or paralysis in a limb. *Plumbum met.* is also used for neuralgic pains that appear suddenly and radiate in all directions or shoot from the toes to the hips.
Symptoms better With warmth; from a massage or pressure on the affected area.
Symptoms worse At night; with movement.

MUSCLE WEAKNESS

Symptoms Weakness, spasms, and trembling in the muscles, which feel tired, heavy, and aching. There is a sense of retraction, for example as if the eyes are being pulled back into the head or the testicles or penis are being pulled up into the body. There may be wrist drop due to weakness in the wrist muscles.
Symptoms better With warmth; from a massage or pressure on the affected area.
Symptoms worse At night; with movement.

CONSTIPATION

Symptoms Colicky pains in the stomach and constipation There is a constant urge to defecate, but often only small, black, ball-shaped stools are passed. Painful urine retention and a sensation as if the navel is being pulled into the backbone are further possible symptoms.
Symptoms better With warmth; from bending over; firm pressure on the abdomen; from massaging the abdomen.

Symptoms worse From fasting; in the evening and at night; with movement.

DUPUYTREN'S CONTRACTURE

Symptoms Thickened and shortened tissues or tendons in the fingers or the palms of the hands. One or more fingers may become fixed in a bent position. Either or both hands may be affected
Symptoms better From a massage of the affected area.
Symptoms worse Trying to grasp smooth objects.

SOURCE DETAILS

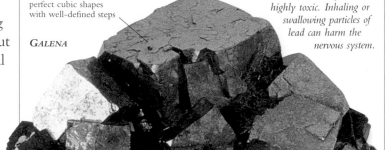

Galena forms as perfect cubic shapes with well-defined steps

GALENA

LEAD
Usually mined as galena, a common lead ore, lead is widely used but highly toxic. Inhaling or swallowing particles of lead can harm the nervous system.

ORIGIN
Most commonly occurring in galena, a lead ore that is found in Australia, the US, Africa, and Europe.

BACKGROUND
Soft and malleable, and has been used to make everyday objects, from plumbing to hairpins, since Roman times.

PREPARATION
For the mother tincture, pure lead is extracted from galena and finely ground until it becomes soluble in alcohol.

KEY SYMPTOMS

MENTAL DULLNESS ◆ HARDENING OF ATTITUDE AND STATE OF MIND ◆ HARDENING OR THICKENING OF TISSUES AND ARTERIES ◆ EXTREME CHILLINESS ◆ SHOOTING PAINS

SEE ALSO

Multiple sclerosis, *page 179*; Diabetes, *page 191*; Vaginismus, *page 260*

Silicea terra syn. *Acidum silicicum*

SILICA

SILICA IS A FORM of the nonmetallic element silicon, which is one of the major elements of the Earth's crust and a vital constituent in the structure of plants. In the human body, it strengthens teeth, hair, and nails and is also found in connective tissue. *Silica,* proved by Hahnemann in 1828 and given more for slow-developing conditions than for acute ailments, has the unusual feature of reputedly being able to help expel foreign bodies such as splinters from the skin.

SOURCE DETAILS

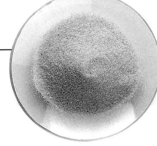

SILICON DIOXIDE

FLINT

SILICA
A principal constituent of sandstone and other rocks, silica is found in many forms, from colorless rock crystal to stonelike flint and semiprecious stones such as opal.

REMEDY PROFILE

People who respond best to *Silica* typically lack mental and physical stamina. Their over-conscientious attitude to work can often lead to exhaustion or insomnia. They may feel anxious and "in two minds" about things, and fear pointed objects, such as needles. Their outlook and aspirations are limited by fear of failure. Very shy as children, they are self-conscious and unassertive as adults, but can be extremely stubborn and may relieve their frustrations on subordinates.

Chilliness is a typical physical symptom, along with a marked tendency for profuse, smelly sweat. Digestive problems and a weakened bone structure, due to poor absorption of food and undernourishment, may occur, along with recurrent infections caused by a weak immune system. Skin and bone problems are slow to heal and any wounds tend to suppurate.

Many symptoms appear at an early age: the fontanelles (membrane-covered spaces between the bones of a baby's skull) close slowly, for instance, and the bones and teeth form more slowly and are weaker than those of other children.

SKIN, TEETH, NAIL & BONE CONDITIONS
Symptoms Slow eruption of teeth, wisdom teeth problems, and defects in skin, hair, and nails, due to poor absorption of minerals in the diet. Brittle, distorted, infected nails and

ingrown toenails are also common symptoms. Wounds, even scratches, suppurate and heal slowly; abscesses may form anywhere, including in the roots of teeth. There may be itchy scars or keloids after larger wounds, persistent acne, and copious, smelly sweating. Backache is common, brittle, poor-quality bones are slow to mend if broken, and there may be curvature of the spine.
Symptoms better In summer; lying down; from being well wrapped up.
Symptoms worse In cold and dampness; menstruating; from pressure on the painful area.

EAR, NOSE & THROAT CONDITIONS
Symptoms Recurrent colds, swollen glands, ear infections, and tonsillitis leading to quinsy (abscess on the tonsil). Chronic phlegm may cause sinusitis, and glue ear (fluid in the middle ear) may cause earaches and hearing problems.
Symptoms better Lying down; from being well wrapped up; from warm drinks.
Symptoms worse In cold and dampness; in drafts; from suppressing perspiration.

COUGHS
Symptoms A persistent, dry, irritating cough that takes the form of severe, exhausting coughing bouts. Inflammatory conditions such as bronchitis may be accompanied by foul-smelling sputum.

ORIGIN
Hahnemann prepared *Silica* from mountain crystal; homeopaths later made it from flint. Chemically prepared silicon dioxide (silica sand) is now used.

BACKGROUND
Used as silica sand in industry in the making of cement and concrete as well as ceramics and glass. It is also used to grind and polish glass and stone.

PREPARATION
Made by triturating silicon dioxide, grinding the sand repeatedly with lactose sugar until it becomes soluble in water, then diluting and succussing it.

KEY SYMPTOMS

LACK OF ASSERTIVENESS AND STUBBORNNESS ◆ LACK OF STAMINA ◆ CHILLINESS, BUT WITH OFFENSIVE-SMELLING PERSPIRATION ◆ SUSCEPTIBILITY TO RECURRENT INFECTIONS

Symptoms better From being well wrapped up; lying down; from warm drinks.
Symptoms worse In cold and dampness; in drafts; from suppressing perspiration.

DIGESTIVE DISORDERS
Symptoms A weak digestive system, with intolerance of particular foods, especially fat and milk; in babies this may even include mother's milk. There may be poor absorption of essential minerals into the body and a preference for cold foods. Symptoms may include constipation, with an inability to expel stools so that they slip back into the rectum, which may develop painful cracks (fissures) or abscesses. Painful abdominal cramps and smelly flatulence are other symptoms.

Symptoms better In summer; from being well wrapped up.
Symptoms worse In cold and dampness; at a new moon; from suppressing perspiration.

HEADACHES
Symptoms Severe pain, starting at the back of the head and extending over to the forehead, with dizziness and visual disturbance.
Symptoms better With warmth; with closed eyes; in dark, quiet rooms.
Symptoms worse In cold; in light; near noise.

SEE ALSO
Tuberculosis, *page 182;* Diabetes, *page 191;* Skin, *page 192;* Osteoarthritis, *page 196;* Reproduction, *page 198*

Stibium sulfuratum nigrum syn. *Antimonium crudum*

ANTIMONIUM CRUD.

ANTIMONY OCCURS NATURALLY in crystalline form as the mineral stibnite, which was used (as kohl) by women in ancient Rome and the Middle East as a cosmetic. Prepared chemically for various industrial purposes, it is often used to coat the tips of matches, since it ignites when struck against red phosphorus. The homeopathic remedy was proved by Hahnemann and his colleague, Caspari, in 1828. It is prescribed primarily for skin problems and digestive disorders.

SOURCE DETAILS

ANTIMONY
This substance can be derived from the prismatic crystals of stibnite, which are opaque with a metallic luster.

STIBNITE

ORIGIN
Found naturally in the mineral stibnite, which forms as crystals in quartz veins throughout many parts of the US and Europe.

BACKGROUND
Used to treat horses with damaged hooves, and to fatten pigs and cattle. Industrially, used to purify gold and to line brass instruments.

PREPARATION
Stibnite is roasted and heated with carbon to extract the antimony, which is then triturated with lactose sugar, diluted, and succussed.

REMEDY PROFILE

Antimonium crud. is associated with sentimental people who yearn for the past. They can be withdrawn, sulky, irritable people, prone to experiencing grief, serious depression, or despondency after a failed romance. They often dislike being touched or even spoken to. When ill, children who fit this profile cannot bear being looked at and have a tendency to cry. Both adults and children of this disposition may have insatiable appetites, yet in some cases there is a strong aversion to food, which can eventually lead to emaciation.

Typical physical symptoms include recurring digestive problems and the appearance of a thick, white coating on the tongue. The feet tend to be sensitive and prone to ailments such as corns and callouses, which make walking painful.

Antimonium crud. is typically prescribed for certain skin conditions and infections, as well as for toothaches, digestive problems, and gout.

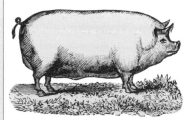

FATTENING THE SOW
Legend relates that a monk, pleased with antimony's ability to fatten his pigs, tried the same approach when feeding his fellow monks. Sadly, his efforts proved fatal, hence the name antimony – antimonk!

SKIN & NAIL CONDITIONS
Symptoms Callouses, warts, and corns that may form on the hands, under the fingernails (especially if the nails are damaged), on the soles of the feet, and on the tips of the toes. The skin may thicken, chap, or roughen easily, and cracked patches may form, particularly around the nostrils and the corners of the mouth. The nails may split repeatedly.
Symptoms better With rest; in the evening.
Symptoms worse In cold; from strong heat; if touched.

SKIN INFECTIONS WITH A RASH
Symptoms A rash on the trunk, arms, and legs, inside the mouth or, in the case of chicken pox, behind the ears, with mild fever. There may be eczema, hives (urticaria), or rashes that resemble measles, with itching that becomes worse in a warm environment such as a bed. Fluid-filled blisters, often due to impetigo, may appear in patches, usually around the nose and mouth.
Symptoms better With rest; in the evening.
Symptoms worse In cold; from strong heat; if touched.

TOOTHACHE
Symptoms Persistent, gnawing toothaches, usually caused by decaying teeth. The pain can extend to the head.

KEY SYMPTOMS
SENTIMENTALITY ♦ DISLIKE OF BEING TOUCHED OR LOOKED AT ♦ INSATIABLE APPETITE ♦ THICK, WHITE COATING ON THE TONGUE ♦ DIGESTIVE PROBLEMS

Symptoms better In fresh air; with rest.
Symptoms worse At night; from eating; from cold foods and drinks.

DIGESTIVE DISORDERS
Symptoms Indigestion, with burping, nausea, and possibly vomiting of bile. The abdomen feels either bloated or empty, and stomach ulcers may have formed. Diarrhea alternates with constipation. The tongue has a thick, white coating, and there may be a headache. The digestion is highly sensitive, yet there may be cravings for sour foods that aggravate it, such as pickles, vinegar, and wine. Overindulgence and pregnancy often trigger the symptoms. The remedy is given to babies who vomit breast milk and will not suckle, or to their mothers.

Symptoms better With rest.
Symptoms worse During the night; if touched; from sour or starchy foods; from cold foods and drinks.

GOUT
Symptoms Inflammation and redness in affected joints (often in the big toe). Joint pain impedes walking if the leg or foot are affected. A mild fever may set in, and there may be unease and restlessness, with tense and jumpy muscles.
Symptoms better With rest.
Symptoms worse In cold; from strong heat; if touched.

SEE ALSO
Toothache, *page 232*; Indigestion, *page 234*; Skin, *page 240*

Sulfur
SULFUR

COMMON NAMES
Sulfur, flowers of sulfur, brimstone, sublimated sulfur

I N THE 9TH CENTURY BCE the Greek poet Homer used vapors of burning sulfur to purify his house. Long used in Chinese and Western medicine for skin problems and as an antiseptic, sulfur was also given to children in the West as brimstone and molasses, a popular tonic to "cleanse" the blood and keep the bowels regular. Hahnemann proved the remedy and published it in his *Materia Medica Pura* (1821–34). It is used chiefly for skin and digestive complaints.

REMEDY PROFILE

Those best suited to *Sulfur* are imaginative and inventive, but inept practically. A key problem is being unable to channel their disorganized, philosophical thoughts, which tend to spin off in different directions. With a strong desire for recognition, they may expend a great deal of energy on ideas and speculations but fail to harness it, losing resolve and appearing egocentric and lazy. Friends are exasperated by their impatience, irritability, and self-absorption, yet charmed by their generosity, naivety, and good humor.

Sensitive to warmth, these people have a tendency to become overheated and strip off layers of clothing. Sweat, stools, and other discharges are often strong-smelling. Heat, eating, standing, and washing usually aggravate symptoms.

Sulfur is prescribed to treat a broader range of ailments than any other remedy in the homeopathic repertory. It is also given to any type of person to boost vitality and clear up lingering illnesses.

SKIN CONDITIONS
Symptoms Patches of itchy, red, weepy skin, but generally dry, dirty-looking skin. *Sulfur* is used for many skin problems, including diaper rash, cradle cap, acne, psoriasis, eczema, ringworm, and scabies. It is given for bacterial infections such as erysipelas, cellulitis, impetigo, and boils; for viral infections such as oral and genital herpes; and for measles and chicken pox.
Symptoms better In fresh, warm, dry air; lying on the right side.
Symptoms worse In a stuffy environment; from being in a hot bed; from scratching; from wearing wool; from washing.

DIGESTIVE DISORDERS
Symptoms A bloated stomach with burning pains, burping, flatulence, indigestion, and a tendency to regurgitate food. Any vomiting or diarrhea is worse at 5 A.M. and typically alternates with constipation. The anus is sore and itchy after passing stools and may develop hemorrhoids. Hunger pains and a sinking feeling in the stomach may strike at around 11 A.M. Discharges such as stools and flatulence have an offensive smell.
Symptoms better From cold foods and drinks; flatulence.
Symptoms worse From over-exertion; from milk.

WOMEN'S HEALTH
Symptoms Painful or irregular menstruation, with a burning feeling in the vulva and vagina. The vagina may itch, and there may be a white or yellow discharge typically caused by candida. There may be headaches, irritability, and insomnia that are linked with premenstrual syndrome. *Sulfur* may ease the burning pain of cystitis and help treat menopausal dizziness, hot flashes, and strong-smelling sweats, particularly if these symptoms are accompanied by vaginal itching.
Symptoms better In fresh, warm, dry air; lying on the right side.
Symptoms worse In a stuffy environment; at night.

MEN'S HEALTH
Symptoms Impotence or erectile failure accompanied by sharp pains in the penis and itching in the tip of the penis. Penis or prostate inflammation may be helped by the remedy.
Symptoms better In fresh, dry, warm air; with movement.
Symptoms worse With heat; at night; with rest.

RESPIRATORY ILLNESS
Symptoms A dry, sore throat with a choking feeling, swollen tonsils, and hoarseness. Colds and coughs are marked by thick, smelly, yellow or green phlegm. Coughing disrupts sleep. Colds may develop into bronchitis, pleurisy, or pneumonia with chest pains.
Symptoms better In the open air; from dry heat; lying on the right side.
Symptoms worse At night; in the morning; reclining.

SOURCE DETAILS

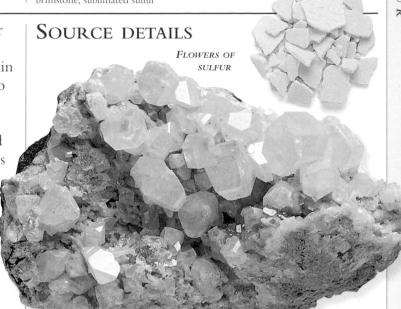

FLOWERS OF SULFUR

SULFUR

SULFUR
The mineral is refined into flowers of sulfur which, when burned, produce sulfur dioxide, a powerful disinfectant.

ORIGIN
Produced by volcanic activity, and found near hot springs and volcanic craters in Sicily and the US, and on the Italian peninsula.

BACKGROUND
Used traditionally as a disinfectant, laxative, and purgative, to treat skin complaints, clear up bronchial phlegm, and ease rheumatic pains.

PREPARATION
Sulfur is chemically purified. The mineral is then triturated by grinding it into a fine powder that is soluble in water and alcohol.

KEY SYMPTOMS
LAZINESS ◆ TENDENCY TO OVERHEAT ◆ SELF-CENTEREDNESS ◆ PHILOSOPHICAL STATE OF MIND ◆ ITCHING ◆ BURNING PAINS

SEE ALSO
Skin & bones, *pages 192, 240, 268*; Reproduction, *page 198*; Children's health, *page 246*; Women's health, *page 256*

Tartarus stibiatus syn. *Antimonium tartaricum*

ANTIMONIUM TART.

COMMON NAMES
Antimony potassium tartrate, tartar emetic

ALCHEMISTS CALLED this compound "tartar emetic," and it was traditionally prescribed as a powerful emetic. Known as the "prince of evacuants," it caused severe vomiting and was taken to expel intestinal worms. The remedy *Antimonium tart.* was proved in various separate trials by Drs. Hahnemann, Stapf, and Hencke and published in Allen's *Encyclopedia of Pure Materia Medica* (1874–79). It is commonly prescribed for strength-sapping illness in the young or elderly.

REMEDY PROFILE

Antimonium tart. is appropriate for rather attention-seeking people who respond well to rest, comfort, and reassurance. The remedy also suits children who tend to complain unless they are carried around.

Illness often exhausts these individuals, making them feel restless, generally apathetic, and drowsy. Their energy levels may be so low that they are unable to cough up mucus and seem in danger of suffocating in their own secretions. They become irritable and averse to being bothered or disturbed by others, and dislike being touched or examined.

Typical symptoms include a lack of thirst and profuse, cold sweat. *Antimonium tart.* is used for chest complaints, such as whooping cough, which are marked by the sound of mucus rattling in the chest. It is also given for headaches, nausea and vomiting, and skin problems such as acne, impetigo, and chicken pox.

RESPIRATORY ILLNESS
Symptoms Severe respiratory infection or chronic bronchitis with wheezing and rattling in the throat and chest due to a buildup of mucus. Coughing up mucus becomes difficult due to severe fatigue. Fits of coughing may alternate with gasping or rapid, shallow breathing accompanied by a sensation of suffocation. Symptoms may be aggravated by irritability or anger.

Symptoms better In cold air; from sitting up; from coughing up mucus.
Symptoms worse With warmth; in dampness and cold; lying down.

WHOOPING COUGH
Symptoms Breathlessness and coughing spasms primarily in infants, followed by sleep or nausea and vomiting (*see below*). Mucus causes congestion and a rattling sound in the chest.
Symptoms better From sitting up; from coughing up mucus; from vomiting.
Symptoms worse With warmth; from being too hot or cold; lying down; with movement; from tantrums.

NAUSEA
Symptoms Persistent nausea with trembling, weakness, and fainting. The nausea seems to center in the chest or may be felt as a weight on the chest; it may be accompanied by coughing. There may be vomiting, ineffectual retching, and a thick, white coating or red streaks on the tongue.
Symptoms better In cold air; from sitting up; from burping; from vomiting.
Symptoms worse With warmth; in dampness and cold; lying down.

SKIN CONDITIONS
Symptoms Pustular skin eruptions that leave a purplish mark when healed. There may be warts, or acne with

SOURCE DETAILS

ANTIMONY POTASSIUM TARTRATE
This compound is commonly used as an insecticide and fix to bind dyes to textiles and leather.

Crystals of antimony potassium tartrate are poisonous

ORIGIN
Prepared by combining potassium tartrate with oxide of antimony, which is formed by the reaction of moist air and antimony (*see page 98*).

BACKGROUND
Traditionally used for medicinal purposes in the West for treating intestinal worms and fungal infections, and as an expectorant.

PREPARATION
The remedy is prepared by triturating antimony potassium tartrate with lactose sugar and then repeatedly diluting and succussing the mixture.

KEY SYMPTOMS

LOUD RATTLING OF MUCUS IN THE CHEST AND A SUFFOCATING SENSATION ◆ INCREASING WEAKNESS ◆ DISLIKE OF PHYSICAL EXAMINATION ◆ LACK OF THIRST

---

pea-sized pustules. Small, fluid-filled blisters and reddened skin may be caused by impetigo.
Symptoms better In cold air; from sitting up.
Symptoms worse From bathing in cold water; in the evening; from lying down.

CHICKEN POX
Symptoms Large, blistering, bluish skin eruptions that leave a purple scar. The remedy is particularly apt when the skin symptoms have not developed strongly but associated chest or digestive symptoms have appeared, such as a chesty cough with rattling mucus or diarrhea. The tongue is coated white, and there may be extreme irritability.
Symptoms better In cold; from coughing up mucus.

Symptoms worse With warmth; from bathing in cold water; becoming heated in bed; in the evening; lying down.

HEADACHES
Symptoms Pain as if a tight band is constricting the head, heightened by coughing. There may be weariness and a longing to close the eyes.
Symptoms better In the open air; from bathing in cold water; with movement.
Symptoms worse With warmth; at night; in the morning; from overeating.

SEE ALSO
Asthma, *page 181*

Zincum metallicum
ZINC. MET.

A SOFT, BLUE–WHITE METAL that does not corrode, zinc is used to make galvanized roofing and alloys such as brass, a melding of copper and zinc that is used for many purposes, including musical instruments. Zinc stimulates the production of many proteins in the body and is a vital trace element. In conventional medicine, zinc-oxide cream is applied to ulcers, and given as a supplement for tetanus, neuralgia, and convulsions. The remedy was proved by Hahnemann in 1828.

REMEDY PROFILE

Hard-working individuals who find it hard to relax are most suited to *Zinc. met.* They take on too much responsibility then become stressed. A state of nervous excitement follows, which makes them sensitive, especially to noise, irritable, and complaining. This over-stimulation saps their vitality and can lead to mental and physical exhaustion.

These people tend to be forgetful, feel the cold keenly, are prone to anemia, and are notorious for complaining when ill. Symptoms tend to worsen at night, and twitching persists during sleep. Drinking alcohol, especially wine, and eating also aggravate symptoms, which tend to improve after expelling natural discharges through urination, defecation, and menstruation.

Typical physical symptoms are extreme fatigue, weakness, and restless, twitchy, trembling limbs, particularly the legs. The remedy is used for these conditions, for nervous and urogenital disorders, and for itchy skin eruptions with fatigue and twitching limbs.

NERVOUS EXHAUSTION
Symptoms A state of collapse due to overwork, stress, or overstimulation, marked by mental and physical weakness. The mind is either excitable or confused and slow – if asked a question, the person may repeat it once or twice before its meaning sinks in. Bursting

headaches may be a feature (*see below, right*). There may be incessant trembling in the limbs due to weakness and restless feet in constant motion. The soles of the feet may feel painful. Nervous exhaustion may lead to depression marked by moodiness, introversion, and irritability. Noise and chatter may be intolerable, and anger tends to provoke tears.
Symptoms better Rubbing the body; with movement.
Symptoms worse If touched; with jarring; from wine.

TWITCHING LIMBS
Symptoms Involuntary jerking, twitching, or even convulsions, and a pale face. The legs may be restless and fidgety, despite great weariness, and there may be numb, cold feet and a desire to keep the legs moving. Severe spasms may be due to chorea or Parkinson's disease.
Symptoms better Rubbing the body; with movement.
Symptoms worse If touched; with jarring; from wine.

UROGENITAL PROBLEMS
Symptoms Involuntary urine leakage while coughing, laughing, or straining in any way, due to stress incontinence. There may be complete loss of bladder control during severe convulsions (*see above*). Urine retention due to nervousness or prostate enlargement may also be helped by the remedy,

SOURCE DETAILS

ZINC
This trace element, found in sphalerite, is vital for a healthy body, although excess consumption can cause anemia, weaken the immune system, and impair the healing process.

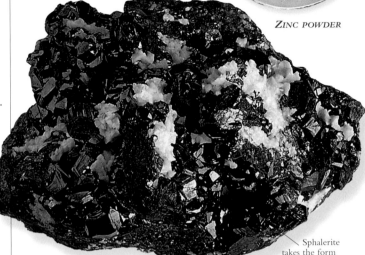

ZINC POWDER

SPHALERITE

Sphalerite takes the form of black crystals

ORIGIN
Refined from the ore sphalerite, formed in hydrothermal mineral veins in South America, the US, and Australasia.

BACKGROUND
Used traditionally as an antiseptic and astringent in calamine and other lotions, and now in sun-screens to block UV rays.

PREPARATION
Zinc is heated and then ground into a fine powder. This is followed by trituration with lactose sugar.

KEY SYMPTOMS

NERVOUS FATIGUE OR EXHAUSTION ♦ RESTLESS FEET ♦ TWITCHING AND TREMBLING ♦ PERSON FEELS BETTER FOR EXPELLING DISCHARGES AND DEVELOPING SKIN ERUPTIONS

---

as may premature ejaculation.
Symptoms better With movement.
Symptoms worse Near noise; in the evening; at night.

ECZEMA & VIRAL SKIN INFECTIONS
Symptoms Red, itchy, weepy, or crusty patches of eczema, particularly on the insides of the limb joints. Childhood viral infections such as chicken pox, measles, and German measles may also be helped by *Zinc. met.* if the rash is slow to appear, if the child is mentally and physically weak, and if there is involuntary twitching.
Symptoms better Allowing the rash to weep and discharge

its fluids; with movement.
Symptoms worse Near noise; if touched; at night.

HEADACHES
Symptoms Pounding, bursting, possibly one-sided pain in the forehead or the temples, due to overwork or nervous exhaustion (*see left*).
Symptoms better In fresh air; with movement.
Symptoms worse Near noise; if touched; from wine.

SEE ALSO
Restless legs, *page 230*

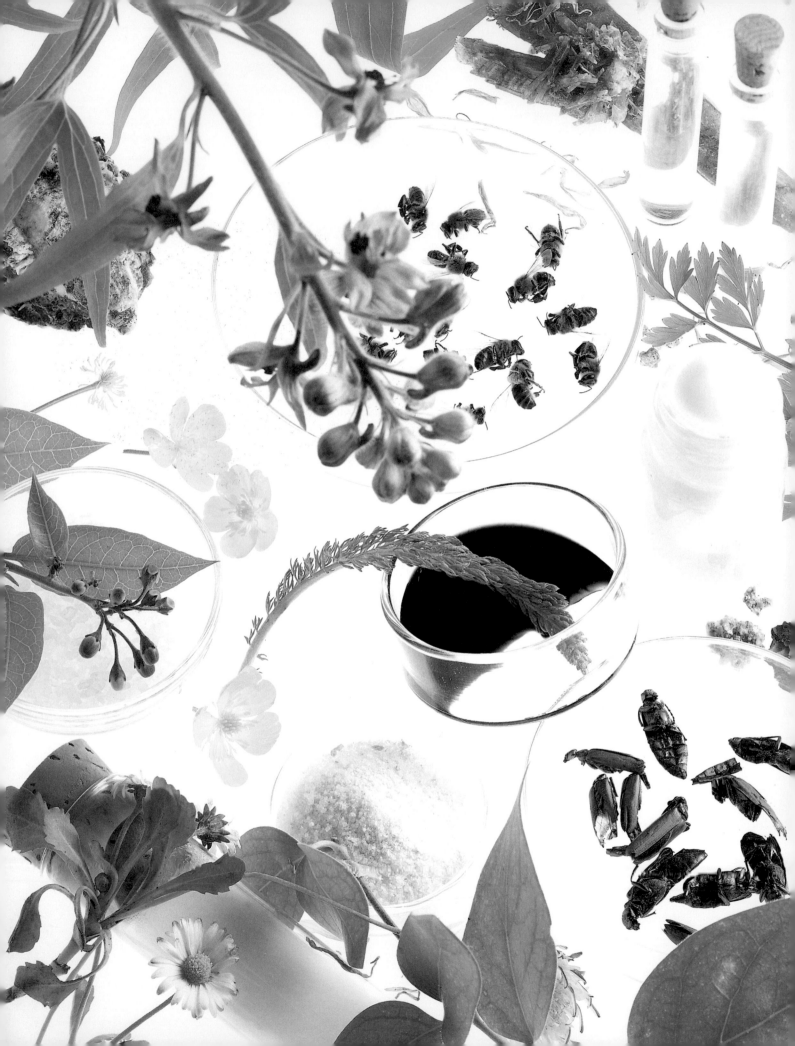

MAJOR ANIMAL REMEDIES

THIS SMALL BUT IMPORTANT COMPONENT OF THE

HOMEOPATHIC MATERIA MEDICA INCLUDES REMEDIES

MADE FROM ANIMALS, INSECTS, ANIMAL PRODUCTS

OR SECRETIONS, AND STERILIZED BACTERIA TAKEN

FROM DISEASED TISSUE. THE MAJOR ANIMAL-BASED

REMEDIES ARE FEATURED IN THIS SECTION.

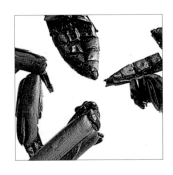 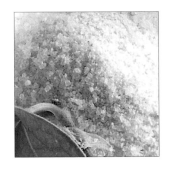 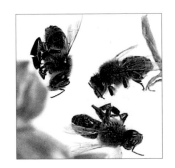

Apis mellifica
APIS

COMMON NAME
Honey bee

A 9,000-YEAR-OLD CAVE PAINTING depicting a figure taking honey from a hive is the oldest record of our relationship with the honey bee. Bees provide us with more than just honey, however: Beeswax is refined and used in ointments and polishes; propolis (a resin collected by bees from tree buds) is used medicinally; and royal jelly is taken as a nutritional supplement. The homeopathic remedy, proved in 1852 by Dr. Frederick Humphries, is often used to treat insect bites and stings.

REMEDY PROFILE

Homeopaths easily recognize people likely to benefit from *Apis* because, in some ways, their behavior echoes that of bees. They tend to be fussy, restless, irritable and hard to please. Frantic hours spent tidying and sorting, sometimes clumsily, often accomplish little. A vulnerable side reveals oversensitivity, sadness, weepiness, and an aversion to being alone. This need for company gives this type of person a reputation as a "queen bee" who organizes everyone. Such people reserve a sting for those who upset them. Fiercely territorial, they can be highly jealous or suspicious of newcomers.

Apis is prescribed generally for symptoms that start on the right side and move to the left side. Ailments treated with *Apis* include urticaria (hives), insect bites or stings, and burns. It is used for urinary infections such as cystitis, and for edema or urine retention, especially in newborn babies. Inflammation of the eyes, mouth, or throat, and fever may also be helped.

URTICARIA, BITES & STINGS

Symptoms The skin is itchy, swollen, and highly sensitive to touch, with stinging pain. It may be puffy and blotchy, with raised bumps that seem full of water. Urticaria may develop after a chill or fever (*see right*).
Symptoms better In cool surroundings; from washing; cold compresses on the skin.
Symptoms worse With heat; in hot, stuffy rooms; at night; from touch or pressure on the affected area.

CYSTITIS

Symptoms Burning, stinging pain in the urethra and bladder on urination. The need to urinate is frequent, but only meager amounts of urine are passed. Kidney inflammation with puffy eyes and a lack of thirst may also respond to *Apis*
Symptoms better In cool surroundings.
Symptoms worse With heat; from pressure on the bladder.

EDEMA

Symptoms Swelling of body tissues due to fluid retention. The swelling may be associated

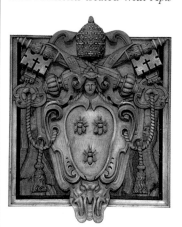

SYMBOLIC SIGNIFICANCE
Symbols of immortality and diligence, bees also represented Pope Urban VIII's family on his 17th-century coat of arms.

SOURCE DETAILS

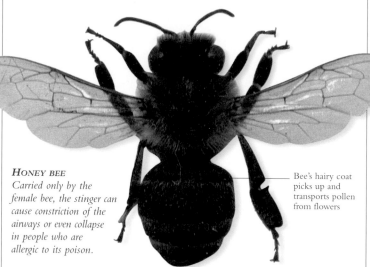

HONEY BEE
Carried only by the female bee, the stinger can cause constriction of the airways or even collapse in people who are allergic to its poison.

Bee's hairy coat picks up and transports pollen from flowers

ORIGIN
Made from the native European honey bee, which can today be found throughout Europe and in Canada, the US, and many other countries.

BACKGROUND
Bee-derived substances such as beeswax and honey have long been used in many medicinal traditions, including ancient Greek, Western, Chinese, and Unani.

PREPARATION
The remedy is made from the whole female, including the stinger, or from the stinger alone. The insect is crushed, dissolved in alcohol, diluted, and succussed.

KEY SYMPTOMS
BURNING, STINGING PAINS ♦ SWELLING OF AFFECTED AREAS ♦ ALLERGIC REACTIONS ♦ ANXIOUS RESTLESSNESS ♦ JEALOUSY

---

with arthritis (accompanied by the typical burning or stinging pain), meningitis, pleurisy, or peritonitis.
Symptoms better From cold compresses on the affected area.
Symptoms worse With heat; from touch or pressure on the affected area.

INFLAMMATION OF THE EYES, LIPS, MOUTH, OR THROAT

Symptoms Inflammation of the eyes, mouth, or throat. The eyes are red, sore, and sensitive to the light. They may water profusely with hot tears. The mouth and throat are swollen, and are subject to burning pains. Any swelling in the throat may obstruct breathing. There is a marked lack of thirst.
Symptoms better From cold compresses on the affected

area; from inhaling cool air.
Symptoms worse With heat; in hot, stuffy rooms; if touched.

FEVER

Symptoms Fever with a total lack of thirst and possible sore throat. There may be a severe headache with stabbing pains, in which the head feels hot. There may also be chills, and the skin is dry and sensitive.
Symptoms better In cool surroundings; from uncovering; from cold compresses.
Symptoms worse With heat; in hot, stuffy rooms; with sleep; from touch or pressure on the affected area.

SEE ALSO

Circulation, *page 184*; Osteoarthritis, *page 196*; Prostate problems, *page 202*; Allergies, *page 206*; Urticaria, *page 242*

Cantharis vesicatoria syn. *Lytta vesicatoria*

CANTHARIS

THE IRIDESCENT BODY of this beetle contains an irritant called cantharidine, which has a long, if dubious, reputation in traditional medicine, due in part to its alleged aphrodisiac properties. If taken in large doses, cantharidine is a powerful poison that attacks the urinary system. It causes vomiting, diarrhea, burning pain in the stomach and throat, and kidney damage, and can lead ultimately to death. The remedy *Cantharis*, proved by Hahnemann in 1805, is given for complaints accompanied by burning pain.

REMEDY PROFILE

Those who benefit most from *Cantharis* usually have high sex drives, which may become uncontrollable during certain illnesses. They can be restless, querulous, and difficult to get along with when ill. Irritability or insolence can even explode into paroxysms of violence or rage. In extreme cases, this may escalate into psychological problems such as intense mental confusion or mania.

Cantharis is prescribed for conditions that deteriorate very rapidly. Typical symptoms are loss of appetite, burning pain in the throat or stomach, and raging thirst with an aversion to drinking, since even a small amount of water makes the bladder pain worse.

Burning cystitis and urinary tract inflammation are the main disorders for which *Cantharis* is used. Tenderness in the area of the kidneys, renal colic, kidney inflammation such as nephritis and pyelonephritis, and some other urinary disorders may also be eased by the remedy. It is given for sunburn, scalds, and burns if the skin has blistered, and is also used for insect bites and stings. Some digestive tract disorders, such as gastritis, severe diarrhea, or dysentery, may respond to the remedy, as may an excessive libido.

SEVERE CYSTITIS
Symptoms Constant, urgent desire to urinate, with violent, spasmodic pains in the lower abdomen. Urine is scant, hot, and bloody, and is passed drop by drop, with violent burning or cutting pains in the bladder and urethra. After urinating there is a sensation that the bladder is not actually empty. There may be long-term urine retention, which results in a loss of muscle tone in the bladder. Inflammation of the genital area may overly stimulate the libido (*see right*).
Symptoms better With warmth; at night.
Symptoms worse Before, during, and after urination; from coffee; from cold drinks.

BURNS & SCALDS
Symptoms Burns, sunburn, and scalding, if the skin blisters. *Cantharis* is also prescribed for blisters that resemble burns.

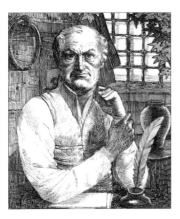

MARQUIS DE SADE
This 18th-century Frenchman, infamous for his perverse sexual practices, gave his victims Spanish fly as an aphrodisiac.

SOURCE DETAILS

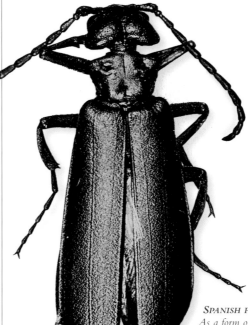

SPANISH FLY
As a form of defense, this beetle secretes cantharidine if touched. This active chemical causes the skin to blister.

ORIGIN
Found in southern Europe, notably in Spain and southern France, as well as in western Asia. Feeds on the leaves of white poplar, ash, privet, elder, and lilac trees.

BACKGROUND
Traditionally used for warts, baldness, arousing the libido, and inducing miscarriage. The Greek "father of medicine," Hippocrates, advocated Spanish fly for dropsy in the 5th century BCE.

PREPARATION
Whole, live beetles are killed by heating. They are then macerated in alcohol and left to stand for five days before being filtered, diluted, and succussed.

KEY SYMPTOMS

BURNING, CUTTING PAINS ◆ URINE THAT PASSES IN DROPS ◆ VERY HIGH LIBIDO WITH URINARY PROBLEMS ◆ VIOLENT BEHAVIOR ◆ PERSON FEELS WORSE FROM COFFEE

Symptoms better From cold compresses on the affected area.
Symptoms worse With warmth; if touched.

INSECT BITES & STINGS
Symptoms Unusually sharp pain at the site of a sting or bite, which has a black center. Anger, restlessness, excitability, or aggravation may also be evident after the bite or sting.
Symptoms better From cold compresses on the affected area.
Symptoms worse With warmth; from coffee.

GASTRITIS, DIARRHEA & DYSENTERY
Symptoms Violent, burning pain, distended abdomen, and possibly diarrhea accompanied by a scalding sensation. There may be an urge to empty the bowels when urinating, a loss of appetite, and irritability.

Symptoms better At night; With warmth; bending double.
Symptoms worse During urination; from drinking.

EXCESSIVE LIBIDO
Symptoms Uncontrollable, inappropriate sexual arousal. An inflamed genital area, due to urinary tract infection, may stimulate sexual activity (*see left*). Sexual fantasies may be strong enough to disturb sleep.
Symptoms better With warmth; with rest; from rubbing the genitalia.
Symptoms worse During urination; during sexual intercourse.

SEE ALSO
Irritable bowel syndrome, *page 189*; Ulcerative colitis, *page 190*; Cystitis, *page 260*

Carcinosinum
CARCINOSIN

THIS HOMEOPATHIC REMEDY is made from cancerous tissue, usually obtained from the breast. Cancer is the second most common cause of death in the Western world (after heart disease). The development of a homeopathic remedy derived from cancerous tissue is attributed to two British homeopaths, Dr. Compton Burnett and Dr. Clarke, who first proved the remedy in the late 19th century. Its uses have widened considerably following research published by the American homeopath Dr. Jonathan Shore in 1989. *Carcinosin* is thought to be particularly beneficial for noncancerous conditions in people who have a strong family history of cancer.

REMEDY PROFILE

Carcinosin is best suited to people who were shy, highly sympathetic, and hypersensitive during childhood. Such children typically suppress their emotions, dislike being criticized or scolded, and are easily offended. During puberty they may find it difficult to contain their sexual feelings. As adults, they tend to be passionate, and often become workaholics, continually pushing themselves to the limit. They may have a great desire for travel and excitement. Their yearning for deep fulfillment may lead to exhaustion and illness.

People who benefit most from the remedy may have a strong craving for fatty foods, especially butter and chocolate. Physical symptoms may be positively or negatively affected by being at the beach. These people generally feel better when they dance or listen to music. Their symptoms may be relieved by lying with the knees drawn up to the elbows.

Carcinosin may be prescribed for those who have a personal or family history of cancer, diabetes, or tuberculosis. In some cases the remedy may even be used in the treatment of the actual diseases. The remedy also has an affinity with those who have a history of emotional stress, or who are recovering from chronic fatigue syndrome or mononucleosis.

CHRONIC FATIGUE SYNDROME
Symptoms Weakness and exhaustion, associated with tenderness in the muscles. This is often accompanied by dizziness, numbness, and nausea. Frequent colds and recurrent acute illnesses are common characteristic traits. There may be depression and a loss of concentration. This condition may arise following a bout of mononucleosis.
Symptoms better With short naps; in the evening; at the beach; lying with the knees drawn up to the elbows.
Symptoms worse In damp, clammy surroundings; from physical exertion; undressing.

INSOMNIA
Symptoms Chronic inability to sleep soundly, especially if the pattern has been apparent since childhood. This insomnia is particularly associated with prolonged periods of emotional stress, and some form of rejection is often the root of the problem. Stimuli such as thunderstorms may cause excitement and prevent sleep.
Symptoms better In the evening; with short naps.

SOURCE DETAILS

Malignant cancer cell exists as parasite in body

CANCER
The potential of cancer tissue, which is used curatively just in the field of homeopathy, is only now being fully explored.

Cancer cell divides more rapidly than normal body cells

ORIGIN
Carcinosin is a nosode, a remedy made from diseased tissue (*see page 20*). It is prepared from cancerous tissue, which is commonly taken from the breast.

BACKGROUND
Breast cancer is the most common form of cancer in women. Most malignant breast tumors are found in the upper, outer part of the breast.

PREPARATION
The prepared specimen of cancerous tissue is sterilized and then dissolved in purified water. This mixture is then repeatedly diluted and succussed.

KEY SYMPTOMS
WORKAHOLIC, PASSIONATE NATURE ◆ CONDITIONS THAT ARE AFFECTED BY BEING AT THE BEACH ◆ DESIRE FOR TRAVEL ◆ DESIRE FOR BUTTER AND CHOCOLATE ◆ SLEEPING DIFFICULTIES

Symptoms worse With physical exertion; during thunderstorms.

RESPIRATORY ILLNESS
Symptoms Bronchitis with a cough that develops from a tickle in the throat. There may also be asthma and a feeling of constriction in the chest.
Symptoms better In the evening; with short naps.
Symptoms worse In cold air; from talking; from laughing; from running; from undressing.

ABDOMINAL PAIN
Symptoms Abdominal pain with dry, hard stools and burning pain on the right side of the colon. There may be constipation, which is typically associated with a desire for fatty foods such as chocolate.

Symptoms better From pressure on the abdomen; bending forward; hot drinks.
Symptoms worse Between 4 P.M. and 6 P.M.

SKIN GROWTHS & BLEMISHES
Symptoms Multiple moles and blemishes, acne on the back and chest, or boils. There may be itching and a tendency to bruise or bleed easily.
Symptoms better In the evening.
Symptoms worse From undressing.

SEE ALSO
Allergies, *page 206*

Crotalus horridus horridus

CROTALUS

COMMON NAMES
Rattlesnake, pit viper

THE LATIN NAME FOR THE rattlesnake derives from the Greek *krotalon*, meaning "rattle" or "castanet." This is due to the distinctive rattling sound made by the snake's tail, which vibrates at 50 beats per second as the creature prepares to strike its prey. The remedy, proved by the US homeopath Dr. Constantine Hering in 1837, is prescribed primarily for a range of serious disorders, including hemorrhaging, angina, strokes, and infection.

REMEDY PROFILE

Those who respond best to *Crotalus* tend to be sluggish and melancholic. They are prone to forgetfulness, and may lose their way in their own neighborhood, or even forget the names of close friends. An aversion to family members is typical of these people, and a desire for meat, especially pork, is common.

 Crotalus is considered to help stop bleeding from any orifice, making it highly useful for hemorrhaging. It is given following the onset of a state of total collapse, which may be due to a severe septic state, a stroke, or a heart attack. In addition, it may help cases of delirium or throat infection.

BLEEDING

Symptoms Copious bleeding from any orifice. The remedy is especially effective for slow bleeding, or for thin, dark blood that does not clot well. It may seem as though blood is present in the perspiration or tears. The bleeding may be associated with a state of collapse or severe infection.

THE RATTLER
Once it has reached sexual maturity, the rattlesnake adds a new segment to its tail each time it sheds its skin.

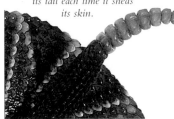

Crotalus is used for septicemia with hemorrhaging where the breakdown of red blood cells is so great that the liver becomes overwhelmed, leading to the onset of serious conditions such as jaundice.
Symptoms better In fresh air; from light; from movement.
Symptoms worse Lying on the left side; from wearing tight clothes.

STROKE

Symptoms Weakness or total collapse after a stroke. There may be paralysis or impaired function in the limbs, which is generally right-sided and accompanied by pain that extends down to the left hand. Other symptoms may include retinal hemorrhaging and nosebleeds. There may be signs of delirium (*see below, right*).
Symptoms better In fresh air; from light.
Symptoms worse Lying on the left side.

HEART DISORDERS

Symptoms Partial or total collapse following angina or a heart attack. There may be weakness, fainting, and pain that is worse on the left side of the body and that possibly extends down the arm to the left hand. There may be great reluctance to move due to a feeling that something is going to burst underneath the breastbone.
Symptoms better From light.

SOURCE DETAILS

RATTLESNAKE
This venomous snake is also called the pit viper, due to the heat-sensitive pit between its eyes and nostrils that it uses to locate its prey.

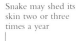
Snake may shed its skin two or three times a year

ORIGIN
Native habitat, like that of many other species of rattlesnake, is Canada, the US, and South America. Found in arid terrain and desert areas.

BACKGROUND
Venom "milked" from live snakes is used to make antivenin, which triggers production of antibodies that neutralize the poison from a snakebite.

PREPARATION
Venom obtained from a live snake by "milking" it is dropped onto lactose sugar. The resulting mixture is then triturated.

KEY SYMPTOMS
BLEEDING, POSSIBLY FROM EVERY ORIFICE ◆ SEPTICEMIA OR EVEN SEPTIC SHOCK ◆ AVERSION TO TIGHT COLLARS

Symptoms worse Lying on the left side; from climbing up steps, or walking up a hill or slope.

DELIRIUM

Symptoms Confused and disordered thoughts as a result of a serious infection, stroke, or heart attack. There may be irritability, anxiety, and an inability to answer questions. Insomnia is another possible symptom: those affected may suddenly jump out of bed and try to run away, muttering and babbling. These symptoms may also be associated with the delirium tremens caused by alcoholism.
Symptoms better From light; with movement.
Symptoms worse Falling asleep; from alcohol; waking.

THROAT INFECTIONS

Symptoms Inflammation or infection of the throat, often from laryngitis or tonsillitis. The pain is particularly sharp on the left side of the throat, and is often accompanied by a dry, irritating cough. Another characteristic symptom linked with *Crotalus* is soreness in the throat with associated difficulty in swallowing.
Symptoms better From being in fresh air.
Symptoms worse Lying on the left side; from clothing that is tight around the neck.

SEE ALSO
Cancer, *page 208*

Lac caninum

LAC CAN.

SINCE THE ERA OF ancient Rome the milk of nursing female dogs has been put to medicinal use. In the 1st century CE the Roman naturalist Pliny the Elder advocated it for allaying certain disorders of the female reproductive system. The Greek physician Sextus used it in the 3rd century CE for treating intolerance of light and inflammation of the inner ear. The homeopathic remedy *Lac. can.* was proved in 1888 by Drs. Swan and Berridge.

REMEDY PROFILE

Those who benefit most from *Lac can.* tend to lack self-confidence. Often restless and nervous, they may be highly sensitive to sensory stimulation. An active imagination and excitable nature combine to engender irrational fears that may develop into phobias. They may be prone to bouts of depression.

A typical symptom in those who respond to *Lac can.* is a feeling of "otherworldliness," as if the self is floating just above or behind the body, or a sensation that is often described as "floating on air."

Lac can. is used for irrational phobias and for acute sensory hypersensitivity. The remedy is also considered particularly effective for the throat, the nervous system, and the female reproductive system. In all conditions, symptoms tend to move from site to site around the afflicted area of the body.

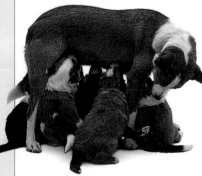

FEEDING MOTHER
The calmness of a nursing bitch is often seen as motherly love, but her behavior is actually due to a hormonal reaction designed to stimulate the release of milk.

THROAT INFECTIONS
Symptoms Excessive dryness in the throat. Burning pain makes swallowing difficult. The pain alternates from side to side, and may extend to the ears. The saliva is of a viscous consistency, and the back of the throat may be lined with a silvery film. Symptoms may coincide with menstruation if they are caused by tonsillitis.
Symptoms better From being in fresh air; from cold drinks.
Symptoms worse If touched.

PHOBIAS
Symptoms Irrational fears, usually of snakes, storms, dogs, or disease. The fear of snakes is particularly strong, and may be associated with a sensation of snakes crawling all over and around the body. There may be hypochondria and a constant desire to wash the hands. Anxiety and fear may trigger hysteria, with possible aggressive behavior.
Symptoms better From being in fresh air.
Symptoms worse If touched.

BREAST PROBLEMS
Symptoms Swollen, sore breasts prior to menstruation. Pain switches from side to side. In breast-feeding mothers, breast milk may be lacking or suppressed, or milk production may be excessive. The breasts are painful and feel as though they are full of hard lumps. There may be a desire to hold the breasts firmly.

SOURCE DETAILS

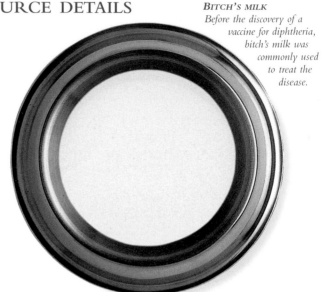

BITCH'S MILK
Before the discovery of a vaccine for diphtheria, bitch's milk was commonly used to treat the disease.

ORIGIN
The milk from any nursing bitch may be used, although in practice mongrels are used most often.

BACKGROUND
Ancient Romans used remedies derived from bitch's milk for ovarian pains, and for uterine and cervical problems.

PREPARATION
Fresh milk from a nursing mongrel bitch is expressed and diluted in a mix of alcohol and water for the tincture.

KEY SYMPTOMS
PAIN THAT ALTERNATES FROM SIDE TO SIDE ◆ FEAR OF SNAKES ◆ GREAT SENSITIVITY ◆ LACK OF CONFIDENCE ◆ SWOLLEN BREASTS BEFORE MENSTRUATION ◆ SENSITIVITY TO TOUCH

Symptoms better With warmth; in fresh air; with rest.
Symptoms worse If touched; with the slightest movement; from going up and down stairs.

VAGINAL BLEEDING & DISCHARGE
Symptoms Bleeding between menstrual periods or following sexual intercourse. A vaginal discharge may accompany bleeding, particularly before menstruation. The genitalia are very sensitive to touch or pressure, including that of washing or the friction of clothes. Sexual intercourse may be painful, and during orgasm hysteria may develop. The libido may be sharply increased or reduced.
Symptoms better With warmth; in fresh air; with rest.
Symptoms worse If touched; with movement.

HYPERSENSITIVITY
Symptoms Mental hypersensitivity due to an overactive imagination. A hysterical state may develop; this may involve seeing faces and hearing noises that do not exist. Parts of the body, such as the genitalia, are also physically hypersensitive. Touch is felt acutely, and there may be an urge to keep the legs or fingers apart to avoid skin-to-skin contact. Absent-mindedness and hypochondria may accompany this state.
Symptoms better With warmth; in fresh air; with rest.
Symptoms worse If touched; with movement; in cold air.

SEE ALSO
Phobias, page 211;
Sore throat, page 226;
Breast pain, page 258

Lachesis muta syn. *Trigonocephalus lachesis*

LACHESIS

KNOWN AS "SURUCUCU" by indigenous South American peoples, the bushmaster is a highly poisonous snake whose venom inhibits nerve impulses in the heart, destroys red blood cells, and interferes with clotting. One bite directly into a vein can cause almost instant death. The remedy, proved by Dr. Constantine Hering in 1828, is given mainly for vascular and circulatory conditions.

SOURCE DETAILS

BUSHMASTER SNAKE
Unlike other members of the rattlesnake family, the bushmaster is an aggressive hunter, with an extremely loud rattle and highly lethal venom.

Snake grows up to 10 ft (3 m) in length

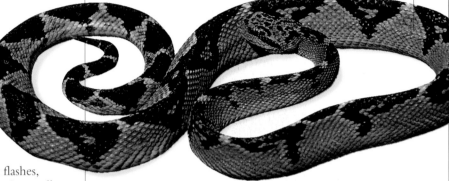

ORIGIN
A deadly member of the rattlesnake family. Native habitat is South America, and preferred territory tends to be the wooded areas of tropical regions.

BACKGROUND
"Milked" from the live snake, the bushmaster's venom is used to make an antivenin for people bitten by it. The anti-venin helps counteract the effects of the bite.

PREPARATION
Venom is "milked" from the bushmaster snake before being dissolved in alcohol. The mixture is then repeatedly diluted and succussed.

KEY SYMPTOMS

**ZEALOUS TEMPERAMENT ♦ LOQUACITY ♦ CONDITIONS
THAT GENERALLY APPEAR ON THE LEFT SIDE ♦
PERSON FEELS BETTER FROM EXPELLING DISCHARGES**

REMEDY PROFILE

Those most responsive to this remedy tend to be ambitious, creative, perceptive, talkative people who live life to the full. If they believe in an ideology, they have a tendency to follow it dogmatically. Their intensity may cause them to become fanatical about religion or sex. Being confined in any way is anathema to them, whether physically by tight, restrictive clothing, or emotionally by commitment in a relationship. A tendency to become over-stimulated by their intense lifestyle may lead to physical and mental "congestion" that makes it hard to control their emotions. Egocentric, cruel, and wildly jealous behavior may result. They also slip easily into depression and extreme loquacity.

Conditions treated by this remedy usually appear on the left side. The symptoms tend to develop or worsen during sleep. Energy levels fluctuate. Physical symptoms are eased by expelling natural discharges such as menstrual blood or gas (while suppressing them can cause discomfort or pain). Similarly, releasing "emotional discharges" brings relief.

Lachesis is often used for hot flashes that occur during menopause, premenstrual syndrome, and certain nervous disorders. The remedy is also prescribed for a sore throat, poor circulation, varicose veins, and certain vascular conditions such as angina.

WOMEN'S HEALTH
Symptoms Menopausal hot flashes, perhaps with fainting spells, palpitations, and hot sweats. *Lachesis* is also used for painful menstruation or premenstrual syndrome with hot flashes, a left-sided headache, and violent mood swings. The symptoms may disrupt sleep and improve with the onset of menstruation.
Symptoms better In fresh air; from menstruating; expelling natural discharges; from eating.
Symptoms worse With heat; with sleep; on waking; if touched; from tight clothing.

SPASMS & TREMORS
Symptoms Muscle spasms, tremors, and weakness in the limbs. Spasms may be triggered by the slightest touch, and may be accompanied by fainting or convulsions. These symptoms may be linked to alcoholism, fever, multiple sclerosis, petit mal epilepsy, or even brain damage following a stroke.
Symptoms better In fresh air; from expelling natural discharges; with movement.
Symptoms worse With heat; with sleep; if touched; on the left side; from menopause; from alcohol or hot drinks.

POOR CIRCULATION & VARICOSE VEINS
Symptoms Poor circulation that turns the face, ears, and extremities blue or purple. Any wounds bleed very easily; even a pin-prick will ooze large drops of blood. *Lachesis* may also be used for varicose veins that are engorged and bluish purple in color.
Symptoms better In fresh air; from expelling natural discharges; from eating.
Symptoms worse Lying on the left side; if touched; from the pressure of tight clothes.

SORE THROAT
Symptoms Swollen, dark purple throat, predominantly on the left side, with splinter-like pain that may spread to the ears. Air or liquids seem more painful to swallow than solids.
Symptoms better In fresh air; from expelling natural discharges; loosening clothing.
Symptoms worse With heat; with sleep; on waking; from constriction around the neck; from swallowing fluids.

HEART DISORDERS
Symptoms Cramping pains in the chest, with a rapid, irregular, weak pulse and possible palpitations. There may be a strange sensation as though the heart has swollen and become too large for the body. Further accompanying symptoms typically include anxiety and cyanosis (bluish lips, tongue, and extremities).
Symptoms better In fresh air; from expelling natural discharges; from eating.
Symptoms worse With heat; lying on the left side; from any constriction around the throat or chest; if touched.

SEE ALSO
Multiple sclerosis, *page 179*; Palpitations, *page 186*; Rosacea, *page 193*; Reproduction, *page 198, 258*; Emotions, *page 210*

Medorrhinum

MEDORRHINUM

COMMON NAME
Gonorrhea

GALEN, THE FAMOUS GREEK physician active in the 2nd century CE, gave gonorrhea its name, from *gonos*, or "seed," and *rhoia*, or "flow." It is thought that the disease predates ancient Greece, however, and was known in ancient Egypt and China. Widespread by the 18th century, gonorrhea was considered a major underlying cause of illness, described by Hahnemann as a "miasm" (*see page 20*). The remedy, derived from a "nosode" (*see page 20*) of the infection itself, was proved by Dr. Swan and published in Allen's *Materia Medica of Nosodes* (1880–90).

REMEDY PROFILE

Medorrhinum is best suited to people who feel hurried and anxious, yet simultaneously isolated and empty, in a dream-like, detached state. They are passionate and experience life to the limit. Behavioral extremes are not uncommon, ranging from a withdrawn, aesthetically sensitive state to an egotistical, selfish one.

Physical symptoms typically center on mucous membranes, which are prone to infection. Symptoms are generally better from a discharge of mucus, in salt air, and in the evening. In damp weather, and between 3 A.M. and 4 A.M., they tend to worsen. A thirst for cold drinks and cravings for meat, fish, salt, candy, and unripe foods are common, as is an aversion to "slimy" foods such as eggplant or oysters.

Medorrhinum is prescribed for infections of the urinary tract, reproductive system, genitals, and respiratory tract. It is also a remedy for asthma, and may be especially effective for those who have a personal or family history of gonorrhea or early heart disease.

URINARY TRACT INFECTIONS
Symptoms Sharp, burning pain on urinating, perhaps with a yellow, pus-filled discharge or blood in the urine (indicative of nonspecific urethritis), or with a frequent urge to urinate,

if cystitis is the cause. In severe cases kidney infections such as renal colic may follow. In men, if accompanied by pain in the abdomen, lower back, rectum, or testicles, fever, and a urinal discharge, symptoms may be due to prostatitis (*see below*).
Symptoms better From kneeling on all fours; lying on the abdomen; in the evening.
Symptoms worse In hot weather; from passing urine; with movement.

WOMEN'S HEALTH
Symptoms Profuse, foul-smelling menstrual flow, and an acrid, thick vaginal discharge with a fishy odor. There may be marked sensitivity near the cervix, tenderness in the breasts and nipples, and even sterility.
Symptoms better From kneeling on all fours; lying on the abdomen; in the evening.
Symptoms worse In hot weather; from urinating; with movement.

TESTICULAR PAIN
Symptoms Prostatitis with an enlarged, painful, heavy prostate gland. The urethra may be inflamed and tender with a foul-smelling discharge, and there may be impotency.
Symptoms better From kneeling on all fours; lying on the abdomen; in the evening.
Symptoms worse In hot weather; from urinating; with movement.

SOURCE DETAILS

Bacterium called *Neisseria gonorrhoeae* transmits infection

GONORRHEA
Transmitted via sexual contact, this infection invades the reproductive system and can cause sterility if left untreated.

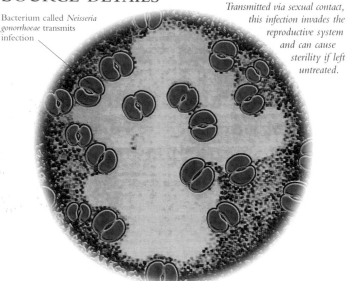

ORIGIN
Discharge from the gonorrhea bacterium, *Neisseria gonorrhoeae*, which commonly infects the mucous membranes of the vagina or urethra.

BACKGROUND
Worldwide one of the most common sexually transmitted diseases, now treated with antibiotics; earlier forms of treatment included silver nitrate injections.

PREPARATION
Urethral discharge from a male patient infected with gonorrhea is diluted in purified water and succussed to make the homeopathic remedy.

KEY SYMPTOMS
BEHAVIORAL EXTREMES ♦ HURRIED FEELING ♦ EXTREMELY PASSIONATE NATURE ♦ PERSON FEELS BETTER FROM LYING ON THE ABDOMEN AND IN THE EVENING

GENITAL WARTS & HERPES
Symptoms Cauliflower-like, pink warts on the genitals. A sore, itchy rash of small genital blisters bursting to leave painful ulcers is indicative of herpes.
Symptoms better From kneeling on all fours; lying on the abdomen; in the evening.
Symptoms worse In hot weather; from urinating; with movement.

RHINITIS, SINUSITIS & ASTHMA
Symptoms Burning, profuse mucus associated with inflammation of the mucous membranes in the nose. There may be rhinitis, with postnasal drip (mucus that drips down the back of the throat) and frequent sneezing. Pressure

and aching in the sinuses may develop into sinusitis. Asthma may occur, and typically is better from lying on the abdomen and sticking out the tongue. There may be a cough that is also better from lying on the abdomen, and aggravated by sweet foods and drinks. A further symptom is sore, watering eyes that may develop conjunctivitis.
Symptoms better In salt air; lying on the abdomen and sticking out the tongue.
Symptoms worse With cold; with dampness; in daytime.

SEE ALSO
Asthma, *page 181*; Rheumatoid arthritis, *page 197*; Candidiasis, *page 200*

Psorinum
PSORINUM

I N LATIN, *scabere* means "to scratch." From this is derived the name of the scabies mite, which tunnels into the skin and causes an itchy, blistering infection. Hahnemann believed that scabies infection reflected a more deep-seated, underlying disease, or "miasm," in his patients (*see page 20*), which could be revealed and healed by treatment. He proved the homeopathic remedy, *Psorinum*, from a "nosode" (*see page 20*) of the infection, although it was not published until it was reproved by Hering in 1831. *Psorinum* is given mainly for skin, bowel, and respiratory-tract complaints.

REMEDY PROFILE

There is characteristically an anxious, rather unambitious air to those for whom *Psorinum* is best suited. They are prone to feeling somewhat abandoned, forsaken, and pessimistic.

Lack of stamina is typical. These people generally possess weak constitutions and are easy prey to infections and viruses. Recovery from any illness is slow. Often worse in the winter, they tend to feel the cold strongly, even in summer, wrapping warmly to avoid the chill that aggravates their symptoms, but they can also feel worse from intense heat. Despite a huge appetite, they are usually thin. They have an increased sense of well-being just before the onset of illness, but when ill are prey to morbid fears that they will not recover.

Skin, bowel, or respiratory tract disorders are the primary conditions for which *Psorinum* is prescribed, generally when the underlying vitality is poor.

SKIN CONDITIONS
Symptoms Pus-filled spots, crusting, scaly eruptions, or itchy, blistered patches of skin. The skin always looks dirty, even afterwashing. Pus-filled acne often appears on the face, neck, scalp, and hairline. Prevalence is especially common in teenagers (acne vulgaris) and middle-aged women (acne rosacea). Scaly eruptions are typically caused by eczema, producing large areas of weeping skin or itchy, scaly patches of skin that may blister and are prone to infection and suppuration, with a foul-smelling yellow discharge.
Symptoms better From washing; from warm clothing.
Symptoms worse From overheating due to exertion.

DIARRHEA
Symptoms Diarrhea with spasmodic abdominal cramps, and a strong appetite but no weight gain. If accompanied by a distended abdomen, excessive flatulence, and a feeling of incomplete evacuation during bowel movements, symptoms may indicate irritable bowel syndrome (IBS), and may also include bouts of constipation. Stools are foul-smelling, fluid, gushing, dark, and bloody. Accompanying symptoms may include a headache, and mucus and a burning sensation in the rectum.
Symptoms better In moderate temperatures.
Symptoms worse With cold; with heat; in the early morning; from coffee.

RESPIRATORY ILLNESS
Symptoms Recurrent acute respiratory infections with offensive-smelling phlegm and breathlessness. Sinus infection is common, as is bronchitis or a cough accompanied by great

SOURCE DETAILS

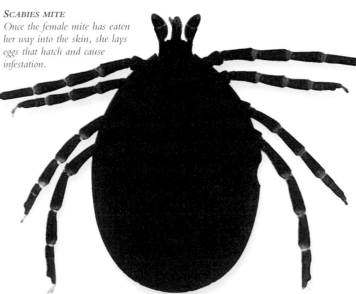

SCABIES MITE
Once the female mite has eaten her way into the skin, she lays eggs that hatch and cause infestation.

ORIGIN
Scabies mite, or *Sarcoptes scabiei*, eats into the skin to lay eggs. Its saliva is highly irritant, causing fluid-filled blisters on the skin. This fluid is used for the remedy.

BACKGROUND
Transmitted via skin contact, scabies is highly contagious and found worldwide. It is treated by applying insecticide lotion to the entire surface area of the skin.

PREPARATION
Fluid is drawn by syringe from a scabies blister on the skin of an infected person. It is sterilized, dissolved in purified water, then diluted and succussed.

KEY SYMPTOMS
DESPAIR AND PESSIMISM ◆ **SENSE OF BEING FORSAKEN** ◆
CHILLINESS ◆ **OFFENSIVE-SMELLING DISCHARGES** ◆
CONSTANT HUNGER

---

fatigue. Symptoms typical of the hay fever and asthma that may respond to *Psorinum* are coughing, breathlessness, and wheezing, often exacerbated by exercise or cold weather. There may be an associated eye or ear infection (*see below*).
Symptoms better In moderate temperatures; lying on the back with the arms outstretched.
Symptoms worse With cold; in open air; from cold drinks.

EYE & EAR INFECTIONS
Symptoms Painful sties with yellow pus, or an eye infection such as conjunctivitis, which causes inflamed eyelids and a yellowish discharge. Ear infections such as otitis media or otitis externa may also be helped by the remedy if there is a foul-smelling discharge.
Symptoms better In moderate temperatures.
Symptoms worse With cold; in the open air.

DEPRESSION
Symptoms Profound fear of personal failure, poverty, and death, with a pessimistic belief that life holds no promise. Feelings of intense loneliness and abandonment may lead to despair and suicidal thoughts.
Symptoms better In warm surroundings; from eating.
Symptoms worse With cold;

SEE ALSO
Rosacea, *page 193*; Severe eczema, *page 194*; Phobias, *page 211*; Skin problems, *page 268*

Sepia officinalis
SEPIA

COMMON NAME
Cuttlefish

CUTTLEFISH INK, ALSO KNOWN AS SEPIA, is used to make a dark brown pigment traditionally used by painters and printers. In 1834 Hahnemann proved the homeopathic remedy, after observing the apathy and depression experienced by an artist friend who frequently licked his sepia-soaked paintbrush while painting. *Sepia* is predominantly prescribed to treat women's health problems, especially during or before menstrual periods, or throughout menopause.

SOURCE DETAILS

CUTTLEFISH
Related to the octopus and squid, this mollusk camouflages itself by changing color and protects itself by squirting its brownish black ink when threatened.

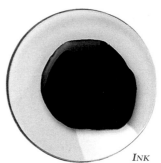

INK

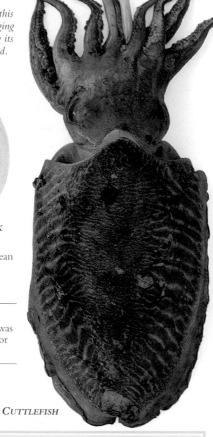

CUTTLEFISH

ORIGIN
Found mainly in the Mediterranean Sea, the preferred habitat of the cuttlefish is near the bottom of waters close to the shore.

BACKGROUND
In ancient Greece cuttlefish ink was used medicinally as a treatment for gonorrhea and kidney stones.

PREPARATION
Cuttlefish ink is dried to a crystalline form and then triturated with lactose sugar.

REMEDY PROFILE

Sepia is best suited to people who are irritable with loved ones but extroverted with others. Often appearing opinionated, detached, and hard, detesting sympathy, they disguise their vulnerability. A sense of sagging or drooping is typical. Despite weepiness, crying does not bring relief.

These individuals typically prefer sour foods and drinks, sweet foods, and alcohol, but dislike milk and pork.

Sepia is chiefly linked with the vagina, uterus, and ovaries. It is used for menopause, premenstrual syndrome (PMS), and some pregnancy-related ailments. Indigestion and headaches, phlegm, discolored, itchy skin, and circulatory problems may also be helped.

indicator of a prolapsed uterus.
Symptoms better In fresh air; with exercise; from crossing the legs; from being occupied; with sleep; from eating.
Symptoms worse In the early morning; in the early evening; in thundery weather; lying on the left side; with fatigue.

FATIGUE
Symptoms Emotional and physical exhaustion. The back and sides may ache, and the muscles may feel weak.
Symptoms better With warmth; in fresh air; with sleep; from being occupied; from vigorous exercise.
Symptoms worse In the early morning; in the early evening; in thundery weather; before menstruation.

WOMEN'S HEALTH
Symptoms *Sepia* may be used for hormone imbalances linked to PMS, and for candida, heavy, painful menstruation, and menopause. Typical symptoms may include a dislike of being touched, particularly before menstruation, during menopause, or if there are associated emotional problems. Before, during, and after pregnancy, emotional and physical ailments such as nausea and fatigue may be helped by the remedy. Sexual intercourse may seem painful, prompting an aversion to it. There may be intense abdominal pressure and stress incontinence on laughing or coughing, which may be an

DIGESTIVE DISORDERS
Symptoms Indigestion and flatulence, with an abdomen that feels tender and empty, even after eating. There may be constipation, with a feeling of a lump in the rectum. Vomiting and nausea may also occur, notably in pregnancy.
Symptoms better With warmth; vigorous exercise.
Symptoms worse With fatigue; lying on the left side.

HEADACHES
Symptoms Headaches that are particularly prevalent on the left side, possibly with nausea, dizziness, and hair loss.
Symptoms better With warmth; from being in fresh

air; with sleep; from eating.
Symptoms worse In the early morning; in the early evening; lying on the left side; before menstruation.

PHLEGM
Symptoms Salty-tasting phlegm caused by an allergy or a cold with a cough.
Symptoms better With warmth; in fresh air.
Symptoms worse At night; during sleep.

SKIN CONDITIONS
Symptoms Discolored, itchy patches, and a yellowish or brownish "saddle" (chloasma) on the nose and cheeks, especially during pregnancy.

Symptoms better In fresh air.
Symptoms worse Before menstruation; in pregnancy.

POOR CIRCULATION
Symptoms Varicose veins, or hot and cold flashes, especially during menopause.
Symptoms better In fresh air; with exercise; from eating.
Symptoms worse In the early morning; in the early evening; before menstruation; during menopause.

KEY SYMPTOMS
CHILLINESS ◆ WEEPINESS ◆ IRRITABILITY ◆
INDIFFERENCE ◆ AVERSION TO SEXUAL INTERCOURSE ◆
CRAVING FOR SOUR FOODS

SEE ALSO
Palpitations, *page 186*; Skin, *pages 192, 242*; Reproduction, *page 198*; Emotional problems, *page 210*; Women's health, *page 256*

Syphilinum
SYPHILINUM

LEGEND RELATES THAT syphilis takes its name from a 16th-century poem by the Italian poet Fracastoro, which portrayed a shepherd named Syphilus as the first victim of the disease. Also known as the "French disease," the incidence of syphilis reached epidemic proportions at the end of the 15th century, then fell dramatically after the development of penicillin in the 20th. After initial infection, symptoms may disappear for years, but left untreated will eventually ravage the body. The remedy *Syphilinum* was proved by the homeopath Dr. Samuel Swan and published in Henry C. Allen's *Materia Medica of Nosodes* (1880–90).

REMEDY PROFILE

Syphilinum is most effective for people with poor memory and concentration. Often highly anxious, possibly with obsessive or compulsive tendencies, they may also have a dependency on alcohol, drugs, or tobacco. Great destructiveness is a key factor, as is a strong fear of disease, possibly culminating in suicidal feelings. Symptoms of physical damage may be evident, often with ulcers and bone pains and distortions. Generally, symptoms appear and disappear gradually, and are worse at night. Alcohol is often craved.

Physical ailments most often treated with *Syphilinum* include ulcers, asthma, constipation, menstrual problems, eye inflammation, and headaches.

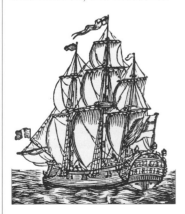

EXPLORERS OF THE AMERICAS
Explorers in the wake of Columbus are thought to have brought syphilis from America to Europe in the 15th century.

ULCERS
Symptoms Recurrent boils, abscesses, and suppurations linked to chronic ulceration, often appearing on the groin. They discharge pus but are relatively painless. Mouth ulcers with excessive salivation may be helped by the remedy.
Symptoms better During the day.
Symptoms worse At night; in extreme heat or cold.

ASTHMA
Symptoms Wheezing and breathlessness, which may be accompanied by a dry cough and tightness in the chest.
Symptoms better For warm, wet, damp weather; during thunderstorms; from breathing mountain air; lying down.
Symptoms worse At night.

CONSTIPATION
Symptoms Obstinate, sluggish bowels, recurring over many years. There may be spasms in the rectum, possibly with a feeling that the rectum is too tight to pass stools.
Symptoms better For walking slowly.
Symptoms worse At night.

OBSESSIVE-COMPULSIVE BEHAVIOR
Symptoms Obsessive or compulsive behavior, such as obsessively washing the hands,

SOURCE DETAILS

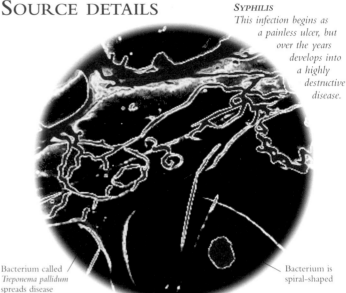

SYPHILIS
This infection begins as a painless ulcer, but over the years develops into a highly destructive disease.

Bacterium called *Treponema pallidum* spreads disease

Bacterium is spiral-shaped

ORIGIN
Caused by the *Treponema pallidum* bacterium, the disease is often spread by sexual intercourse, via mucous membranes or broken skin.

BACKGROUND
Originally treated using mercury and arsenic, which were ineffective and almost as dangerous as syphilis itself. Now treated with penicillin.

PREPARATION
A swab of the serum that coats a syphilis chancre (ulcer) is first sterilized and dissolved in purified water, then diluted and succussed.

KEY SYMPTOMS
COMPULSIVE BEHAVIOR ◆ ULCERS AND DESTRUCTION OF BODY TISSUES ◆ CONDITIONS THAT ARE WORSE AT NIGHT ◆ CRAVING FOR ALCOHOL

---

and generally great anxiety. Substance abuse may be an associated feature. There may be destructive tendencies that extend to the self, possibly leading to suicidal thoughts.
Symptoms better During the day.
Symptoms worse At night.

MENSTRUAL PROBLEMS & MISCARRIAGE
Symptoms Painful, scanty menstrual periods. Menstrual blood has an offensive odor. A vaginal discharge may also be evident, and it is generally unpleasant-smelling, watery, acrid, and profuse. Frequent miscarriage is another ailment for which *Syphilinum* may be prescribed.
Symptoms better During the day.
Symptoms worse At night.

EYE INFLAMMATION
Symptoms Inflamed iris or conjunctiva, perhaps from an ulcer on the cornea. Discharges with pus or mucus may occur.
Symptoms better During the day.
Symptoms worse At night.

HEADACHES
Symptoms An ache that feels as if it is deep in the brain, accompanied by pain over the right eye. The pain is worse when sticking out the tongue.
Symptoms better During the day.
Symptoms worse At night.

SEE ALSO
Asthma, *page 181*; Mouth ulcers, *page 233*; Constipation, *page 238*; Painful periods, *page 256*

Tarentula hispanica syn. *Lycosa tarentula*

TARENTULA

COMMON NAMES
Tarantula, wolf spider, Spanish spider, hunting spider

OFTEN CONFUSED WITH THE formidable American arachnid, which belongs to a different family, this European spider is not deadly. However, its bite was once thought to cause tarantism, a disease marked by either mania or melancholy. The name tarantula is derived from Tarento, a port on the coast of southeast Italy that was particularly associated with the spider. The common names "wolf spider" and "hunting spider" arose from this species' habit of chasing its prey rather than trapping it in a web. *Tarentula* was proved in 1864 by the Spanish homeopath Dr. Nunez, and is used for overstimulation of the nervous system.

SOURCE DETAILS

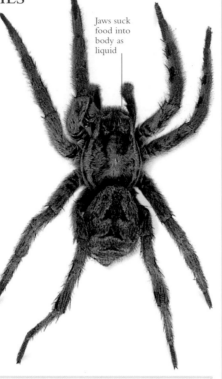

Jaws suck food into body as liquid

TARENTULA
Despite its fearsome reputation, probably based on the link with tarantism and on confusion with the deadly North American tarantula, the bite of this spider is about as toxic as a bee sting.

ORIGIN
Found in many parts of southern Europe.

BACKGROUND
Not used medicinally outside homeopathy, although a related species, the trapdoor spider (*Cteniza fodiens*), is used for swellings and skin ulcers in traditional Chinese medicine.

PREPARATION
The whole, live spider is macerated in alcohol and left to dissolve. The resulting solution is then succussed and diluted.

REMEDY PROFILE

Those who respond best to *Tarentula* often exhibit signs of hyperactivity, overstimulation, and extreme sensitivity to music. They are full of energy, with a constant sense of hurry, impatience, and physical and mental restlessness. A classic symptom is mood swings, where laughter and happiness are rapidly replaced by violent, destructive rage and a marked tendency to be manipulative.

When ill, these people tend to roll from side to side in an attempt to ease the symptoms. Their constant restlessness makes them unable to remain still for any length of time. They often crave salty or spicy foods, and may have a strong aversion to meat.

Tarentula is most commonly prescribed to treat extreme anger and mood swings, restless limbs and chorea (also called St. Vitus' dance), and certain heart problems. It is also given for some ailments affecting women's health.

THE TARANTELLA
This frenetic Italian peasant dance was said to be linked to tarantism, a nervous disorder causing wild, uncontrollable body movements that was popularly thought to be caused by a bite from the wolf spider.

MOOD SWINGS
Symptoms Sudden mood changes switching from gaiety to starkly negative moods that are marked by argumentative, angry, ungrateful behavior. There is a tendency to exhibit extreme sensitivity to music, erratic behavior, or sudden, violent, destructive actions such as smashing something, laughing, and then apologizing.
Symptoms better From music; with relaxation; from massage; from smoking a cigarette.
Symptoms worse If touched; near noise; after menstruation.

RESTLESS LIMBS & CHOREA
Symptoms Constant jerking and trembling of the hands and legs. There may be constant movement, a compulsion to hurry, and frenetic, excess energy, although walking and kneeling may be difficult. The twitching and jerking movements are random and unpredictable, possibly with pins and needles or numbness. Sleep is restless, and there may be a headache that feels as though needles are pricking the brain. There may be great irritability and impatience.
Symptoms better In fresh air; from seeing bright colors; from music; from smoking a cigarette.

KEY SYMPTOMS
SENSITIVITY TO MUSIC ◆ MOOD SWINGS ◆ EXTREME RESTLESSNESS ◆ ROLLING FROM SIDE TO SIDE ◆ PROMISCUITY AND HEIGHTENED LIBIDO ◆ CRAVING FOR SPICY FOODS

Symptoms worse If touched; with movement; near noise; at the same time each year; from witnessing the suffering and pain of others.

ANGINA & HEART DISORDERS
Symptoms Trembling, starts, and thumping in the heart, which feels twisted and out of position. The pulse is irregular and infrequent, and there may be chorea (*see left*).
Symptoms better In fresh air; with rest; from music.
Symptoms worse If touched; near noise; with exertion; putting hands in cold water.

WOMEN'S HEALTH
Symptoms Sensitive genitalia with severe vulval itching. The vagina may feel hot, dry, and raw. Symptoms may be associated with excessive sexual activity and fibroids.
Symptoms better From rolling from side to side.
Symptoms worse If touched; from scratching; after heavy menstruation; on the left side.

CYSTITIS
Symptoms Intense burning and stinging on urinating, a frequent urge to urinate, and incontinence when laughing and coughing. Urine smells foul and has a sandy sediment.
Symptoms better From rolling from side to side; with rest.
Symptoms worse With cold; in the evening; if touched; after menstruation.

SEE ALSO
Multiple sclerosis, *page 179*; Diabetes, *page 191*

Tuberculinum Koch & T. bovum

TUBERCULINUM

COMMON NAME
Tuberculosis

O NE QUARTER OF ALL DEATHS in Europe in the mid-19th century were due to tuberculosis (TB). It was a major killer worldwide, particularly in areas subject to poverty, malnutrition, or disease, until the German bacteriologist Robert Koch identified the bacillus in 1882, and discovered that a preparation of tuberculinum (dead tuberculosis bacilli) could be used to treat and prevent it. The British homeopath Dr. James Compton Burnett began a series of tests on lung tissue from infected patients in 1885, and by 1890 was able to prove the homeopathic remedy, which is given mainly for respiratory tract complaints.

REMEDY PROFILE

Intensity and yearning are two traits that characterize people most suited to *Tuberculinum*. There is typically a longing for constant stimulation and change that may manifest itself, for example, in a desire to change partners, to change jobs, to travel, or to frequently change the decor of the home.

These tendencies can have negative consequences. For example, a deep, romantic longing unfulfilled by a string of partners may ultimately lead to disillusionment. This and a lack of fulfillment may result in maliciousness, cruelty, and destructive anger, and may even lead to alcohol or drug addiction. Many 19th-century Romantic composers and artists were of this disposition: Their works display the bittersweet quality and underlying dissatisfaction typical of this temperament.

Although the remedy is not used for TB itself, many people suited to *Tuberculinum* have a family history of TB infection. Common symptoms include a susceptibility to colds and persistent tiredness. Symptoms improve in fresh, dry air, such as mountain air. There is a desire for candy, cold milk, and smoked meats, and a tendency to perspire heavily during the night.

COUGHS & ACUTE BRONCHITIS
Symptoms A dry, hard, possibly recurrent cough, with fever and night sweats. Sharp pains may be felt in the upper left lung. The lymph glands in the neck may be enlarged. If symptoms are associated with bronchitis, there is shortness of breath, wheezing, and a persistent cough with yellow phlegm. Eventually, illness may lead to emaciation.
Symptoms better In fresh air; in cool winds; in dry surroundings.
Symptoms worse With heat; in dampness and humidity; in stuffy surroundings; with physical exertion.

COLDS
Symptoms A recurrent, persistent chest cold, with solid, yellow phlegm, a slight fever, and aching muscles. The eyes have a tendency to water, and the throat is sore.
Symptoms better In fresh air;

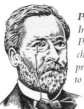
PASTEURIZATION
In the 1860s Louis Pasteur, a French chemist, developed a process of heating milk to kill harmful bacteria, leaving it safe to consume. Before he invented this process, called pasteurization, TB was regularly contracted through milk from infected cows.

SOURCE DETAILS

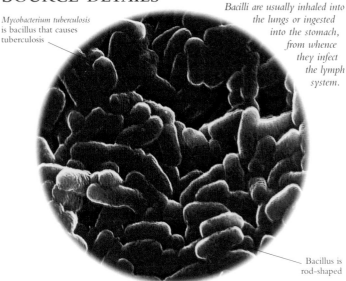

Mycobacterium tuberculosis is bacillus that causes tuberculosis

TUBERCULOSIS
Bacilli are usually inhaled into the lungs or ingested into the stomach, from whence they infect the lymph system.

Bacillus is rod-shaped

ORIGIN
Prepared from human sputum (*Koch*) or bovine lymph gland tissue (*bovum*) infected with *Mycobacterium tuberculosis*.

BACKGROUND
Once a major killer, TB fell in incidence through vaccination, but is now rising again, partly due to the prevalence of HIV.

PREPARATION
Bacilli from infected tissue or sputum are sterilized, dissolved in purified water, diluted, and succussed.

KEY SYMPTOMS
CONSTANT DESIRE FOR CHANGE ♦ IRRITABLE, MALICIOUS TEMPERAMENT ♦ ROMANTIC NATURE ♦ SUSCEPTIBILITY TO RECURRENT RESPIRATORY ILLNESS ♦ DESIRE FOR OPEN AIR

in cool, dry surroundings.
Symptoms worse In dry cold; in dampness and humidity; in stuffy rooms.

ARTHRITIC PAINS
Symptoms Aching joint and limb pains that move from one part of the body to another. There may also be initial stiffness that loosens with movement. The limbs are weary and restless.
Symptoms better In fresh air; in cool, dry surroundings.
Symptoms worse With cold; in dampness and humidity; with physical exertion.

HAY FEVER
Symptoms A runny nose with constant sneezing, nasal congestion, and watery mucus. The eyes tend to water.
Symptoms better In fresh air; in cool, dry surroundings.

Symptoms worse With cold; in dampness and humidity; with physical exertion.

NEUROTIC BEHAVIOR
Symptoms Irritable, malicious behavior, with a strong sense of discontent. This can cause a compulsive urge to change job, move home, or travel. A sense of lack of fulfillment is often combined with an incurably romantic nature. There is a tendency to suffer insomnia.
Symptoms better In fresh air; in cool, dry surroundings.
Symptoms worse With cold; in damp and humidity; with physical exertion.

SEE ALSO
Asthma, *page 181*; Tuberculosis, *page 182*; Osteoarthritis, *page 196*; Allergies, *page 206*

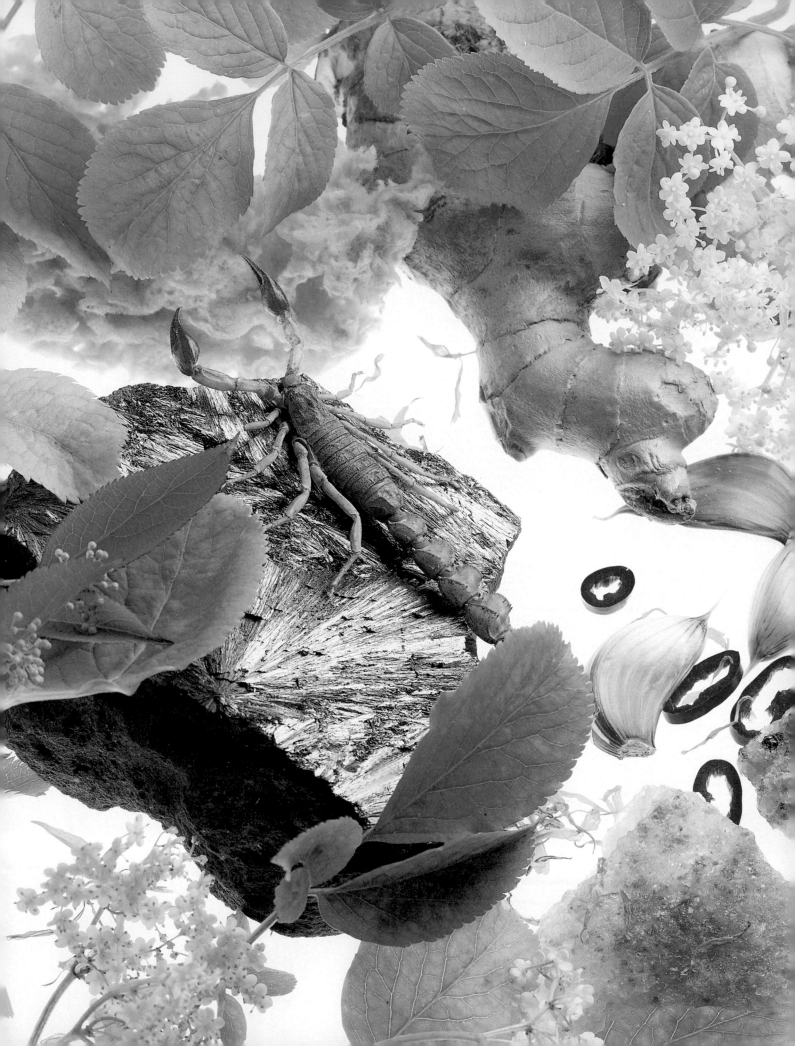

MINOR REMEDIES

THE FULL HOMEOPATHIC MATERIA MEDICA CONTAINS

OVER 2,000 REMEDIES MADE FROM A WIDE

VARIETY OF MATERIAL FROM THE PLANT, MINERAL,

AND ANIMAL KINGDOMS, SOME OF WHICH

ARE MORE COMMONLY USED THAN OTHERS. THIS

SECTION PROVIDES PROFILES OF APPROXIMATELY 250

OF THE MOST IMPORTANT MINOR REMEDIES.

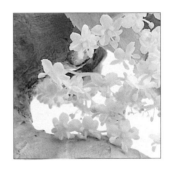
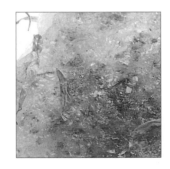
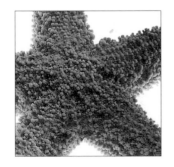

Abies canadensis syn. *Tsuga canadensis*

ABIES CAN.

COMMON NAMES Hemlock spruce, Canada pitch, Canada spruce.
ORIGIN Native to North America and eastern Asia.
BACKGROUND As early as 1535 Native Americans used this plant internally for indigestion, and externally (mixed with castor oil) for gonorrhea.
PREPARATION The fresh bark and young buds are macerated in alcohol.

REMEDY PROFILE

Abies can. is best suited to people who tend to be either fretful or quiet and careful. Often weak, nervous, and light-headed, they may lie down frequently, especially with their legs drawn up, to avoid fainting.

Classic physical characteristics include chilliness and clammy skin, a sensation that the blood has turned to cold water, or a feeling that there is a wet cloth between the shoulder blades.

Abies can. is given primarily to treat digestive disorders associated with inflamed mucous membranes in the stomach and poor absorption of food. Overeating is common in such cases; even after eating there are hunger pains and rumbling in the bowels. Nausea, bloating, and severe burning pain in the abdomen may cause palpitations to develop in the heart.
Symptoms better From pressure on the affected area; from passing gas.
Symptoms worse After standing for long periods; from sitting; from drinking tea.

Acanthia lectularia
syn. *Cimex lectularius*

CIMEX

COMMON NAME Bedbug.
ORIGIN Found in unsanitary environments in temperate regions.
BACKGROUND The ancient Greeks and Romans crushed bedbugs with salt and human milk to make an eye ointment. When powdered they were used for fevers and as a preventive remedy for plague.
PREPARATION Live bedbugs are steeped in alcohol, diluted, and succussed.

REMEDY PROFILE

Cimex is most appropriate for those who are prey to anxiety, especially after a chill or drinking alcohol. They may adopt a crouching position, desiring to creep into their own body because they are unable to curl themselves up sufficiently. A chilly stage may develop prior to fever, during which they may be violent, wanting to tear everything to pieces or clenching their hands in rage.

Cimex is typically prescribed for certain types of joint or muscle aches accompanied by a strong compulsion to stretch and, sometimes, chills and fever. Muscles and tendons may feel too short for the limbs.
Symptoms better From sitting huddled up; from passing gas; from avoiding alcohol.
Symptoms worse With movement; with stretching.

Achillea millefolium

MILLEFOLIUM

COMMON NAMES Yarrow, milfoil, woundwort, stanchweed, nosebleed.
ORIGIN Native to Europe and western Asia, yarrow grows wild in meadows and waste ground in temperate regions.
BACKGROUND The Latin name of this plant derives from the warrior Achilles, the Greek hero of the Trojan war, who

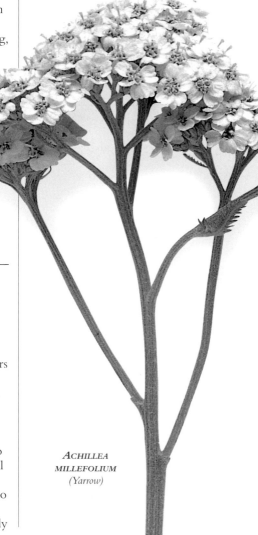

**ACHILLEA
MILLEFOLIUM**
(Yarrow)

used yarrow to stanch the wounds of his soldiers. The plant has also been used for centuries in Europe as a bitter tonic.
PREPARATION The fresh, flowering aerial parts are chopped and steeped in alcohol.

REMEDY PROFILE

Millefolium best suits those who tend to be most irritable in the evening. Longing for rest but going to bed late, they wake feeling unrefreshed, confused, dizzy, and stupefied, as if drunk. When irritable, they may become overly excitable and violent. Children who fit this profile tend to moan and sigh.

Millefolium is used chiefly for bleeding from injuries, and for internal bleeding and menstrual irregularities, such as delayed or absent menstruation that may lead to convulsions, or heavy menstrual periods that impair fertility. *Millefolium* may also be given in pregnancy for severe colicky pain, diarrhea, and painful varicose veins, or for recovery from miscarriage. It is used for profuse, painless uterine bleeding following childbirth or an abortion, and for sore nipples and suppressed breast milk after childbirth.

The other key symptom for *Millefolium* is congestion, associated with piercing pains in the ears, teeth, and temples. There may be congestion in the ears, eyes, nose, and chest.
Symptoms better From bleeding; if regular menstruation is reestablished; from wine.
Symptoms worse With sleeping or lying down; from bending double; from lifting; from violent exertion; from injury; from coffee.

Acidum aceticum

ACETIC AC.

COMMON NAMES Acetic acid, glacial acetic acid, ethanoic acid.
ORIGIN Chemically prepared.
BACKGROUND Dilute acetic acid is a principal component of vinegar, and is used in the herbal and culinary traditions of many diverse cultures.
PREPARATION Acetic acid is dissolved in alcohol, diluted, and succussed.

REMEDY PROFILE

People who benefit most from *Acetic ac.* often sigh because they feel depressed, anxious, or irritable, and are also prone to forgetfulness. They are often anemic, with pale, waxy, clammy skin and intense thirst. Despite profound sleepiness, they may find it difficult to sleep.

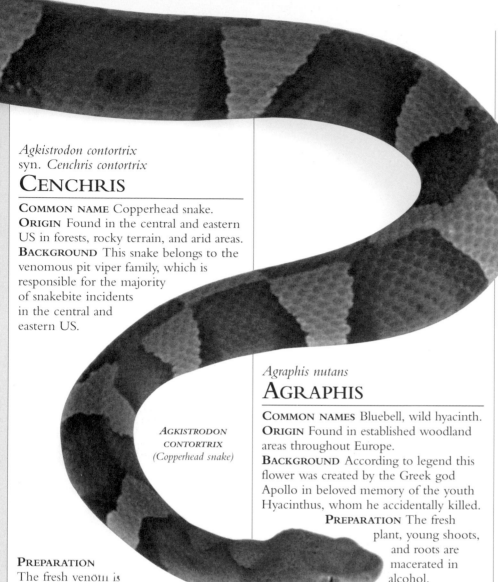

**AGKISTRODON
CONTORTRIX**
(Copperhead snake)

CENCHRIS

Agkistrodon contortrix
syn. *Cenchris contortrix*

COMMON NAME Copperhead snake.
ORIGIN Found in the central and eastern US in forests, rocky terrain, and arid areas.
BACKGROUND This snake belongs to the venomous pit viper family, which is responsible for the majority of snakebite incidents in the central and eastern US.

PREPARATION
The fresh venom is triturated with lactose sugar.

REMEDY PROFILE

Cenchris is particularly suitable for people who experience great mental restlessness, jealousy, suspicion, and abandonment. They have a general tendency to be rather absentminded, moody, and dreamy, often experiencing vivid, horrible dreams that continue in their thoughts once they are awake. Their anxieties may include a fear of rape, pins and pointed objects, going to sleep, and sudden death.

The classic symptom picture for *Cenchris* is of breathlessness, mental and physical restlessness, and a desire to drink small quantities of water. Another classic symptom is a need to loosen the clothing, triggered by congestion in the blood vessels. Complaints are usually right-sided. There may be a susceptibility to allergies, especially in the spring.
Symptoms better In the morning.
Symptoms worse In the afternoon, in the evening, and all night; lying down; on waking; from pressure on the affected area.

122

AGRAPHIS

Agraphis nutans

COMMON NAMES Bluebell, wild hyacinth.
ORIGIN Found in established woodland areas throughout Europe.
BACKGROUND According to legend this flower was created by the Greek god Apollo in beloved memory of the youth Hyacinthus, whom he accidentally killed.
PREPARATION The fresh plant, young shoots, and roots are macerated in alcohol.

REMEDY PROFILE

People for whom *Agraphis* is best suited are low in vitality and prone to catching colds. The classic symptom picture is of ear, nose, and throat infections linked to phlegm and deafness, particularly during childhood. There may be phlegm in the bridge of the nose, obstructing the nostrils, and discharges from all the mucous membranes. Chills develop easily after exposure to cold winds, accompanied by diarrhea with mucus. During infection the tonsils and adenoids may be swollen.
Symptoms better With shelter from winds; lying on the stomach.
Symptoms worse In heat and humidity.

AILANTHUS

Ailanthus altissima

COMMON NAMES Tree of heaven, shade tree, Chinese sumac, copal tree.
ORIGIN Native to China and India, but can now also be found growing in North America, Europe, and Australia.

BACKGROUND In Australia and Asia the tree's bark was used for profuse vaginal discharge, gonorrhea, worms, malaria, and asthma. Chinese herbalists use it to treat diarrhea and dysentery.
PREPARATION The fresh, budding flowers are macerated in alcohol.

REMEDY PROFILE

Ailanthus is best suited to those who feel extremely weak when ill, and frequently behave in a stupid, dull, and confused way. They may feel anxious, odd, or even insane. Key symptoms indicating that this remedy is suitable are fevers with great weakness and congestion of the blood, which typically gives the skin a purple, mottled, swollen appearance. It is often given for acute bouts of infectious mononucleosis with swollen tonsils and neck glands. Pain extends from the neck glands to the ears when swallowing. The tonsils on the left side are mainly affected, and may develop oozing mucus or ulcers.
Symptoms better Lying on the right side; from hot drinks.
Symptoms worse From skin eruptions that fail to develop; with any movement; from sitting up; from the sight of food.

SEE ALSO Infectious mononucleosis, *page 254*

ALLIUM SAT.

Allium sativum

COMMON NAME Garlic.
ORIGIN Native to central Asia, and now grown worldwide.
BACKGROUND Garlic is one of the most ancient of herbs, used by the Babylonians as early as c. 3000 BCE. A popular culinary herb and an important medicinal plant, it is valued for its antibiotic properties.
PREPARATION The fresh garlic bulbs are minced and macerated in alcohol.

REMEDY PROFILE

Allium sat. is most appropriate for people who are oversensitive and need company. Although subject to many fears, they have a particular fear of being poisoned. They generally enjoy a rich, gourmet diet, especially one that includes meat, but are prone to indigestion and phlegm problems.

The remedy is primarily associated with indigestion caused by a rich diet or by dietary change. The digestive process is accompanied by pressure in the upper abdomen, foul-smelling gas, and colicky pains around the navel. Dull pains in the bowels and either constipation or diarrhea may be present. *Allium sat.* is also used to treat tearing pains in the hip area and abdomen.

Adonis vernalis
ADONIS

COMMON NAMES False hellebore, yellow pheasant's eye.
ORIGIN Native to Russia and the Black Sea region, and now found in much of Europe, growing on mountain pastures.
BACKGROUND The plant takes its name from Adonis, a Greek mythological figure linked to the seasonal renewal of plant life. In Russia it is used as a heart remedy.
PREPARATION The chopped aerial parts of the plant are steeped in alcohol.

REMEDY PROFILE
People for whom *Adonis* is suitable tend to be apprehensive and prone to horrible dreams and restless sleep. They generally feel "waterlogged" and uncomfortable.

The classic symptom picture for *Adonis* is of heart degeneration, perhaps following a severe bout of the flu or rheumatic fever. There may be pain and palpitations in the area around the heart. The heart rhythms may be abnormally rapid or slow and faltering, possibly because of diseased valves or fatty degeneration. Edema (an irregular accumulation of fluid in the body tissues or cavities), which develops as a result of poor circulation and is accompanied by scant urine flow, may be treated by *Adonis*.

The remedy is also used to treat asthma with breathlessness, discomfort, or heart disease. Further symptoms may include headaches that move from the back of the head around the temples to the eyes.
Symptoms better From exertion.
Symptoms worse With cold; lying down.

Aesculus hippocastanum
AESCULUS

COMMON NAMES Horse chestnut, conker.
ORIGIN Native to southeastern Europe, and grown in temperate areas worldwide.
BACKGROUND The common name is thought to originate from the traditional Turkish custom of feeding the nuts to horses as an antidote to flatulence.
PREPARATION The fresh, ripe, peeled, and finely chopped horse chestnuts are macerated in alcohol.

REMEDY PROFILE
This remedy is best suited to people who are very low, depressed, and irritable, with poor concentration. They may lose their temper easily, tending to brood afterward.

The remedy is given primarily for treating hemorrhoids, especially when the rectum feels dry and uncomfortable, as

though it is full of small sticks, or when the hemorrhoids are internal and associated with constipation and pain in the lower back. Often the anus feels hot, dry, and itchy. Lumpy stools may occur, with stabbing, tearing, or splinterlike pains in the anus. Distension in the bowels may develop, with colicky pain and foul-smelling gas. There may be varicose veins, and a feeling of congestion and tenderness in the liver. The hemorrhoids may be associated with pains and chills in the spine, and a dull, constant backache that makes bending down or rising after sitting difficult, and walking almost impossible.

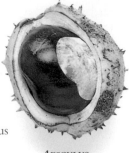

AESCULUS HIPPOCASTANUM
(Horse chestnut)

In addition, the remedy is given for a dry, rough, burning throat accompanied by sneezing and profuse phlegm.
Symptoms better In cool air (unless it is directly inhaled).
Symptoms worse From bending or getting up from a seat; walking; standing; from breathing deeply; from swallowing; from passing stools; after eating.

SEE ALSO Hemorrhoids, *page 238*

Aethusa cynapium
AETHUSA

COMMON NAME Fool's parsley.
ORIGIN Found throughout Europe.
BACKGROUND The poison from this plant is thought to produce marked dullness and stupor, hence its common name of fool's parsley.
PREPARATION The whole flowering plant, with the root and unripe fruits, is chopped and macerated in alcohol.

REMEDY PROFILE
People who respond best to *Aethusa* are often characterized by poor concentration and a tendency to be easily distracted. They are generally reserved, alienated, reclusive, and irritable.

Key symptoms associated with *Aethusa* include a confused state of mind with scattered thoughts; those affected may talk to themselves and behave foolishly. Other typical symptoms can include marked dullness and a sluggish mental state, possibly linked with an inability to study. These symptoms may be

accompanied by prostration with a sense of staleness, or anxiety with associated nervous diarrhea.

Aethusa is also appropriate for children with milk intolerance, notably babies who are prone to sudden vomiting after feeding, and who may have diarrhea. Lack of nutrition may set up a cycle of hunger, frequent feeding, and subsequent violent vomiting. This may result in a state of extreme exhaustion and collapse, causing the baby's face to appear drawn, agonized, and aged. It may also seem as though the baby's whole body has enlarged, particularly in the heart area.
Symptoms better In open air; from walking; from company and conversation; with rest.
Symptoms worse With warmth and hot weather; between 3 A.M. and 4 A.M.; from overexertion; from eating frequently; from milk.

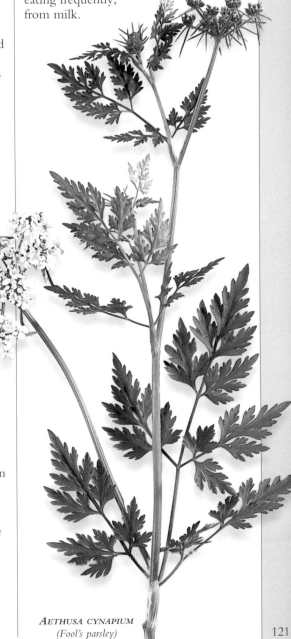

AETHUSA CYNAPIUM
(Fool's parsley)

Debilitation and emaciation are the key factors linked to this remedy. It is often prescribed to treat fainting, breathlessness, water retention, diabetes, or great exhaustion following an injury, an operation, or hemorrhaging.

Severe burning pains and tenderness in the stomach can also be treated using *Acetic ac.*, if they are accompanied by symptoms such as sour-tasting burps, vomiting, and profuse salivation, or by the classic debilitation symptoms.

Symptoms better Lying on the stomach; from burping; from eating potatoes.

Symptoms worse In the morning; with movement; with overexertion; lying on the back; from bread and butter; from vegetables; from cold drinks; from wine.

Acidum benzoicum
BENZOIC AC.

COMMON NAME Benzoic acid.
ORIGIN Chemically prepared.
BACKGROUND Found naturally in Siam benzoic resin, this acid was first produced synthetically in the 1860s from coal tar. It is widely used as a food preservative.
PREPARATION Benzoic acid is dissolved in alcohol, diluted, and succussed.

REMEDY PROFILE

Benzoic ac. is best suited to those who tend to alternate between excitable behavior and a state of deep, stuporous sleep, general dullness, and weariness. A preoccupation with unpleasant topics may cause them to dwell on their own and other people's misfortunes. They are often extremely sensitive to noise, especially if they have Ménière's disease (a disorder of the inner ear). Babies who respond well to *Benzoic ac.* like to be picked up and held, but dislike being laid down.

Wandering pains are the key symptoms associated with this remedy, such as pains that move from the leg joints to the internal organs, especially the heart, and then radiate to the joints of the extremities. Other symptoms may include joints that crack, with redness and swelling that may be linked to acute gout, and sharp, tearing pains in the joints of the big toe.

The remedy is used particularly if symptoms include profuse, dark brown, strong-smelling urine and incontinence at night, or if there are frothy, white stools that smell offensive.

Symptoms better With warmth; with rest; from passing large quantities of urine.

Symptoms worse With cold; in damp weather; in drafts; with movement; from scanty flow of urine; from chocolate, candy, alcohol, coffee, and wine.

Acidum boricum
BORIC AC.

COMMON NAMES Boric acid, boracic acid, orthoboric acid.
ORIGIN Chemically prepared.
BACKGROUND Used as a mild antiseptic in conventional medicine, boric acid is more commonly utilized in the nuclear industry.
PREPARATION Powdered or crystallized boric acid is triturated with lactose sugar.

REMEDY PROFILE

Low spirits, sighing and weeping, and a state of mental and physical collapse are all indications of the suitability of *Boric ac.* All parts of the body feel cold, although paradoxically the remedy may be used for menopausal hot flashes.

Typical symptoms treated by *Boric ac.* include a heavy, nauseous feeling in the stomach, with profuse, cold saliva and a dry, furred tongue and throat. It is also prescribed for headaches accompanied by nausea, for dizziness, and for eyes that are prone to swelling and conjunctivitis, and aggravated by light.

Boric ac. is also taken for its antiseptic properties. It is used to halt putrefaction in wounds, and for skin eruptions that are accompanied by flaking, itching, and hard, red, swollen patches.

Symptoms better Walking in open air.

Symptoms worse No specific factors.

Acidum carbolicum
CARBOLIC AC.

COMMON NAMES Carbolic acid, phenol.
ORIGIN Chemically prepared.
BACKGROUND In 19th-century Europe and the US this acid was used to sterilize surgical equipment. It is an antiseptic and disinfectant, although prolonged contact can lead to health problems.
PREPARATION Carbolic acid is dissolved in purified water, diluted, and succussed.

REMEDY PROFILE

This remedy is most suited to those who tend to be restless, irritable, forgetful, and bewildered. Often exhausted, they yawn and stretch constantly, and have a very acute sense of smell. Perplexing dreams leave them unrefreshed after sleep.

Carbolic ac. is used for sudden burning, prickling, stinging pains, typically with marked collapse, such as the anaphylactic shock that may follow a bee sting. It is also prescribed for malignant or septic wounds, particularly if these are linked to compound fractures. Another use of the remedy is for treating increased urine production with or without burning

pain, possibly associated with diabetes or other diseases that may affect urine production. Urine is typically dark black or green in color, and is accompanied by putrid, strong-smelling discharges, notably from the anus.

The remedy may additionally be used to treat vomiting caused by sea sickness, pregnancy, or cancer. The vomiting is accompanied by a constant thirst for water, a tendency to burp, and abdominal pain. Offensive-smelling diarrhea, dysentery, or cholera may also be treated, as may constipation with foul breath.

Symptoms better From rubbing and binding up painful areas; from smoking; from strong tea.

Symptoms worse During pregnancy; from jarring and walking; with mental exertion.

Acidum hydrochloricum
syn. *A. muriaticum*
MURIATIC AC.

COMMON NAME Hydrochloric acid.
ORIGIN Chemically prepared.
BACKGROUND Discovered by alchemists in the 13th century, hydrochloric acid is present in the stomach's gastric juices. In excess it can cause gastric ulcers to develop, while a deficiency leads to poor food absorption and anemia.
PREPARATION The acid is dissolved in alcohol, diluted, and succussed.

REMEDY PROFILE

People for whom *Muriatic ac.* is most appropriate tend to feel too weak to move. Drowsy by day, but restless in bed, they have anxious dreams and are prone to talking in their sleep. They may be either sad and reserved or loquacious. Often irritable and fretful, their minds may be crowded with thoughts.

This remedy is typically prescribed for weakness or physical collapse, such as that associated with chronic fatigue syndrome, or developing after a feverish illness such as infectious mononucleosis or typhoid. The muscles, especially those of the heart, tongue, bladder, and anus, may be weak, exhausted, or partially paralyzed.

Muriatic ac. is given when the collapsed state is associated with dryness, bleeding, and ulceration of the mucous membranes of the mouth and digestive tract. A heavy tongue and dry mouth may make talking difficult, and deep-seated canker sores or small tumors may develop on the tongue.

Symptoms better With warmth; with movement; lying on the left side.

Symptoms worse In wet weather; from touch; from swimming in the ocean; during menstruation; from cold drinks.

Acidum oxalicum
OXALIC AC.

COMMON NAME Oxalic acid.
ORIGIN Chemically prepared.
BACKGROUND Identified as a constituent of wood sorrel in the 17th century, this acid was first made synthetically in 1776.
PREPARATION Oxalic acid crystals are dissolved in alcohol, diluted, and succussed.

REMEDY PROFILE
Oxalic ac. is used for those whose pains occur violently and briefly in localized areas of the body, and who generally feel worse from dwelling on them. They are nervous, confused, dizzy people, who often have trouble sleeping.

Usually the remedy is given for angina with palpitations that worsen when lying down. When those affected think about their heart, it seems to make it flutter or beat intermittently. In men, other symptoms that can be treated by *Oxalic ac.* include throbbing, crushing pain in the testes, and pain in the spermatic cord.
Symptoms better After passing stools; from changing position.
Symptoms worse With cold; from mental exertion; from dwelling on symptoms; from light; in the early morning; in the evening or at night; with movement; from being touched on the left side; from shaving; from grapes, strawberries, or sour fruit; from sugar; from coffee; from wine.

Acidum picrinicum
PICRIC AC.

COMMON NAMES Picric acid, trinitrophenol.
ORIGIN Chemically prepared.
BACKGROUND This acid derives its name from the Greek *pikros*, meaning "bitter." It is used as a yellow dye and in explosives.
PREPARATION The crystals are dissolved in alcohol, diluted, and succussed.

REMEDY PROFILE
Picric ac. is best suited to people who are prone to intellectual collapse and nervous exhaustion – perhaps students who have worked too hard for examinations. They have a tendency to be indifferent, listless, and unmotivated, and the slightest exertion makes them want to lie down. Exhaustion and poor concentration are other common symptoms.

The classic symptom picture for *Picric ac.* is of indifference with great mental and physical fatigue, which may develop into actual paralysis. Muscular pains in the limbs may accompany fatigue, and there may be weak, heavy sensations in the limbs and back, and burning along the spine, particularly from exertion. The hands and feet may feel cold.
Symptoms better From bandaging sore areas; with rest; in the sun and open air; from cold air; from bathing in cold water.
Symptoms worse With movement; from mental exertion; from any secretion, such as semen, blood, or vaginal discharge.

Acidum salicylicum
SALICYLIC AC.

COMMON NAME Salicylic acid.
ORIGIN Obtained originally from the bark of the willow tree, but now commercially prepared from phenol.
BACKGROUND Salicylic acid is the main ingredient of aspirin. It was first used to prepare aspirin by the Italian chemist R. Piria in 1838.
PREPARATION Salicylic acid crystals are triturated with lactose sugar.

REMEDY PROFILE
This remedy is most appropriate for those who are prone to extreme prostration, weakness, and fainting, often due to post-viral fatigue. They may be mild-natured, restless, or anxious, and tend to be either highly excited or stupefied and dull. They are sleepy and yawn often, but wake frequently from sleep thinking that they hear music.

Key symptoms associated with *Salicylic ac.* are weakness, ulceration, and ear problems such as tinnitus, vertigo, and progressive deafness, possibly due to Ménière's disease (a disorder of the inner ear). The remedy may also be used for severe headaches with piercing pains that start at the top or back of the head. Any ulceration tends to focus on the mucous membranes: canker sores, for instance, may be treated with *Salicylic ac.*
Symptoms better From hot compresses, especially dry compresses.
Symptoms worse In cold air; at night; from the slightest touch; with movement.

SEE ALSO Tinnitus, *page 222*

Acidum sulfuricum
SULFURIC AC.

COMMON NAMES Sulfuric acid, oil of vitriol.
ORIGIN Chemically prepared.
BACKGROUND This oily, corrosive liquid was first discovered by alchemists in the 13th century. It is used to manufacture dyes, drugs, and fertilizers.
PREPARATION Sulfuric acid is dissolved in alcohol, diluted, and succussed.

REMEDY PROFILE
People for whom *Sulfuric ac.* is best suited are hurried, mentally restless, and excitable, despite great exhaustion, weakness, and trembling. Usually mentally sharp, they are prone to nervous exhaustion, becoming absentminded and dull when ill.

The classic symptom picture for this remedy is of extreme fatigue following an injury, concussion, or operation, especially if healing is slow, with bruising, bleeding, ulceration, gangrene, or other symptoms of decay. There is often a marked sensitivity to pollutants such as smoke. The remedy may also be prescribed for diabetes.
Symptoms better In moderate temperatures; lying on the affected side; with hot drinks.
Symptoms worse In the open air; during menopause; from injuries; from the smell of coffee; from air pollution and tobacco smoke.

SEE ALSO Diabetes, *page 191*

Actaea spicata
ACTAEA SPIC.

COMMON NAMES Baneberry, herb Christopher.
ORIGIN Native to Eurasia, although now found in many temperate regions of the northern hemisphere.
BACKGROUND Herbalists use this plant to treat rheumatic symptoms, especially those occurring in minor joints. Its purplish black berries are used in dyes.
PREPARATION The fresh root, collected after the shoots emerge and before bloom, is chopped and macerated in alcohol.

REMEDY PROFILE
Actaea spic. is most suited to sad, absent-minded people who are easily startled and often prey to fear or anxiety. They are prone to a fear of death, particularly when in bed at night. Their judgment is generally poor, and they may feel hopeless, confused, impatient, and restless, especially if they experience a shock. They may even think that they are going insane.

Actaea spic. is usually given for this state of mind in conjunction with rheumatoid arthritis that is accompanied by tearing pains, especially if minor joints such as the wrists are affected. The pain may be so severe that the limbs actually feel paralyzed, causing crying out, weariness, and possibly eventual lameness.
Symptoms better No specific factors.
Symptoms worse From changes in the weather or temperature; from cold air; at night; if touched; from the slightest fatigue; from the slightest exertion; from mental exertion.

Adonis vernalis
ADONIS

COMMON NAMES False hellebore, yellow pheasant's eye.
ORIGIN Native to Russia and the Black Sea region, and now found in much of Europe, growing on mountain pastures.
BACKGROUND The plant takes its name from Adonis, a Greek mythological figure linked to the seasonal renewal of plant life. In Russia it is used as a heart remedy.
PREPARATION The chopped aerial parts of the plant are steeped in alcohol.

REMEDY PROFILE

People for whom *Adonis* is suitable tend to be apprehensive and prone to horrible dreams and restless sleep. They generally feel "waterlogged" and uncomfortable.

The classic symptom picture for *Adonis* is of heart degeneration, perhaps following a severe bout of the flu or rheumatic fever. There may be pain and palpitations in the area around the heart. The heart rhythms may be abnormally rapid or slow and faltering, possibly because of diseased valves or fatty degeneration. Edema (an irregular accumulation of fluid in the body tissues or cavities), which develops as a result of poor circulation and is accompanied by scant urine flow, may be treated by *Adonis*.

The remedy is also used to treat asthma with breathlessness, discomfort, or heart disease. Further symptoms may include headaches that move from the back of the head around the temples to the eyes.
Symptoms better From exertion.
Symptoms worse With cold; lying down.

Aesculus hippocastanum
AESCULUS

COMMON NAMES Horse chestnut, conker.
ORIGIN Native to southeastern Europe, and grown in temperate areas worldwide.
BACKGROUND The common name is thought to·originate from the traditional Turkish custom of feeding the nuts to horses as an antidote to flatulence.
PREPARATION The fresh, ripe, peeled, and finely chopped horse chestnuts are macerated in alcohol.

REMEDY PROFILE

This remedy is best suited to people who are very low, depressed, and irritable, with poor concentration. They may lose their temper easily, tending to brood afterward.

The remedy is given primarily for treating hemorrhoids, especially when the rectum feels dry and uncomfortable, as though it is full of small sticks, or when the hemorrhoids are internal and associated with constipation and pain in the lower back. Often the anus feels hot, dry, and itchy. Lumpy stools may occur, with stabbing, tearing, or splinterlike pains in the anus. Distension in the bowels may develop, with colicky pain and foul-smelling gas. There may be varicose veins, and a feeling of congestion and tenderness in the liver. The hemorrhoids may be associated with pains and chills in the spine, and a dull, constant backache that makes bending down or rising after sitting difficult, and walking almost impossible.

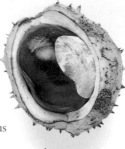

AESCULUS HIPPOCASTANUM
(Horse chestnut)

In addition, the remedy is given for a dry, rough, burning throat accompanied by sneezing and profuse phlegm.
Symptoms better In cool air (unless it is directly inhaled).
Symptoms worse From bending or getting up from a seat; walking; standing; from breathing deeply; from swallowing; from passing stools; after eating.

SEE ALSO Hemorrhoids, *page 238*

Aethusa cynapium
AETHUSA

COMMON NAME Fool's parsley.
ORIGIN Found throughout Europe.
BACKGROUND The poison from this plant is thought to produce marked dullness and stupor, hence its common name of fool's parsley.
PREPARATION The whole flowering plant, with the root and unripe fruits, is chopped and macerated in alcohol.

REMEDY PROFILE

People who respond best to *Aethusa* are often characterized by poor concentration and a tendency to be easily distracted. They are generally reserved, alienated, reclusive, and irritable.

Key symptoms associated with *Aethusa* include a confused state of mind with scattered thoughts; those affected may talk to themselves and behave foolishly. Other typical symptoms can include marked dullness and a sluggish mental state, possibly linked with an inability to study. These symptoms may be accompanied by prostration with a sense of staleness, or anxiety with associated nervous diarrhea.

Aethusa is also appropriate for children with milk intolerance, notably babies who are prone to sudden vomiting after feeding, and who may have diarrhea. Lack of nutrition may set up a cycle of hunger, frequent feeding, and subsequent violent vomiting. This may result in a state of extreme exhaustion and collapse, causing the baby's face to appear drawn, agonized, and aged. It may also seem as though the baby's whole body has enlarged, particularly in the heart area.
Symptoms better In open air; from walking; from company and conversation; with rest.
Symptoms worse With warmth and hot weather; between 3 A.M. and 4 A.M.; from overexertion; from eating frequently; from milk.

AETHUSA CYNAPIUM
(Fool's parsley)

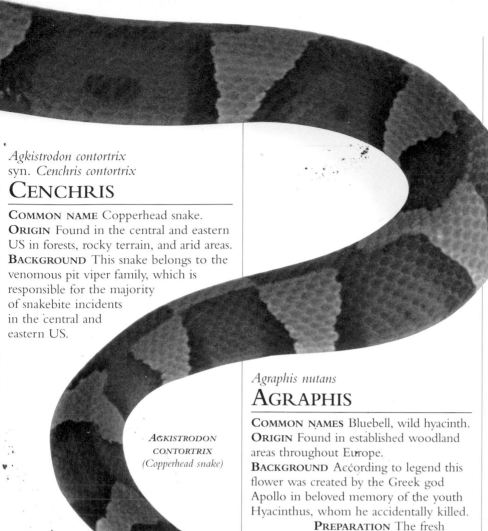

AGKISTRODON
CONTORTRIX
(Copperhead snake)

Agkistrodon contortrix
syn. Cenchris contortrix

CENCHRIS

COMMON NAME Copperhead snake.
ORIGIN Found in the central and eastern US in forests, rocky terrain, and arid areas.
BACKGROUND This snake belongs to the venomous pit viper family, which is responsible for the majority of snakebite incidents in the central and eastern US.

PREPARATION
The fresh venom is triturated with lactose sugar.

REMEDY PROFILE
Cenchris is particularly suitable for people who experience great mental restlessness, jealousy, suspicion, and abandonment. They have a general tendency to be rather absentminded, moody, and dreamy, often experiencing vivid, horrible dreams that continue in their thoughts once they are awake. Their anxieties may include a fear of rape, pins and pointed objects, going to sleep, and sudden death.

The classic symptom picture for *Cenchris* is of breathlessness, mental and physical restlessness, and a desire to drink small quantities of water. Another classic symptom is a need to loosen the clothing, triggered by congestion in the blood vessels. Complaints are usually right-sided. There may be a susceptibility to allergies, especially in the spring.
Symptoms better In the morning.
Symptoms worse In the afternoon, in the evening, and all night; lying down; on waking; from pressure on the affected area.

Agraphis nutans

AGRAPHIS

COMMON NAMES Bluebell, wild hyacinth.
ORIGIN Found in established woodland areas throughout Europe.
BACKGROUND According to legend this flower was created by the Greek god Apollo in beloved memory of the youth Hyacinthus, whom he accidentally killed.
PREPARATION The fresh plant, young shoots, and roots are macerated in alcohol.

REMEDY PROFILE
People for whom *Agraphis* is best suited are low in vitality and prone to catching colds. The classic symptom picture is of ear, nose, and throat infections linked to phlegm and deafness, particularly during childhood. There may be phlegm in the bridge of the nose, obstructing the nostrils, and discharges from all the mucous membranes. Chills develop easily after exposure to cold winds, accompanied by diarrhea with mucus. During infection the tonsils and adenoids may be swollen.
Symptoms better With shelter from winds; lying on the stomach.
Symptoms worse In heat and humidity.

Ailanthus altissima

AILANTHUS

COMMON NAMES Tree of heaven, shade tree, Chinese sumac, copal tree.
ORIGIN Native to China and India, but can now also be found growing in North America, Europe, and Australia.

BACKGROUND In Australia and Asia the tree's bark was used for profuse vaginal discharge, gonorrhea, worms, malaria, and asthma. Chinese herbalists use it to treat diarrhea and dysentery.
PREPARATION The fresh, budding flowers are macerated in alcohol.

REMEDY PROFILE
Ailanthus is best suited to those who feel extremely weak when ill, and frequently behave in a stupid, dull, and confused way. They may feel anxious, odd, or even insane. Key symptoms indicating that this remedy is suitable are fevers with great weakness and congestion of the blood, which typically gives the skin a purple, mottled, swollen appearance. It is often given for acute bouts of infectious mononucleosis with swollen tonsils and neck glands. Pain extends from the neck glands to the ears when swallowing. The tonsils on the left side are mainly affected, and may develop oozing mucus or ulcers.
Symptoms better Lying on the right side; from hot drinks.
Symptoms worse From skin eruptions that fail to develop; with any movement; from sitting up; from the sight of food.

SEE ALSO Infectious mononucleosis, *page 254*

Allium sativum

ALLIUM SAT.

COMMON NAME Garlic.
ORIGIN Native to central Asia, and now grown worldwide.
BACKGROUND Garlic is one of the most ancient of herbs, used by the Babylonians as early as c. 3000 BCE. A popular culinary herb and an important medicinal plant, it is valued for its antibiotic properties.
PREPARATION The fresh garlic bulbs are minced and macerated in alcohol.

REMEDY PROFILE
Allium sat. is most appropriate for people who are oversensitive and need company. Although subject to many fears, they have a particular fear of being poisoned. They generally enjoy a rich, gourmet diet, especially one that includes meat, but are prone to indigestion and phlegm problems.

The remedy is primarily associated with indigestion caused by a rich diet or by dietary change. The digestive process is accompanied by pressure in the upper abdomen, foul-smelling gas, and colicky pains around the navel. Dull pains in the bowels and either constipation or diarrhea may be present. *Allium sat.* is also used to treat tearing pains in the hip area and abdomen.

Symptoms better From sitting bent over.
Symptoms worse In the evening; at night; from walking; from pressure on the affected area.

Aluminum potassium sulfuricum
ALUMEN

COMMON NAMES Potash alum, double sulfate of aluminum and potassium.
ORIGIN Chemically produced from sulfates of aluminum and potassium.
BACKGROUND Potash alum is used in the making of chamois leather, and as a dye in the paint industry. It is used medicinally for minor bleeding cuts and canker sores.
PREPARATION Pure crystals of potash alum are triturated with lactose sugar.

REMEDY PROFILE
People for whom *Alumen* is best suited are extremely anxious and sad. They are usually very nervous, experiencing tremors on hearing bad news, or palpitations on thinking about any illness that may affect them. They have a fear of falling, and may mistrust others. Sleep is light or elusive, and they tend to stay in bed more than necessary. Illness tends to develop during sleep. *Alumen* is often given to the elderly.

The typical symptom picture for *Alumen* is of bowel problems and paralytic, sluggish weakness of the muscles. Disturbances of the bowel include dysentery and bloody diarrhea, painful ulceration in the rectum, bleeding hemorrhoids, and a deep anal ache. There may be severe constipation, possibly due to uterine or rectal cancer.
Symptoms better In open air.
Symptoms worse With cold; when asleep; lying on the right side; from bad news.

Ambrosia artemisifolia
AMBROSIA

COMMON NAMES Ragweed, Roman wormwood, hogweed.
ORIGIN Found in Europe, Mexico, Brazil, and North America.
BACKGROUND This plant's green, tassel-like flowers produce large amounts of pollen that can trigger severe hay fever.
PREPARATION A tincture is made from the fresh flower heads and young shoots.

REMEDY PROFILE
Ambrosia is generally given for hay fever. The entire respiratory system may be affected. The nose and head feel congested, and there is sneezing, watery phlegm, and possible nosebleeds. The eyes water, smart, burn, and itch. There may be a wheezy cough, asthmatic irritation, or whooping cough. These symptoms may also be associated with diarrhea, notably in the summer months.
Symptoms better From being indoors.
Symptoms worse From being outside.

Ammonium bromatum
AMMONIUM BROM.

COMMON NAME Ammonium bromide.
ORIGIN Chemically prepared.
BACKGROUND This compound exists as colorless prismatic crystals with a salty taste. It is not used commercially.
PREPARATION The crystals are dissolved in alcohol, diluted, and succussed.

REMEDY PROFILE
People who respond best to *Ammonium brom.* tend to be timid and lack self-confidence. They fear failure and criticism, and are often resentful of other people. They have a tendency to bite their nails.

Key symptoms linked with this remedy include neuralgic headaches, sore eyes, ovarian problems, and epilepsy. Symptoms may appear concurrently or individually. The constrictive head pains are like a band above the ears. During the aura (the warning sensation) preceding an epileptic fit, there may be feelings of suffocation and faintness, along with sighing and a need to walk around the room.

Eye symptoms typically include sore, irritated eyes that feel as if they contain sand. There may be mucus bathing the eyes, swollen eyelids, and possibly a pterygium (a wing-shaped thickening of the conjunctiva). In the evening the eyes feel large, with constantly blurred vision.

In women symptoms may be associated with the ovaries. They may include nagging, neuralgic pains, bleeding of the uterus, and hard swelling, especially of the left ovary, possibly in conjunction with eye irritation. *Ammonium brom.* may also be prescribed for a tormenting, tickly, spasmodic cough, such as whooping cough, or it may be given for a strangling cough with mucus that tends to occur in the morning. Coughing may be incessant at night.
Symptoms better With warmth; from warm drinks.
Symptoms worse In open air or cold air.

Ammonium chloratum
AMMONIUM MUR.

COMMON NAMES Sal ammoniac, ammonium chloride.
ORIGIN Until the 19th century the only source of this mineral was in central Asia, but now it is also chemically prepared.
BACKGROUND Sal ammoniac is used industrially as an electrolyte in dry cells. Medicinally it is found in many over-the-counter cold and cough medicines.
PREPARATION The compound is dissolved in alcohol, diluted, and succussed.

REMEDY PROFILE
This remedy is typically given to people who are grieving, sad, depressed, and tearful, yet are unable to weep. Usually reserved and self-pitying, they may resent feeling alone in the world.

Ammonium mur. is generally used for these symptoms in conjunction with liver complaints, particularly if they are accompanied by pinching, shooting pains in the stomach, phlegm, and a violent cough that is dry and scraping or loose and profuse. Inflammatory eye conditions, menstrual disorders, enlarged glands, joint pains, and sciatica are other possible symptoms that may appear, and for which the remedy may be prescribed. Further respiratory symptoms typically associated with *Ammonium mur.* include a congested nose, sneezing, a reduced sense of smell, a sore throat, hoarseness, and thick, slimy mucus in the nose and throat.
Symptoms better In open air; from rapid movement; from walking bent over.
Symptoms worse From walking erect; from chronic sprains; in the morning (in the case of head and chest symptoms); in the afternoon (in the case of abdominal pains); in the evening (in the case of joint pains).

SEE ALSO Sciatica, *page 218*

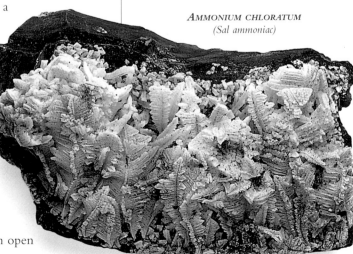

AMMONIUM CHLORATUM
(Sal ammoniac)

123

Amylium nitrosum
AMYL NIT.

COMMON NAME Amyl nitrite.
ORIGIN Chemically prepared.
BACKGROUND A powerful drug that dilates the blood vessels, amyl nitrate is often used in illegal recreational drugs such as "poppers."
PREPARATION Amyl nitrite is dissolved in purified water, diluted, and successed.

REMEDY PROFILE

Amyl nit. is most appropriate for people who are hot and red, feel constricted by their clothes, and have a desire for fresh air. They may be weak, anxious, restless, and weary, often due to disturbed sleep.

The classic symptom picture is of flushing that spreads rapidly over the skin, followed by drenching sweats and great exhaustion. The remedy may be used for these symptoms in conjunction with menopause, sunstroke, or heart problems.

Typical heart symptoms treated with *Amyl nit.* include sharp pains in the heart area and a feeling of oppression, with pain radiating down the right arm.
Symptoms better In open air; from exercising outside; with rest; from drinking cold water.
Symptoms worse From the slightest emotion; from physical or mental exertion; during menopause.

Anacardium occidentale
ANACARDIUM OCC.

COMMON NAME Cashew nut.
ORIGIN Native to the West Indies.
BACKGROUND The juice inside the shell is a skin irritant that causes blistering. In 19th-century Europe it was used to burn off warts and corns.
PREPARATION The black juice between the outer and inner shell is dissolved in alcohol, then diluted and successed.

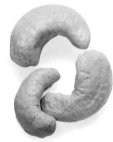

ANACARDIUM OCCIDENTALE (Cashew nuts)

REMEDY PROFILE

Anacardium occ. is most appropriate for people who are prone to poor memory and willpower, and who feel mentally and physically apathetic and numb. They are prone to exam nerves and phobias.

The remedy is given for the above state of mind in conjunction with skin and muscle complaints. Skin eruptions initially itch and burn, then become swollen and sore before producing blisters that may become infected. The ears and face may itch and burn. *Anacardium occ.* may also be prescribed for warts or leprosy.
Symptoms better No specific factors.
Symptoms worse On beginning to move.

SEE ALSO Phobias, *page 211*; Exam nerves, *page 254*

Anamirta cocculus syn. *Cocculus indicus*
COCCULUS

COMMON NAME Indian cockle.
ORIGIN Found in India and southeast Asia.
BACKGROUND Fishermen in southern India use this plant as a poison to stun fish and catch them easily. It was once added to beer to make it more intoxicating.
PREPARATION The powdered seeds are macerated in alcohol.

REMEDY PROFILE

Cocculus is most effective for those whose concern for others makes them feel at the end of their tether. They may become severely exhausted, possibly leading to fainting, insomnia, and stupor. This state is common in those who have spent long periods of time nursing a sick relative.

This remedy has a strong affinity with central nervous system disorders, especially vertigo, dizziness, nausea, sea and motion sickness, vomiting, and hypersensitivity to touch. Nervous oversensitivity may lead initially to agitation and dizziness, and possibly develop into more serious conditions such as muscle weakness, spasms in the legs, and gradual paralysis.
Symptoms better From sitting in a warm room; from lying quietly.
Symptoms worse With cold; from lack of sleep; with movement; movement in vehicles; from anxiety; emotional stress.

Anhalonium lewinii syn. *Lophophora williamsii*
ANHALONIUM

COMMON NAMES Mescal buttons, peyote, sacred mushroom.
ORIGIN Native to the southwestern US and Mexico.
BACKGROUND For over 3,000 years it has been used throughout North America as a hallucinogenic means of deepening spiritual experiences in religious rites.
PREPARATION Boiling water is poured at two intervals on the fresh, chopped root.

REMEDY PROFILE

This remedy is best suited to people who have lost all conception of time and feel separated from ordinary life. They may be introverted, lethargic, depressed, and resentful and distrustful of others, and can experience irrational changes in mood. A general loss of identity and willpower may affect them, along with an impression that life is meaningless. They may have the strange feeling that their whole being has become transparent, enabling them to see their internal organs.

The symptom picture for *Anhalonium* is of mental exhaustion, hallucinations with brilliant-colored vision, migraines, and lack of coordination. Headaches or migraines may occur in the front of the head, or there may be a persistent aching, tired sensation at the back of the head. There may be blurred vision, dilated pupils, or grotesque, multicolored, distracting visual disturbances. Listening to music may trigger the feeling that each note is surrounded by a halo of color that pulses to the music.

Severe lack of coordination is also associated with *Anhalonium*; it may be accompanied by muscle tremors, nausea, faintness, and giddiness, and neuralgic pains and paralysis in the face. The brain is often overactive and prevents sleep.
Symptoms better Lying down.
Symptoms worse From closing the eyes; with movement.

Apocynum cannabinum
APOCYNUM

COMMON NAMES Indian hemp, American hemp, hemp dogbane.
ORIGIN Found in North America.
BACKGROUND This plant has long been known by Native Americans as a treatment for chronic heart disease. Its fibers are also made into rope, twine, mats, and baskets.
PREPARATION The fresh underground parts are chopped and steeped in alcohol.

REMEDY PROFILE

Apocynum is most suitable for people who feel confused, low-spirited, and distressed. The remedy is prescribed primarily as a treatment for edema (a collection of watery fluid in the body cavities or under the skin). The edema is characteristically associated with diseased organs, and may be linked with Hodgkin's lymphoma or Bright's disease. There is often great weakness, irritation in the digestive system, a slow or irregular pulse, and considerable thirst. Secretions such as perspiration and urine may be reduced, and breathing patterns may become uneasy.
Symptoms better With warmth; from sitting up; after passing stools.
Symptoms worse With cold of any kind; from uncovering the body; after sleep.

Aqua sanicula
SANICULA

COMMON NAME Sanicula water.
ORIGIN Found in northern Illinois.
BACKGROUND The Sanicula Springs that provide this particular mineral water are located near Ottawa in the state of Illinois.
PREPARATION The springwater is mixed with alcohol, diluted, and succussed.

REMEDY PROFILE
Irritation is common in those for whom *Sanicula* is most suited. In children, behavior alternates between playfulness and bad temper, during which they will throw themselves backward. Intolerance of the slightest jarring movement, particularly downward motion, such as that of an escalator, is another typical feature of this remedy profile. The classic symptom picture is of low vitality due to undernourishment and slow digestion. The physique is usually slim and the skin condition is poor, possibly with eczema. Symptoms tend to change frequently. There is often perspiration where body parts touch. In women there may be menstrual disorders and an uncomfortable feeling that the pelvic contents are going to drop out.

Digestive symptoms associated with *Sanicula* include large, heavy, painful stools. The body tends to remain thin despite great appetite, and eating causes bloating, sour-tasting burps, and an urge to pass stools. There may be halitosis and a bad taste in the mouth.
Symptoms better From vomiting; in open air; with rest; lying down.
Symptoms worse With movement; from jarring; from strain; eating and drinking.

Araneus diadematus
ARANEA DIADEMA

COMMON NAMES Papal cross spider, European garden spider, diadem spider.
ORIGIN Found in Europe and the US.
BACKGROUND The name of this spider derives from the yellow-and-white crosses on its back. After mating the female usually binds, kills, and eats the male.
PREPARATION The whole, live spider is crushed and macerated in alcohol.

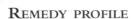
*ARCTOSTAPHYLOS
UVA–URSI
(Uva-ursi)*

REMEDY PROFILE
People who respond best to this remedy tend to be irritable, uneasy, nervous, and restless. Feelings of claustrophobia or confusion may also be present.

Aranea diadema is most appropriate for problems that affect the nervous system and are accompanied by coldness and a susceptibility to dampness. A sensation of great chilliness may occur, as if the bones themselves are frozen, and there may be a fever. All parts of the body may feel heavy, numb, and enlarged (especially on waking); for example, the hands may feel as if they are twice their normal size, and there may be pains that feel like electric shocks. Symptoms tend to occur or recur periodically, or at the same time each day, and are usually on the right side.
Symptoms better From smoking; in open air; from pressure on the affected area.
Symptoms worse With cold; with dampness; from rain; from getting wet; at exactly the same time each day.

Arctostaphylos uva-ursi
UVA–URSI

COMMON NAMES Uva-ursi, bearberry.
ORIGIN Found in Europe, the US, Mexico, and northern Asia.
BACKGROUND Bears like to eat the fruits of this plant, hence the name uva-ursi, which is derived from the Latin for "bear's grape."
PREPARATION The fresh leaves and young shoots are chopped and steeped in alcohol.

REMEDY PROFILE
Uva-ursi is generally used for inflammation and stones in the kidneys. There may be chronic bladder irritation with blood in the urine, or pain with straining to urinate, possibly accompanied by a weak, irregular pulse, breathlessness, vomiting, nausea, and cyanosis (bluish mucous membranes and skin caused by too much deoxygenated hemoglobin in the blood). Sharp pains may pass from hip to hip. In men the prostate gland may become enlarged. Further symptoms that may accompany urinary conditions include flushing of the face, phlegm, a tight sensation in the chest, slight dizziness, and a headache. *Uva-ursi* may also be given for certain digestive, respiratory, or childbirth symptoms, but the primary focus of the remedy is on urinary problems.
Symptoms better After urination; from lying back.
Symptoms worse During urination; in the evening.

Argentum metallicum
ARGENTUM MET.

COMMON NAME Silver.
ORIGIN Deposits are widely distributed throughout the world, but are often small.
BACKGROUND This precious metal has been found in ornaments and decorations dating from 4000 BCE, and has long been used to make coins and jewelry.
PREPARATION Ground silver is triturated with lactose sugar.

REMEDY PROFILE
Anxious, restless, hurried, impulsive people who often act on a whim respond best to *Argentum met.* When ill, having to concentrate usually makes these people feel worse, and their thoughts are chaotic, so that they constantly flit from subject to subject when talking. Often changeable and deceitful, although normally cheerful and lively, they may be unusually depressed by small upsets.

Argentum met. is generally used for joint and bone disorders associated with the connective tissues, especially the cartilage.

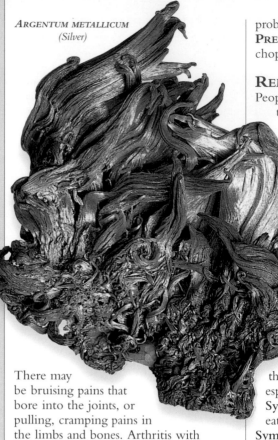

ARGENTUM METALLICUM
(Silver)

There may be bruising pains that bore into the joints, or pulling, cramping pains in the limbs and bones. Arthritis with paralytic pain and weakness may be present. The remedy may also be prescribed to treat nervous complaints involving spasmodic movements and convulsive shocks in the body.

Disorders of the reproductive organs may also be treated by *Argentum met.*, especially if they are accompanied by thick, profuse secretions of the related mucous membranes. In men frequent seminal emissions without sexual excitement at night may be treated. In women the remedy is given for ovarian pain, possibly caused by cysts or tumors, and for bleeding between menstrual periods or heavy hemorrhaging during menopause. *Argentum met.* may also be helpful in treating throat inflammation and voice loss.
Symptoms better From wrapping up; with movement.
Symptoms worse With warmth; in sun; from mental strain; from using the voice.

Arisaema triphyllum syn. *A. atrorubens*, *Arum triphyllum*

ARUM TRIPH.

COMMON NAMES Indian turnip, jack-in-the-pulpit, wild turnip.
ORIGIN Found in North America.
BACKGROUND Indian turnip was used medicinally by Native Americans. The fresh root is a severe skin irritant, but when dried it was used for a variety of ailments, including headaches, chest

problems, and rheumatoid arthritis.
PREPARATION The fresh tuber is chopped and macerated in alcohol.

REMEDY PROFILE

People who respond best to *Arum triph.* tend to be excitable and nervous. They are often restless and irritable and may also bore their heads into their pillows. Key conditions associated with *Arum triph.* involve irritation and inflammation of the mucous membranes and skin, such as allergic skin reactions, eczema, scarlet fever, or hay fever. Typical symptoms include raw, red, itchy skin, particularly on the face, and a raw, burning mouth and throat, with acute or chronic hoarseness. The lips may be chapped or cracked at the corners. Picking the lips and the nose are further common symptoms, especially if accompanied by delirium.
Symptoms better With warmth; from eating breakfast and dinner.
Symptoms worse In cold and wet; with heat; from cold, northeasterly winds; from overusing the voice; lying down.

SEE ALSO Allergies, *page 206*

Arsenicum iodatum

ARSEN. IOD.

COMMON NAMES Arsenic iodide, iodide of arsenic.
ORIGIN Chemically prepared.
BACKGROUND These orange-red crystals are highly toxic and must be protected from light to prevent the loss of iodine.
PREPARATION Pure arsenic iodide crystals are dissolved in alcohol.

REMEDY PROFILE

This remedy is most appropriate for people who are irritable and restless. Excitable and impatient, they may have sudden, violent impulses. Their bodies are warm.

The classic symptom picture for *Arsen. iod.* is of either great restlessness or total exhaustion, possibly associated with chronic chest infection and burning discharges from the mucous membranes. There may be a history of allergic and respiratory conditions.

Arsen. iod. is most often used for hay fever, a case of the flu that is accompanied by the classic burning discharge, soreness of the mucous membranes, and frequent sneezing. There may be a loose, short, hacking cough or a burning, sore throat associated with inflammation. The

remedy may also be given for asthma and shortness of breath with rapid breathing that gradually becomes a wheeze.
Symptoms better In open air; after eating.
Symptoms worse In dry, windy, cold, or foggy weather; from the heat of the bed; from exertion; from tobacco smoke.

SEE ALSO Hay fever & allergic rhinitis, *page 224*

Artemisia abrotanum

ABROTANUM

COMMON NAMES Southernwood, lady's love, old man.
ORIGIN Native to southern Europe.
BACKGROUND Containing a strong, volatile oil that repels insects, this plant's leaves have long been used as a moth repellent when placed among clothes.
PREPARATION The fresh, finely chopped leaves and shoots are steeped in alcohol.

REMEDY PROFILE

People for whom *Abrotanum* is best suited tend to be anxious and depressed. They may feel dull-minded and become easily fatigued when speaking or studying. Alternatively, they can be irritable, excited, and violent, and have an urge to shout.

Key symptoms include emaciation and debilitation of the lower limbs, possibly in children who fail to thrive, or have had polio. A classic feature of *Abrotanum* is that certain symptoms die away rapidly and are immediately replaced by other symptoms. For example, chest symptoms may develop after skin eruptions have failed to come out, heart disease develops following the suppression of rheumatic symptoms, or mumps is transferred from the parotid glands to the testes.
Symptoms better From passing loose stools; with movement.
Symptoms worse In cold and damp air; if secretions are suppressed (for instance, by taking drugs to suppress diarrhea).

Artemisia absinthium

ABSINTHIUM

COMMON NAMES Common wormwood, green ginger.
ORIGIN Native to Europe, but now grows wild in central Asia and the eastern US, and is widely cultivated in temperate areas.
BACKGROUND Common wormwood was originally a primary flavoring in vermouth, and the basis of absinthe, an addictive drink popular in 19th-century France but now illegal in many countries.
PREPARATION The fresh flowers, young leaves, and shoots are steeped in alcohol.

REMEDY PROFILE

Those who respond best to *Absinthium* are prone to nervous overexcitement, experiencing terrifying, horrible dreams and dreadful hallucinations. A kind of brutish stupor or stupidity may even be apparent in them.

Absinthium is primarily associated with the nerves, and key symptoms include trembling, grimacing, and unsteadiness, possibly linked to alcoholism. In children the remedy may be given for terrible dreams, nervousness, insomnia, vertigo, fits or seizures, and epilepsy.

Symptoms better With movement.
Symptoms worse When rising from bed or from a seat; when staying still.

*ARTEMISIA
ABSINTHIUM
(Common wormwood)*

Artemisia vulgaris
ARTEMISIA

COMMON NAMES Mugwort, wormwood, sailor's tobacco.
ORIGIN Found in temperate regions of the Northern Hemisphere.
BACKGROUND Mugwort was traditionally kept in medieval homes to ward off the devil. Chinese doctors use the herb in moxibustion, a traditional treatment.
PREPARATION The fresh root is dug up at the beginning of winter, chopped, and macerated in alcohol.

REMEDY PROFILE

The classic symptom picture for *Artemisia* is of nervous disorders, possibly triggered by bad news, grief, or a blow to the head.

The nervous conditions for which this remedy is used include sleepwalking, fits or seizures, chorea (involuntary rapid, jerky body movements), and epilepsy. There may be absentmindedness and stupor. Seizures may be brought on by cooling after exertion, or by flickering lights. Children who benefit from *Artemisia* may tend to experience petit mal fits or absences rather than full seizures, possibly during teething. They may have been born to mothers who felt great grief during their pregnancy.

Symptoms better At night; from rubbing the eyes; from deep breathing.
Symptoms worse From fright; from grief; from a head injury; from menstrual problems; from prolonged dancing.

Arum maculatum
ARUM MAC.

COMMON NAMES Cuckoopint, lords and ladies.
ORIGIN Native to central and western Europe, growing in woods and hedges.
BACKGROUND The arrow-shaped leaves and bright red flowers of this plant are poisonous. Insects are trapped by the flowers and digested by the plant.
PREPARATION The fresh, finely chopped tuber is macerated in alcohol.

REMEDY PROFILE

Arum mac. is associated with severe, violent inflammation or irritation of the mucous membranes, and is frequently used for respiratory-tract problems. Typical respiratory symptoms treated by the remedy include asthma, phlegm, nasal polyps, and constant swallowing. The gums may bleed, and the tongue and throat may be swollen and sore, so that swallowing becomes difficult. There may be tickling in the throat, hoarseness, and a desire to cough. The chest may feel tight, and there may be a violent cough and profuse, possibly blood-streaked phlegm.

Symptoms better No specific factors.
Symptoms worse With pressure on the affected area; from stretching; on the left side of the body.

Arundo mauritanica
ARUNDO

COMMON NAMES Reed, cannizzola.
ORIGIN Found in southern Europe, Africa, and Asia.
BACKGROUND This genus is used in reeds for wind instruments, in wickerwork, and to make windbreaks to control erosion.
PREPARATION The root sprouts are macerated in alcohol.

REMEDY PROFILE

The mental state for which *Arundo* is most appropriate is one in which laughter comes easily, as do lascivious thoughts. Allergic problems are the key symptoms treated by this remedy. Typical problems include hay fever with sneezing, phlegmy inflammation, and extreme itching inside the nose, accompanied by excessive salivation. There may be a reduced sense of smell, and itching and burning in the back palate of the mouth. Pain at the back of the head may extend to the right eye, with deep-seated pain on either side of the head. The hay fever symptoms may extend to the eyes, causing prickling, itching, and burning of the conjunctiva. The remedy may be used to treat blepharitis (inflammation of the eyelids).

Arundo may also be prescribed for a wet cough with breathlessness. Bluish-tinged mucus may be coughed up, with a sensation of bruising in the throat and burning pain in the stomach.

Symptoms better In open air.
Symptoms worse With movement.

SEE ALSO Allergies, *page 206*

Asarum europaeum
ASARUM

COMMON NAMES Hazelwort, European snakeroot, wild nard, public-house plant.
ORIGIN Native to woods and shady sites in northern and eastern Europe.
BACKGROUND Introduced medicinally by the ancient Greek physician Dioscorides, this plant was used chiefly as an emetic. Also a stimulant, it was once an ingredient of tobacconists' "head-clearin' snuff."
PREPARATION The fresh, finely chopped underground parts are steeped in alcohol.

REMEDY PROFILE

People who respond best to *Asarum* are nervous, excitable, and oversensitive. They are usually weak, often feel chilly, and are unable to live robust, ordinary lives. Often they are overly ambitious, and exhausted by a stressful occupation. *Asarum* is also given to recovering alcoholics.

The classic symptom picture for this remedy is of nervous hypersensitivity and edgy, hysterical behavior; even the sound of scratching on cloth becomes unbearable. Other symptoms commonly include nervous exhaustion, restlessness, wringing of the hands, severe insomnia, and a sensation of floating and dizziness. Noise may trigger pain in the ears and teeth.

Digestive problems with an aversion to eating, possibly associated with anorexia, may accompany this disturbed state. There is often alcoholism or a desire for alcohol, and an aversion to sexual intercourse.

Symptoms better In damp weather; from bathing in cold water.
Symptoms worse In cold, dry weather; from any noise or even the thought of noise; from penetrating sounds.

127

Asclepias tuberosa
ASCLEPIAS TUB.

COMMON NAMES Pleurisy root, butterfly weed.
ORIGIN Native to the southern US.
BACKGROUND Traditionally considered a cure-all in Native American herbalism, pleurisy root was often used to treat fevers.
PREPARATION The fresh root is chopped and macerated in alcohol.

REMEDY PROFILE
Those for whom *Asclepias tub.* is most appropriate tend to be depressed, languid, and unable to concentrate.

Asclepias tub. is associated particularly with rheumatic pain and congestion, both tending to arise in damp weather. The rheumatic pain is characterized by stitchlike pains in the muscles and joints. The remedy may be prescribed for many forms of respiratory inflammation, such as bronchitis, the flu, pleurisy, or other feverish conditions with a painful, dry, hacking cough. The chest may feel warm with sharp pains, especially when breathing deeply. The above symptoms are often accompanied by copious perspiration, phlegm, and restless, uneasy sleep.
Symptoms better From bending forward, which eases pain in the lungs.
Symptoms worse With movement; from deep breathing; lying down; in the morning; in winter.

Astacus fluviatilis
ASTACUS

COMMON NAMES Freshwater crayfish, river crab.
ORIGIN Found in the Gulf of Mexico and along the coast of the Atlantic Ocean.
BACKGROUND The common name of this crustacean derives from the old French word *crevice*, perhaps because it lives in the crevices between stones.
PREPARATION The live crayfish is pounded and then steeped in alcohol.

REMEDY PROFILE
Astacus is best suited to people who feel unprotected and vulnerable during transitional phases in their lives. They are often taciturn loners who desire calmness and clarity, but tend to be vague and absentminded, their heads feeling full of spiderwebs.

Astacus has a strong affinity with the liver, digestion, glands, and skin. It is well known as a remedy for hives (urticaria), particularly if the rash is accompanied by cramps and pain, or inflammation in the liver area that feels worse when pressed. There may be stinging pains in the temples, ears, and kidneys, and the glands may be enlarged and inflamed, especially in children and the elderly.
Symptoms better From walking; from sitting; after crying.
Symptoms worse From uncovering the affected area or exposing it to the air; from eating fish or meat.

Asterias rubens
ASTERIAS

COMMON NAME Red starfish.
ORIGIN Found around the coastline of western Europe.
BACKGROUND Dating back to the earliest geological age, the Precambrian era, this species has amazing regenerative powers: If one of its five arms is lost, for instance, a new one grows in its place.
PREPARATION The whole, live animal is chopped up and macerated in alcohol.

REMEDY PROFILE
Tearfulness is typical of those who respond best to *Asterias*, and they feel better after crying. They like to have people around them, yet prefer to retain a degree of independence. If contradicted they may become angry and irritable, especially in hot weather. *Asterias* is generally used in the treatment of left-sided symptoms that occur particularly in women, as well as for circulatory problems in both sexes. It also

ASTERIAS RUBENS (Red starfish)

has the unusual feature of apparently making old scars, particularly those in the breast area, become painful again.

Asterias may benefit women who experience an increased sex drive so intense that it causes restless sleep, erotic dreams, a bad temper, and weepiness. Further symptoms that may respond to *Asterias* include obstinate constipation, particularly during menopause; hard, swollen glands in the armpits; or sharp pains in the breasts at night with a drawing sensation in the nipples, especially in the left breast. These symptoms may be accompanied by a high libido.

The remedy is also used for circulatory disorders such as strokes, especially if they are preceded by great impatience, dizziness, and muscle spasms in the limbs.
Symptoms better After a headache; after crying; from cold drinks.
Symptoms worse With heat; in cold, damp weather; at night; on the left side of the body; from menstruating; from being contradicted; from coffee.

Aurum chloratum
AURUM MUR.

COMMON NAME Gold chloride.
ORIGIN Chemically prepared.
BACKGROUND The glass traditionally made from this reddish yellow crystal was called "ruby glass" by alchemists. It was also noted as a treatment for syphilis by the 16th-century scientist Paracelsus.
PREPARATION The crystals are dissolved in alcohol, diluted, and succussed.

REMEDY PROFILE
Aurum mur. is best suited to those who are restless, easily depressed, sensitive to humiliation, and anxious about developing diseases. These feelings may be eased by company, but can spiral into suicidal thoughts if left unchecked. The remedy may be prescribed for heart conditions such as palpitations and a sense of constriction in the chest, possibly associated with high blood pressure. *Aurum mur.* is also used for edema (an irregular accumulation of fluid in the tissues or cavities of the body), with a feeling of congestion in the liver, kidneys, and genitals. Fibroids or cancer may also be helped.
Symptoms better In cold weather; from bathing in cold water; with gentle movement.
Symptoms worse With warmth; at night; from music.

SEE ALSO Fibroids, *page 199*; Cancer, *page 208*

Avena sativa
AVENA

COMMON NAME Oats.
ORIGIN Native to northern Europe, but now grown worldwide in temperate areas.
BACKGROUND Oats have a long history of medicinal use in Europe for a wide range of ailments.

They are most often used in herbalism for general debility, eczema, and nervous conditions.
PREPARATION The fresh, green aerial parts in flower are expressed for their juice, which is mixed with alcohol.

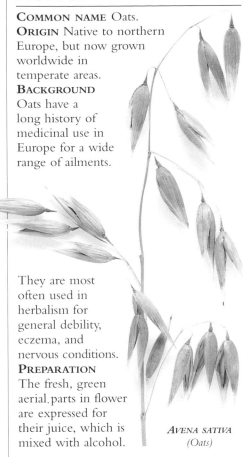

AVENA SATIVA
(Oats)

REMEDY PROFILE
People for whom *Avena* is considered most appropriate are prone to mental and physical exhaustion accompanied by poor concentration. These people typically tend to be nervous or elderly. Alternatively, they may be feeling the effects of a drug or alcohol addiction.

Nervous exhaustion, great weakness, and a tendency to suffer chronic insomnia are key symptoms associated with the remedy. There may be a very low libido or male impotence, possibly linked with excessive sexual activity. The tincture is often prescribed as herbal drops rather than homeopathic pills.
Symptoms better In open air.
Symptoms worse When convalescing.

Bacillinum pulmo
BACILLINUM

COMMON NAME Tubercular lung tissue.
ORIGIN Tissue from a lung infected with tuberculosis.
BACKGROUND See information under *Tuberculinum* (see page 115).
PREPARATION Sterilized lung tissue is dissolved in purified water, diluted, and succussed.

REMEDY PROFILE
Melancholy and depression are typical in those who respond best to *Bacillinum*. They tend to be taciturn, irritable, and snappy, and often whine and complain. Generally they feel weak and do not want to be disturbed. They often start one task before completing another, and may have a fear of dogs.

The remedy has an affinity with the respiratory organs, and may be given constitutionally to those with a personal or family history of respiratory problems. It is typically prescribed for weak lungs, possibly involving shortness of breath, hacking coughs that disrupt sleep, purulent mucus, asthma, and sharp pain in the heart area that may be triggered by deep breathing.

Bacillinum is also used for certain skin conditions, such as eczema on the eyelids, pimples that develop on the left cheek, ringworm on the scalp, alopecia areata (patchy loss of hair), and a susceptibility to fungal skin infections. Symptoms may occur independently or in conjunction with respiratory problems.
Symptoms better In summer; with heat; in dry climates; with rest; from tight bandaging.
Symptoms worse In cold air; in the early morning; at night.

SEE ALSO Asthma, *page 181*; Tuberculosis, *page 182*; Pneumonia, *page 183*

Barium chloratum
BARYTA MUR.

COMMON NAME Barium chloride.
ORIGIN Chemically prepared from barium carbonate and hydrochloric acid.
BACKGROUND Barium chloride is mixed with sodium sulfate to form a white filler and pigment (*blanc fixe*) used in the manufacture of leather, rubber, cloth, and photographic paper.
PREPARATION The compound is dissolved in alcohol or triturated with lactose sugar.

REMEDY PROFILE
Baryta mur. has strong links with the nervous system. It is most appropriate for people with a predisposition to develop an aneurysm (ballooning of an artery).

The remedy is generally used for nervous symptoms, which may develop into manic nervous states. It is best suited to adults who behave "childishly" and to children who cannot play or interact with others because of their dullness or retarded mental development. *Baryta mur.* may be prescribed for mental disability in children whose development is delayed, and for elderly people with retardation. Principal physical symptoms treated with this remedy include disorders of the nervous system such as seizures, perhaps occurring periodically, with stiffness, restlessness, and a loss of sensibility. The hands and feet may swell, and the limbs may feel paralyzed and heavy, with trembling and twitching.

Baryta mur. is additionally used for acutely swollen glands, possibly the cervical or parotid glands, accompanied by a sore throat and possibly tonsillitis. Stroke symptoms or severe eczema may also respond to the remedy.
Symptoms better No specific factors.
Symptoms worse In wet weather; in spring; in autumn.

SEE ALSO Stroke, *page 187*; Severe eczema, *page 194*

Bellis perennis
BELLIS

COMMON NAMES Common daisy, garden daisy, European daisy, bruisewort.
ORIGIN Found throughout Europe.
BACKGROUND In the 16th century the English herbalist John Gerard noted this plant as a treatment for gout. It has a long tradition of use as a medicinal herb, and is currently being tested as a treatment for HIV infection.
PREPARATION The whole, fresh plant, including the root, is gathered when in flower and steeped in alcohol.

REMEDY PROFILE
Bellis best suits people who are prone to restlessness, insomnia, and angry dreams. They are often sensitive to the cold.

Key conditions treated by *Bellis* include muscle strain, sprains, and bruises, including deep bruising to the muscles such as that produced by sports injuries to the thighs. It is also given to ease pain after surgery, or prolonged pain after injury. The remedy is appropriate when a tumor forms on the site of an old injury or scar.

Bellis is also used to treat varicose veins and congestion of the veins, possibly when they are associated with physical labor. During pregnancy or following an abortion or miscarriage, the remedy may help ease pain and bruising in the uterus.
Symptoms better With heat; from cold compresses; with continuous movement; from pressure on the painful area; eating.
Symptoms worse From getting chilled when hot; from the warmth of the bed; before storms; from touch; from exertion; from childbirth; from injuries; from surgery; on the left side; from cold drinks.

Bismuthum metallicum
BISMUTH MET.

COMMON NAMES Bismuth, precipitated subnitrate of bismuth.
ORIGIN Found widely in nature, in hydrothermal veins and igneous rock.
BACKGROUND First discovered by a German monk called Basil Valentine in 1450, bismuth is widely used industrially in alloys, and its compounds are also used for medicinal purposes.
PREPARATION Bismuth is mixed with lactose sugar and triturated.

REMEDY PROFILE
Bismuth met. is most suited to those who are experiencing great anguish, fear, and restlessness, with poor concentration. They have a desperate need for company and cannot bear to be alone. They often crave cold drinks.

This remedy is generally used for violent abdominal pains, possibly with burning and ulceration in the stomach, bowels, and throat. The pains may be accompanied by frequent burping and rumbling flatulence. Sleep is restless, with frequent waking and feelings of fright or a sensation of falling.
Symptoms better From cold compresses; from company; with movement; from bending backward; from cold drinks.
Symptoms worse From being alone; from eating.

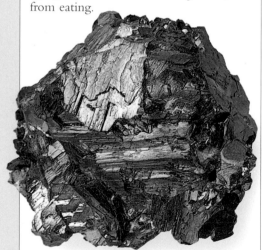

BISMUTHUM METALLICUM
(Bismuth)

Bothrops lanceolatus
syn. Lachesis lanceolatus
BOTHROPS

COMMON NAMES Yellow pit viper, fer-de-lance.
ORIGIN Found from Mexico to Brazil and on many West Indian islands.
BACKGROUND The name fer-de-lance derives from this snake's flat, lance-shaped mouth. A bite from the snake causes immediate swelling and intense pain.
PREPARATION Fresh venom is triturated with lactose sugar.

REMEDY PROFILE
People who crave attention, have a strong desire to appear attractive, and possibly the feeling that they have been forsaken by others are most suited to *Bothrops*. They may be either loquacious or, conversely, find it difficult to talk, forgetting words when they are speaking.

The characteristic symptom picture for *Bothrops* is of problems of the blood or blood vessels. Symptoms include bruising, hemorrhaging of thin blood that will not clot, or severe premenstrual syndrome. The face may be bluish or dark red and bloated, and the right hand may turn blue. Sharp pain may radiate from the right nipple to the back, which becomes worse when raising the left arm or breathing deeply.
Symptoms better No specific factors.
Symptoms worse On the right side; after midnight; at sunrise; from walking; from taking a deep breath.

Brassica nigra syn. Sinapis nigra
SINAPIS

COMMON NAME Black mustard.
ORIGIN Native to the Middle East.
BACKGROUND This pungent, warming herb stimulates the digestive system and circulation. A mustard footbath is an old folk cure for colds and headaches.
PREPARATION Mustard seeds are ground to a powder and macerated in alcohol.

REMEDY PROFILE
Sinapis is given mainly to people who are irritable and become angry for no reason. They have poor concentration, although studying and mental exercise make them feel better and focus their minds.

Classic conditions linked with *Sinapis* are hay fever, colds, and pharyngitis, with hot, dry mucous membranes. Further characteristic symptoms include sweat that forms on the upper lip and forehead, phlegm or mucus that feels cold, intense sneezing that is worse at night, and a feeling that the blood vessels are filled with hot water. Colds tend to affect the left nostril in particular.
Symptoms better From concentrating or studying; from sitting erect; from lying down at night; from shutting the eyes; from eating a good meal.
Symptoms worse In a warm room; in damp weather; in summer; if touched or from pressure on the affected area; from sitting forward and stooping; between 4 P.M. and 6 P.M. and 7 P.M. and 9 P.M.

Bromum
BROMUM

COMMON NAME Bromine.
ORIGIN Chemically prepared.
BACKGROUND The name bromine comes from the Greek *bromos*, or "bad smell." An acrid, brownish red, smoking fluid, it is used as a water purifier, disinfectant, and bleach, and in the production of tear gas.
PREPARATION Bromine is dissolved in alcohol, then diluted and succussed.

REMEDY PROFILE
Bromum is best suited to people with an underlying restlessness who tend to stay on the move or run away from situations. They are prone to anxiety and subject to the delusion that someone is behind them.

Respiratory problems treated by *Bromum* include colds that start in the larynx and travel upward or down to the chest. The nose and larynx may be irritated, with sneezing, phlegm, and hoarseness. An overheated room may cause hoarseness and an inability to speak.

A stony hardness is the most typical gland symptom treated by *Bromum*. It is most likely to affect the thyroid, ovary, or testicle on the left side of the body.
Symptoms better After nosebleeds; from shaving; from being on the seashore; with movement; from riding a horse.
Symptoms worse With warmth; in damp; from overheating; getting chilled while hot; swimming in the ocean; dust; drafts; in the evening until midnight; from tobacco smoke; after eating.

Bufo bufo syn. Rana bufo
BUFO

COMMON NAMES Common toad, Brazilian toad.
ORIGIN Found in North America, Japan, southern Asia, and Europe.
BACKGROUND During the 19th century native Brazilian women were known to give the toad's venom to their husbands in food or drink to lower sexual vitality.
PREPARATION Venom secreted by the dorsal glands on the toad's back is mixed with lactose sugar and triturated.

REMEDY PROFILE
Those prone to immature, childish behavior respond best to this remedy. They have a tendency to be emotionally underdeveloped or potentially even educationally subnormal. Their faces may be characterized by a stupid and besotted expression. Particularly thick lips, which they may lick constantly, are another classic feature.

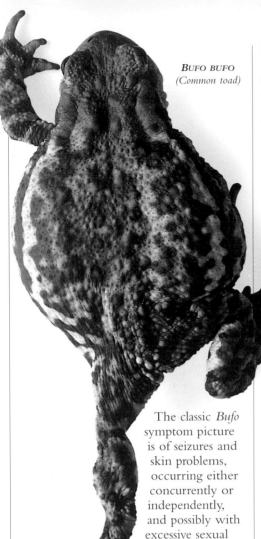

BUFO BUFO
(Common toad)

The classic *Bufo* symptom picture is of seizures and skin problems, occurring either concurrently or independently, and possibly with excessive sexual activity. Typical skin symptoms include blisters and itching, burning pustules. The sexual element of this remedy involves symptoms such as an extremely high sex drive, frequent masturbation, poorly developed sexual relationships, and even sexual depravity.
Symptoms better In cool air; from bathing and putting the feet in hot water; from bleeding, especially in saliva or as a bloody discharge from the nipples.
Symptoms worse During sleep; in warm surroundings; from the slightest movement; after an injury.

Cadmium metallicum
CADMIUM MET.

COMMON NAME Cadmium.
ORIGIN Found naturally in small quantities in minerals and ores, such as zinc, but prepared chemically for commercial use.
BACKGROUND This bluish white element was discovered by Frederick Stromeyer, a German chemist, in 1817. It is used in alloys, batteries, metal-plating, and magnets.
PREPARATION Cadmium is mixed with lactose sugar and triturated.

REMEDY PROFILE
People for whom *Cadmium met.* is best suited tend to be irritable, hypersensitive, and indifferent, and may avoid company.

The classic symptom profile associated with this remedy is of great fatigue, with dull aches all over the body, flulike symptoms, a poor memory, and difficulty in concentrating. Since these are symptoms associated by homeopaths with the effects of aluminum on the body (*see page 72*), this remedy is often used as an antidote to aluminum exposure. There may be accompanying nausea or diarrhea with soft stools and a sensation of a foreign body in the rectum. More serious gastrointestinal symptoms may be helped by this remedy, such as painful abdominal bloating, colitis, or hernias in the diaphragm. It may also be used for constipation and hemorrhoids that tend to be aggravated by passing stools.

A feature of the remedy is that as the fatigue lessens, skin eruptions may appear on the skin, causing it to redden, burn, and itch, and perhaps develop pimples, blisters, or nonweeping eruptions.
Symptoms better From pressure on the affected area; from cold compresses; from the development of skin eruptions; from eating.
Symptoms worse In the morning; with movement; from mental exertion; on the left side of the body.

Cadmium sulfuricum
CADMIUM SULF.

COMMON NAME Cadmium sulfate.
ORIGIN Chemically prepared.
BACKGROUND This mineral derives its name from the Greek word *kadmia*, meaning "earth." It is used as a pigment in oil paints and printing ink.
PREPARATION Cadmium sulfate is triturated with lactose sugar.

REMEDY PROFILE
Cadmium belongs to the same family on the periodic table as zinc and mercury, and the *Cadmium* remedy shares some of the traits associated with the remedies based on those elements. When ill, these people are often chilly, exhausted, anxious, irritable, depressed, and have a fear of death. The more their illness progresses, the more they want to stay still, perhaps becoming faint when rising.

The remedy is typically used to treat stomach problems accompanied by sharp, cutting pains in the abdomen, a feeling of constriction, intense burning, and vomiting. There may be nausea so severe that the slightest touch to the lips will trigger abdominal pain and the retching of black or yellowish green vomit.
Symptoms better With rest; from eating.
Symptoms worse In the open air; from getting up; with the slightest movement; after sleep.

SEE ALSO Depression, *page 212*

Caladium seguinum
CALADIUM

COMMON NAMES American arum, dumb cane, poison arum.
ORIGIN Found in the Caribbean islands, Guyana, and northern Brazil.
BACKGROUND This plant's poison causes muteness and impotence: In the 17th and 18th centuries the men of the West Indian Maroons applied it to their wives' sexual organs to suppress their libido and cause impotence in any man who seduced them.
PREPARATION The whole, fresh plant, including the root, is macerated in alcohol.

REMEDY PROFILE
Caladium is most appropriate for people who feel debilitated, nervous, restless, and forgetful, perhaps following a feverish illness. Illness depletes their energy levels and libido, despite a prior history of high sexual energy and a susceptibility to lascivious thoughts. Other symptoms include rough, dry, itchy skin and a marked craving for tobacco.
Symptoms better After sweating; from sleeping in the daytime.
Symptoms worse With movement.

Calcium fluoratum syn. *Calcarea fluorica*
CALC. FLUOR.

COMMON NAME Calcium fluoride.
ORIGIN Made originally from fluorspar (fluorite) found in Mexico, the US, and the UK, but now chemically prepared.
BACKGROUND This gray-white powder is odorless, tasteless, and luminous when heated. Dr. Schüssler originally developed the remedy as one of his "biochemic" tissue salts (*see page 90*).
PREPARATION Calcium fluoride is mixed with lactose sugar and triturated.

REMEDY PROFILE
Anxiety is typical in those for whom this remedy is most appropriate, especially anxiety about health. They fear poverty and may be miserly or envious of others.

Calc. fluor. is primarily used to treat disorders of the bones, teeth, joints, and musculoskeletal system. Key conditions associated with the remedy include bone malnutrition and deformity, tumors and growths, possibly on the bones or the tendons, and swollen, inflamed joints that crack or dislocate easily on moving. Further symptoms associated with *Calc. fluor.* include teeth that are prone to crumbling or breaking easily, and hard lumps that develop on the skull and jaw.

The remedy may also be prescribed for the treatment of varicose veins.

Symptoms better With heat; from rubbing the affected area; with continued movement.

Symptoms worse With cold; dampness; on beginning to move; from sprains.

CALCIUM FLUORATUM
(Fluorspar)

Calcium iodatum syn. Calcarea iodata
CALC. IOD.

COMMON NAME Calcium iodide.
ORIGIN Chemically prepared.
BACKGROUND In large doses this white, soluble powder may irritate the bowels, but it is also thought to prevent "rotting in the bowels" and to deodorize the stools.
PREPARATION Calcium iodide is dissolved in alcohol, diluted, and succussed.

REMEDY PROFILE
This remedy is most suitable for people who feel light-headed, as if their head "isn't there." They may be indifferent to life and disinclined to work.

Key conditions linked with the *Calc. iod.* remedy are enlarged tonsils honeycombed with pits, glandular swellings, and fibroids. Adenoid complaints accompanied by frequent colds in children may respond to the remedy, as may thyroid enlargement during puberty. In certain cases the glandular swellings, such as those in the breast, may become cancerous.

Symptoms better In the open air.
Symptoms worse With warmth; from the heat of the bed; at night; in cold weather.

SEE ALSO Fibroids, *page 199*

132

Calcium silicatum syn. Calcarea silicata
CALC. SIL.

COMMON NAME Calcium silicate.
ORIGIN Occurs naturally as woollastonite, but usually prepared chemically.
BACKGROUND Calcium silicate is a vital constituent of glass and cement. In the food industry it is used in salt, rice, and candies to counteract sticking.
PREPARATION The compound is mixed with lactose sugar and triturated.

REMEDY PROFILE
Those for whom *Calc. sil.* is most suited tend to feel weak and cold, although overheating makes them feel worse. They may seem obsessed with dead friends and relatives, and may talk to the dead in their imaginations. Thrift and a lack of confidence are also typical of these people.

The remedy is used primarily for this state of mind in conjunction with skin conditions, especially severe acne or acne rosacea, boils, warts, or abscesses.

Symptoms better Lying down, especially on the back.
Symptoms worse With cold; if touched; from jarring; in the evening; at night.

Calcium sulfuricum syn. Calcarea sulfurica
CALC. SULF.

COMMON NAMES Gypsum, calcium sulfate.
ORIGIN Found widely in nature, forming in hot springs and clay beds.
BACKGROUND Gypsum is used to make plaster of Paris, which can be formed into a protective sheath to immobilize injuries. Dr. Schüssler developed the remedy as one of his "biochemic" tissue salts (*see page 90*).
PREPARATION Gypsum is mixed with lactose sugar and triturated.

REMEDY PROFILE
Calc. sulf. is best suited to people who tend to be timid and fearful, especially of birds. They may compensate for their timidity by being argumentative and bossy, and can be terribly jealous.

Suppurating, yellow discharges of pus are typically associated with this remedy. *Calc. sulf.* is generally prescribed once the pus has "found a vent." The pus may affect wounds and other skin conditions, such as eczema, as well as the mucous membranes, glands, and bones. Healing generally occurs slowly or not at all. Typical mucous-membrane discharges

include thick, yellow-colored phlegm accompanying a cold, or thick, yellow, lumpy mucus with a cough.

Symptoms better In open air; with heat; from uncovering; from swimming.
Symptoms worse In cold and dampness; in drafts; from walking rapidly.

SEE ALSO Severe eczema, *page 194*

Calendula officinalis
CALENDULA

COMMON NAMES Marigold, pot marigold.
ORIGIN Native to southern Europe, but now found throughout the world.
BACKGROUND The antiseptic and anti-inflammatory properties of calendula have made it one of the longest established popular herbal remedies. Large amounts are grown in Russia, and it has been nicknamed "Russian penicillin."
PREPARATION The finely chopped, fresh flowers and leaves are steeped in alcohol.

REMEDY PROFILE
Calendula is usually given to heal and soothe cuts and broken skin. It may prevent the development of disfiguring scars from torn and jagged wounds. In addition, nonalcohol-based preparations of the remedy may soothe eczema.

Calendula is prescribed internally and externally for leg and varicose ulcers, postoperative wounds, and ruptured muscles or tendons. It may be used to treat torn perineal tissues following childbirth, joint wounds where there is loss of synovial fluid, and bleeding in the gums after a tooth extraction.

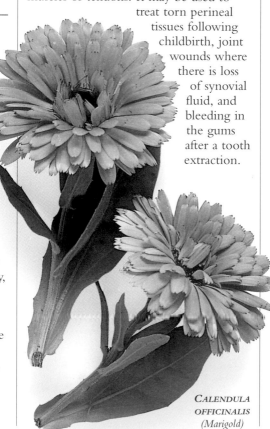

CALENDULA OFFICINALIS
(Marigold)

Symptoms better Lying completely still; from walking.
Symptoms worse In damp, cloudy weather; in drafts; from eating.

Camellia sinensis syn. *Thea sinensis*

THEA

COMMON NAME Tea.
ORIGIN Native to China, although now cultivated commercially, particularly in India, Sri Lanka, and China.
BACKGROUND Long established in many cultures as a beverage, tea is also used in Indian Ayurvedic medicine as a tonic for the digestive system and nerves.
PREPARATION The leaves are dried, then steeped in alcohol, diluted, and succussed.

REMEDY PROFILE
Thea is associated chiefly with an overactive nervous system. Those who respond best to it tend to be in a rather overwrought frame of mind, and are inclined to argue over the slightest things. *Thea* is given for extreme forms of behavior in children and adults, including irritability, mental restlessness, violent impulses, and even psychiatric problems. Adults may have murderous desires, perhaps toward their own children, or they may feel suicidal, especially at night when they are unable to sleep because of a highly active mind.

This overactivity of the nervous system causes physical symptoms such as insomnia, indigestion, and palpitations or other heart problems, which may be helped by *Thea*.
Symptoms better With warmth; from bathing in warm water.
Symptoms worse From walking in the open air; at night; after meals.

Cannabis sativa

CANNABIS SAT.

COMMON NAMES European hemp, American hemp, marijuana, pot, weed.
ORIGIN Native to northern India, China, and Iran, but now cultivated worldwide.
BACKGROUND This plant is cultivated legally for its fiber and seeds and illegally as a recreational drug. It is closely related to *Cannabis sativa* 'Indica' (*see page 43*).
PREPARATION The tops of the male and female flowers are macerated in alcohol.

REMEDY PROFILE
People for whom *Cannabis sat.* is considered most suitable have a tendency to be rather dreamy, absentminded, and detached. They often have the feeling that everything is slightly unreal, and are easily debilitated.

The remedy is prescribed primarily for problems of the urinary and reproductive systems. It may be used for urogenital symptoms such as infections in the urinary tract, and cystitis with severe, burning pains and spasms that interrupt the flow of urine. Typical reproductive system disorders associated with the remedy include discharges from or narrowing of the urethra, inflammation of the penis, and acute gonorrhea.
Symptoms better With warmth and rest.
Symptoms worse From urinating; from being approached by anyone; from looking at bright objects; if touched.

Capsella bursa-pastoris syn. *Thlaspi bursa-pastoris*

THLASPI

COMMON NAME Shepherd's purse.
ORIGIN Native to Europe and Asia.
BACKGROUND This plant's common name derives from its seedpods, which resemble heart-shaped purses. It was used in World War I to treat hemorrhaging.
PREPARATION The aerial parts, dried when in flower, are finely chopped and macerated in alcohol.

REMEDY PROFILE
Predominantly a remedy given for problems of the female reproductive system, *Thlaspi* is especially associated with fibroids and with hemorrhaging, particularly during pregnancy. The hemorrhaging is characteristically accompanied by great pain and violent cramping in the uterus. It may occur between menstrual periods, during pregnancy, following labor, or after a miscarriage or abortion. Menstrual flow tends to be excessively profuse and frequent, causing great exhaustion. Frequent nosebleeds are also a possible symptom during pregnancy.
Symptoms better From bending over.
Symptoms worse No specific factors.

Capsicum annuum var. *annuum*

CAPSICUM

COMMON NAMES Chili pepper, cayenne pepper, sweet pepper, bell pepper.
ORIGIN Native to tropical America, and cultivated throughout Africa and India.
BACKGROUND The dried pods have long been used both as a hot spice in cooking and as a stimulant and irritant in herbalism. The indigenous tribes of tropical America also used it as a local painkiller.
PREPARATION The dried pods are steeped in alcohol, then diluted and succussed.

REMEDY PROFILE
Capsicum is best suited to those who are "peppery," discontented, and rather pessimistic. Homesickness or nostalgia often prevents them from fully engaging in their daily lives.

The classic symptom picture for this remedy is of low vitality, perhaps in the elderly or those debilitated by alcoholism or prostate conditions. Weakness is usually accompanied by slow healing processes, infections that tend to suppurate, and great sensitivity to drafts. Further typical symptoms include a raw, red, burning throat that stings, as if from eating the pepper itself.

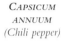

CAPSICUM ANNUUM (Chili pepper)

Symptoms better With heat; with continued movement; from eating.
Symptoms worse In cold air; from the least draft; from uncovering the affected area; from drinking; bathing in cold water.

SEE ALSO Prostate problems, *page 202*

Carbo animalis

CARBO AN.

COMMON NAME Animal charcoal.
ORIGIN Charcoal made from ox hide.
BACKGROUND To make animal charcoal, ox hide is heated until luminescent, then transferred to an airtight environment.
PREPARATION Charcoal ash is triturated with lactose sugar.

REMEDY PROFILE
Carbo an. is typically prescribed for elderly people with strong nostalgia for the past and an aversion to modern life. They tend to feel chilly, feeble, abandoned, and that "everything was better in the old days."

The remedy is mainly used for painful, slow-developing symptoms associated with old age, poor nutrition, and decay, such as swollen, painful veins, poor circulation with blue extremities, cancer, and great fatigue. Pains typically feel as if they are burning, cutting, or stabbing.

Carbo an. is used particularly in the treatment of cancer, especially cancers of the glands or the uterus.
Symptoms better In warm rooms; from rubbing the eyes; from pressing the hand on the uncomfortable area.
Symptoms worse In dry, cold air; after midnight; from shaving; from eating; from fatty foods and milk.

SEE ALSO Cancer, page 208

Carbonium sulfuratum
CARBON SULF.

COMMON NAMES Carbon bisulfide, carbon disulfide.
ORIGIN Chemically prepared.
BACKGROUND Carbon bisulfide is used as an industrial solvent in rubber works, and in the manufacture of synthetic fibers such as viscose, rayon, and cellophane.
PREPARATION The compound is dissolved in purified water, diluted, and succussed.

REMEDY PROFILE
People for whom *Carbon sulf.* is best suited seem unable to think clearly. They may either be loquacious or respond slowly to others, forgetting words. In severe cases, they can be affected by dementia alternating with excitement, associated with fear, biting, sudden rage, or delusions of grandeur. At the ultimate extreme they progress to complete breakdown, especially in their relationships, with a loss of dignity and confused sense of self. They may even attempt suicide and require restraining.

This pattern of breakdown is reflected in the physical conditions for which *Carbon sulf.* is chiefly used. The body systems become "disorganized," leading to muscle-wasting, jerking pains, visual disturbances with progressive loss of vision and color blindness, widespread nerve inflammation, and digestive upsets. These symptoms may occur concurrently or in isolation.

Other important symptoms that may respond to the remedy include tinnitus, chronic sciatic pain and twitching, recurrent breathing difficulties, skin irritation, loss of sensation, and diarrhea or constipation.
Symptoms better In the open air; from warm drinks.
Symptoms worse From bathing; during and after eating.

SEE ALSO Tinnitus, *page 222*

Castoreum
CASTOREUM

COMMON NAME Castoreum.
ORIGIN Secretion from glands in the genitals of the beaver.
BACKGROUND This brownish red resinous substance was once used in its dried form as a fixative in the perfume industry.
PREPARATION Castoreum is macerated in alcohol, filtered, diluted, and succussed.

REMEDY PROFILE
Castoreum is primarily associated with women, particularly those with an angry, irritable, and argumentative state of mind that is especially evident during menstrual periods. Nervous and discontented, they tend to have anxious dreams, and to shout out angrily when they are asleep.

Castoreum is generally used for this nervous state in conjunction with profuse sweats and a weird sensation that the tongue is being pulled back by a thread from its base to the hyoid bone in the neck. There is a tendency not to recover fully from any bout of illness, and the remedy is frequently given for chronic fatigue syndrome in women. Further symptoms may include sudden spasms of pain in the abdomen.
Symptoms better From pressure on affected areas.
Symptoms worse With cold; during menstruation; after debilitating diseases; from emotional stress.

Caulophyllum thalictroides
CAULOPHYLLUM

COMMON NAMES Blue cohosh, squaw root, papoose root.
ORIGIN Native to eastern North America.
BACKGROUND Native Americans valued this plant highly for women, using it as a contraceptive, to regulate menstrual flow, to induce labor, and for children's colic.
PREPARATION The fresh root is macerated in alcohol, diluted, and succussed.

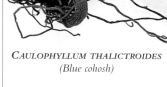

CAULOPHYLLUM THALICTROIDES
(Blue cohosh)

REMEDY PROFILE
This remedy is exclusively prescribed for symptoms in women. Those for whom it is most appropriate tend to be prone to restlessness, nervousness, and insomnia, as if they have drunk too much coffee. In severe cases they may be unable to speak.

Caulophyllum is used primarily for problems of the uterus, such as excessive bleeding and lack of tone in the uterine muscles. There may be erratic or absent uterine muscle action during menstruation or during or following labor. Inner trembling may also occur.

The remedy is also used for rheumatic joint pains affecting the small joints, particularly if they occur in conjunction with menstruation or uterine problems. The fingers, toes, and ankles may be stiff, and the wrists may ache.
Symptoms better With warmth.
Symptoms worse With movement; from coffee.

Ceanothus americanus
CEANOTHUS

COMMON NAME New Jersey tea.
ORIGIN Native to eastern North America.
BACKGROUND Native Americans used the root to make a tea for fevers, congestion, and sore throats. During the American Revolution, the leaves were used as a substitute for tea.
PREPARATION The dried leaves are steeped in alcohol, diluted, and succussed.

REMEDY PROFILE
Ceanothus is most suitable for people who feel apathetic and lack energy. They may be depressed by a fear of being unable to work due to illness.

The classic symptom picture is one of lethargy, with swelling, tenderness, and pain in the spleen. There may be such deep pain on the left side of the body that it is impossible to lie on this side. Further symptoms include palpitations, chilliness, a right-sided headache, and shortness of breath. The symptoms may be associated with serious blood or lymph disorders such as leukemia or Hodgkin's disease. The remedy is also used for those who experience great nervous excitement, with chilliness and a loss of appetite. Their nerves may be so badly shaken that they can barely hold a knife and fork. They may find it difficult to sleep, and may experience dreams of snakes and robbers.
Symptoms better In warm weather.
Symptoms worse In cold, damp weather; with movement; lying on the left side.

Centella asiatica syn. *Hydrocotyle asiatica*
HYDROCOTYLE

COMMON NAMES Gotu kola, Indian pennywort, tiger grass.
ORIGIN Native to India, and found in Sri Lanka, south China, and southwest Asia.
BACKGROUND Gotu kola has long been used in India as a meditation aid. It is also an important herbal remedy in Indian Ayurvedic medicine, notably for leprosy and as a "tonic" herb.
PREPARATION The dried aerial parts of the plant are macerated in alcohol.

REMEDY PROFILE

Hydrocotyle is best suited to people who alternate between lively, talkative behavior and dull sadness, with a desire to be alone. They may sleep heavily, sometimes with persistent dreaming all night long.

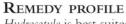

CENTELLA ASIATICA (Gotu kola)

Classic features associated with this remedy are overgrowth and hardening, which often manifests itself as thickening or hardening of the connective tissue, or scaly, thickening skin conditions. Typical skin conditions treated include psoriasis, with hardening and scaling of the affected area, lupus (red, scaly patches that leave dull white scars), and leprosy with no ulceration. The remedy may even be used for excessive skin thickening, swelling, and distortion, like that occurring in elephantiasis (a chronic disease of the lymphatic system).

Symptoms better From rubbing the affected area.

Symptoms worse In summer; at night; with movement; from pressure on the affected area; on the left side.

Chamaelirium luteum syn. *Helonias dioica*

HELONIAS

COMMON NAMES False unicorn root, devil's bit, fairy wand, blazing star.
ORIGIN Native to eastern North America.
BACKGROUND The plant was long used by Native Americans to prevent miscarriage, and herbalists still consider it invaluable for many gynecological disorders.
PREPARATION The fresh, finely chopped root and rhizome are steeped in alcohol.

REMEDY PROFILE

Characteristically, those who respond best to *Helonias* are melancholy and depressed, and have a tendency to feel better when mentally or physically occupied.

Helonias is used primarily for women's problems accompanied by severe fatigue. This exhaustion or enervation is often caused by excessive physical or mental exertion or is, conversely, the result of

a hedonistic lifestyle. It may also be associated with the extreme physical demands of frequent pregnancies or terminations. There is extreme sensitivity to and awareness of the uterus. Problems of the female reproductive system that may be treated with *Helonias* include suppressed menstruation, uterine prolapse with a sensation of weakness and dragging in the sacrum and pelvis, and a congested feeling in the kidneys, as if the menstrual flow had moved to that area. The remedy may also be used to treat edema (retention of fluid in the tissues) after uterine hemorrhage.

Symptoms better From being busy; from holding the abdomen.

Symptoms worse From fatigue; if touched; with movement; from stooping; from the pressure of clothes; in pregnancy.

Chenopodium ambrosioides var. *anthelminticum*

CHENOPODIUM

COMMON NAMES American wormseed, Jesuit's tea, Mexican tea, Jerusalem oak.
ORIGIN Native to the Caribbean and to Central and South America, and cultivated in China and the US.
BACKGROUND This plant was widely used from the middle of the 18th century by Native Americans to expel worms.
PREPARATION The seeds or whole, fresh plant are macerated in alcohol, or the oil from the seeds is diluted with alcohol.

REMEDY PROFILE

The classic use of *Chenopodium* is in treating the effects of a stroke, particularly if they involve right-sided paralysis.

Typical symptoms include repeating words or using inappropriate words, or repeating the same actions over and over again. The limbs may spasm and contract, and the hands may flex. These symptoms may be accompanied by very heavy breathing with a rattling sound, as if a ball were rolling loose in the trachea. The remedy is also used to treat right-sided migraines with giddiness, loss of sight, roaring in the ears, and dull pain in the liver area that may extend to the right shoulder blade.

Symptoms better No specific factors.

Symptoms worse With movement.

Chimaphila umbellata

CHIMAPHILA

COMMON NAMES Pipsissewa, Prince's pine, ground holly, umbellate wintergreen.
ORIGIN Found in North America, Asia, and Europe.
BACKGROUND By the 19th century this Native American remedy for sweating and fevers was adopted by European settlers for rheumatic pain and urinary problems.
PREPARATION The whole, fresh plant or aerial parts in flower are steeped in alcohol.

REMEDY PROFILE

Those who respond best to this remedy tend to feel restless and hot but seem unable to sweat. They tremble inwardly, yet are emotionally calm and stable.

Chimaphila is used chiefly for urinary tract problems such as painful urination and obstructed urine flow. It is given for cystitis with blood in the urine and a great urge to urinate despite an empty bladder. In men it is also prescribed for an enlarged prostate, urine retention, and a feeling of a ball in the pelvis.

Symptoms better From walking.

Symptoms worse In cold and damp; from sitting on cold stone; on starting to urinate.

SEE ALSO Prostate problems, *page 202*

Chininum arsenicosum

CHINA ARS.

COMMON NAME Quinine arsenite.
ORIGIN Chemically prepared.
BACKGROUND This compound of quinine (*see page 49*), arsenious acid, and potassium carbonate is little used outside homeopathy.
PREPARATION Quinine arsenite is mixed with lactose sugar and triturated.

REMEDY PROFILE

People for whom *China ars.* is appropriate tend to be exhausted and drained, and to feel that they cannot endure their state for much longer. They are either restless and on edge or completely relaxed.

The key symptom treated by *China ars.* is great fatigue, perhaps following chronic fatigue syndrome, or serious illness such as malaria or a debilitating epileptic attack. The fatigue tends to recur at specific times, possibly with burning pains, stiff joints, and fluttering "electric" pulses in the body. The remedy may also be given to treat asthma with a sensation of suffocation, oppressed breathing, and anxiety.

Symptoms better In the open air; from pressure on the affected area; from bending forward; sitting up; yawning.

Symptoms worse In the morning; with movement; from hunger.

Chininum sulfuricum
CHINA SULF.

COMMON NAME Quinine sulfate.
ORIGIN Chemically prepared.
BACKGROUND This compound is one of the quinine salts used in conventional medicine to treat malaria (*see page 49*).
PREPARATION The compound is dissolved in alcohol, diluted, and succussed.

REMEDY PROFILE

A great fear of impending misfortune or extreme anxiety about the future is typical in those most responsive to *China sulf.* They often seem bad-tempered, nervous, indifferent, weepy, and depressed. They may have difficulty naming objects.

Classic physical symptoms linked to *China sulf.* include heavy, aching limbs, joint pains, and a tender, sensitive spine that feels worse from pressure. There may be a sinking sensation when lying down, as if falling through the bed. The remedy may also be used for tinnitus, severe head pain, and recurrent fever, possibly due to malaria. Symptoms often recur at the same time each day, particularly around 3 P.M.
Symptoms better From cold compresses; from yawning; from bending forward; from pressure on the area (except the spine).
Symptoms worse In cold; if touched; at particular times of day; around 3 P.M.

SEE ALSO Tinnitus, *page 222*

Chionanthus virginicus
CHIONANTHUS

COMMON NAME Fringe tree.
ORIGIN Native to the US but now also found in eastern Asia.
BACKGROUND Traditionally used to treat canker sores, spongy gums, and eye inflammation by Native Americans and early European settlers in the 18th century.
PREPARATION The chopped bark of the fresh root is macerated in alcohol.

REMEDY PROFILE

Chionanthus is most appropriate for those who are insular, melancholic, and gloomy, with hypochondriac tendencies. They feel "played out," apathetic, and listless, and may develop nervous exhaustion.

The remedy is generally used for liver problems such as jaundice, gallstones, and biliary colic, with the characteristic fatigue. Liver pain is usually accompanied by colic, cramps, vomiting, and the feeling that the intestines are being spasmodically squeezed. The stools may be pale due to lack of bile.

Another key use of *Chionanthus* is for headaches, especially those associated with nervous tension or menstruation,

or accompanied by digestive upsets.
Symptoms better From lying on the abdomen.
Symptoms worse With movement; from jarring.

Chocolatum
CHOCOLATE

COMMON NAME Chocolate.
ORIGIN Made from the fruits of the *Theobroma cacao* tree, native to Central America and grown in other tropical areas.
BACKGROUND Used for centuries by the Maya and Aztecs in a bitter drink called *xocolatl*, cocoa was taken to Europe by Christopher Columbus in 1502. The Europeans then gradually developed this import into the chocolate that has become so popular in modern times.
PREPARATION Dark chocolate, high in cocoa, is triturated with lactose sugar.

THEOBROMA CACAO
(Cacao pod and seeds)

REMEDY PROFILE

This remedy is primarily used for a classic state of mind rather than a set of physical symptoms. People for whom *Chocolate* is best suited tend to lack concentration and to feel anxious, vulnerable, and self-conscious, as if they are being watched. They are prone to fears of cars, accidents, illness, dogs, or being attacked. They may feel estranged from loved ones, and believe that they do not belong anywhere. This state of mind can develop into withdrawal and antisocial behavior, associated particularly with a reluctance to talk and a desire to be alone in the evening.

Although used chiefly for emotional states, the symptom picture for *Chocolate* may include physical symptoms such as constriction in the chest or head, and nervous disorders associated with great clumsiness and heaviness in the limbs.
Symptoms better With warmth; from being covered up.
Symptoms worse In the evening; on waking; from eating chocolate or candies; from drinking tea.

Cicuta virosa
CICUTA

COMMON NAMES Water hemlock, cowbane.
ORIGIN Found in swamps and wet places in Kashmir and the Arctic.
BACKGROUND The name cowbane derives from the fact that grazing on the plant can transmit a potentially fatal disease to cattle.
PREPARATION The fresh root, gathered when the plant is in bloom, is chopped and macerated in alcohol.

REMEDY PROFILE

Cicuta has an affinity with the nervous system and is used both for nervous temperamental conditions and for physical disorders of the nervous system. It is generally given to people who behave childishly and do absurd things. They may be wild, delirious, and overexcited, or exhibit great sensitivity to sad stories and to the happiness of other people. Alternatively, they may be distrustful, despise other people, and have an aversion to society. Their memories can go blank for long periods. Classic physical symptoms associated with *Cicuta* focus on spasmodic effects on the nervous system, ranging from stammering and hiccups to sudden, strong jerks and spasms. Petit mal fits with long absences may be treated with the remedy, as may epilepsy or violent convulsions accompanied by facial contortions and severe backward twisting and arching of the head and neck.

The remedy may also be used for some skin disorders, often involving pustules that leave yellowish scabs, such as eczema or impetigo. The head and face may be most affected, or the whole body may develop chronic eruptions that itch and burn. A craving for chalk may occur, as may an inability to distinguish what is edible.
Symptoms better With warmth; from arching the head, neck, and spine backward; dwelling on pain; after eating.
Symptoms worse In cold; from being touched or jarred; during sleep; from noise; if skin symptoms are suppressed or diminished but not cured; from intestinal worms; after a concussion.

SEE ALSO Severe eczema, *page 194*

Cinnamomum camphora
syn. *Laurus camphora*
CAMPHORA

COMMON NAME Camphor.
ORIGIN Native to Indochina and Japan, but now found in tropical and subtropical regions throughout the world.
BACKGROUND Commonly used as a

moth repellent, camphor is also a strong narcotic, and was praised by the famous 16th-century scientist Paracelsus for its "cooling" effect on brain disorders.
PREPARATION The gum of the tree is dissolved in alcohol, diluted, and succussed.

REMEDY PROFILE
Contradictory symptoms, contrariness, and emotional and physical coldness are typical in those who respond best to *Camphora*. They crave sympathy, but may be quarrelsome, aggressive, and depressed.

Camphora made its reputation as a treatment for cholera (*see pages 16 and 65*), but is now used primarily for the initial stages of a cold with chills and sneezing. There may be great heat and perspiration with a desire to remain covered up, or chilliness with a desire to be uncovered. Other possible accompanying symptoms include insomnia and restless sleep or, conversely, deep, comatose sleep.
Symptoms better From thinking about symptoms, especially pain; from sweating.
Symptoms worse In cold; in drafts; from suppressing discharges.

Cistus canadensis
CISTUS

COMMON NAMES Frostweed, Canadian rock rose.
ORIGIN Found in North America.
BACKGROUND Frostweed is named for the early winter frost on its roots that helps it thrive.
PREPARATION The whole, fresh plant and root are macerated in alcohol.

REMEDY PROFILE
Cistus is most appropriate for those who are frightened and stressed. Mental stress often aggravates their physical symptoms. Extremely sensitive to cold air, they tend to feel cold sensations all over the body. Their illnesses are generally affected by the seasons, becoming worse in winter.

Cistus is used mainly for frequent colds, tonsillitis, upper respiratory tract infections, chronic or recurrent sinusitis, and allergic rhinitis. Typical symptoms include thick phlegm, a runny nose, and violent sneezing. The throat is dry and feels sore if even small amounts of cold air are inhaled.

Another key symptom associated with *Cistus* is glandular swelling and hardening, particularly in the neck, and possibly with concurrent respiratory symptoms. It may result from infection or even cancer.
Symptoms better From coughing up mucus; from swallowing; from eating.
Symptoms worse In cold; in drafts; if touched; in winter.

Clematis recta
CLEMATIS

COMMON NAMES Clematis, upright virgin's bower.
ORIGIN Native to central and southern Europe.
BACKGROUND This plant irritates the skin on contact, but is used by herbalists to treat sores, skin ulcers, and itchy rashes.
PREPARATION The fresh leaves and stems of the plant are macerated in alcohol.

REMEDY PROFILE
People for whom *Clematis* is best suited tend to be peevish, dissatisfied, and prone to melancholy or homesickness. Despite apathy toward friends, they generally fear being alone. They often feel confused in stuffy rooms, and improve in open air.

Clematis is strongly indicated for skin complaints and swollen glands, especially if they arise simultaneously or if there is a history of both conditions. The remedy is given for moist, itchy, sensitive pustules that erupt on the back of the head or skull.

Gland symptoms that indicate *Clematis* include hardness, swelling, and pain. The prostate, testes, ovaries, or breasts are most often affected. Further related symptoms may include urethral inflammation, which causes an aversion to sexual intercourse, and abnormal urine flow. The right side of the body is usually particularly affected.
Symptoms better From sweating; in the open air; during a waning moon.
Symptoms worse At night; from cold air; from bathing in cold water; from the heat of the bed; if touched; with movement; during a new moon.

Colchicum autumnale
COLCHICUM

COMMON NAMES Meadow saffron, autumn crocus.
ORIGIN Found wild in Europe and Africa, and cultivated in North America.
BACKGROUND During classical times the plant was considered too toxic for use. Arabian physicians used it in the Middle Ages for joint pain and gout.
PREPARATION The fresh bulb, dug up in spring, is chopped and steeped in alcohol.

REMEDY PROFILE
Those who respond well to *Colchicum* are typically weak and restless. They may be depressed or irritable, and have poor concentration and memory, so that they appear dazed even though they may answer questions correctly. There is a marked absence of any apprehension and no discernable fear of death.

The key symptoms linked with *Colchicum* focus on the muscle tissues and joint membranes, especially the membranes in the small joints. The joints may be painful, hot, and swollen, and the muscles extremely relaxed and even limp. Arthritic joint pain or gout may be so severe that it causes screaming if the joints are touched or jolted. There may be a twitching, tingling sensation all over the body.

Colchicum is also considered a useful remedy for ulcerative colitis and for nausea with colicky pains and painful distension of the abdomen. Illness is typically accompanied by a feeling of icy coldness in the stomach.

In addition to any other symptoms, the body may feel cold inside, with extreme oversensitivity to external stimuli such as bright lights, strong odors, physical contact, and even other people's behavior.
Symptoms better With warmth; from rest; after passing stools.
Symptoms worse In cold and dampness; in changeable weather; from vibrations or jarring.

SEE ALSO Ulcerative colitis, *page 190*; Rheumatoid arthritis, *page 197*

Collinsonia canadensis
COLLINSONIA

COMMON NAMES Stoneroot, horsebalm, richweed.
ORIGIN Native to moist woodlands in eastern North America.
BACKGROUND Stoneroot named for its hard, knotted root. It is used herbally in a poultice for bruises and sores.
PREPARATION The fresh root is chopped and macerated in alcohol.

REMEDY PROFILE
Collinsonia is best suited to people who have a gloomy temperament. They tend to experience strange bodily sensations, including the feeling that the body is being pricked by needles, that it is enlarged, and that the lower limbs are disembodied.

The classic symptom picture for this remedy is of sore, bleeding hemorrhoids, with a sensation of sharp sticks, constriction, and pricking pain in the rectum, which is prone to fissures.

Collinsonia is also used for menstrual pain, pelvic aches, and labor or pregnancy problems such as an itchy vulva during pregnancy, or diarrhea after labor. It is especially appropriate if symptoms occur in conjunction with rectal or bowel disorders.
Symptoms better With heat; in the morning.
Symptoms worse At night; in cold; during pregnancy; from emotional stress.

Comocladia dentata
COMOCLADIA

COMMON NAMES Guao, bastard Brazil wood.
ORIGIN Native to Cuba.
BACKGROUND This tree exudes a milky sap that turns black on contact with air and stains clothes and skin. It causes a violent skin reaction in people who have sensitive skin.
PREPARATION The fresh leaves and bark are chopped and macerated in alcohol.

REMEDY PROFILE
Comocladia is most appropriate for irritable people who are prone to maliciousness, gloomy behavior, and restlessness while awake. Sleep refreshes them, however, and they enjoy vivid, pleasant, and perhaps even clairvoyant dreams. The key physical symptoms associated with this remedy include nerve sensitivity and skin problems such as extreme itching, burning, inflammation, and blistering. The skin may flake or begin to shed, or it may redden, possibly forming stripes. There may be ulceration or other swelling, which may be fever-related.
Symptoms better In the open air; from scratching; with movement.
Symptoms worse With heat; if touched; with rest; in the evening.

Convallaria majalis
CONVALLARIA

COMMON NAME Lily-of-the-valley.
ORIGIN Native to Europe, but also found across North America and in northern Asia.
BACKGROUND The 16th-century herbalist John Gerard praised this plant for its success in treating gout and heart problems. It is used in modern herbalism, particularly for heart disorders.
PREPARATION The fresh, flowering aerial parts are macerated in alcohol.

REMEDY PROFILE
People who respond best to *Convallaria* have difficulty in thinking, because their brains feel dull. They often find themselves unable to concentrate when reading, and tend to become irritable when questioned. There is a tendency to experience feelings of depression.

Convallaria is prescribed primarily for heart problems. Typical heart symptoms treated by the remedy include palpitations triggered by the slightest exertion. The heartbeat may seem to reverberate through the whole chest and rib cage, or it may become fluttery and irregular after exercise, possibly causing nausea and breathlessness. Water retention may accompany heart problems, as may poor circulation. It is often given for heart palpitations that occur in conjunction with soreness of the uterus.
Symptoms better In the open air.
Symptoms worse In warm rooms; lying on the back.

CONVALLARIA MAJALIS
(Lily-of-the-valley)

Copaifera officinalis
COPAIVA

COMMON NAME Balsam of copaiva.
ORIGIN Native to tropical South America, but also found in southern Africa.
BACKGROUND This traditional native Brazilian remedy for healing wounds and removing scars was first recorded in 1625 by a Portuguese monk, Manoel Tristaon.
PREPARATION A tincture of balsam is made from oleoresin (a semisolid mixture of resin and essential oil) from the plant.

REMEDY PROFILE
Copaiva is given to restless, overwrought people who are prone to burning pains and a feeling of heaviness or pressure on any part of the body. Their nervous system is extremely sensitive, and they tend to startle when they hear noises, and to weep on hearing piano music. A key symptom associated with the remedy is excessive discharge from the mucous membranes. This includes urinary-tract discharges, phlegm during a cold, and profuse, greenish gray, offensive-smelling mucus during a bout of chronic bronchitis. The remedy is also used as a treatment for mucus discharges associated with leucorrhea (abnormal discharge from the vagina), urethritis (inflammation of the urethra), and gonorrhea.
Symptoms better From pressure on the affected area; from walking; from bending double; from perspiring.
Symptoms worse In the morning; from catching cold; from starchy foods.

Corallium rubrum
CORALLIUM

COMMON NAMES Red coral.
ORIGIN The *Gorgonia nobilis* species of coral, which is found mainly in the waters of the Mediterranean and Japan.
BACKGROUND Coral is the skeleton of a tiny animal called the coral polyp. Red coral's delicate, pink skeleton is largely comprised of calcium, and is commonly used to make jewelry and prayer beads.
PREPARATION Pieces of skeleton are mixed with lactose sugar and triturated.

REMEDY PROFILE
Corallium is most appropriate for critical, peevish, angry people who tend to swear and curse when they are in pain. They may have a craving for sour foods, and like wine but easily become stupefied and drunk. Prone to extreme tiredness, they may even fall asleep when standing up.

The remedy is used chiefly for whooping and spasmodic coughs, which tend to occur in rapid, frequent fits, accompanied by violent paroxysms, exhaustion, a smothering sensation, and the bringing up of blood. The face may become purple and congested. The air passages may feel cold on breathing in deeply, and there may be profuse phlegm. The throat is very sensitive, especially to air.
Symptoms better With heat; from covering up; in the afternoon and evening; from sitting.
Symptoms worse From inhaling in the open air; from moving from a warm to a cold room; from eating.

Crataegus laevigata syn. *C. oxyacantha,* or *C. monogyna*
CRATAEGUS

COMMON NAMES Hawthorn, May tree, whitethorn.
ORIGIN Found in all temperate regions of the Northern Hemisphere.
BACKGROUND Hawthorn is an extremely valuable medicinal herb, used since the Middle Ages as a heart remedy. Modern trials have shown that it improves the heart rate and lowers blood pressure.
PREPARATION The fresh, ripe berries are chopped and macerated in alcohol.

REMEDY PROFILE
Crataegus is most appropriate for irritable, grumpy, melancholic people who are prone to heart complaints. They tend to feel weak, fragile, and despairing. Their brains feel dull and confused, with possible periods of quiet and calm.

The characteristic symptom picture for the remedy is of a weak heart, palpitations, and a rapid heartbeat with a sense of hurry and urgency. The pulse is fast, feeble, and intermittent. Fainting and collapse may accompany palpitations, and the area around the heart can feel as

CRATAEGUS LAEVIGATA
(Hawthorn)

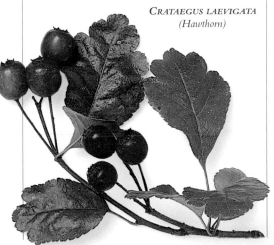

though it were bursting from congestion or overexertion.
Symptoms better In fresh air; from quiet; rest; washing; during menstruation.
Symptoms worse With heat; from sweating; in the morning; in the evening.

Crocus sativus
CROCUS

COMMON NAME Saffron crocus.
ORIGIN Native to India and the Balkans, and now cultivated in Spain, France, Italy, and the Middle East.
BACKGROUND It takes roughly 150,000 flowers and 400 hours' work to make 2.2 lb (1 kg) of dried saffron, making it the most costly spice known.
PREPARATION The dried stigmas of the plant are macerated in alcohol.

CROCUS SATIVUS
(Saffron crocus)

REMEDY PROFILE
The range of key symptoms for which *Crocus* is generally prescribed includes nervous excitement, alternating moods, a sensation of something moving inside the abdomen, and hemorrhages with dark, clotted, stringy blood, usually in the form of nosebleeds or uterine bleeding.

Crocus is taken for rapidly alternating mental and physical states. The nervous system is overexcited, causing mood swings and hysterical, excited behavior. The feeling that something is moving inside the abdomen may be linked to general nervous hyperactivity. Hopping or jumping sensations may be felt inside the abdomen; these may be linked to a false pregnancy.
Symptoms better In the open air; from yawning; after breakfast.
Symptoms worse With movement; during pregnancy; during puberty; from changes of the moon.

Crotalus durissus terrificus syn. *C. cascavella*
CROTALUS CASC.

COMMON NAME South American rattlesnake.
ORIGIN Found in South America.
BACKGROUND This snake can grow up to 59 in (1.5 m) long. It has a deadly venom that primarily affects the nervous system.
PREPARATION Fresh venom is mixed with lactose sugar and then triturated.

REMEDY PROFILE
This remedy is most appropriate for people who feel jealous and forsaken. They fear being alone and love crowds and activity. They are frequently hypochondriacs who are sensitive to the cold. Characteristically they tend to be preoccupied by death and dying, and their dreams may feature corpses. They may feel that they are being haunted by ghosts. Right-sided symptoms are generally predominant.

Crotalus casc. is typically used for this state of mind in conjunction with a sense of constriction, which is sometimes felt as a band around the throat or abdomen; wearing clothes may cause discomfort.
Symptoms better In the open air.
Symptoms worse With cold; at night; on the right side; from washing; during menopause; from drinking.

Croton tiglium
CROTON

COMMON NAME Croton.
ORIGIN Found in subtropical and tropical forests from India to Malaysia.
BACKGROUND Croton oil, made from the pressed seeds, has been used as a drastic purgative. An overdose of this carcinogenic oil may cause shock, while contact with the skin may lead to blistering.
PREPARATION The oil from the seeds is percolated in alcohol.

REMEDY PROFILE
People for whom *Croton* is most suitable tend to be "pent-up" emotionally. Often they feel anxious, as if some personal misfortune is about to befall them. They tend to be exhausted, dissatisfied, and morose, with an inability to work or think of anything except themselves.

Mirroring the uses of the oil itself, which is strongly purgative and irritating, *Croton*'s main affinities are with the skin and digestion. The remedy is typically used for allergic skin conditions with extreme itching, such as eczema on the scrotum, or blistering rashes on the scrotum and penis. *Croton* is also given for digestive problems such as nausea and urgent diarrhea immediately after eating or drinking.

A key symptom is the strange sensation that a string has been attached to the eyes or the nipples and is pulling them inward. The eyes feel as if they are being drawn backward into the head, and there is tense pain over the right eye, causing headaches.
Symptoms better After sleep; from rubbing the affected area; from warm milk.
Symptoms worse If touched; in summer; while skin eruptions are disappearing; from drinking; from eating.

Cuprum arsenicosum
CUPRUM ARS.

COMMON NAMES Copper arsenite, Scheele's green.
ORIGIN Chemically prepared.
BACKGROUND This toxic, yellow-green pigment was used in wallpapers until a link was established between it and a multitude of health problems, especially digestive disorders and cramps.
PREPARATION The compound is mixed with lactose sugar and triturated.

REMEDY PROFILE
Those who respond best to *Cuprum ars.* are often confused, restless, and in anguish. Their bodily functions are also confused and disturbed, with chilliness and periods of irregular or weak heart function. Their bodies tremble, especially when walking, or they may be prostrated.

A key condition associated with *Cuprum ars.* is poor kidney function. Typical symptoms include burning pain on urinating, dark red, discolored urine with a strong odor, perhaps of garlic, and diarrhea. The remedy may also be given to those who have experienced prolonged fluid loss, perhaps after injury or an operation.

Symptoms better From hard pressure on the affected area.
Symptoms worse In damp; if touched; with movement; during bouts of diarrhea.

Cyclamen europaeum
CYCLAMEN

COMMON NAMES Cyclamen, sowbread.
ORIGIN Found throughout Europe.
BACKGROUND In the 1st century CE Pliny the Elder noted the use of this plant as an arrowhead poison in ancient Rome. The name sowbread refers to the medieval practice of feeding the roots to swine.
PREPARATION The fresh root, gathered in spring, is chopped and steeped in alcohol.

REMEDY PROFILE
Cyclamen is best suited to rather dutiful, conscience-stricken people who tend to find fault with themselves and others. Prone to drowsiness, gloominess, and depression, they may wish to be alone and cry or weep silently, or they may have a sense of joy that alternates with irritability.

The symptom picture for *Cyclamen* typically focuses on menstrual problems and indigestion. The remedy is used when the menstrual flow is irregular, possibly too frequent, or absent. Blood flow may be profuse and black, or the blood may clot too rapidly, and there may be severe

pains resembling those felt during labor. Visual disturbances, migraines, or a squint may accompany these symptoms.

Extreme indigestion that is aggravated by eating fats is another condition suitable for treatment with *Cyclamen*.

Symptoms better With movement; from rubbing the affected area; from weeping; during menstruation.
Symptoms worse With cold; in open air; before menstruation; from suppression of menstrual flow due to shock or extreme cold; from sitting; from standing.

Dactylopius coccus syn. *Coccus cacti*
COCCUS CACTI

COMMON NAME Cochineal beetle.
ORIGIN Found in Spain, Mexico, and the West Indies.
BACKGROUND The dried bodies of the female insects are used as a scarlet dye and food coloring, and in cosmetics, inks, artists' pigments, and medicines.
PREPARATION The fertilized females are killed by heat, then dried and macerated in alcohol.

REMEDY PROFILE
Coccus cacti is generally prescribed for spasmodic coughing associated with congestion, and for urinary problems with pain in the kidneys, particularly in those who are anxious and confused.

The remedy is used for spasmodic coughing, especially whooping cough, and for asthma. Symptoms are usually worse in the mornings, and include frequent, violent, ticklish coughing fits accompanied by vomiting and retching up of clear, ropy mucus that may hang from the mouth. There is a sensation of a thread hanging down the back of the throat. The mucous membranes in the throat may feel so sensitive that even brushing the teeth causes retching and vomiting.

Symptoms better From washing in cold water; from walking; from cold drinks.
Symptoms worse On the left side of the body; lying down; after sleep; if touched; from the pressure of clothing; with the slightest exertion; from brushing the teeth; from rinsing the mouth.

SEE ALSO Asthma, *page 181*

Daphne mezereum
MEZEREUM

COMMON NAMES Mezereon, spurge olive.
ORIGIN Native to Eurasia and found in North America, Europe, and north Africa.
BACKGROUND Herbalists in northern Europe once used the plant to treat skin

ulcers and cancers, but today mezereon is considered too toxic for common use.
PREPARATION The fresh bark, gathered just before the plant blooms, is chopped and steeped in alcohol.

REMEDY PROFILE
Mezereum is most appropriate for people who are prone to despondency, apathy, and detachment. They have a tendency toward hypochondria.

Key conditions associated with this remedy are suppurating skin complaints that form a thick crust or cause cracking. Skin symptoms typically affect the scalp, usually manifesting as eczema or psoriasis with oozing discharge that smells offensive and causes the hair to mat. Eruptions on the face are usually around the hairline or eyebrows. The skin is intensely itchy, and may feel cold and clammy. The remedy is also used for shingles affecting the chest.

Neuralgic pains around the teeth or face, and pains in the long bones, are also usually linked with *Mezereum*. Symptoms include erratic, jerking, sharp pains, and a sensation of lightness or enlargement in the body.

In addition *Mezereum* is prescribed for digestive system disorders that are anxiety-related and involve symptoms such as diarrhea and a discharge from the anus.
Symptoms better In open air; from eating.
Symptoms worse At night; lying down; from the warmth of the bed; if skin eruptions are suppressed by ointments; from drafts; with movement; if touched.

SEE ALSO Severe eczema, *page 194*

Digitalis purpurea
DIGITALIS

COMMON NAMES Common foxglove, purple foxglove.
ORIGIN Native to western Europe, and cultivated in India, southern and central Europe, Norway, Madeira, and the Azores.
BACKGROUND The 18th-century English doctor William Withering first established this flower's importance as a heart remedy, and its active constituents are still used in herbal and conventional heart medicines.
PREPARATION The fresh leaves are picked before the plant blooms in its second year. The juice is expressed from the leaves, then mixed with alcohol and diluted.

REMEDY PROFILE
Digitalis is associated primarily with the heart. It is prescribed for people who are prone to heart and circulatory disorders. The remedy is considered particularly appropriate if symptoms are accompanied by a fear of death, or a fear that moving –

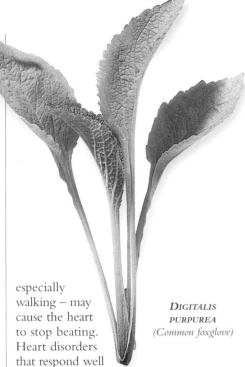

DIGITALIS PURPUREA
(Common foxglove)

especially walking – may cause the heart to stop beating. Heart disorders that respond well to treatment with *Digitalis* are typically accompanied by pains in the region of the heart, a slow pulse, faintness, and nausea. The remedy is also used for liver problems, particularly if they occur in conjunction with heart symptoms.

Symptoms better In cool air; with rest; lying on the back; with an empty stomach; from frequent urination.

Symptoms worse With heat; from standing up; exertion; with movement; lying on the left side; from sexual excess.

SEE ALSO Palpitations, *page 186*

Dioscorea villosa
DIOSCOREA

COMMON NAME Wild yam.

ORIGIN Native to North and Central America.

BACKGROUND A traditional Aztec remedy for pain, wild yam was commonly used in Central America for colic and menstrual pain. It was also used in the production of the first contraceptive pill.

PREPARATION The fresh root is dug up after the plant has flowered. It is then chopped and macerated in alcohol.

REMEDY PROFILE
People for whom this remedy is most appropriate are prone to irritability, stress, and nervousness.

Key symptoms associated with *Dioscorea* are neuralgic and colicky pains, primarily affecting the gastrointestinal system. The pains are typically severe, cutting, cramping, and grinding, and radiate out in all directions from a central point that may shift location. They may affect the

area of the liver, radiating upward to the right nipple. In women, the pains may occur during menstruation. In men, *Dioscorea* is typically prescribed to treat renal colic associated with kidney stones, sharp pains radiating down the testicles and legs, and cold, clammy perspiration.

Symptoms better From stretching out; from bending backward; from standing erect; with movement; from firm pressure on the affected area; from burping.

Symptoms worse From doubling up; lying down; from 2 A.M. onward; from eating; from drinking tea.

Drosera rotundifolia
DROSERA

COMMON NAMES Sundew, common sundew, round-leaved sundew, red rot, youthwort, moorgrass.

ORIGIN Grows in Europe, Asia, and North America.

BACKGROUND Sundew was taken in the 16th and 17th centuries for melancholia. In 1735 the *Irish Herbal* advised that it could be used to "eat away rotten sores."

PREPARATION The whole, fresh, flowering plant is macerated in alcohol.

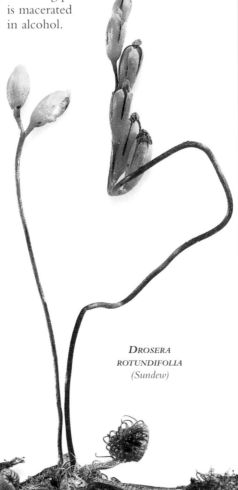

DROSERA ROTUNDIFOLIA
(Sundew)

REMEDY PROFILE
Drosera is usually prescribed to treat a deep, violent, spasmodic cough, especially whooping cough. Associated symptoms may include restlessness, anxiety, retching, vomiting, cold sweats, and nosebleeds. There may also be a feeling that there is a feather or crumb in the larynx, which triggers coughing. The voice is often toneless, hoarse, and deep.

There is some indication that *Drosera* may be helpful in treating behavioral problems, particularly in children. It is best suited to children who are restless, anxious, peevish, and distrustful. Their emotions seem unbalanced, and they often have difficulty concentrating. Their anxiety may increase when they are alone, and can be associated with a fear of ghosts.

Drosera may also be given for childhood growing pains, especially if they are accompanied by emotional imbalance. Symptoms may include stiff ankles and pains in the joints and bones, particularly affecting the hips and thighs.

Symptoms better In the open air; with movement; from walking; from sitting up; from pressure on the affected area.

Symptoms worse With warmth; after midnight; lying down; from cold foods.

SEE ALSO Whooping cough, *page 250*

Echinacea angustifolia
ECHINACEA

COMMON NAMES Echinacea, coneflower.

ORIGIN Native to North America, and now cultivated in Europe and the US.

BACKGROUND Native Americans used echinacea for toothaches and sore throats. Long considered an herbal "cure-all" and thought to stimulate the immune system, it is currently being researched as a treatment for HIV and AIDS.

PREPARATION The fresh plant, including the root, is pulped and steeped in alcohol.

REMEDY PROFILE
Echinacea is typically prescribed for its antiseptic properties, to treat abscesses, boils, carbuncles, swollen glands, animal and insect bites and stings, septicemia, and diphtheria. The remedy is also given to treat cancer, especially as an analgesic in the late stages of the illness. Typical physical symptoms include chilliness, tiredness, and weakness, with aching muscles, considerable weight loss, debility, and foul-smelling discharges.

Symptoms better With resting or lying down; after physical or mental exertion.

Symptoms worse With cold; in cold air.

Equisetum hyemale & E. arvense
EQUISETUM

COMMON NAMES Rough horsetail, field horsetail, bottlebrush.
ORIGIN Found mainly in Asia, particularly China, and in Europe and North America.
BACKGROUND This primitive genus has been used to heal wounds since at least the 1st century CE. Strongly abrasive, it was used between the Middle Ages and the 18th century for scouring pots.
PREPARATION The fresh plant of either species, including the root, is first pulped, then steeped in alcohol.

EQUISETUM ARVENSE (Field horsetail)

REMEDY PROFILE
Those who respond best to this remedy are irritable and easily tired. *Equisetum* is used chiefly for painful irritation of the bladder, which is aching, full, and tender. There is a sensation of painful pressure on either side of the lower abdomen and bladder. The pain becomes worse at the end of urination. There may be a constant desire to urinate, possibly with dribbling of urine, or mucus in the urine. It is also given to children who wet their bed during nightmares or other dreams.
Symptoms better Lying on the back; from walking.
Symptoms worse From being touched; with movement; from pressure on the painful area.

SEE ALSO Bedwetting, *page 248*

Erythroxylum coca
COCA

COMMON NAME Coca.
ORIGIN Native to Peru and Bolivia, but now also cultivated elsewhere in South America and in Asia, usually illegally.

BACKGROUND Early European travelers to the Andes noted that the indigenous people chewed coca leaves as a stimulant. Coca contains cocaine, a narcotic drug that has spawned a huge illegal industry.
PREPARATION The leaves are dried, powdered, and macerated in alcohol.

REMEDY PROFILE
Coca is most appropriate for people who alternate between complete exhaustion and great mental excitement. They may be timid and antisocial, and have a sense of impending death and auditory hallucinations, or they may be extremely talkative and experience blissful visions. Their brains may feel muddled, and they can lose their sense of right or wrong and neglect their appearance. The remedy is a very successful antidote for altitude sickness. Athletes and elderly people with symptoms of breathlessness or asthma may also be treated with *Coca*, since the classic physical symptom picture includes breathlessness.
Symptoms better With rapid movement; in the open air; after sunset; from wine.
Symptoms worse With cold; from ascending to high altitudes; with physical and mental exertion.

Eupatorium perfoliatum
EUPATORIUM PER.

COMMON NAMES Boneset, agueweed, thoroughwort, sweating plant.
ORIGIN Native to North America.
BACKGROUND Native Americans used a boneset infusion for colds, fever, arthritis, and rheumatic pain. Its ability to stimulate the immune system against fever made it popular with European settlers.
PREPARATION The fresh aerial parts in flower are macerated in alcohol.

REMEDY PROFILE
When people for whom this remedy is best suited are ill, they may moan with pain and feel that they are going out of their minds. They tend to feel anxious and restless, wishing that they could keep still. They may have a sensation of their bones as broken.
Eupatorium per. is usually given for the flu or malarial fever accompanied by pain in the limbs. Fever typically starts as a chill, then generates heat, sweating, and a strong thirst, accompanied by pains in the bones and great restlessness. Further symptoms that may be treated include vomiting of bile, and headaches that feel worse during the sweating phase.
Symptoms better From conversation; after vomiting bile.

Symptoms worse In cold air; after a recurring interval of time; with movement; from the smell or sight of food.

Euphorbia resinifera 'Berger'
EUPHORBIUM

COMMON NAMES Spurge, gum euphorbia.
ORIGIN Native to Morocco.
BACKGROUND In classical times spurge was used as a purgative, until recognition of the danger of poisoning from an overdose led to disuse. In Europe its milky, irritating sap was used to burn off warts until the 19th century.
PREPARATION The hardened, resinous sap is macerated in alcohol.

REMEDY PROFILE
A key symptom linked with *Euphorbium* is burning pain in the bones, as if live coals were in or on the bones. The limbs may feel weak and dislocated, with sharp, cramping pains and weakness in the joints.
Another classic problem treated by this remedy is itching, burning skin, possibly with warts, slow-healing ulcers, or yellow blistering. These symptoms may be due to erysipelas (a bacterial infection) on the face.
Symptoms better With movement; from applying oil to the affected area.
Symptoms worse From sitting; if touched; on beginning to move.

Euphrasia officinalis
EUPHRASIA

COMMON NAME Eyebright.
ORIGIN Native to Europe, but now also found in Asia and North America.
BACKGROUND This herb has been used to treat eyestrain and inflammations since the Middle Ages. Modern herbalists use it for infections and allergic conditions of the eyes, middle ear, sinuses, and nasal passages.
PREPARATION The whole, fresh, flowering plant, including the root, is chopped and macerated in alcohol.

REMEDY PROFILE
People who respond well to *Euphrasia* are typically taciturn, indolent, melancholic, and prone to daydreaming.
Euphrasia has a classic affinity with the eyes. Common physical symptoms include irritation in the eyes, with cutting, burning, pressing pains and sticky mucus. There is typically heightened sensitivity to light, with burning, swollen eyelids and frequent blinking. The eyes tend to water profusely, a symptom that is exacerbated

EUPHRASIA OFFICINALIS
(Eyebright)

by open air, lying down, or coughing. The remedy is used mainly for allergies or infections affecting the eyes and nose, such as colds, hay fever, or conjunctivitis. It may also be prescribed if eye symptoms occur after an injury.
Symptoms better In open air; from blinking; wiping the eyes.
Symptoms worse With warmth; from wind; from sunlight; from being indoors.

SEE ALSO Conjunctivitis, *page 220;* Hay fever & allergic rhinitis, *page 224*

Euspongia officinalis

SPONGIA

COMMON NAME Common sponge.
ORIGIN Traditionally gathered from waters of the Mediterranean, near Syria and Greece.
BACKGROUND It is thought that roasted sponge was first used as a remedy in the 13th century, by the alchemist Arnold von Villanova as a treatment for goiter.
PREPARATION Sponge is carefully cleaned of sand, then toasted in a metal drum before being powdered and triturated.

REMEDY PROFILE

Spongia is most appropriate for those who have a marked fear of heart disease and of death, particularly by suffocation. They may feel uncomfortable in clothes.

There is a strong focus on the heart with this remedy. Typical physical symptoms that it is used to treat include palpitations and an uneasy feeling in the area of the heart. There may be congestion, with a sensation of blood rushing into the chest and face. A fear of suffocation and a sense of the heart being forced upward out of the chest can disrupt sleep after midnight. There is great exhaustion and the body feels heavy, so that even the slightest exertion causes complete prostration.

Spongia is also prescribed for upper respiratory tract infections that tend to settle in the larynx, such as a dry, hollow, barking, croupy cough. There

is typically a feeling of dryness in the mucous membranes, and inflammation, enlargement, and hardening of the glands, especially the thyroid gland. There may be a sensation of a plug in the larynx, which may feel very sensitive to touch. Pain in the larynx typically becomes worse from swallowing, singing, or talking.
Symptoms better Lying with the head low; from bending forward; eating small amounts; from warm foods and drinks.
Symptoms worse In dry, cold winds; from waking up.

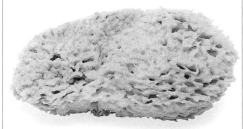

EUSPONGIA OFFICINALIS
(Common sponge)

Fagopyrum esculentum

FAGOPYRUM

COMMON NAME Buckwheat.
ORIGIN Native to central and northern Asia, and cultivated in temperate regions, especially in the US and eastern Europe.
BACKGROUND This major grain crop may have been taken to Europe during the 11th and 12th centuries. Medicinally, the leaves were used for high blood pressure, cold sensitivity, and frostbite.
PREPARATION The aerial parts are picked after flowering and before the fruits ripen, then chopped and macerated in alcohol.

REMEDY PROFILE

Confusion and alternating states of mind are typical in those for whom *Fagopyrum* is best suited. These people also tend to be depressed and irritable.

Fagopyrum is generally associated with eczema and itching skin, possibly on the genitals, scalp, eyelids, and ears, or in the folds of the skin of infants and the elderly. The inside of the nose may become sore and crusted. Foul-smelling secretions may accompany itching.

Heart complaints associated with visibly pulsing arteries, either with or without concurrent skin conditions, may also be treated with *Fagopyrum*. Other symptoms linked to this remedy include a rapid, irregular pulse and a strong sensation of oppression in the heart area.
Symptoms better From cold compresses; from pressure on the affected area; coffee.
Symptoms worse From sunlight; from scratching; with movement.

Ferula assa-foetida
syn. *Narthex assa-foetida*

ASAFETIDA

COMMON NAMES Asafetida, devil's dung.
ORIGIN Native to Iran, Afghanistan, and Pakistan.
BACKGROUND In the 7th century BCE the *Charaka Samhita*, an Ayurvedic medicine book, advocated this foul-smelling plant for bloating and flatulence, for which it is still used in India and the Middle East.
PREPARATION Gum resin from the living roots is macerated in alcohol.

REMEDY PROFILE

People who respond best to this remedy tend to be in a rather nervous, hysterical, hypersensitive, and hypochondriacal state. This nervous state extends to the physical symptoms, which generally focus on digestive disorders and on nervous twitching. The stomach may feel as if it is pushing upward so that everything will burst into the mouth, or there may be a sensation of a lump in the stomach rising upward into the throat.
Symptoms better In the open air; with movement; from pressure on the affected area; from scratching.
Symptoms worse At night; with rest; from sitting; if touched.

Fraxinus americana

FRAXINUS

COMMON NAME White ash.
ORIGIN Native to eastern North America.
BACKGROUND In Norse mythology the ash tree was considered sacred. In Europe its nutritious sap has traditionally been used as a gentle laxative.
PREPARATION The bark of the tree is chopped and macerated in alcohol.

REMEDY PROFILE

A need to talk is common in those who respond best to this remedy, and they tend to be depressed, nervous, and anxious. Illness may be accompanied by uneasy sleep and frightening dreams.

Fraxinus is chiefly used for uterine problems. Typical symptoms include a uterus that is relaxed in tone, or possibly prolapsed, with a watery, nonirritating vaginal discharge and a heavy, painful, bearing-down sensation. The remedy is also given for heavy, painful menstruation, and for fibroids and other tumors.
Symptoms better No specific factors.
Symptoms worse From injury; from sprains; from lifting.

SEE ALSO Fibroids, *page 199*

Galipea officinalis syn. *G. cusparia*
ANGUSTURA

COMMON NAME Angustura.
ORIGIN Native to the Caribbean and tropical South America.
BACKGROUND The bitter bark of this tree was long used by Native Americans as a tonic, and to stun fish and hence increase the catch. Taken to Europe in 1759, it was originally used for aromatic bitters.
PREPARATION Dried bark from the tree's branches is macerated in alcohol.

REMEDY PROFILE

Angustura is best suited to people who are either timid and weak, or highly sensitive, touchy, and "filled with bitterness." They are often very restless at night, waking for no reason, and unable to get back to sleep. Their dreams are vivid, anxious, and unsettling, and they may crave coffee.

The remedy is typically prescribed for rheumatic conditions and nervous system disorders, especially those affecting the nerves in the spine or causing paralysis. Symptoms include tension and stiffness in the muscles and joints, making them feel sore and bruised. There may be tearing pains in the bones that lead to difficulty in walking. The tissues may even decay due to painful ulcers that penetrate the bone marrow and cause the bones to crumble, particularly the long bones of the body.
Symptoms better From applying cold fingers or a cold compress to the affected area; from sitting up; with rest.
Symptoms worse From exertion; from stooping; from sitting bent over; from touching the affected area; from noise.

Gelsemium sempervirens
GELSEMIUM

COMMON NAMES Carolina jasmine, yellow jasmine, false jasmine.
ORIGIN Native to the southern US and Central America, and now grown worldwide.
BACKGROUND Carolina jasmine came into regular use from the middle of the 19th century, chiefly as a treatment for nervous disorders such as sciatica and neuralgia.
PREPARATION The fresh bark of the root is finely chopped and macerated in alcohol.

REMEDY PROFILE

People for whom *Gelsemium* is most suited fear losing control. They dislike being disturbed, especially while feverish, when they feel dull, drowsy, and dizzy, but want to be held. Their faces are flushed dark red, with a dull, confused expression.

A general state of mental and physical paralysis, with weakness and an inability to perform, are key symptoms linked to this remedy. At times the remedy has been given to strengthen courage on the battlefield, and it is often used for phobias, exam nerves, stage fright, and other anticipatory terrors, which cause trembling, weakness, diarrhea, and frequent urination. In the long term these symptoms may lead to more complicated, serious neurological disorders and possibly even paralysis, which the remedy may help.

Gelsemium is also used to treat acute bouts of the flu or sore throats, with weakness, limp limbs, chills, fever, headaches with double vision, and heavy, drooping eyelids. There may be a lack of thirst, even during fever. In addition the remedy can be given for hay fever if accompanied by these symptoms.
Symptoms better From profuse urination; from sweating; from shaking; from alcoholic drinks.
Symptoms worse In humid weather, especially during spring; from extreme emotions; from dread or ordeals; from surprises or shocks.

SEE ALSO Phobias, *page 211*; The flu, *page 224*; Sore throat, *page 226*; Exam nerves, *page 254*

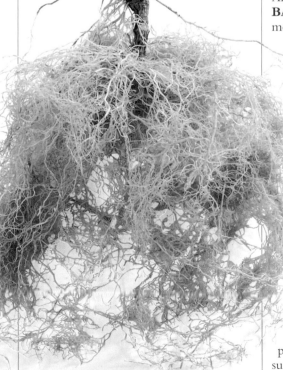

GELSEMIUM SEMPERVIRENS
(Carolina jasmine)

Gnaphalium polycephalum
GNAPHALIUM

COMMON NAMES Sweet-scented everlasting flower, cudweed.
ORIGIN Native to North America.
BACKGROUND This plant has been used in herbal medicine to treat colds, fevers, and respiratory and intestinal mucus, and has been applied as a poultice to bruises.
PREPARATION The whole, fresh plant is macerated in alcohol.

REMEDY PROFILE

This remedy is used mainly for intense sciatic pains alternating with or followed by numbness. Lumbago with numbness and heaviness in the affected area may also be treated, as may joint pains and rheumatic complaints. In addition, foul-smelling diarrhea with colic that is worse in the morning may respond to the remedy, as may scant menstrual periods that are most painful on the first day.
Symptoms better From sitting in a chair; from flexing the limbs.
Symptoms worse With cold; in dampness; with movement; from walking; from stepping up or down; lying down.

Gratiola officinalis
GRATIOLA

COMMON NAMES Hedge hyssop, herb of grace.
ORIGIN Found in central Europe, North America, and Australia.
BACKGROUND Originally esteemed medicinally for jaundice and other liver or spleen complaints, this herb is now rarely used due to its toxicity.
PREPARATION The fresh bulb is dug up prior to flowering and steeped in alcohol.

REMEDY PROFILE

Gratiola is most suited to those who appear irritable, haughty, and possibly excessively proud. They may develop mental symptoms if they drink coffee regularly over a long period of time, as well as physical symptoms such as migraines, sciatica, and a high libido. A high sex drive, frequent masturbation, and nymphomania are primary conditions that may be helped by *Gratiola*, particularly in women. In addition, the remedy is prescribed for gastrointestinal problems such as cramps in the pit of the stomach, and, after eating, the sensation of a stone rolling from side to side in the stomach.

Eating may be followed by a strange sense of emptiness in the stomach. There may be green, frothy, watery diarrhea that is expelled with great force.

Symptoms better In the open air.
Symptoms worse In summer; from eating; from drinking excessive amounts of water; from coffee.

Guaiacum officinale
GUAIACUM

COMMON NAME Lignum vitae.
ORIGIN Native to the South American and Caribbean Islands.
BACKGROUND In the 16th century Native Americans were found to be using lignum vitae for venereal disease and syphilis, and it became popular in Europe until discredited in the 18th century.
PREPARATION The resin obtained from the tree is macerated in alcohol.

REMEDY PROFILE

Guaiacum is most appropriate for narrow-minded people who tend to be obstinate, overcritical, and inflexible. This mental rigidity is mirrored by a fixation of the joints. The remedy is most commonly used for great arthritic or rheumatic joint pain, especially in the wrists. Arthritic pain may feel worse with heat, and there may also be a sensation of swelling, tension, and tautness in the muscles, as if they were too short. There is a strong desire to yawn and stretch. Children with this remedy profile may have growing pains.
Symptoms better In cold, wet weather; from cold compresses; from apples.
Symptoms worse With heat; in wet weather; if touched; with movement; from exertion; from rapid growth.

Hamamelis virginiana
HAMAMELIS

COMMON NAME Virginia witch hazel.
ORIGIN Native to Canada and eastern and central US, and grown in Europe.
BACKGROUND Native Americans used witch hazel in poultices for tumors and inflammations. It is used as an herbal first-aid remedy for its astringent properties.
PREPARATION Fresh, chopped bark from the twigs and root is steeped in alcohol.

REMEDY PROFILE

People who respond best to *Hamamelis* often feel a lack of appreciation and respect from others prior to illness, which tends

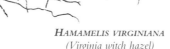

HAMAMELIS VIRGINIANA
(Virginia witch hazel)

to make them become depressed and solitary. When ill they are prone to feelings of restlessness and irritability.

The remedy's primary use is in treating hemorrhoids and varicose veins. The veins are typically inflamed and weak. There is susceptibility to hemorrhaging, such as heavy periods in women or nosebleeds. Bleeding is generally slow to stop, and is usually accompanied by calm.
Symptoms better In fresh air; from reading; from thinking; from talking.
Symptoms worse In warm, damp air; from pressure on the affected area; with movement.

SEE ALSO Varicose veins, *page 230*; Hemorrhoids, *page 238*

Hecla lava
HECLA

COMMON NAME Hecla lava.
ORIGIN Volcanic ash from the immediate vicinity of Mt. Hecla in Iceland.
BACKGROUND Mt. Hecla last erupted in 1970. Its lava contains aluminum silicate, magnesium, calcium, and iron oxide.
PREPARATION Ash is triturated with lactose sugar to make the tincture.

REMEDY PROFILE

Hecla is best suited to people who are rather volcanic in temperament. They usually suppress any anger, but after a certain point they erupt.

The remedy is typically used for bone disorders, such as exostosis (benign bony outgrowths) or osteitis (inflammation of the bone). It is considered particularly suitable for treating sarcoma (cancer of the connective tissue) and osteosarcoma

(a malignant bone tumor), especially if they occur in the jaw, head, or legs. Glandular swellings, particularly those in the neck, can also be treated with *Hecla*, as can toothaches.
Symptoms better With continued movement; toward 3 P.M.
Symptoms worse From pressure on the affected area; from sitting; on beginning to move.

SEE ALSO Cancer, *page 208*

Hippomane mancinella
MANCINELLA

COMMON NAMES Manchineel, manzanilla.
ORIGIN Found in the West Indies.
BACKGROUND The sap of this tree, or even just the smoke from its wood when burning, is so acrid that it can cause blindness on contact with the eyes.
PREPARATION The fresh fruits, leaves, and bark of the tree are chopped and steeped in alcohol.

REMEDY PROFILE

Mancinella is used primarily for mental rather than physical symptoms. It is most appropriate for people who fear that they may become insane and lose control of their minds, due to the intrusion of evil thoughts or possession by evil spirits. Their feelings are intensified by watching horror movies, and their anxieties may become obsessive or even lead to a psychological breakdown. An advanced breakdown may cause the memory to deteriorate, with forgetfulness from one minute to the next. *Mancinella* is also prescribed for confused feelings about sexuality that are bound up with the fear of being possessed by evil spirits, especially if these feelings occur during puberty or menopause.

Physical symptoms typically associated with *Mancinella* include skin problems such as dermatitis. They are generally accompanied by an oozing, sticky serum, which may form crusts or blisters, or stinging blisters on the soles of the feet, with acrid, sticky foot perspiration.

The sense of smell may be affected by strange illusions, such as phantom smells of gunpowder or dung. There may be a peppery, burning sensation in the mouth, along with a taste of blood and copious yellow saliva.
Symptoms better From rubbing the affected area; from walking.
Symptoms worse In cold and dampness; if touched; with puberty; menopause.

LUPULUS

Humulus lupulus syn. *Lupulus humulus*

COMMON NAME Hops.
ORIGIN Native to Europe and Asia.
BACKGROUND Hops have been cultivated in Europe since at least the 11th century to make beer. Medicinally, hops are used mainly as a sedative, often sewn into a bed pillow to aid sleep at night.
PREPARATION The fresh hops are finely chopped and macerated in alcohol.

REMEDY PROFILE

Appropriately enough for a remedy based on a plant used to make beer, *Lupulus* is often used to treat hangovers or the aftereffects of drinking alcohol, such as nausea, dizziness, and headaches. It may also be given for nervous twitches or delirium associated with drunkenness.

Muscles affected by twitching, nervous tremors may also be treated by *Lupulus*, as may rheumatic pains that shift from place to place, mainly in the shoulders, arms, and hands. There may be a sensation of churning in the stomach, accompanied by nausea and vomiting. Burning in the urethra when urinating and overexcitability are further possible symptoms, as is greasy, clammy, profuse perspiration.
Symptoms better In the open air.
Symptoms worse From coffee; from alcohol.

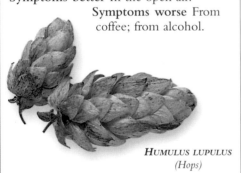

HUMULUS LUPULUS
(Hops)

MERC. CORR.

Hydrargyrum bichloratum
syn. *Mercurius sublimatus corrosivus*

COMMON NAME Mercuric chloride.
ORIGIN Chemically prepared.
BACKGROUND Mercuric chloride is a powerful disinfectant with rapid, violent effects, especially on the rectum, if ingested.
PREPARATION The compound is mixed with lactose sugar and triturated.

REMEDY PROFILE

People who respond best to *Merc. corr.* are prone to anxiety and restlessness, which may develop into delirium and stupor during illness. They often feel detached or disconnected from others, and may stare blankly at people when they are talking, without comprehending what they are saying.

Symptoms linked to *Merc. corr.* tend to be excessive, rapid, and violent, often centering on the digestion. The remedy is used for colitis or dysentery with hot, foul-smelling stools, cutting pains, and constant straining, even after passing a stool. Great straining may be needed to empty the bladder. Burning in the throat, stomach, rectum, and bladder, with great susceptibility to the cold, may be linked to throat complaints treated by *Merc. corr.*, such as swollen glands, a constant need to swallow despite pain, and ulcerated tonsils.
Symptoms better With rest.
Symptoms worse In the open air; from urinating; from passing a stool; at night.

SEE ALSO Ulcerative colitis, *page 190*

MERC. IOD. RUBER.

Hydrargyrum biiodatum
syn. *Mercurius biiodatus*

COMMON NAME Mercuric iodide.
ORIGIN Chemically prepared.
BACKGROUND This red, odorless powder has a faintly metallic taste. It is used as an antiseptic and disinfectant for the skin.
PREPARATION Mercuric iodide is mixed with lactose sugar and triturated.

REMEDY PROFILE

Those who respond best to *Merc. iod. ruber.* tend to be weepy, low in spirits, and irritable, particularly in the morning. Toward evening they often feel better and become more cheerful.

The classic symptom picture for this remedy is of an ulcerated sore throat with swollen glands, especially on the left side. The throat may be painful and dark red, and neck and throat muscles may be stiff.
Symptoms better In the open air; in the evening.
Symptoms worse With sleep; in the morning.

MERC. DULC.

Hydrargyrum chloratum
syn. *Mercurius dulcis*

COMMON NAMES Mercurous chloride, calomel.
ORIGIN Chemically prepared, although it occurs naturally in Germany, the former Yugoslavia, Mexico, and Texas.
BACKGROUND This compound was used medicinally from the 16th century as a cathartic, but has since fallen out of favor because of its toxicity.
PREPARATION Mercurous chloride is mixed with lactose sugar and triturated.

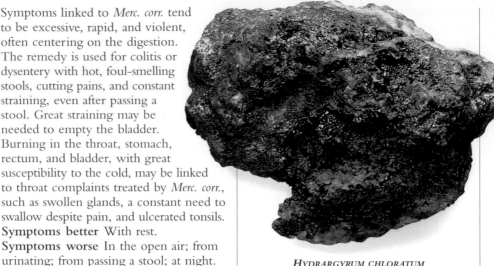

HYDRARGYRUM CHLORATUM
(Mercurous chloride)

REMEDY PROFILE

Apprehension, restlessness, and agitation are common in those for whom *Merc. dulc.* is most suitable.

Key symptoms associated with *Merc. dulc.* include congested inflammation in the ears and eustachian tubes, leading to deafness and chronic fluid in the ear. The condition is predominant in children, and *Merc. dulc.* is particularly appropriate for those who appear pale and ill-nourished.
Symptoms better From cold drinks.
Symptoms worse From acidic foods and drinks.

MERC. CYAN.

Hydrargyrum cyanatum
syn. *Mercurius cyanatus*

COMMON NAME Mercurous cyanide.
ORIGIN Chemically prepared.
BACKGROUND This highly poisonous substance has no history of use in medicine, except in homeopathy.
PREPARATION Mercurous cyanide is mixed with lactose sugar and triturated.

REMEDY PROFILE

Merc. cyan. is given most often to people who are talkative, highly emotional, and overexcited. They may have frequent spells of unconsciousness or fainting, depending on the severity of their illness.

The remedy is typically used for acute infectious diseases with rapidly sinking strength and a tendency to hemorrhage. It is strongly associated with throat and mouth conditions such as tonsillitis and diphtheria. The throat is typically red with a white coating, and there may be pain on swallowing, with inflammation of the uvula. The tongue, lips, and cheeks tend to ulcerate, the saliva tastes metallic, and the breath smells offensive.

These symptoms are usually accompanied by weakness, great sensitivity to the cold, nausea, and cold, damp, sweaty skin.
Symptoms better From drinking milk.
Symptoms worse From swallowing; from speaking; from eating.

Hydrargyrum iodatum flavatum
syn. *Mercurius iodatus flavatus*
MERC. IOD. FLAV.

COMMON NAME Mercurous iodide.
ORIGIN Chemically prepared.
BACKGROUND In Western conventional medicine this compound has traditionally been used to make an ointment that is applied externally for eye diseases.
PREPARATION Mercurous iodide is mixed with lactose sugar and triturated.

REMEDY PROFILE
Merc. iod. flav. is most appropriate for people who tend to alternate rapidly between depression and high spirits.

The classic symptom picture for *Merc. iod. flav.* is of right-sided complaints, particularly throat infections with swollen glands and a coated tongue. If pharyngitis, tonsillitis, or ear infections affect the right side, *Merc. iod. flav.* is strongly indicated. Common symptoms include a sensation of a lump in the throat, throat inflammation, and ulcerated patches in the throat that exude a cheeselike mucus. Sharp, throbbing pains may affect the right ear, becoming worse on swallowing.
Symptoms better In the open air; from physical exertion; during the day.
Symptoms worse In cold, damp weather; at night; with gentle movement.

Hydrargyrum sulfas
syn. *Mercurius sulfuricus*
MERC. SULF.

COMMON NAMES Mercuric sulfate, turpeth mineral.
ORIGIN Chemically prepared.
BACKGROUND This heavy, odorless, tasteless, lemon yellow powder has no medicinal uses, except in homeopathy.
PREPARATION Mercuric sulfate is mixed with lactose sugar and triturated.

REMEDY PROFILE
Eating tends to make people for whom *Merc. sulf.* is best suited feel irritable. They may be chilly, pale, and anxious.

Key conditions associated with this remedy include digestive complaints and respiratory difficulties. *Merc. sulf.* is given for breathing that tends to be rapid and short, with burning in the chest, pain in the region of the heart, and weakness that may feel better from sitting up.

An irritated stomach, with vomiting, burning in the anus, hot, copious urine, and watery, soft, or violently expelled stools are characteristic of the digestive symptoms treated by *Merc. sulf.* In some cases, symptoms may be combined: For instance, fluid in the lungs may be accompanied by watery or violent diarrhea and other digestive symptoms.
Symptoms better From sitting up; from profuse diarrhea (in the case of breathing difficulties).
Symptoms worse Lying down; in the morning; at night.

Hydrargyrum sulfuratum rubrum
syn. *Cinnabar*
CINNABARIS

COMMON NAMES Mercuric sulfide, sulfide of mercury, quicksilver.
ORIGIN Found mainly in Spain, and also in Peru, Italy, and California.
BACKGROUND In traditional Chinese medicine this mineral is used to treat sore throats, canker sores, and palpitations. Its bright scarlet pigment is called vermilion.
PREPARATION Mercuric sulfide is triturated with lactose sugar.

REMEDY PROFILE
Cinnabaris is best suited to people who are nervous, uneasy, sad, weak, and weary. They do not want to use their brains, and may become forgetful, often feeling that their heads are "full" from mental use. At night a stream of constantly changing

HYDRARGYRUM SULFURATUM RUBRUM
(Mercuric sulfide)

thoughts runs through their heads. They are usually sensitive to touch and to the slightest noise, preferring to be left alone.

This remedy has a classic affinity with genital and rectal ulceration and warts, and its profile is similar to that of *Merc. sol.* (*see page 85*). Key symptoms include fiery red ulcers on the skin and the mucous membranes, warts that bleed easily, pimples, pustules, and red skin eruptions that tend to itch violently.

The head is a focus for other symptoms that may be helped by the remedy. These include headaches with congestion; red, inflamed eyes; phlegm in the nose and throat; and a dry, sore throat. Sleep patterns may be disrupted, with noticeable restlessness and sleeplessness, although there is often a marked lack of tiredness.

Cinnabaris may also be used to treat women who experience very painful menstruation and pregnancy, or great pains during labor.
Symptoms better In the open air; from sunshine; after dinner.
Symptoms worse With dampness; if touched; in the evening; at night; from light; before menstruation.

Hydrastis canadensis
HYDRASTIS

COMMON NAMES Goldenseal, orange root, yellow puccoon.
ORIGIN Native to North America.
BACKGROUND Native Americans used goldenseal's root for its intense yellow dye, and medicinally for cancer, fevers, indigestion, and heart or liver disorders. It was introduced to Europe in 1760.
PREPARATION The dried underground parts of the plant are steeped in alcohol.

REMEDY PROFILE
People who benefit from *Hydrastis* tend to be weary, exhausted, thin, and elderly, often with degenerative conditions.

The classic symptom picture for this remedy is of problems of the mucous membranes. It is associated with phlegm, sinusitis, a sore throat, and an abnormal taste in the mouth. There may be copious, thick, yellowish, stringy mucus affecting the mucous membranes of the respiratory system. The remedy is also used for stomach problems, possibly occurring in conjunction with the classic problems of the mucous membranes. Characteristic symptoms include poor digestion, a sensation of emptiness in the stomach that remains even after eating, and constipation with no urge to pass stools.

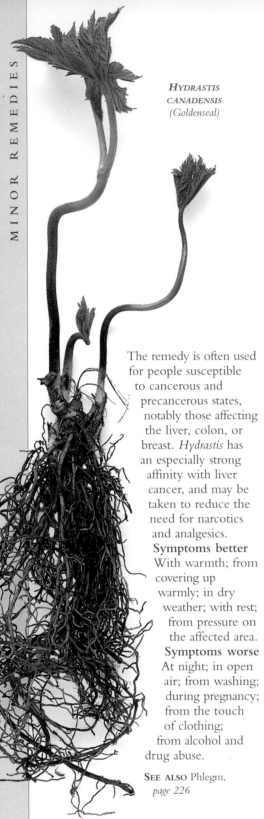

*HYDRASTIS
CANADENSIS*
(Goldenseal)

The remedy is often used for people susceptible to cancerous and precancerous states, notably those affecting the liver, colon, or breast. *Hydrastis* has an especially strong affinity with liver cancer, and may be taken to reduce the need for narcotics and analgesics.

Symptoms better With warmth; from covering up warmly; in dry weather; with rest; from pressure on the affected area.

Symptoms worse At night; in open air; from washing; during pregnancy; from the touch of clothing; from alcohol and drug abuse.

SEE ALSO Phlegm, *page 226*

Hypericum perforatum
HYPERICUM

COMMON NAME St. John's wort.
ORIGIN Native to Europe and Asia, but now found in temperate areas worldwide.
BACKGROUND Renowned medicinally since classical times, St. John's wort was long thought to have magical importance too. An extract of it is given for depression.
PREPARATION The whole, fresh plant is finely chopped and macerated in alcohol.

REMEDY PROFILE
Hypericum is prescribed for people who are depressed, frightened, or shocked following an injury or accident. They may be nervous, overexcited, constantly drowsy, talk while asleep, and forgetful when speaking. These people may also experience a constant sensation of elevation or falling.

Key physical symptoms associated with this remedy are injuries or wounds that feel more painful than they appear, with extremely sharp pains, perhaps in nerve-rich areas such as the fingertips or the base of the spine. The remedy may be used to relieve pain following operations, accidents, puncture wounds, and animal bites, and is also given to help prevent tetanus. Nervous pains in phantom limbs after amputation, and toothaches or discomfort after dental treatment may also be helped by the remedy.
Symptoms better Lying quietly; lying face down; from bending the head backward; from rubbing the affected area.
Symptoms worse In cold, damp weather; from injury; from jarring; from shock.

Iridium metallicum
IRIDIUM MET.

COMMON NAME Iridium.
ORIGIN Obtained from osmiridium, an alloy of iridium, osmium, and platinum.
BACKGROUND This metal is named after the Greek goddess of the rainbow, Iris, due to its colorful salts. It is used in fountain-pen nibs and syringe needles.
PREPARATION Iridium is triturated with lactose sugar.

REMEDY PROFILE
Those who respond most effectively to *Iridium met.* are generally well presented and confident. If not successful in their plans or projects, or if they become ill and exhausted, they may experience confusion, with poor concentration and the feeling that their minds are empty.

Classic physical symptoms linked to *Iridium met.* include exhaustion and anemia following a bout of illness, and muscle pain and stiffness with tender, swollen joints. There may be nervous, pinching pains in the wrists, fingers, and limbs. In the hip joints there may be scraping, stinging pains and a crawling sensation; sciatic nerve pain may radiate down the legs. Neuralgic pains, perhaps in the back of the head, may be treated with *Iridium met.*, as may lameness or partial paralysis, especially in the elderly. The remedy is also used to help prevent suppurating abscesses in the armpits.

Symptoms better With cold; from being indoors; from pressure on the affected area; with continued movement.
Symptoms worse From talking; on the left side of the body.

Iris versicolor
IRIS

COMMON NAME Blue flag, wild iris.
ORIGIN Native to North America, and now also grown widely in Europe.
BACKGROUND Native Americans used blue flag to treat stomach complaints, wounds and sores, colds, and earaches, and as a diuretic. Modern herbalists use the plant in detoxification treatments.
PREPARATION The fresh root, dug up and chopped in summer, is steeped in alcohol.

REMEDY PROFILE
The mood of people who respond best to *Iris* is generally low. They often feel restless and discouraged.

Key symptoms related to the remedy are headaches and migraines accompanied by digestive disorders such as nausea, severe diarrhea, or cholera. Warning signals that precede a migraine include great exhaustion and blurring or loss of vision. Migraines are typically right-sided but may alternate from side to side. They usually center in the temple or around the eyes, and involve throbbing pain, severe nausea, vomiting, and profuse salivation. The head pain is typically aggravated by vomiting.
Symptoms better With gentle movement.
Symptoms worse In hot weather; at night; from mental exhaustion.

Juniperus communis
JUNIPER

COMMON NAME Juniper.
ORIGIN Found in Europe and North America, and from southwestern Asia to the Himalayas.
BACKGROUND Juniper has been used since classical times, both medicinally and in cooking. Traditionally, sprigs were flung into fires to ward off evil spirits, and burned to protect against the plague. The berries are used to flavor gin.
PREPARATION Alcohol is added to the finely chopped, fresh, ripe berries.

REMEDY PROFILE
Classically this remedy has a reputation for increasing urine production, and is used to treat water retention, possibly with advanced kidney disease. The urine may contain blood and have a strange

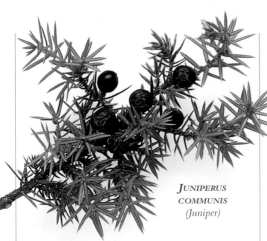

JUNIPERUS
COMMUNIS
(Juniper)

scent of violets, and there may be a feeling of heaviness in the region of the kidneys. *Juniper* is also used separately as a stimulant for the uterine muscles and to ease menstrual pain. It is usually given as a tincture rather than in tablet form.
Symptoms better No specific factors.
Symptoms worse No specific factors.

Juniperus sabina
SABINA

COMMON NAME Savin.
ORIGIN Grows in temperate regions of the northern hemisphere.
BACKGROUND Savin was used internally in 19th-century Europe to induce abortions, though generally it has been little used in herbal medicine due to its high toxicity.
PREPARATION The fresh, young branch tops and leaves are chopped before being macerated in alcohol.

REMEDY PROFILE
This remedy is best suited to people who are dejected and hypochondriacal. They may be irritable and find that even music makes them nervous. They often dislike being talked to, especially when walking in the open air. They may sob or weep and have weak memories.

Sabina is strongly associated with the reproductive organs, and is commonly used for problems such as genital warts or itching, burning external genitalia. In men it is also prescribed for phimosis (constriction of the foreskin), swelling of the upper penis, and gonorrhea.

The remedy may be given to women for uterine problems featuring pale red, clotting hemorrhages that become worse with the slightest movement and better from walking. The uterus may seem to quiver, as if a fetus were moving inside it. Further symptoms include itchy nipples with a voluptuous, crawling sensation, sharp pains shooting up the vagina, and violent hot flashes and pulsations in the body. Menstrual flow is often profuse and

premature, with pains similar to those felt during labor. *Sabina* is a classic remedy in pregnancy for those who are prone to miscarriages, especially during the third month of pregnancy. It is also prescribed following labor, if the placenta has been retained and there is intense pain.

A craving for acidic foods and drinks, especially lemonade, may be apparent, and everything – especially coffee and milk – may taste bitter. There may be violent, hot flashes, pulsations in the body, and an urge to throw open a window.
Symptoms better With cold; in the open air; from breathing out.
Symptoms worse With heat; from warm air; from the heat of the bed; with the slightest movement; in foggy weather; at night; during pregnancy and menopause; from music; if touched.

SEE ALSO Infertility, *page 203*

Kalium arsenicosum
KALI. ARS.

COMMON NAMES Potassium arsenate, Fowler's solution.
ORIGIN Chemically prepared.
BACKGROUND The form of potassium arsenate used is Fowler's solution, which consists of tincture of lavender, potassium carbonate, arsenous acid, and pure water.
PREPARATION The compound is triturated with lactose sugar.

REMEDY PROFILE
Kali. ars. is most suitable for people who are very anxious, especially about their health, and is similar in profile to *Arsen. alb. (see page 68)*. Those affected may experience great mental and physical restlessness, with nervousness, depression, anemia, and hypersensitivity to touch and noise. They have a tendency to be either argumentative and excitable, or withdrawn, timid, and indifferent.

Key physical symptoms associated with this remedy are chronic or malignant skin problems. The skin typically burns and itches, becoming worse when undressing and from the cold; cracks may develop in the bends of the knees and arms. This is usually symptomatic of eczema, psoriasis, acne, or ulcers. The remedy may be used to ease skin cancer, and for varicose veins on the legs that have become ulcerous.

In addition, the remedy may be given for asthma with rapid, anxious breathing, which may become worse after midnight.
Symptoms better On rainy days.
Symptoms worse From noise; with cold feet; if touched; between 1 A.M. and 3 A.M.

SEE ALSO Mild acne, *page 240*

Kalium bromatum
KALI. BROM.

COMMON NAME Potassium bromide.
ORIGIN Chemically prepared.
BACKGROUND Potassium bromide is used in photography to make gelatin papers and plates, and was used medicinally in the past as a sedative and antiepileptic.
PREPARATION Solid potassium bromide is triturated with lactose sugar.

REMEDY PROFILE
Poor memory, sadness, and loss of mental capabilities is often noted in those for whom *Kali. brom.* is most appropriate. The remedy has an affinity with the nervous system, and may be prescribed following a stroke, epilepsy, or other seizures. Great physical restlessness, with characteristic traits such as frequent wringing of the hands or fidgeting of the feet, is a typical accompanying symptom, as is numbness in the skin and the mucous membranes, especially those of the throat.

At its most extreme, the state of mind associated with this remedy can develop into depressive delusions with a sense of being pursued for imagined wrongdoings. Fear of insanity and feelings of suspicion and rage may occur, developing in extreme cases to psychosis, mania, paranoia, autism, and retardation, which *Kali. brom.* may alleviate. It may also ease intense sexual feelings that progress to sexual addiction.

In addition to its association with nervous symptoms, *Kali. brom.* is used for skin symptoms such as acne (especially on the forehead), psoriasis, rosacea, pustules, cysts, eczema on the legs, cold, numb skin, and crops of small boils. The skin tends to be blue and mottled in appearance, and may scar following skin eruptions.

The remedy may also be used to treat female reproductive organs that develop ovarian cysts, tumors, or fibroids, and for symptoms triggered during menstrual periods, such as

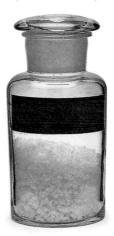

KALIUM BROMATUM
(Potassium bromide)

epilepsy. In men, *Kali. brom.* may be given for excessive sexual appetite or impotence.
Symptoms better From being occupied, mentally and physically.
Symptoms worse From sexual excess; during puberty or pregnancy; with mental overexertion.

SEE ALSO Rosacea, *page 193*

Kalium chloratum
KALI. MUR.

COMMON NAME Potassium chloride.
ORIGIN Obtained from the mineral sylvine, which is found mainly in North America and Germany.
BACKGROUND Dr. Schüssler introduced this compound to homeopathy, using it for one of his tissue salts (*see page 90*).
PREPARATION Potassium chloride is triturated with lactose sugar.

REMEDY PROFILE
People who respond best to *Kali. mur.* tend to be optimistic and hardworking. They alternate between cheerfulness and sadness, being sensitive to sadness in others and in themselves, which may make them seem self-pitying.

Key symptoms treated by this remedy include chronic mucus and congestion in the nose. It is particularly appropriate if symptoms affect the middle ear, causing earaches, pain behind the ears, snapping noises in the ears, blockage of the eustachian tube, and possibly deafness. The nasal congestion is due to profuse, whitish mucus, and is characteristically accompanied by nosebleeds.

Kali. mur. is also an important remedy for tonsillitis or swollen throat glands, for chronic sore throats with crusts of phlegm in the throat, and for cancer. Inflammation in the membranes and joints may also respond to the remedy.
Symptoms better From rubbing the affected area; from letting the hair down.
Symptoms worse In the open air; from fats and rich foods; from cold drinks.

SEE ALSO Cancer, *page 208*; Blockage of the eustachian tube, *page 222*; Phlegm, *page 226*

KALIUM CHLORATUM
(Sylvine)

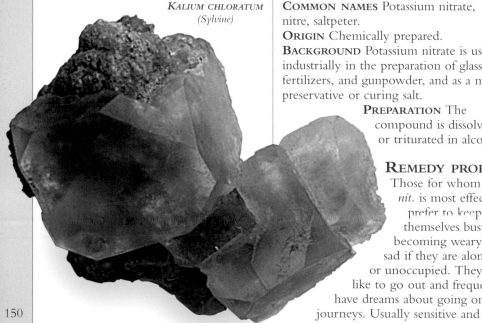

Kalium iodatum
KALI. IOD.

COMMON NAME Potassium iodide.
ORIGIN Chemically prepared.
BACKGROUND Potassium iodide is added regularly to table salt and animal feed to protect against iodine deficiency.
PREPARATION Potassium iodide is triturated with lactose sugar.

REMEDY PROFILE
Those for whom *Kali. iod.* is best suited have strong tempers, and know that they can be cruel and difficult for others to cope with, especially their families.

Classic symptoms indicating the *Kali. iod.* remedy include chronic phlegm, recurring sinusitis, swellings, abscesses, or atrophy of the glands. Symptoms are characteristically long-standing, and tend to be accompanied by great weakness, sensitivity, and soreness that is difficult to pinpoint on the body. There is frequently water retention and swelling, and a desire to move around in the open air.

Kali. iod. is often prescribed for the treatment of discharges that are copious and watery, possibly with chronic allergic rhinitis and pain in the sinuses. It is also prescribed for thick, chronic phlegm, accompanied by an unpleasant smell and susceptibility to nosebleeds.
Symptoms better In cold air; in the open air; with movement.
Symptoms worse With heat; with warmth from clothes or a hot room; at night; with rest; from pressure or touch.

Kalium nitricum
KALI. NIT.

COMMON NAMES Potassium nitrate, nitre, saltpeter.
ORIGIN Chemically prepared.
BACKGROUND Potassium nitrate is used industrially in the preparation of glass, fertilizers, and gunpowder, and as a meat preservative or curing salt.
PREPARATION The compound is dissolved or triturated in alcohol.

REMEDY PROFILE
Those for whom *Kali nit.* is most effective prefer to keep themselves busy, becoming weary and sad if they are alone or unoccupied. They like to go out and frequently have dreams about going on journeys. Usually sensitive and

dutiful, they become increasingly anxious and melancholic when ill, and may feel physically and mentally numb, as if they were made of wood.

Sharp pains and numbness are typically associated with *Kali. nit.*, in conjunction with respiratory problems. The remedy is used for conditions such as asthma, croup, and bronchitis. Further symptoms may include faintness, nausea, an inability to drink due to breathing difficulties, and a sensation of coldness around the area of the heart. There may be labored breathing caused by tightness in the larynx, the throat may be hoarse and rough, and the nose may develop polyps, chronic irritation, phlegm, and sinusitis.
Symptoms better From gentle movement; from drinking sips of water.
Symptoms worse From cold and dampness; from getting cold; from walking; from veal; from wine or beer.

Kalium sulfuricum
KALI. SULF.

COMMON NAMES Potassium sulfate, sulfate of potash, Vesuvian salt, glaserite.
ORIGIN Chemically prepared.
BACKGROUND This compound is used as an ingredient in fertilizers and in the manufacture of glass, and was chosen by Dr. Schüssler to be one of his "biochemic" tissue salts (*see page 90*).
PREPARATION Potassium sulfate is triturated with lactose sugar.

REMEDY PROFILE
Kali. sulf. is most appropriate for people who tend to be conservative and anxious to do things right, even to the last detail. They are often hurried, anxious, restless, easily startled, and irritable. Dutiful in loving relationships, they may be self-sacrificial because of the connection this gives them with others.

The remedy's classic affinities are with the skin and the respiratory system. It is commonly prescribed for peeling skin conditions such as eczema and psoriasis, and may also be appropriate for ringworm, polyps, oily skin problems, and skin cancer. The skin is characteristically chapped, scaly, or peeling, and there may be sore areas with thin, yellow, watery discharges.

Chronic respiratory problems are a further key affinity of *Kali. sulf.* It is used for chronic phlegm, or mucus in the ear, nose, larynx, or bronchi, and for asthma. The nose is typically highly congested, with rattling mucus in the lungs and loss of the sense of smell. There may be smelly, long-standing discharges in the ears, with frequent inflammation.

Symptoms better In the open air; in cold air; from walking; from fasting.
Symptoms worse In warm air; in warm, stuffy rooms; in the evening; from noise; from sympathy; from eggs.

Kalmia latifolia
KALMIA

COMMON NAMES Mountain laurel, calico bush, ivy bush, lambkill.
ORIGIN Native to eastern North America.
BACKGROUND This plant is notoriously poisonous: Grazing on the leaves can kill cattle and sheep and cause the meat from the animals to become too toxic to eat.
PREPARATION The fresh leaves of the plant in flower are chopped and macerated in alcohol.

REMEDY PROFILE
People for whom *Kalmia* is most suitable feel fine when lying down, but become dizzy and disoriented on trying to move.

The remedy is usually given for severe, sharp neuralgic pains in the muscles and joints, and for general muscle pain. The pains are sharp and darting, and generally radiate downward. They are frequently accompanied by great weakness, stiffness, numbness, trembling, and a tingling sensation. Heart disease, especially if it develops after a history of neuralgic pain and stiffness, may also be treated with the *Kalmia* remedy.
Symptoms better From eating; from remaining still.
Symptoms worse From becoming cold; with movement; from sunrise to sunset.

Kreosotum
KREOSOTUM

COMMON NAME Creosote.
ORIGIN Distilled from beechwood tar.
BACKGROUND Creosote has long been used as a wood preservative, and its name derives from the Greek *kreas*, or "flesh," and *soter*, or "preserver." A Moravian chemist, Reichenbach, introduced it to medicine in the 19th century, but it fell out of favor with all except homeopaths.
PREPARATION Creosote is dissolved in alcohol, diluted, and succussed.

REMEDY PROFILE
A temperamental state is typical of people who respond best to *Kreosotum*. They may also be forgetful, peevish, sensitive to music, and restless at night. A tendency to dwell on the past is characteristic, as are dreams of sexual intercourse and a fear of being raped.

The classic symptom picture associated with *Kreosotum* is of mucous membranes that become inflamed, suppurate, and then break down and bleed, particularly in the vagina, the cervix, and the uterus. The remedy is given for offensive-smelling discharges from the mucous membranes that burn the skin and cause itching and swelling, and it may help when urine burns the skin on contact. It may be prescribed for particular problems before and after menstruation, such as bleeding between cycles and heavy, offensive-smelling menstrual flow that burns the skin on contact. Candidiasis may also respond to the remedy.
Symptoms better With warmth; with movement; after sleep; from pressure on the affected area.
Symptoms worse With cold; from bathing in cold water; with rest; during pregnancy.

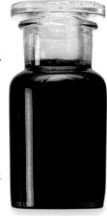

KREOSOTUM
(Creosote)

SEE ALSO Candidiasis, *page 200*

Lac vaccinum defloratum
LAC DEFL.

COMMON NAME Skimmed cow's milk.
ORIGIN Skimmed cow's milk.
BACKGROUND Milk has had a checkered history. It has been lauded as being full of healthy vitamins and minerals, yet is also linked to causing phlegm, tuberculosis, and Crohn's disease.
PREPARATION The milk is dissolved in purified water, diluted, and succussed.

REMEDY PROFILE
Lac defl. is most effective for people who are claustrophobic, chilly, listless, and forgetful. They often have either an aversion to milk, or a tendency to drink large amounts, but show signs of lactose intolerance, which affects their nutrition and tends to make them thin or obese.

Key symptoms associated with *Lac defl.* are weakness and anemia after chronic disease. Diabetes, water retention related to heart disease, and chronic liver disease may respond to the remedy, and it may also help headaches, particularly those associated with menstruation.
Symptoms better With rest; from profuse urine flow.
Symptoms worse With cold; from the slightest draft; during menstruation and pregnancy; from milk.

Lachnanthes tinctoria
LACHNANTHES

COMMON NAMES Red root, spirit weed.
ORIGIN Native to eastern North America.
BACKGROUND A red dye is derived from the plant's root, hence one of its common names. When eaten, the root causes cerebral stimulation or narcosis.
PREPARATION The whole, fresh, flowering plant, with the root, is steeped in alcohol.

REMEDY PROFILE
Lachnanthes is most appropriate for those who are prone to hilarious, overexcited, talkative behavior followed by stupid, irritable moods. They are restless both night and day, and sleepy, although they often have difficulty falling asleep and may experience distressing dreams.

The main focus of the remedy rests on the circulation, especially in relation to the head and chest. There is typically a sensation of heat bubbling and boiling up from the heart and chest to the head. Right-sided headaches accompanied by great chilliness may also be treated with this remedy, as may tuberculosis.
Symptoms better From being in bed; from being warmed.
Symptoms worse On the right side; from noise; on waking during the night.

Lathyrus sativus
LATHYRUS

COMMON NAME Chickpea.
ORIGIN Found in the Mediterranean area, Africa, and central Asia.
BACKGROUND These edible, pealike seeds have long been used in cooking, though there is little tradition of medicinal use.
PREPARATION The dried, green seed pods are macerated in alcohol.

REMEDY PROFILE
This remedy focuses predominantly on the spine and lower limbs. Characteristic symptoms treated include pain in the lower back, urinary incontinence, tremors, and total loss of sexual function. Sharpened reflexes are further possible symptoms, as are burning heat in the legs and icy cold feet. *Lathyrus* has also been used for weakness and heaviness in the aftermath of the flu and other viral illnesses, and for multiple sclerosis. Symptoms may worsen rapidly following exposure to cold, damp night air.
Symptoms better From undressing.
Symptoms worse In damp, cold weather; at night; if touched.

SEE ALSO Multiple sclerosis, *page 179*

Latrodectus mactans
LATRODECTUS MAC.

COMMON NAME Black widow spider.
ORIGIN Found throughout North America, mainly in the southern US.
BACKGROUND The name of this highly poisonous spider comes from the female's habit of eating the male after mating.
PREPARATION The live spider is steeped in alcohol, diluted, and succussed.

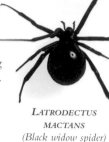

LATRODECTUS MACTANS
(Black widow spider)

REMEDY PROFILE
Latrodectus mac. is best suited to people who are tense and easily fatigued. They are often chilly but prone to hot flashes, and may dream of flying.

The remedy is typically prescribed for heart problems, particularly angina, with cramping, unbearable pain in the heart area. The pain is violent, sharp, numbing, and radiates to the arms or shoulders on both sides of the body, although it is worse on the left side. There may also be extreme restlessness that is particularly associated with an acute attack of angina.
Symptoms better From sitting quietly.
Symptoms worse In damp weather; before thunderstorms; from changes in the weather; with the slightest movement; from light.

SEE ALSO Angina, *page 185*

Ledum palustre
LEDUM

COMMON NAMES Marsh tea, wild rosemary.
ORIGIN Found in the northern hemisphere, especially Canada, the US, Scandinavia, and Ireland.
BACKGROUND Marsh tea has traditionally been used in Scandinavia to eliminate lice. After the infamous tea tax of 1773, it was used briefly in the US as a tea substitute.
PREPARATION As the plant comes into flower, the tips of the leafy shoots are collected, dried, and steeped in alcohol.

REMEDY PROFILE
Those who respond best to *Ledum* have a tendency to be angry, dissatisfied, anxious, antisocial, or even demented when ill.

Ledum is best known as a first-aid remedy for cuts, grazes, puncture wounds, insect stings, and black eyes and other eye injuries. It is used to prevent infection in open wounds, especially in severe wounds with bruising, puffy, purplish skin, and

stinging pains. It may help treat a slow-healing black eye. *Ledum* is also used for bleeding into the eye chamber after an iridectomy (removal of part of the iris). Other symptoms treated with *Ledum* include rheumatic pains that arise in the feet and move upward, and stiff, painful joints that feel hot inside despite being cold to the touch. The pain may be relieved by cold compresses.
Symptoms better From cold compresses.
Symptoms worse With warmth; at night; if touched.

SEE ALSO Osteoarthritis, *page 196*

Lithium carbonicum
LITHIUM CARB.

COMMON NAME Lithium carbonate.
ORIGIN Occurs naturally in some mineral waters in Europe and the US, but is prepared chemically for homeopathic use.
BACKGROUND This compound is used in conventional medicine as a treatment for manic depression and hypomania.
PREPARATION Lithium carbonate is triturated with lactose sugar.

REMEDY PROFILE
People for whom this remedy is best suited are prone to anxious, excitable, and confused behavior.

The classic symptom picture for *Lithium carb.* is of hip pain, gout, distorted joints, and arthritic conditions, possibly with associated heart problems. The limbs may feel stiff, as if they have been beaten, and the bones, joints, and muscles are sore. The joints, particularly the small joints, tend to be swollen, tender, and red.
Symptoms better With movement; from urinating; from eating.
Symptoms worse At night; during and after menstruation; if menstruation ceases.

Lobaria pulmonaria
STICTA

COMMON NAME Tree lungwort.
ORIGIN Found throughout Europe.
BACKGROUND This lichen has been used in Europe for thousands of years to treat conditions such as chronic respiratory congestion, bronchitis, and coughing.
PREPARATION The whole, dried lichen is macerated in alcohol.

REMEDY PROFILE
Sticta is most effective for lively people who tend to be loquacious, and who may feel as if they are floating on air. They may experience sleeplessness or confusion.

Sticta is most appropriate for respiratory problems associated with hay fever or other allergic reactions, the flu, or bronchitis. There may be repeated sneezing, which tends to become worse at night. *Sticta* may also be used for pneumonia, and for chronic phlegm that is difficult to expel and causes stuffiness, a dull, heavy feeling in the head, and a dry, tickly throat.
Symptoms better In the open air; from expelling phlegm or mucus.
Symptoms worse At night; from changes in temperature; lying down; with movement.

SEE ALSO Pneumonia, *page 183*

Lobelia inflata
LOBELIA

COMMON NAMES Indian tobacco, puke weed.
ORIGIN Found in North America, especially the eastern and central US.
BACKGROUND This plant was used by Native Americans as a tobacco substitute, and to induce vomiting or expectoration.
PREPARATION The whole, fresh plant in flower, including the seeds and roots, is finely chopped and macerated in alcohol.

REMEDY PROFILE
This remedy is most appropriate for people who are profoundly anxious about their health, particularly those who fear death from a disease of the heart or lungs. It is commonly prescribed for breathlessness and asthma accompanied by great anxiety. Characteristic symptoms include a rattling sound in the chest, despite the presence of little or no mucus, and a feeling of oppression and constriction in the chest. Further symptoms may include excessive salivation, retching, hiccuping, a sensation of having a lump in the throat, nausea, and a sinking feeling in the stomach. Nausea with giddiness, and vomiting with profuse perspiration, may also be helped by this remedy.
Symptoms better With warmth; with rapid movement; from small amounts of food.
Symptoms worse After sleep; with the least movement; from bathing in cold water; from beer; smoking tobacco.

LOBELIA INFLATA
(Indian tobacco)

Lycopus virginicus
LYCOPUS

COMMON NAMES Bugleweed, Virginia horehound.
ORIGIN Found in eastern North America.
BACKGROUND Bugleweed has been used in herbal medicine for various ailments, such as hyperthyroidism, tuberculosis, coughing, and heavy menstruation.
PREPARATION The whole, fresh, finely chopped plant in flower, including the root, is macerated in alcohol.

REMEDY PROFILE
People who respond best to *Lycopus* tend to be irritable when ill unless spoken to very softly. Their minds often wander from one thing to another, and they may experience increased mental and physical activity in the evening.

Lycopus is associated chiefly with the heart, and is used to treat a weak heart and erratic pulse or heart disease. Additional symptoms may include a tendency to hemorrhage, and overactivity of the thyroid gland, particularly during menopause. Respiratory complaints may develop in conjunction with the heart problems. These include violent coughing in the evening or at night during sleep, with sweet-tasting mucus that recurs in cold weather, especially following exposure to cold winds. In addition, there may be an increase in appetite.
Symptoms better From warm surroundings; lying in bed.
Symptoms worse In cold winds; toward sunset; in the morning; in the evening; with movement; with exercise; from walking; from climbing stairs.

Lyssin hydrophobinum
LYSSIN

COMMON NAME Rabies.
ORIGIN Saliva from a rabid dog.
BACKGROUND Rabies is an acute viral infection that affects both wild and domestic animals and, more rarely, humans. Transmitted by saliva, it is almost always fatal in humans.
PREPARATION The saliva is rendered sterile, then dissolved in purified water, diluted, and succussed.

REMEDY PROFILE
Lyssin is most appropriate for people who tend to be mentally excited and hyperactive, and have extreme sensitivity to stimuli such as light, noise, and odors. They may be affected by phobias and compulsive disorders associated with ritualistic behavior patterns and violence. There may be a personal or parental history of rabies vaccination in those who suit *Lyssin*.

Physical symptoms generally affect the nervous system, throat, and sexual organs. Typically, the sight or sound of running water may cause fear, irritability, and a desire to pass stools or urinate, possibly involuntarily. On trying to swallow there is a choking sensation, with profuse saliva that is spat out. In addition, the sight of glistening objects may cause distress.

Further conditions that may be associated with *Lyssin* include excessive sexual energy and vaginal pain during sexual intercourse. There may also be uterine prolapse.
Symptoms better From gentle rubbing; from steam baths.
Symptoms worse From the heat of the sun; from the sound or sight of running water; from emotional stress; bad news.

Magnesium carbonicum
MAG. CARB.

COMMON NAME Magnesium carbonate.
ORIGIN Chemically prepared.
BACKGROUND This compound is widely used in industry, especially in the making of bricks, paper, plastics, and paints. It is used medicinally as an antacid.
PREPARATION Magnesium carbonate is triturated with lactose sugar.

REMEDY PROFILE
Mag. carb. is best suited to long-suffering people who feel worn down and who crave quiet calm, being highly sensitive to noise or touch. They are peacemakers

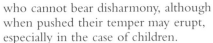

MAGNESIUM CARBONICUM
(Magnesium carbonate)

who cannot bear disharmony, although when pushed their temper may erupt, especially in the case of children.

A key symptom associated with *Mag. carb.* is acidity in the digestive system with sour-smelling stools and perspiration, and poor digestion of milk. The remedy may be used for diarrhea or constipation with abnormal, discolored, fatty stools that contain undigested matter. It may also be prescribed for exhaustion or chronic fatigue syndrome with swollen glands, lax muscles, and susceptibility to hernias.
Symptoms better In open air; in warm air; with movement; after passing stools.
Symptoms worse With cold; from changes in the weather; at night; with rest; during pregnancy; from warm foods.

Magnesium chloratum
MAG. MUR.

COMMON NAME Magnesium chloride.
ORIGIN Chemically prepared.
BACKGROUND The bitter taste of this compound can be detected in many mineral waters and in sea water. It is used in wall-plastering and as a fireproofing agent for wood.
PREPARATION Magnesium chloride is triturated with lactose sugar.

REMEDY PROFILE
Mag. mur. is most suitable for people who feel deep distress on witnessing arguments and crave peace and harmony. Reserved, sad, and self pitying, they often show a long-suffering face to the world. Nervous oversensitivity is typical, with restlessness in bed: They find it hard to sleep well, waking unrefreshed and needing a long time to recover each morning. The liver, nerves, uterus, and rectum are often greatly affected. Conditions treated are usually chronic, involving great weakness, swollen glands, and a susceptibility to colds. Chronic fatigue syndrome, for example, may be helped by the remedy. Digestive complaints such as nausea, indigestion, and constipation are all strongly associated with the remedy if they are accompanied by the characteristic nervous state of mind. Children who are prone to digestive problems and whose parents regularly argue, for instance, may benefit from *Mag. mur.*
Symptoms better In cool, open air; from firm pressure on the affected area; with gentle movement.
Symptoms worse At night; near noise; if touched; lying on the right side of the body; from swimming in the sea; from eating, especially salt; from milk.

Magnesium sulfuricum
MAG. SULF.

COMMON NAMES Magnesium sulfate, epsom salts.
ORIGIN Occurs naturally in some mineral waters, but is chemically prepared for use in homeopathy.
BACKGROUND Magnesium sulfate is found in many spa waters, such as those in Epsom, in England, which were often drunk for their mild laxative effect.
PREPARATION Magnesium sulfate is triturated with lactose sugar.

REMEDY PROFILE
Mag. sulf. is best suited to those who fly into rages and overreact, yet also have the typical *Magnesium* desire for peace. They tend to be restless and uneasy, fearing evil or a terrible event. Often concerned about relationships, they are prone to jealousy.

The remedy is usually prescribed for urinary disorders, possibly with digestive, skin, or menstrual problems and awkward limb movements. The urinary disorders are characterized by an intermittent stream on urinating, and burning pain after urinating.

Mag. sulf. may also be used to treat exhaustion or chronic fatigue, dry skin, and nausea. Sleep may occur in the early evening, followed by insomnia at night. It may be restless as a result of anxious, disagreeable dreams.
Symptoms better From rubbing the affected area; from walking.
Symptoms worse In the morning; on waking.

Malandrinum
MALANDRINUM

COMMON NAME Grease.
ORIGIN Specimen of the oily secretion taken from an infected horse.
BACKGROUND Grease is a disease that affects horses, causing inflammation of the fetlocks, which become covered by an oily secretion.
PREPARATION The specimen is rendered sterile, dissolved in purified water, then diluted and succussed.

REMEDY PROFILE
Malandrinum is commonly used for skin problems characterized by greasy, pustular eruptions, rough, unhealthy-looking skin, or dry, scaly, itchy skin with cracks or fissures, especially on the hands and feet during cold weather. The remedy may also be given as an antidote to any adverse effects of a smallpox vaccination.
Symptoms better No specific factors.
Symptoms worse In the evening.

Mandragora officinarum
MANDRAGORA

COMMON NAME Common mandrake.
ORIGIN Native to the Mediterranean region of Europe.
BACKGROUND Legend attributed magical aphrodisiac properties to the mandrake root. It is highly toxic and narcotic, and is no longer used herbally.
PREPARATION The root is dried and macerated in alcohol.

REMEDY PROFILE
People for whom *Mandragora* is best suited are prone to changeable moods, such as crying spells alternating with feelings of euphoria. They may be in a state of "aroused exhaustion," simultaneously sleepy and hyperactive. There is general hypersensitivity, particularly to noise, but also to smell.

The classic symptom profile associated with *Mandragora* focuses on abdominal pain that is worse on the upper right side and better from bending backward. The remedy may also help limbs that feel heavy, bruised, and sore, as if from muscular exertion, and may ease sciatica with burning pain that is worse on the right side. A further use is for congestive headaches that are better in cold air and from applying cold compresses.
Symptoms better From urinating; from bending backward; with rest; continuous movement; from warm compresses (except in the case of headaches).
Symptoms worse In damp and stormy weather; between 3 A.M. and 5 A.M.

Manganum metallicum
MANGANUM MET.

COMMON NAME Manganese.
ORIGIN Occurs primarily in pyrolusite and rhodonite.
BACKGROUND This metal was discovered in 1774. After iron it is the second most common metal in Earth's crust. It is most often used for industrial purposes to make alloys of steel and copper.
PREPARATION Manganese is triturated with lactose sugar.

REMEDY PROFILE
Manganum met. is most appropriate for those who are open, friendly, and helpful. They are orderly and conscientious and, if unable to be of help to others, tend to feel restless and lost.

The remedy is most commonly given when the bones are extremely sensitive, especially in children who have been experiencing rapid growth. Symptoms are usually better when lying down. *Manganum met.* is also prescribed for ear conditions such as earaches, temporarily reduced hearing, tinnitus, and great sensitivity to noise and wind. Earaches seem to begin elsewhere in the body and travel to the ear.
Symptoms better From a change of air; lying down; from sad music.
Symptoms worse In cold and damp; at night; if touched; from speaking.

Medicago sativa
ALFALFA

COMMON NAMES Alfalfa, lucerne.
ORIGIN Native to Asia, northern Africa, and Europe.
BACKGROUND Cultivated for thousands of years as a fodder plant, alfalfa is highly nutritious and detoxifying, and has long been used herbally and in cooking.
PREPARATION The fresh aerial parts are finely chopped and macerated in alcohol.

REMEDY PROFILE
Alfalfa is usually given in the mother tincture form as a tonic for conditions associated with malnutrition or great weight loss, such as cancer, anorexia, nervous indigestion, insomnia, and chronic fatigue syndrome. There may be constant hunger or an increased appetite, particularly in the middle of the morning, and a craving for sweet foods. Further symptoms may include a left-sided headache or a heavy, dull sensation in the back of the head.
Symptoms better No specific factors.
Symptoms worse In the evening.

Melilotus officinalis syn. *M. arvensis*
MELILOTUS

COMMON NAMES Melilot, yellow melilot, sweet clover.
ORIGIN Native to Europe, temperate parts of Asia, and northern Africa, and naturalized in North America.
BACKGROUND This sedative herb can be used medicinally to relieve spasms, reduce inflammation, and as a decongestant.
PREPARATION The fresh, flowering tops, without the woody stems, are finely chopped and steeped in alcohol.

REMEDY PROFILE
Melilotus is best suited to people who are highly agitated, talkative, suspicious, insane, and possibly even suicidal. They often worry about being poisoned, fear the police, and fail to recognize familiar people and places.

The remedy is used mainly as a treatment for throbbing headaches with a feeling of violent blood congestion in the head, as if blood is going to burst out of it. A red face, bloodshot eyes, and dizziness are further common symptoms that occur in conjunction with the headaches, while weariness, a feverish sensation, and a hot face may precede them. The feeling of congestion may be eased by nosebleeds. *Melilotus* may also be prescribed to treat circulatory problems with a sensation of engorgement in other parts of the body.
Symptoms better From bleeding, such as nosebleeds or menstruation; from profuse urination; from changes in position.
Symptoms worse From changes in the weather; from the approach of a storm; during menopause.

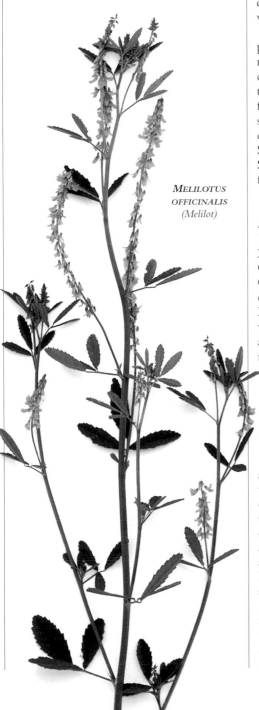

MELILOTUS OFFICINALIS (Melilot)

Micrurus corallinus syn. *Elaps corallinus*
ELAPS

COMMON NAME Brazilian coral snake.
ORIGIN Found in Brazil.
BACKGROUND This poisonous snake has roughly 200 rings on its belly, which are colored alternately bright black and red.
PREPARATION Venom from a live snake is triturated with lactose sugar.

REMEDY PROFILE
People who respond best to *Elaps* tend to be rather intense, haughty, and suspicious. They are often depressed and long to be alone, yet also fear being left alone in case something horrible happens. In addition, they fear developing a serious illness such as a stroke, and feel afraid and miserable during wet weather. Generally, they are very sensitive to the cold.

The blood is commonly affected in people who benefit from *Elaps*. There may be hemorrhages or other discharges characterized by black blood. In addition, the remedy is given for right-sided paralysis following a stroke. Despite a chilly sensation in the stomach, there may be a craving for ice, salads, fruits, and yoghurt.
Symptoms better With rest; from walking.
Symptoms worse With cold; at night; from the approach of a storm; if touched.

Moschus moschiferus
MOSCHUS

COMMON NAME Musk deer.
ORIGIN Found in northeastern and central Asia, and in northern India.
BACKGROUND Male musk deer secrete a waxy substance called musk, which has a heady scent that is widely used in the manufacture of perfume. Musk also has a strong reputation as an aphrodisiac.
PREPARATION The musk is dried and macerated in alcohol before being diluted and succussed.

REMEDY PROFILE
Moschus is best suited to people who are bustling, overexcited, and prone to uncontrollable laughter. They tend to be quarrelsome and may express violent anger. Often physically awkward and with confused speech, they may be preoccupied and absentminded. Their feelings of anxiety and fear of death may lead to hysteria, and they may experience intense sexual excitement even if they are elderly.

Key symptoms associated with *Moschus* include heightened physical and mental tension, which may cause spasms, twitches, and seizures in the muscles. General coldness is another characteristic symptom, or a chill in a specific area of the body; for instance, one cheek may be red but cold, the other pale but hot.

The remedy is prescribed chiefly for fainting that is triggered by the slightest excitement, such as scolding or anger, or by eating, menstruation, or heart disease. In addition, *Moschus* is given for chest spasms, and spasms in the abdominal muscles or diaphragm, such as hiccups.
Symptoms better In the open air; with warmth; from rubbing the affected area.
Symptoms worse With cold; from any excitement; from suppressing symptoms; from pressure on the affected area.

Murex purpurea & *M. trunculus*
MUREX

COMMON NAMES Murex, purple fish.
ORIGIN Found off the shores of the Mediterranean and Adriatic seas.
BACKGROUND These mollusks produce a juice that was formerly used to make a rich, dark dye called Tyrian purple.
PREPARATION The juice secreted by either *Murex* species is dried and then triturated with lactose sugar.

REMEDY PROFILE
Murex is given mainly to women. It is most appropriate for those who are thin, wiry, nervous, and affectionate, with a high libido. They may have a tendency to develop deep depression, hypochondria, or a fear of illness.

The remedy is strongly associated with problems of the female reproductive organs, especially intense menstrual pain accompanied by great impatience and a desire to die. It is also used if, prior to menstruation, there is pain so severe that it causes unconsciousness. In addition, breasts that are painful, perhaps developing benign tumors, may respond to *Murex*. Pain typically extends diagonally upward from the right ovary to the left breast. There is a great awareness of the uterus, which may feel constricted, dry, and sore, as if it has been wounded. The genitals feel as if they are being pushed out of the body, and there is nausea and great weakness, which may cause prostration.

Murex may be prescribed for digestive problems in women, particularly if the symptoms include a sinking, empty sensation in the stomach and a desire to eat. It may also be used during menopause if the bowels are very sensitive.
Symptoms better Before menstruation; with pressure and support on the affected area; from sitting and crossing the legs.
Symptoms worse During menstruation; if touched; lying down; after sleep.

Mygale lasiodora
syn. *M. avicularis, Aranea avicularis*
MYGALE LAS.

COMMON NAMES Mygale, Cuban spider.
ORIGIN Found mainly in South America.
BACKGROUND This hairy, bird-catching spider weaves tube-shaped nets between tree leaves to capture its prey.
PREPARATION The whole, live spider is steeped in alcohol, diluted, and succussed.

REMEDY PROFILE
Mygale las. is best suited to people who are restless, anxious, fearful, and delirious. They may talk deliriously about work, fear death, and have a high sex drive.

The remedy is generally prescribed for twitching, convulsive movements, possibly accompanied by nausea, dimmed vision, and heart palpitations. It is also used for chorea, especially when this affects the muscles of the upper body, including the face. The tongue is so dry that words may seem to be "jerked" out on speaking. During sleep there may be restlessness, bizarre dreams, and grinding of teeth.
Symptoms better During sleep.
Symptoms worse In the morning; from sitting; from eating.

Myristica fragrans syn. *Nux moschata*
NUX MOSCH.

COMMON NAME Nutmeg.
ORIGIN Native to the Molucca Islands of Indonesia, but now widely cultivated.
BACKGROUND Although best known now as a culinary spice, nutmeg has long been used medicinally by several cultures, although only in low doses.
PREPARATION The whole, fresh or dried nutmegs are treated with lime before being macerated in alcohol.

MYRISTICA FRAGRANS (Nutmeg)

REMEDY PROFILE
Highly excited intense sensing is typical in those who respond best to *Nux mosch.*, as are rapidly alternating emotions, such as laughing and crying in turn. They may feel as if they have two heads, or as if one part of them is able to watch another part. These people have a sense of detachment from ordinary life, feeling as if they are wrapped in cotton batting.

The classic symptom picture for *Nux mosch.* is of confusion, dizziness, fainting, loss of coordination, and great, even overwhelming, drowsiness. Extreme "dryness" in the digestive system may be treated by the remedy, especially if there is the classic drowsiness. Symptoms typically include chronic constipation with fullness and bloating in the abdomen, unquenchable thirst, and a tongue so dry that it sticks to the roof of the mouth.
Symptoms better With warmth and heat; in the open air.
Symptoms worse In cold weather; from emotional stress and shock; in pregnancy.

Naja naja syn. *N. tripudians*
NAJA

COMMON NAME Indian cobra.
ORIGIN Native to India, although now found in Asia and tropical Africa.
BACKGROUND Indian Ayurvedic doctors have long used the poisonous venom of this snake for nervous and blood disorders.
PREPARATION The venom is dried and triturated with lactose sugar.

REMEDY PROFILE
People who respond best to *Naja* feel unfortunate and deeply wronged, but tend to exaggerate or take their problems out of context. They often feel confused, forgetful, sad, tremulous, weak, and chilly.

Naja is prescribed chiefly for heart symptoms, particularly those affecting the valves. Symptoms typically include heart murmurs, a slow or racing pulse, violent palpitations with choking and an inability to speak, a valvular lesion (abnormality of the structure or function of the valve), and angina with pain extending down the left arm and up to the throat and neck. *Naja* may be used for a heart that has become enlarged from being forced to work harder in order to push blood through damaged valves. The internal organs feel as if they are drawn together or screwed up. Sleep may be restless or inhibited by a sense of suffocation at night.
Symptoms better From driving in the open air; lying on the right side.
Symptoms worse In cold air; from the pressure of clothes, especially collars; from stimulants; lying on the left side.

Natrum arsenicum
NAT. ARS.

COMMON NAME Sodium arsenate.
ORIGIN Chemically prepared.
BACKGROUND These colorless, transparent prismatic crystals are used medicinally only in homeopathy.
PREPARATION The compound is triturated with lactose sugar.

REMEDY PROFILE
A history of grief and suppressed emotions is typical in people for whom *Nat. ars.* is best suited. Despite being high achievers and ambitious perfectionists, they are prone to forgetfulness and poor concentration. Often suspicious, they tend to bottle up their emotions, and are easily frightened or startled. Their sleep may be restless or heavy, and they may wake as if from fright.

The key affinity for *Nat. ars.* is with the chest, which generally feels dry, tight, and oppressed. There may be breathlessness or a dry, hacking cough, great sensitivity to smoke or dust, restlessness, and chilliness with a preference for wrapping up warmly and sitting by a fire.
Symptoms better From bending forward.
Symptoms worse On waking in the morning; with the slightest exertion; from jarring; from pressure on the affected area.

Natrum fluoricum
NAT. FLUOR.

COMMON NAME Sodium fluoride.
ORIGIN Chemically prepared.
BACKGROUND In some countries sodium fluoride is added in minute quantities to the water supply to reduce dental decay.
PREPARATION Sodium fluoride is triturated with lactose sugar.

REMEDY PROFILE
Nat. fluor. is typically given to those who are deeply insecure, needing contact with many different people in order to feel that they "belong." They tend to be highly sensitive, easily hurt, and feel that they do not fit in. Prone to impulsive sexual relationships, they may also develop long-standing, passionate liaisons.

Any physical symptoms typically occur on the right side, and sleeping on the left side is preferred. Symptoms may include cold sweats in the armpits, an aversion to sour-tasting things, and a desire for alcohol.
Symptoms better From being outside; with violent movement.
Symptoms worse From heat; from sun; with warmth; between 11 A.M. and 9 P.M.

Natrum phosphoricum
NAT. PHOS.

COMMON NAME Sodium phosphate.
ORIGIN Chemically prepared.
BACKGROUND These crystals were used in the 18th and 19th centuries for intestinal worms, and chosen by Dr. Schüssler as a "biochemic" tissue salt (*see page 90*).
PREPARATION Sodium phosphate crystals are triturated with lactose sugar.

REMEDY PROFILE

Responsible people who find it difficult to delegate tend to respond most effectively to *Nat. phos.* Despite being generally friendly and sympathetic, they are highly self-contained, finding it hard to talk about their problems and tending to become withdrawn from loved ones. Fears of the dark, insects, storms, illness, and death are typical, as is being easily startled by noise.

Nat. phos. is used primarily to treat digestive disorders characterized by excess acidity and sour discharges. There may be a feeling of emptiness in the abdomen and chest, and a tendency to vomit or produce sour burps. Cravings for strong-tasting, spicy foods, salt, and fried eggs are associated with *Nat. phos.* It may also help bottle-fed babies who are failing to thrive.

Symptoms better With cold.
Symptoms worse From storms; after sexual intercourse; from bitter foods; from fatty foods; from sugar; from milk.

Natrum sulfuricum
NAT. SULF.

COMMON NAMES Sodium sulfate, Glauber's salt, sal mirabile.
ORIGIN Occurs naturally in the mineral waters of some saltwater lakes, but it is chemically prepared for homeopathic use.
BACKGROUND The main mineral salt in many spa waters, such as those in Carlsbad, sodium sulfate was also identified by Dr. Schüssler as one of his "biochemic" tissue salts (*see page 90*).
PREPARATION Sodium sulfate is triturated with lactose sugar.

REMEDY PROFILE

Nat. sulf. is best suited to people who are serious, reserved, responsible, and focused on work, yet paradoxically highly sensitive: music may move them to tears. They may feel isolated from intimate, committed relationships, perhaps after losing a partner.

Nat. sulf. has an affinity with head symptoms, such as headaches caused by injury, or those accompanied by increased salivation or strong intolerance of light. It is prescribed for severe or suicidal depression, and for profound mental changes, possibly with suicidal thoughts, following a head injury.

Nat. sulf. is also a major remedy for asthma brought on by damp conditions. In addition, it has an affinity with the digestive system, liver, gallbladder, pancreas, and spleen. Liver conditions treated by the remedy include hepatitis and gallstones with bitter burping, colicky abdominal pains, and jaundice. There may be watery stools, especially on rising in the morning.

Symptoms better In warm, dry air; from changing position; with movement.
Symptoms worse In dampness; in night air; from head injuries; lying on the left side.

Natrum tetraboracicum
BORAX

COMMON NAMES Borax, tincal, sodium tetraborate.
ORIGIN Chemically prepared.
BACKGROUND In the 19th century borax was a traditional Western medicine for treating canker sores and labor pains.
PREPARATION Borax is triturated with lactose sugar.

REMEDY PROFILE

Those for whom *Borax* is most appropriate are irritable, angry, and passionate. They tend to be very fearful, even of the slightest noise, and prone to phobias. If pregnant, women suited to *Borax* dread labor. Mental activity or stress causes nausea, giddiness, and a fear of falling, which become worse when moving downward, as on an escalator. Children may feel worse when being carried or swung downward.

Classic symptoms associated with *Borax* focus particularly on the mucous membranes of the digestive tract and the skin. In children there may be weight loss and a failure to thrive.

The remedy is used for painful canker sores that develop in the mouth or on the tongue, and for ulceration that extends down through the whole gastrointestinal tract. Further symptoms may include cold sores on the lips, a hot, dry mouth containing a white fungal growth, and increased salivation during teething.

Symptoms better In the morning; from pressing on or holding the painful area.
Symptoms worse In cold and dampness; from sudden noises; from downward or upward movement.

SEE ALSO Phobias, *page 211*

Nerium oleander
OLEANDER

COMMON NAMES Oleander, rose bay.
ORIGIN Native to the eastern Mediterranean or possibly further east, as far as China, but now widely naturalized.

BACKGROUND The plant and its vapors are very toxic: In 1844 some soldiers died after eating meat roasted over a fire of oleander wood. In 19th-century southern Europe, bathing in an oleander decoction was a treatment for killing lice and fleas.

PREPARATION The fresh leaves are gathered before flowering, chopped finely, and steeped in alcohol.

NERIUM OLEANDER (Oleander)

REMEDY PROFILE

Oleander is typically given to people with a dull, sad mental state. They are unable to think clearly, and lack self-confidence.

Skin symptoms are the main focus for *Oleander*, and it may be used to treat dry, itching, flaking eruptions, especially on the scalp: Dandruff, cradle cap, eczema, and psoriasis may all be helped. The skin is violently itchy and burning, as if it is being bitten by lice. The slightest friction on the skin causes soreness and chapping. There may be trembling and weakness, and symptoms are generally made worse by eating oranges and other citrus fruits.

Symptoms better From scratching; lying down.
Symptoms worse From rubbing the affected area; from the friction of clothing on the affected area; from undressing; after breast-feeding.

SEE ALSO Severe eczema, *page 194*

157

Nicotiana tabacum
TABACUM

COMMON NAME Tobacco plant.
ORIGIN Native to tropical America, but now cultivated worldwide.
BACKGROUND Tobacco was a traditional Mayan treatment for asthma, convulsions, and skin complaints, and has long been smoked on the American continent. It is no longer used medicinally, but is still used in cigarettes and as an insecticide.
PREPARATION The dried, unfermented leaves are macerated in alcohol.

REMEDY PROFILE
The remedy is best suited to people who feel wretched and gloomy. They are usually unable to concentrate for long.

Severe nausea is a key symptom treated by *Tabacum*. The nausea is similar to that experienced by someone on inhaling their first cigarette, and causes a deathly, icy cold sensation. It may be used for motion sickness or acute digestive upset, especially during pregnancy or chemotherapy. *Tabacum* is also thought to help ease acute diarrhea or, conversely, habitual constipation with rectal paralysis or spasms. A sensation of obstruction or constriction in the rectum or intestines, with weakness and cramping pain, is typical.
Symptoms better With cold and from cold compresses on the affected area; at twilight; from uncovering the abdomen; from vinegar and sour foods or drinks.
Symptoms worse From extremes of heat and cold; in the evening; lying on the left side; from the movement of a car or boat; from opening the eyes.

Onosmodium virginianum
ONOSMODIUM

COMMON NAME False gromwell.
ORIGIN Found in eastern North America.
BACKGROUND It is thought that this plant, like its close relative *Lithospermum*, may suppress ovulation in women and reduce blood sugar and thyroxine levels.
PREPARATION The whole, fresh plant is macerated in alcohol.

REMEDY PROFILE
This remedy is given primarily to women who are physically and mentally worn out. Confused, indecisive, and aimless, they may feel as if their emotions are working in slow motion. Their memory is often weak, and they are unable to finish sentences when speaking.

Physically *Onosmodium* is associated with exhaustion characterized by trembling, a sensation of heaviness, and lack of

coordination. There may be diminished or absent sexual desire in both men and women. *Onosmodium* may also be given for eyestrain, in cases where the eyes feel tense and strained on reading small print, and distances are misjudged because of slow eye accommodation or adjustment.
Symptoms better From undressing; with sleep; lying on the back; from eating; from cold drinks.
Symptoms worse In warm, humid air; from straining the eyes; from sexual excess.

Origanum majorana
syn. *Majorana hortensis*
ORIGANUM

COMMON NAME Sweet marjoram.
ORIGIN Found in regions bordering the Mediterranean Sea.
BACKGROUND Used mainly as a culinary flavoring, sweet marjoram is also prescribed in herbal medicine for anxiety, flatulence, menstrual pain, and insomnia.
PREPARATION The fresh, finely chopped aerial parts in flower are steeped in alcohol.

ORIGANUM MAJORANA (Sweet marjoram)

REMEDY PROFILE
Women who experience sexual problems, especially those who are obsessed by sexual thoughts and those who have a constant desire to masturbate, are likely to benefit most from *Origanum*. They may be restless, finding it difficult to stay still, and as a result become fanatical about keeping fit, turning to sports such as running to burn off energy. Breasts and nipples may become swollen, itchy, and painful. An intense level of sexual addiction may indicate relationship difficulties or a history of sexual abuse.
Symptoms better From being occupied.
Symptoms worse Lying down; at night.

Paeonia officinalis
PAEONIA

COMMON NAME Peony.
ORIGIN Native to Europe and Asia.
BACKGROUND Culpeper, the 17th-century English herbalist, claimed that the root of this herb would prevent epilepsy in children if hung around their necks.
PREPARATION The fresh, finely chopped root, dug in spring, is steeped in alcohol.

REMEDY PROFILE
This remedy is given mostly for problems of the rectum and anus such as fissures and hemorrhoids, although it may also help to treat terrifying nightmares, particularly those involving ghosts. It is used for intense, burning pain in the anus during and after passing stools, followed by a chilly sensation. The pain may be very severe during the night and eased only by walking, rolling on the floor, or lying for hours with the buttocks spread apart.
Symptoms better From warm compresses on the affected area.
Symptoms worse At night; if touched or from pressure on the affected area.

Palladium metallicum
PALLADIUM MET.

COMMON NAME Palladium.
ORIGIN Found in Columbia, Brazil, Russia, and South Africa.
BACKGROUND First isolated in 1803 by the English physicist William Wollaston, this metal was named in honor of the asteroid "Pallas," which had recently been discovered.
PREPARATION The metal is triturated with lactose sugar.

REMEDY PROFILE
Palladium met. is most suitable for people who need approval and praise. They tend to interpret things in a self-centered light and constantly feel neglected, insulted, and unappreciated. Usually enjoying company, they behave in an attention-seeking, excited way, but may later collapse from exhaustion and fear of imagined slights.

The classic symptom picture for this remedy focuses on the uterus and ovaries. Ovarian pains and cysts tend to be right-sided. The pains are worse from jarring, after menstruation, and with excitement; bending the legs and lying on the left side is beneficial. The uterus may prolapse or become displaced, and an infection may develop in the abdomen.

Palladium met. may also be used to treat pains in the head and limbs, including headaches that develop across the top of the head from one ear to the other. They are often accompanied by irritability and impatience. Tired, cold, or tense limbs may respond well to the remedy. In addition it is prescribed to ease the pain of sprained limbs.
Symptoms better With sleep; from passing stools; from rubbing the affected area; touch or pressure on the affected area.
Symptoms worse From emotional excitement; after social functions; from standing; exertion; after menstruation.

Panax pseudoginseng
PANAX GINSENG

COMMON NAMES *San qi* ginseng, *tienchi* ginseng.
ORIGIN Native to Bhutan and northeastern India.
BACKGROUND In Chinese medicine this herb is reputed to clear the mind and make the limbs elastic and dynamic. It is considered to be a tonic and aphrodisiac.
PREPARATION The dried root is steeped in alcohol, diluted, and succussed.

REMEDY PROFILE
Panax ginseng is typically given to people who are experiencing a general sense of stiffening up in the body. The limbs tend to feel heavy, and the joints contract and stiffen. Paralytic weakness, rheumatic pain, and sciatica may be helped by the remedy. People who benefit from it often feel worse in the open air, and are prone to respiratory problems. Generally there is a sensation of weakness in the sexual organs, possibly as a result of excessive sexual intercourse, although there may be no diminishing of sexual desire.
Symptoms better From walking.
Symptoms worse In the open air; at night; from bending and turning.

Pareira brava
syn. *Chondrodendron tomentosum*
PAREIRA

COMMON NAMES Pareira, pareira brava.
ORIGIN Found in Panama, Brazil, Bolivia, and Peru.
BACKGROUND Notoriously used by Native South Americans to make curare, an arrow poison, the root of this plant is also used herbally as a diuretic, to increase menstrual flow, and to reduce fever.
PREPARATION The fresh root is steeped in alcohol, diluted, and succussed.

REMEDY PROFILE
People for whom *Pareira* is best suited tend to have a constant urge to urinate, with great straining and painful urination. There is typically severe pain radiating down the thigh, and it may be possible to urinate only in certain positions. In men there may be severe pain in the penis. Excruciating pains may develop on the left side of the lower back. The urine may contain thick, stringy, white mucus or a red precipitate. *Pareira* may also be helpful for itching in the urethra, kidney colic, an enlarged prostate gland, and prostate disorders with urine retention.

Symptoms better From being on the hands and knees; from pressing the head against the floor.
Symptoms worse After midnight; after urinating.

Passiflora incarnata
PASSIFLORA

COMMON NAME Passionflower.
ORIGIN Native to the southern US and Central and South America, and now cultivated worldwide.
BACKGROUND This plant has long been used by indigenous tribes in Central and North America for its valuable sedative and tranquilizing properties.
PREPARATION The fresh or dried leaves, gathered in spring, are finely chopped and steeped in alcohol.

REMEDY PROFILE
The classic symptom linked with *Passiflora* is insomnia. Those who respond best to the remedy tend to lie awake at night and

PASSIFLORA INCARNATA (Passionflower)

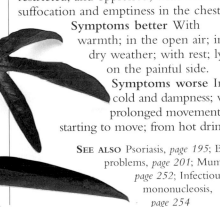

become exhausted. They are prone to odd sensations; they may feel that their eyeballs are protruding, as if being pushed out of their heads, or that the tops of their heads are lifting off. Lying down they may feel that their heels are rising up in the air. *Passiflora* is considered particularly effective for alcoholics and screaming children.

The remedy may also help whooping cough that is worse at night, and insomnia accompanied by hemorrhoids, pain in the coccyx, or discomfort during or just before menstruation.
Symptoms better From remaining quiet.
Symptoms worse At night; from mental anxiety and excitement; from exhaustion; after meals.

Phytolacca americana
PHYTOLACCA

COMMON NAMES Virginia pokeroot, reading plant, garget, pocon.
ORIGIN Native to North America, and naturalized in the Mediterranean region.
BACKGROUND Used by Native Americans for a range of complaints from rheumatoid arthritis to hemorrhoids, this plant is highly potent and toxic in excess.
PREPARATION The fresh root is unearthed during the autumn, finely chopped, and macerated in alcohol.

REMEDY PROFILE
This remedy has a strong affinity with the glands. It may be given for mastitis with hardness, burning, and pain in the breasts that radiates through the whole body on breast-feeding. Breast ulcers, hard lumps, and even breast cancer may also be helped, as may psoriasis.

Phytolacca may be used for hard, inflamed neck glands, with pain in the throat on swallowing. The tonsils may be inflamed, painful, and discolored dark red, and the tip of the tongue may be red. Inflamed parotid glands, for example during mumps, may be helped by the remedy, as may mononucleosis. Breathing feels difficult, restricted, and oppressed, with a sense of suffocation and emptiness in the chest.
Symptoms better With warmth; in the open air; in dry weather; with rest; lying on the painful side.
Symptoms worse In cold and dampness; with prolonged movement; on starting to move; from hot drinks.

SEE ALSO Psoriasis, *page 195*; Breast problems, *page 201*; Mumps, *page 252*; Infectious mononucleosis, *page 254*

Piper cubeba
CUBEBA

COMMON NAMES Cubeb, tailed pepper.
ORIGIN Native to Indonesia and widely cultivated in tropical Asia.
BACKGROUND The antiseptic and diuretic properties of the cubeb fruits are used in herbal medicine, and the oil may be used to flavor tobacco, relishes, and sauces.
PREPARATION The dried, unripe fruits are macerated in alcohol.

REMEDY PROFILE

Cubeba is best suited to people who are restless and easily startled. They are often thirsty, and may crave nuts and delicacies. Their libidos may be very high.

The remedy is typically used for mucous membrane inflammation, especially in the urinary tract. The symptom picture is of burning pain on urinating and profuse or frequent urination, possibly out of anxiety. Discolored, smarting urine, possibly containing blood, and a feeling of fullness are further typical symptoms. Infections such as cystitis or prostatitis (inflammation of the prostate gland) may be treated with *Cubeba*, as may gonorrhea.
Symptoms better From getting up and walking around.
Symptoms worse At night; in bed.

Plantago major
PLANTAGO

COMMON NAMES Greater plantain.
ORIGIN Native to Europe and temperate regions of Asia, where it grows wild.
BACKGROUND Greater plantain has antibacterial properties and is sometimes used herbally as a substitute for comfrey to stop bleeding and encourage tissue repair.
PREPARATION The fresh root is finely chopped and macerated in alcohol.

REMEDY PROFILE

People who respond best to *Plantago* are dull, irritable, and impatient. Mental activity exhausts and flusters them, and this is made worse by physical exertion.

Key conditions for which this remedy may be prescribed include earaches and toothaches. Aches are typically caused by sharp, neuralgic pains, often in the head and ears. Twinges of pain may move around the head from front to back, or from ear to ear, and there may be a sensation in the head as if the brain has turned over. *Plantago* is also given for bed-wetting problems.
Symptoms better With sleep; from eating.
Symptoms worse At night; if touched; with extremes of heat and cold.

Podophyllum peltatum
PODOPHYLLUM

COMMON NAMES Mayapple, American mandrake.
ORIGIN Native to northeastern North America.
BACKGROUND Mayapple was used by Native Americans and 19th-century settlers from Europe as a purgative, but was later found to be highly toxic to cells. It is being researched for treating certain cancers.
PREPARATION The fresh rhizome is dug up when the fruits are fully ripe, finely chopped, and macerated in alcohol.

REMEDY PROFILE

Those who benefit most from *Podophyllum* tend to be forgetful, particularly of words, depressed, afraid that they may die, and unrefreshed by sleep, which is restless.

Digestive tract disorders such as gastroenteritis are typically treated with this remedy. Generally the lower part of the digestive tract and the liver are most affected. The appetite often wanes, perhaps because everything suddenly tastes sour or putrid, or because the smell of food is loathsome. Sour burping, vomiting, or diarrhea, particularly after eating or drinking, are typical of this symptom picture. *Podophyllum* may ease abdominal cramps, or profuse, painless diarrhea, preceded by noisy gurgling. Diarrhea may be accompanied by a sinking feeling, as if the pelvic contents are going to prolapse.
Symptoms better With warmth; in the evening; from rubbing or stroking the liver area; from bending forward; lying on the abdomen; from yawning and stretching.
Symptoms worse In the early morning; in hot weather; with movement; while being bathed or washed; from eating.

Polygala senega
SENEGA

COMMON NAMES Seneca snake root, rattlesnake root.
ORIGIN Native to North America and now cultivated in western Canada.
BACKGROUND The Seneca Indians of North America valued this plant as an antidote to snakebites, hence its common name. It was used herbally by Native Americans for bronchitis, asthma, and whooping cough.
PREPARATION The root is unearthed in autumn and dried. It is then powdered and macerated in alcohol.

REMEDY PROFILE
Senega is most appropriate for people whose mood is dull and depressed. They have a tendency to fly into sudden rages.

The remedy has a strong affinity with the respiratory tract, and is typically used for chest and phlegmy conditions such as coughs, bronchitis, and even tuberculosis, particularly in the elderly. The classic symptom picture includes chest pain, profuse clear mucus that is difficult to expel, and a sensation of the lungs being pushed back against the spine. The throat may be raw and sore. There may be mucus in the throat that causes a scraping sensation on talking. Breathing may be short or hurried, with a painful, oppressed feeling in the lungs, as if they are being squeezed.
Symptoms better From perspiring.
Symptoms worse In windy weather; from walking in and breathing in the cold, in the open air; from touch and pressure on the affected area.

Punica granatum
GRANATUM

COMMON NAME Pomegranate.
ORIGIN Native to southwestern Asia, and naturalized in Europe.

PUNICA GRANATUM
(Pomegranate)

BACKGROUND An ancient treatment for intestinal worms, the pomegranate was cited in the Ebers papyrus, written in Egypt in c. 1500 BCE. The fruits, juice, and seeds all have culinary uses.
PREPARATION The dried bark of the root and branches is macerated in alcohol.

REMEDY PROFILE

Granatum is best suited to people who are ill-humored, very impressionable, and sensitive. Often dejected, discouraged, weary, and gloomy, they tend to be melancholy and prone to hypochondria.

The remedy is used primarily for the expulsion of tapeworms. The typical symptom picture may include nausea, excess salivation, dizziness, pale blue rings around the eyes, itching and tickling in the nose, and itching and tingling in the anus. There may be emaciation or a loss of appetite, or ravenous hunger with cravings for coffee and sour or juicy foods such as fruits.

Symptoms better After dinner; after drinking cold water.

Symptoms worse From looking upward; from walking; from the pressure of clothing; from alcohol.

Pyrogenium
PYROGEN.

COMMON NAME Pyrogen.
ORIGIN Decomposed, rotten meat.
BACKGROUND The term pyrogen often applies to proteins produced in response to infection. They are also produced when flesh decomposes.
PREPARATION Chopped, lean beef is soaked in water, sterilized, dissolved in purified water, then diluted and succussed.

REMEDY PROFILE

People who benefit most from *Pyrogen.* have a tendency to be hypersensitive, and have highly active brains. Restless and talkative, they often think and talk rapidly. They may feel insane and have bizarre physical sensations; for instance, that their body is "crowded with arms and legs." These are most common during a fever.

Conditions usually treated by *Pyrogen.* include infections, fevers, suppuration, the flu, and septic states. Characteristic symptoms include aching, bruising, pain, great restlessness, and foul-smelling sweat, diarrhea, breath, and other discharges. Conditions may be acute or due to a prior infection. There may be red streaks on the skin from the limbs to the heart, or sore, recurring abscesses that never fully heal.

The remedy may also be used to treat infection in the genital tract following childbirth or an abortion, and may help women who have a pelvic infection, or who have a fever during menstruation.

Symptoms better With heat; from a hot bath; from stretching; from changing position; from hot drinks.

Symptoms worse In cold and dampness; from sitting.

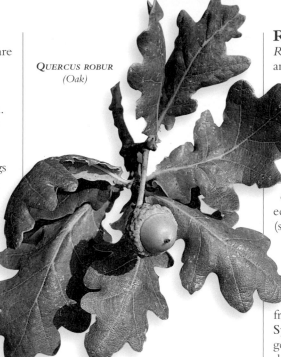

QUERCUS ROBUR
(Oak)

Quercus robur
QUERCUS

COMMON NAMES Oak, common oak, English oak.
ORIGIN Found throughout the Northern Hemisphere and cultivated for its timber.
BACKGROUND Sacred to the Druids and dedicated to the Norse god Thor, the oak has long been important in many cultures, both economically and in herbal medicine.
PREPARATION The acorns are steeped in alcohol until soft, then peeled, crushed, diluted in alcohol, and succussed.

REMEDY PROFILE

People who respond best to *Quercus* tend to be nervous, weepy, and unable to speak clearly or think straight.

Chronic spleen disorders involving fluid retention are primarily associated with *Quercus*. It is used for an enlarged spleen, possibly caused by recurrent malaria or alcoholism. *Quercus* may relieve the effects of acute alcohol poisoning and lessen the desire for alcohol, although it will not cure alcoholism. Recurrent gout may also be helped by the remedy.

Symptoms better No specific factors.
Symptoms worse No specific factors.

Radium bromatum
RADIUM BROM.

COMMON NAME Radium bromide.
ORIGIN Chemically prepared.
BACKGROUND Radium is too unstable to exist in a pure form in nature, and usually combines with chlorine or bromine.
PREPARATION The compound is dissolved in purified water, diluted, and succussed.

REMEDY PROFILE

Radium brom. is best suited to depressed, anxious people who need company and are afraid of being alone in the dark.

Conditions arising from radiation poisoning or treatment, such as ulcers from X-ray burns or skin problems, are typically treated with the remedy. Skin symptoms are characterized by burning, dry, itchy, scaly eruptions, or by thickening or callousing of the skin: Psoriasis, eczema, dermatitis, acne rosacea, nevi (skin blemishes), moles, ulcers, and even cancers may all respond to the remedy. Constricting neuralgic pains, acute rheumatic pains, and numbness may also be helped by *Radium brom.*

Symptoms better In the open air; from hot baths; with sleep; from eating.

Symptoms worse With movement; from getting up after lying down; from shaving; from washing.

Ranunculus bulbosus
RANUNCULUS BULB.

COMMON NAMES Bulbous buttercup, bulbous crowfoot.
ORIGIN Native to Europe, but now also common throughout North America.
BACKGROUND The buttercup has been used medicinally since the time of ancient Greece. Toxic and irritant, it was mostly used externally for skin growths such as warts and blemishes.
PREPARATION The whole plant in flower is finely chopped and steeped in alcohol.

REMEDY PROFILE

This remedy is most suited to those who are irritable, depressed, and contentious. They feel weepy and inadequate, and feel worse when they think about their symptoms. Restlessness and insomnia are common characteristic traits.

The classic symptom picture for *Ranunculus bulb.* includes muscle, joint, and skin problems, possibly occurring simultaneously. Typical muscle problems include soreness and deep, bruising pain, particularly chest pain between the ribs. The classic skin symptoms for this remedy focus on eczema or herpes, especially herpes zoster (shingles), with intense burning and itching.

Symptoms better In warm weather; from warm compresses; with rest; from standing; from sitting bent forward.

Symptoms worse In drafts or open air, especially damp, cold air; in stormy weather; from changes in temperature; with movement, particularly of the arms; when thinking about symptoms; alcohol.

Raphanus sativus var. *niger*
RAPHANUS

COMMON NAME Black radish.
ORIGIN Native to southern Asia, but now widely cultivated worldwide.
BACKGROUND The ancient Romans used radish oil for skin diseases, and radish was a noted digestive stimulant in Chinese medicine by CE 659.
PREPARATION The fresh roots, dug up in spring before flowering, are finely chopped and steeped in alcohol.

REMEDY PROFILE
Those who benefit most from *Raphanus* may feel "collapsed" and lacking in spirit. The remedy has a strong affinity with the digestive tract, and is given for extreme abdominal distension. A classic use of *Raphanus* is for postoperative pain resulting from trapped gas, with gurgling and great swelling in the abdomen.
Symptoms better From walking in the open air.
Symptoms worse At night; from jarring; from coughing; from touch, even of clothing; from laughing.

Resina piceae
ABIES NIG.

COMMON NAME Pine resin.
ORIGIN Resin from the black spruce (*Picea mariana*), found in northern North America from Alaska to Newfoundland.
BACKGROUND The oil distilled from the wood of this tree is used largely in the manufacture of paints.
PREPARATION The resin from the tree is dried and macerated in alcohol.

REMEDY PROFILE
Low-spirited, nervous people who are unable to concentrate or relax are best suited to *Abies nig.* They are lethargic and dull by day, yet cannot sleep at night. *Abies nig.* is mainly associated with a sense of "blockage." It is often used for indigestion with a knotted sensation, as if an egg or stone is lodged in the stomach. The stomach pain always develops after eating and, in an attempt to relieve the discomfort, there may be frequent burping, possibly with constipation, foul-smelling breath, and mild fever with alternating chills and fever. Tea and tobacco are often causative factors behind the *Abies nig.* symptom picture.
Symptoms better With movement; from walking.
Symptoms worse From tobacco; from tea; from eating.

Rheum officinale or *R. palmatum*
RHEUM

COMMON NAME Rhubarb or Chinese rhubarb.
ORIGIN Both species are native to China and Tibet, but are now grown worldwide.
BACKGROUND Long used in Chinese medicine, notably as a laxative, these non-culinary types of rhubarb were adopted by European doctors in the 18th century.
PREPARATION The root of either species is dried and macerated in alcohol.

REMEDY PROFILE
Rheum is most suitable for those with sour moods who tend to be undemanding and withdrawn, yet restless and "quarrelsome in sleep." Children who respond to *Rheum* are full of fears, crying and restless at night. Both adults and children may tire rapidly.

Chronic, sour-smelling diarrhea is a key condition linked with *Rheum*. The stools are sour-smelling, and may be yellow or green, frothy, or fermented. Further typical symptoms include sour-smelling breath and a sour taste to all foods, causing a loss of appetite. The remedy may also be used for nausea or colicky pain that feels worse on standing and is often accompanied by shivering and an urge to pass stools.
Symptoms better From wrapping up; with warmth; from doubling up on lying down.
Symptoms worse In hot weather; from teething; before, during, and after passing stools; from eating sour fruit in summer.

Rhododendron chrysanthum
RHODODENDRON

COMMON NAMES Siberian rhododendron, yellow snow rose.
ORIGIN Found mainly in alpine areas of Siberia, but also in mountainous regions of Asia and Europe.

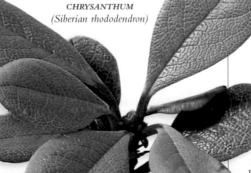

RHODODENDRON CHRYSANTHUM (Siberian rhododendron)

BACKGROUND An infusion of this plant is a traditional Mongolian drink used by hunters to ease weary, painful limbs, and for gout and rheumatic pains.
PREPARATION The leafy shoots are dried and macerated in alcohol.

REMEDY PROFILE
Rhododendron is most suited to nervous, highly sensitive people who are deeply affected by the weather. Prior to a storm they may feel confused, excited, and faint, alternating feverish excitement with chaotic behavior.

The symptom picture for this remedy focuses primarily on joint problems such as gout, arthritis, or rheumatic pain. Symptoms may affect the fibrous tissues, small joints, bones, and nerves, often resulting in swollen joints, with tearing, wrenching pain that causes restlessness, weakness, and stiffness in the limbs. Joint pains may move around the body. The remedy may also be used to ease swelling in the scrotum (hydrocele).
Symptoms better With warmth; with the heat of the sun; after a storm breaks; from wrapping up the head; lying in bed with the limbs drawn up; with movement.
Symptoms worse In rough or windy weather; from getting wet or catching cold; before storms; from temperature changes; with rest; when beginning to move.

SEE ALSO Hydrocele, *page 264*

Rhus toxicodendron
RHUS TOX.

COMMON NAMES Poison ivy, poison oak.
ORIGIN Found widely in North America.
BACKGROUND Native Americans used this plant to treat skin eruptions and nervous paralysis. Contact with its leaves produces redness, swelling, and blistering.
PREPARATION The fresh leaves, gathered at sunset just before the plant comes into flower, are macerated in alcohol.

REMEDY PROFILE
Rhus tox. is particularly beneficial to people who are usually lively yet shy, but restless and agitated when ill. Children who respond to the remedy tend to be overactive, restless, irritable, and malicious. If illness becomes chronic in these people, they may become fixed in their ways. *Rhus tox.* is known primarily as a remedy for skin and joint disorders. It may be helpful for skin eruptions with blisters, followed by burning, red, swollen skin

that tends to scale and flake off. Skin conditions such as chicken pox, shingles, herpes, eczema, rosacea, and diaper rash may all respond to the remedy. Musculo-skeletal problems are another focus of *Rhus tox*. It is used for acute rheumatic or arthritic pain, sciatica, restless legs, cramps, sprains, and strains.

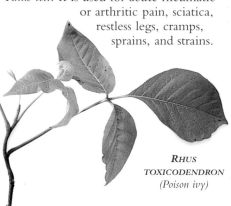

RHUS TOXICODENDRON
(Poison ivy)

Symptoms better With heat; in warm, dry weather; from hot baths; with movement; from nosebleeds. **Symptoms worse** With cold; in winter; from being chilled; in damp conditions; before storms; on beginning to move; during sleep.

SEE ALSO Rosacea, *page 193*; Severe eczema, *page 194*; Osteoarthritis, *page 196*; Rheumatoid arthritis, *page 197*; Sciatica, *page 218*; Restless legs, *page 230*; Diaper rash, *page 246*; Chicken pox, *page 252*

Rhus venenata syn. *R. vernix*
RHUS VEN.

COMMON NAMES Poison sumac, poison elder.
ORIGIN Found throughout North America, from Canada to the Gulf of Mexico.
BACKGROUND More toxic than poison ivy (*see left*), this plant produces a volatile oil that can cause inflamed, blistering lesions, possibly affecting the whole body.
PREPARATION The young, leafy twigs are macerated in alcohol.

REMEDY PROFILE
Gloomy, forgetful people are most likely to benefit from *Rhus ven.*, particularly if they feel unable to connect ideas together and have no interest in life.

The physical symptoms associated with this remedy are similar to those treated by *Rhus tox.*, although the focus is more heavily on skin conditions. The classic symptom picture for *Rhus ven.* includes flaking, itching skin, possibly with patches of thickening or hardening, and a tendency for the skin to crack. All symptoms are markedly worse in the morning.
Symptoms better In the open air; from hot baths; with touch; with mild exercise.

Symptoms worse In damp weather; from getting wet; in the morning; with touch and from pressure on the affected area; with rest; on waking.

Ricinus communis
RICINUS

COMMON NAMES Castor oil plant, Palma Christi, castor bean.
ORIGIN Native to east Africa and grown in hot climates, especially Africa and Asia.
BACKGROUND The seeds of this plant are highly toxic, but the oil made from them has been used medicinally for centuries in many cultures, notably for constipation.
PREPARATION The ripe seeds are steeped in alcohol, filtered, diluted, and succussed.

REMEDY PROFILE
The digestive system is the primary focus of this remedy. Typical symptoms treated include nausea, profuse vomiting, and diarrhea: *Ricinus* is useful for children who are seriously prostrated by diarrhea. Typically, there is severe dehydration and great thirst, but no desire to eat.
Symptoms better No specific factors.
Symptoms worse From pressure on the abdomen.

Rumex crispus
RUMEX CRISPUS

COMMON NAMES Yellow dock, curled dock.
ORIGIN Native to Europe and Africa.
BACKGROUND Long used in Western herbal medicine, yellow dock is a mild laxative and also acts as a stimulant to the liver and gallbladder.
PREPARATION The fresh root is finely chopped and macerated in alcohol.

REMEDY PROFILE
Rumex crispus is best suited to low-spirited, serious people who are very restless in the evening. Their sleep is often wakeful, and unpleasant dreams and fantasies disturb them when asleep or awake. The throat and chest are the main focus of *Rumex crispus*. There may be whooping cough, a dry, tickling cough, croup, or other hard, hacking cough, or asthma that is suffocating and choking on going to bed. There may be great concentration on the breathing and sensitivity to cold air.
Symptoms better From wrapping up, including wrapping the head; from covering the mouth; from drinking; from hard candies.

Symptoms worse In cold air; in the open air; from breathing in cold air; from touch and pressure on the throat; uncovering; with movement; from talking; from eating.

Ruta graveolens
RUTA

COMMON NAMES Rue, herb-of-grace.
ORIGIN Native to dry, sunny regions of Mediterranean countries.
BACKGROUND Rue has been prescribed herbally since the time of ancient Greece and Egypt to induce abortion, strengthen the eyesight, and stimulate menstruation.
PREPARATION The aerial parts, gathered as the plant is beginning to flower, are finely chopped and steeped in alcohol.

REMEDY PROFILE
People who respond best to the *Ruta* remedy are prone to feelings of anxiety and panic and tend to be weepy. They may be argumentative and suspicious, often feeling that they are constantly being deceived or watched.

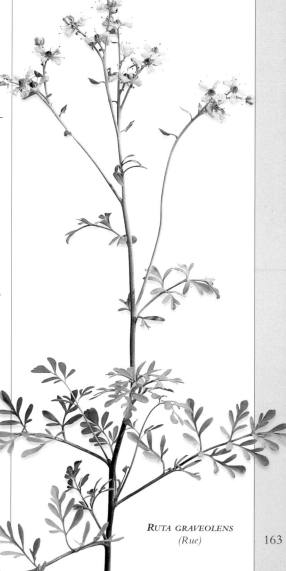

RUTA GRAVEOLENS
(Rue)

163

The classic symptom picture for *Ruta* is of connective tissue problems with marked stiffness and pain in the muscles and tendons, often due to sprains, overuse of the muscles, or injury. The pain is typically sore, bruised, aching, and accompanied by restlessness. Repetitive strain injuries, eyestrain, ganglions, and chronic arthritis may be helped by *Ruta*, as may a stiff, sore lower back or sciatica.

Symptoms better With warmth; lying on the back; with movement; from rubbing or scratching the affected area.
Symptoms worse In cold, damp air; from overexertion, injury, or sprains; from sitting; from menstruating; from eating uncooked or indigestible foods.

SEE ALSO Eyestrain, *page 220*

SAMBUCUS
Sambucus nigra

COMMON NAMES Elder, black elder.
ORIGIN Native to Europe.
BACKGROUND Used medicinally for millennia, elder became known as "nature's medicine chest" and was also strongly linked to much European folklore.
PREPARATION The fresh leaves and flowers are finely chopped and steeped in alcohol.

REMEDY PROFILE
The remedy is best suited to people who are constantly fretful, restless, easily frightened, and prone to trembling. *Sambucus* is used mainly for respiratory problems. General symptoms associated with the remedy include severe weakness, and profuse continuous or intermittent sweating. The remedy may help respiratory conditions such as asthma, croup, whooping cough, or bronchitis. Generally there is hoarseness, with mucus and inflammation in the larynx. During asthma attacks, a lack of oxygen may cause the face to turn blue.

Symptoms better From wrapping up warmly; from sitting up in bed; leaning over a table or chair back; with movement.
Symptoms worse In dry, cold air; with heat; during the night; lying down, especially with the head low; with rest.

SAMBUCUS NIGRA
(Elder)

SANGUINARIA
Sanguinaria canadensis

COMMON NAMES Bloodroot, red puccoon.
ORIGIN Native to eastern North America.
BACKGROUND Native Americans took bloodroot to induce therapeutic vomiting, and used the orange-colored juice of the root as a body paint and clothing dye.
PREPARATION The rhizome, unearthed in autumn, is dried and macerated in alcohol.

REMEDY PROFILE
People who respond best to *Sanguinaria* are confused and full of dread, and feel very weak and stupid. Despite feeling heavy, languid, and drowsy, they cannot sleep at night and the slightest noise wakes them up. An uncomfortable sensation of prickling warmth sometimes spreads over the whole body.

The classic symptom picture for this remedy is of irritation of the mucous membranes, particularly those of the respiratory system. *Sanguinaria* may be given for hay fever accompanied by great sensitivity to grass and flowers, and by burning and dryness in the nose and throat. Other conditions that are typically associated with *Sanguinaria* include asthma with phlegm and raw, burning membranes. Symptoms tend to affect the right side of the body more than the left.

Symptoms better In the evening; lying on the back; lying on the left side; with sleep; from vomiting; from burping.
Symptoms worse In cold and dampness; in sun; with movement and touch; lying on the right side; during menopause; from sweet foods.

SABADILLA
Schoenocaulon officinale

COMMON NAMES Sabadilla, cebadilla.
ORIGIN Found in Mexico, the West Indies, Guatemala, and Venezuela.
BACKGROUND The bitter seeds of sabadilla contain the alkaloids veratridine and veratrine, which are used in insecticides.
PREPARATION The ripe seeds are steeped in alcohol, filtered, diluted, and succussed.

REMEDY PROFILE
Sabadilla is most appropriate for people who are nervous, easily startled, and prone to hysterical paroxysms following a fright.

Key physical symptoms associated with *Sabadilla* include paroxysmal sneezing, an itchy, tingly nose, copious, watery phlegm, and chilliness. There may be throat pain and inflammation, with a constant desire to clear the throat. This remedy is used chiefly for inflammation of the respiratory mucous membranes, possibly due to hay fever, asthma, tonsillitis, or a cold.

Symptoms better In open air; with heat or wrapping up; from warm food or drink.
Symptoms worse In cold air; at periodic, consistent intervals; from cold drinks.

SCORPION
Scorpio europaeus

COMMON NAME Scorpion.
ORIGIN Found in central and southern Europe.
BACKGROUND Scorpions were listed as a medicine in an ancient Egyptian medical papyrus, although their use is not known.
PREPARATION The whole, live animal is macerated in alcohol.

REMEDY PROFILE
Scorpion is most effective for people who feel detached and disconnected from the world. Their mental state is dull and foggy, and they are unable to concentrate on more than one thing at a time. This state of mind may be accompanied by anxiety about health, an aversion to work and to talking, and sensitivity to music. Their moods are usually very changeable, and they may have confused, troubling, vague, angry, or erotic dreams.

Strong fears, especially those of driving and accidents, may be helped by *Scorpion*. A classic symptom is great fear, which is rooted in the abdomen, and may occur with sharp cramps below the ribs.

Symptoms better From crying; walking; with movement; from urinating; eating.
Symptoms worse At night; from bright light; with noise; from sitting; breathing deeply; from pressure on the abdomen.

Scutellaria laterifolia
SCUTELLARIA

COMMON NAME Virginia skullcap.
ORIGIN Native to North America.
BACKGROUND This plant was once used by the Cherokee tribe to promote menstruation, but has more recently been used widely as a sedative, especially for stress and tension.
PREPARATION The whole, fresh plant, excluding the root, is steeped in alcohol.

REMEDY PROFILE
Scutellaria is best suited to people who have a sense of foreboding and feel exhausted, confused, and unable to concentrate.

The typical symptom picture is of nervous exhaustion, possibly as a result of illness, continuous, tiring work, or over-studying. The remedy may help chronic fatigue syndrome, headaches with a sensation of the space in the head being too small for its contents, possible dizziness, twitching muscles, and sensitivity to light.
Symptoms better At night; with movement; in the open air.
Symptoms worse From light; near noise; from smells; from eating.

Secale cornutum
SECALE

COMMON NAME Ergot.
ORIGIN From the fungus *Claviceps purpurea*, which grows mostly on cereal crops in Europe, North America, and Asia.
BACKGROUND This fungus, largely found on rye, is used in a drug prescribed by Western medicine to halt bleeding.
PREPARATION Ergot is collected while still immature, then dried, powdered, and macerated in alcohol.

REMEDY PROFILE
People who benefit most from *Secale* often feel confused, suspicious, and fearful, and may even doubt their own sanity.

A key affinity for *Secale* is with uterine problems in women. It is often used for uterine bleeding and hypercontraction of the muscles in the uterus. *Secale* is given to strengthen weak contractions during labor, and for puerperal sepsis (infection in the genital tract after childbirth). It may also help menstrual cramps with dark, irregular bleeding, and a flow of watery blood between menstrual periods.
Symptoms better With cold; from bathing; stretching; uncovering the body.
Symptoms worse With warmth; if touched; before or after menstruating; in pregnancy; after miscarriage or labor.

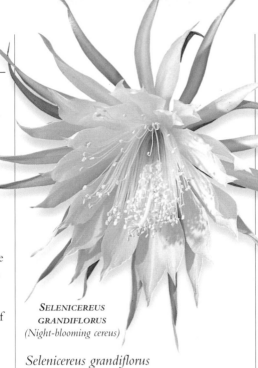

SELENICEREUS GRANDIFLORUS
(Night-blooming cereus)

Selenicereus grandiflorus
CACTUS GRAND.

COMMON NAME Night-blooming cereus.
ORIGIN Native to Central America and the West Indies.
BACKGROUND Widely renowned for its beauty, this plant is also cultivated for use in a conventional rheumatic drug and is valued herbally as a remedy for the heart.
PREPARATION Young, tender stems and flowers are collected in summer, finely chopped, and steeped in alcohol.

REMEDY PROFILE
Sad, distracted people who tend to be anxious about their health are most likely to respond well to *Cactus grand.*

Classic symptoms associated with *Cactus grand.* include constriction in the muscle fibers, and a painful feeling of the body being caged and twisted. The remedy is especially associated with pains in the heart, such as those triggered by angina. Heart conditions relieved by *Cactus grand.* are typified by severe pain in the chest, as if it is being confined and squeezed by an iron band around the torso. The pain may extend into the left arm or hand and be accompanied by numbness.
Symptoms better In the open air; from sitting; with rest.
Symptoms worse From walking; lying on the left side; lying on the back.

SEE ALSO Angina, *page 185*

Selenium metallicum
SELENIUM MET.

COMMON NAME Selenium.
ORIGIN Found in volcanic areas and in sulfide ores such as pyrite.

BACKGROUND Selenium was one of the elements discovered by a Swedish chemist, Berzelius. In 1817 he named it after the Greek *selene*, or "moon," an analogy with tellurium, from *tellus,* or "earth."
PREPARATION The element is triturated with lactose sugar.

REMEDY PROFILE
People who benefit most from this remedy may have difficulties in connecting to or becoming intimate with others and may withdraw, even from close friends. Mental activity may cause them great exhaustion, and they may be very forgetful. Great weakness, particularly if the body temperature increases, is a classic feature associated with this remedy. It is used for conditions such as chronic fatigue syndrome and multiple sclerosis, when there is rapid mental and physical exhaustion, with unhealthy-looking skin, emaciation, constipation, and possible malfunction of the nerves governing the genitourinary tract.
Symptoms better From breathing cold air; after sunset; from drinking cold water.
Symptoms worse On hot days; in drafts of air; with sleep; from talking; from passing stools.

Senecio aureus
SENECIO

COMMON NAMES Life root, squaw weed.
ORIGIN Native to eastern North America.
BACKGROUND Traditionally valued by Native Americans for problems of the female reproductive system, life root is now considered by herbalists to be unsafe for internal use.
PREPARATION The whole plant, including the root, is finely chopped and macerated in alcohol.

REMEDY PROFILE
Senecio is best suited to those who are restless, nervous, low-spirited, and unable to concentrate.

The remedy is typically prescribed for hemorrhaging in the mucous membranes. Bleeding in the lungs or the throat, in congested and inflamed kidneys, or during menstruation may all be helped by *Senecio*, as may nosebleeds. Delayed or absent menstruation, accompanied by a thick vaginal discharge, appetite loss, excitability, and insomnia may also respond well to the remedy.
Symptoms better From menstruation.
Symptoms worse In dampness; in cold air; from sitting; during puberty; from sexual excitement.

Serenoa repens syn. S. serrulata

SABAL

COMMON NAME Saw palmetto.
ORIGIN Native to southeastern North America.
BACKGROUND Native Americans valued this plant as a food source and for its sedative and tonic medicinal properties.
PREPARATION The fresh, ripe fruits are finely chopped and macerated in alcohol.

REMEDY PROFILE

People who benefit most from *Sabal* tend to brood on their symptoms, yet are often angered by sympathy. They may be irritable, apathetic, introverted, depressed, and afraid to go to sleep.

This remedy is given mainly for problems of the genitourinary organs. Typical symptoms treated include frequent urination, especially when this occurs at night, which may be due to cystitis. Urine retention due to prostate enlargement or gonorrhea may be helped by *Sabal*, as may inflammation in the seminal tubes, heavy, aching pains or, occasionally, sharp pains in the bladder that extend to the abdomen or radiate down the thighs. Another typical symptom is a sensation of coldness in the bladder, possibly extending to the external genitals. *Sabal* is also used for sexual or general fatigue.
Symptoms better After sleep.
Symptoms worse In cold, damp weather; before menstruating; from sympathy.

SEE ALSO Prostate problems, *page 202*

Silybum marianum syn. Carduus marianus

CARDUUS

COMMON NAMES St. Mary's thistle, milk thistle.
ORIGIN Native to the Mediterranean region and grown throughout Europe.
BACKGROUND The flower heads were traditionally grown to eat as a substitute for artichokes, and boiled as a spring tonic following the winter months.
PREPARATION The ripe, dried seeds are soaked in water for one to two days and then macerated in alcohol.

REMEDY PROFILE

Carduus is most suitable for people who are completely run down, with the kind of total physical and mental exhaustion, blankness, and indifference that may arise following a hard life of physical labor, or that may be caused by alcoholism.

The classic symptom picture for *Carduus* is of acute or chronic liver problems and lung conditions such as asthma. The remedy may be used for severe liver and abdominal pain that is most marked when lying on the left side, or for gallbladder pain and gallstone colic. The stools are typically discolored and pale due to liver malfunction, or they may be dark due to internal bleeding in the digestive system.
Symptoms better From sitting up in bed; after a nosebleed.
Symptoms worse With movement; lying on the left side; from alcohol.

Simarouba cedron
syn. *Simaba cedron, Quassia cedron*

CEDRON

COMMON NAMES Cedron, rattlesnake beans.
ORIGIN Found in Central America and northern Brazil.
BACKGROUND Known in Panama as an antidote for snakebite and insect stings if chewed immediately after being bitten, cedron was also used for malaria or fever.
PREPARATION Cotyledons (embryonic shoots) from the dried, ripe seeds are macerated in alcohol.

REMEDY PROFILE

People who respond best to *Cedron* tend to be nervous, restless, and even hysterical, possibly experiencing depression following any nervous excitement. They may dread going to bed and fear their friends.

A characteristic of the complaints associated with *Cedron* is that they tend to recur at exactly the same hour each day. The remedy is used for recurrent fevers, such as those associated with malaria, and for neuralgic pains and other nervous system conditions such as spasms or tics. Severe headaches or migraines, perhaps with nausea, fever, or cerebrospinal meningitis, may also respond to *Cedron*.
Symptoms better From standing erect.
Symptoms worse In the open air; at the same time each day; after sleep.

Smilax officinalis
syn. *S. ornata, S. regelii, S. medica*

SARSAPARILLA

COMMON NAMES Sarsaparilla, wild licorice.
ORIGIN Native to Central and South America and Jamaica.
BACKGROUND Long used medicinally by indigenous tribes in South America, sarsaparilla was introduced to Europe in the 17th century as a cure-all. It was later used to flavor root beer.
PREPARATION The dried root is steeped in alcohol, diluted, and succussed.

REMEDY PROFILE

Sarsaparilla is most effective for people who are depressed and anxious, blaming their state of mind on the pain they feel. They tend also to feel the cold.

Sarsaparilla has a strong affinity with the urinary tract. It is prescribed for cystitis characterized by a constant urge to urinate, pain as urination ends, and possibly blood or a sandy or gravelly precipitate in the urine. There may be involuntary dribbling of urine, especially on sitting down, and normal flow may happen only when in a standing position.
Symptoms better From standing; from uncovering the neck and chest.
Symptoms worse In the spring; in wet and cold weather; with movement; as urination ends; during menstruation.

Solidago virgaurea

SOLIDAGO

COMMON NAME Goldenrod.
ORIGIN Native to Europe and Asia and naturalized in North America.
BACKGROUND This herb has traditionally been used externally to heal wounds,

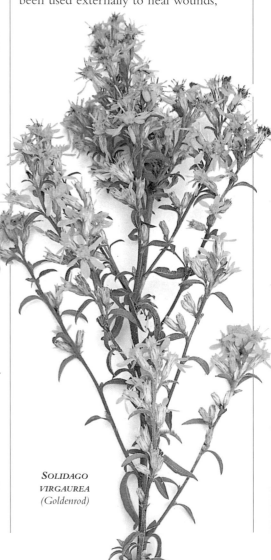

**SOLIDAGO
VIRGAUREA**
(Goldenrod)

yeast infections, ulcers, and insect bites, and internally for urinary tract infections.
PREPARATION The fresh aerial parts are finely chopped and macerated in alcohol.

REMEDY PROFILE
The classic symptom picture for *Solidago* is of kidney disease, possibly with nausea, insomnia, a weak chest, and susceptibility to colds. *Solidago* is used when the kidneys feel distended, sore, aching, and tender, with pain extending down to the thighs, or toward the bladder and abdomen. There are typically difficulties in passing urine, which is scanty and discolored, or clear and foul-smelling. The remedy may also be prescribed to treat fibroids.
Symptoms better From profuse urination.
Symptoms worse From pressure on the affected area.

SEE ALSO Fibroids, *page 199*

Spigelia anthelmia
SPIGELIA

COMMON NAMES Pink root, annual wormgrass.
ORIGIN Native to South America, but now found in the US and the West Indies.
BACKGROUND Pink root contains certain alkaloids that are used in the herbal treatment of heart disease.
PREPARATION The dried aerial parts are macerated in alcohol.

REMEDY PROFILE
A sad, forgetful, "blank" temperament is characteristic of those who respond most effectively to this remedy.

It is given chiefly for problems of the heart and the nervous system, especially if symptoms affect primarily the left side of the body, and if there are intense, violent pains. *Spigelia* may be given for frequent palpitations that are violent, visible, and audible, for heart murmurs or valve disorders, and for rheumatic heart disease. It is also used for angina with constricting chest pains that extend down one or both arms, into the chest, and up to the throat. In addition, the remedy may be used for headaches, migraines, sinus infections, or neuralgic or rheumatic pain, especially if the symptoms are worse on the left side.
Symptoms better From breathing in; lying on the right side with the head higher than the body; from steady pressure on the affected area.
Symptoms worse From changes in the weather; with touch; lying on the left side; with movement; from tobacco.

SEE ALSO Angina, *page 185*; Rheumatoid arthritis, *page 197*; Neuralgia, *page 268*

Spongilla fluviatilis syn. *S. lacustris*
BADIAGA

COMMON NAME Freshwater sponge.
ORIGIN Found in Russia and Europe.
BACKGROUND In Russia this sponge is powdered to make a traditional treatment that causes bruises to disappear overnight.
PREPARATION The fresh sponge is collected in autumn, dried, and triturated with lactose sugar.

REMEDY PROFILE
People for whom *Badiaga* is best suited enjoy mental activity, and feel that their minds are always clear and active, even when ill. Excitement or pleasure may easily bring on palpitations. The body may feel sore to the touch, as if it has been beaten, which may cause restless sleep; frightening dreams may also disturb or disrupt sleep.

Profuse mucus in the respiratory system, with copious phlegm that drips from the nose, possibly due to the flu or hay fever, may respond to *Badiaga*. Sneezing brought on by coughing may be helped, as may hard, swollen glands in the neck and breast, possibly linked to cancer.
Symptoms better With heat; at night.
Symptoms worse With cold; from stormy weather; lying on the right side.

Stannum metallicum
STANNUM MET.

COMMON NAME Tin.
ORIGIN Mined from cassiterite, which is found in England, Nigeria, Thailand, and South America.
BACKGROUND Tin has long been used for household and commercial purposes, and has been used medicinally: In 18th-century Scotland it was taken for intestinal worms.
PREPARATION The metal is triturated with lactose sugar.

REMEDY PROFILE
People who benefit most from *Stannum met.* are suspicious, anxious, uneasy, and sad, possibly with fixed ideas. They may be weak, debilitated, and unable to talk or move, and feel worse during the day.

Stannum met. is used for exhaustion after chronic respiratory problems, or for nervous system disorders. It may be given for weakness in the chest, during or after a serious infection such as bronchitis or pneumonia. The weakness leaves the lungs and bronchi susceptible to inflammation or serious illness, including asthma.
Symptoms better From lying across something hard; from expelling mucus.
Symptoms worse Lying on the right side; with gentle movement; from talking.

Strontium carbonicum
STRONTIUM CARB.

COMMON NAME Strontium carbonate.
ORIGIN Found in strontianite, which occurs mainly in Scotland, Germany, and California.
BACKGROUND This mineral takes its name from Strontian, the village in Argyllshire, Scotland, where strontianite was discovered in 1790.
PREPARATION Strontium carbonate is triturated with lactose sugar.

REMEDY PROFILE
Irritable people who are prone to rage respond to *Strontium carb.* Rage may even provoke violence and destructiveness in them, but they also tend to be forgetful, fearful, particularly of the dark, and easily startled. Although they may seem haughty,

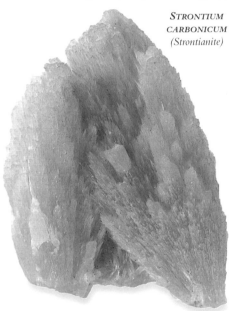

STRONTIUM CARBONICUM (Strontianite)

they are extremely sensitive to the scorn of others. They may jerk involuntarily and violently when asleep, waking themselves.

This remedy is given mainly for acute conditions following an operation or injury, such as fainting, exhaustion, chills, violent palpitations, and collapse, possibly due to severe trauma and bleeding. It may also be used to treat heart conditions, including angina, phlebitis (inflammation of a vein caused by a clot), and terrible pains in the muscles and bones.

The symptom picture for heart problems treated by *Strontium carb.* describes a heavy, smothering sensation in the heart area, or dull, intermittent pressure in the heart.
Symptoms better With heat; from light; from sunlight; from warm compresses; from a hot bath.
Symptoms worse With cold; from loss of blood; from uncovering the affected area; from walking.

Strychnos toxifera
CURARE

COMMON NAMES Curare, woorali root.
ORIGIN Found in South America.
BACKGROUND A paralyzing poison was traditionally extracted by Native South Americans from this and other *Strychnos* species for use on arrows during hunting.
PREPARATION The resin is extracted from the tree and macerated in alcohol.

REMEDY PROFILE

Those who respond best to *Curare* tend to be hurried, irritable, and aggressive. They want to be alone and may behave maliciously toward others. A loss of moral judgment is also possible. They often have a history of self-abuse, perhaps involving biting or hitting themselves, or ripping their clothes. Typically they can eat only small amounts of food at a time.

Classic symptoms associated with *Curare* include weakness, heaviness, numbness, and piercing pains. Progressive muscular paralysis and impaired reflex action may also be treated by the remedy.
Symptoms better No specific factors.
Symptoms worse In dampness; in cold winds; in cold weather; at 2 A.M.; with movement; on the right side of the body.

Sulfur iodatum
SULFUR IOD.

COMMON NAME Sulfur iodide.
ORIGIN Chemically prepared.
BACKGROUND This rather unusual compound is rarely used in medicine other than for homeopathic purposes.
PREPARATION Sulfur iodide is dissolved in a closed vessel, heated to 140°F (60°C), diluted, and succussed.

REMEDY PROFILE

People who benefit most from *Sulfur iod.* tend to be anxious and doubtful, and are unable to string coherent ideas together or to remain calm and composed in a working situation.

The remedy is prescribed primarily for chronic, itchy skin conditions such as weeping eczema, acne, boils, pustules, hives (urticaria), and lichen planus (pink or purple raised spots on the wrists, forearms, and lower legs). The body tends to feel cold on the outside, yet raw and burning hot inside, and symptoms tend to be worse on waking.
Symptoms better In cool air; in winter; from standing.
Symptoms worse With heat; prior to a storm; on waking in the morning; with the slightest exertion.

Symphytum officinale
SYMPHYTUM

COMMON NAMES Comfrey, knitbone.
ORIGIN Native to Europe and now found in temperate regions worldwide.
BACKGROUND This plant had established a reputation as early as the 1st century CE for healing bruises, sprains, fractures, and broken bones.
PREPARATION The fresh root is gathered either before flowering or in the autumn, steeped in alcohol, diluted, and succussed.

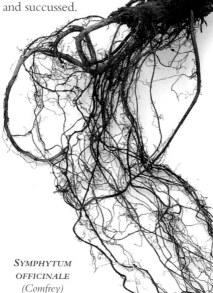

SYMPHYTUM OFFICINALE *(Comfrey)*

REMEDY PROFILE
Symphytum's marked affinity with the bones in herbal medicine is also carried through to its focus in homeopathy. It is used to heal sprains and fractured or badly set bones, as well as to ease any tingling pain from old injuries to the bone, cartilage, and periosteum (the membrane surrounding the bone), or pain on the site of an amputation. Abscesses in the psoas muscle (which links the hip and the pelvis) and malignant bone tumors on the face may also be helped by *Symphytum*.

In addition, the remedy is prescribed to treat painful eye injuries with strange sensations – for example, on closing the eyelids, the eyeballs may feel raised, although there is no visible sign of injury. There is frequently a marked tendency to rub the eyes and great difficulty in opening the eyelids.
Symptoms better With warmth.
Symptoms worse From injuries; from a blow to the affected area; if touched or from pressure on the affected area; from sexual excess; with movement.

Taraxacum officinale
TARAXACUM

COMMON NAME Dandelion.
ORIGIN Grows wild in temperate climates worldwide, and is cultivated in France and Germany.
BACKGROUND Used herbally in the traditional medicines of many cultures, including those of the West, Middle East, and China, dandelion is particularly well known for its use as a diuretic.
PREPARATION The whole plant, including the root, is picked as the flowers open, chopped finely, and macerated in alcohol.

REMEDY PROFILE

Those for whom *Taraxacum* is considered most appropriate have a tendency to be depressed and mutter to themselves.

Key conditions that may benefit from the remedy include digestive disorders, gallbladder inflammation, and gallstones. The classic symptom picture includes an enlarged, hardened liver, urinary problems, bilious attacks, cramping pains, headaches associated with gastric problems, and jaundiced skin. Acidic saliva tends to build up in the mouth, causing raw patches to develop on the tongue and a sensation of dullness in the teeth.
Symptoms better From walking; with movement; if touched.
Symptoms worse With rest; from standing; from sitting; from fatty foods.

Tarentula cubensis syn. *Mygale cubensis*
TARENTULA CUB.

COMMON NAME Cuban tarantula.
ORIGIN Found in Cuba and the southern US, particularly South Carolina and Texas.
BACKGROUND This large, hairy, dark brown spider has a bite that can cause blood poisoning in humans, with symptoms first appearing 24 hours after being bitten.
PREPARATION The whole, live spider is steeped in alcohol, diluted, and succussed.

REMEDY PROFILE

People who respond to *Tarentula cub.* may be delirious, restless, and uneasy. They often feel drowsy but sleep restlessly.

The classic symptom picture for this remedy is of severe, painful inflammation, burning, stinging pains, and extreme prostration and weakness. It is given for slow-developing fever, acute infection such as diphtheria, and septic conditions such as carbuncles, septicemia, painful abscesses, especially near the fingernails, ulcers that will not heal, and gangrene.

In addition, the remedy may be used to ease pain experienced during a slow death. The appetite is generally low, and the stomach feels hard and sore. Severe coughs such as whooping cough may also be helped, if there is great prostration.
Symptoms better From smoking.
Symptoms worse At night; from exertion; from cold drinks.

Tellurium metallicum
TELLURIUM MET.

COMMON NAME Tellurium.
ORIGIN Found throughout the world.
BACKGROUND Klaproth named this rare mineral in 1798 from the Greek *tellus*, or "earth," as a counterpart to his discovery in 1789 of uranium (named from the Greek *ouranos*, or "heaven").
PREPARATION Tellurium is triturated with lactose sugar.

REMEDY PROFILE
Tellurium met. is most appropriate for people who are excitable and irritable, with a disposition that is sometimes described as "rough and angular."

Skin disorders are the characteristic focus of *Tellurium met.*, including conditions such as psoriasis, ringworm, herpes, and eczema on the eyelids and behind the ears. A key symptom associated with the remedy is a characteristic smell of garlic in the perspiration, which tends to burn and irritate the skin. Skin symptoms are often circular or ring-shaped, and may occur in conjunction with severe back pain.

The remedy may also be used for back pain that is typically made worse by coughing, sneezing, or straining when passing a stool. It may help back pain after injury, spinal irritation, ruptured intervertebral disks, and pain that radiates down the legs. In addition, it may be effective for eye and ear infections, especially ear infections that produce a discharge that smells like fish brine.
Symptoms better From lying quietly.
Symptoms worse With cold; if touched; lying on the affected area.

Terebinthina laricina
TEREBINTHUM

COMMON NAMES Turpentine, turps.
ORIGIN Resin tapped from the trunks of the *Larix decidua* "Mill" species of larch, which is native to Europe.
BACKGROUND This viscous resin is used in the manufacture of paints. In the past it was used as a treatment for gonorrhea in traditional Western medicine.

PREPARATION The resin is macerated in alcohol, before being filtered, diluted, and succussed.

REMEDY PROFILE
Terebinthum is best suited to people who are tired, delirious, and unable to concentrate. Classic symptoms associated with the remedy include burning pain and bleeding of the mucous membranes, with dark, fetid-smelling blood. The remedy has an affinity with inflammation of the urinary tract or kidneys, accompanied by hemorrhaging, water retention, and edema in the hands and feet. These ailments are often associated with smoky-colored urine that has a strange smell of violets.
Symptoms better With movement; from walking; from stooping.
Symptoms worse With cold; if touched; in the morning; lying on the affected area.

Teucrium marum
syn. *Marum verum*
TEUCRIUM MARUM

COMMON NAME Cat thyme.
ORIGIN Native to Spain and southern Europe, and now found worldwide.
BACKGROUND Cat thyme has traditionally been used by herbalists for its properties as an astringent and stimulant. It has also been used in the treatment of gallbladder and stomach disorders.
PREPARATION The fresh aerial parts without the woody lower branches are finely chopped before being macerated in alcohol.

REMEDY PROFILE
People for whom *Teucrium marum* is considered most effective tend to be highly sensitive and feel worse when hearing or talking about unpleasant things, including their symptoms. They are easily overexcited and exhausted.

TEUCRIUM MARUM
(Cat thyme)

The primary affinity of this remedy is with polyps, which may affect the nose, ears, vagina, and rectum. Nasal polyps may be accompanied by chronic phlegm, dried-up, foul-smelling crusts of phlegm, and loss of smell. Fibrous tumors on the eyelids and fibroids in the uterus may be helped by the remedy, as may lumps in the urethra caused by gonorrhea.

Teucrium marum may also be given for intestinal worms, involving itching and tingling in the anus and rectum.
Symptoms better In the open air; from perspiring.
Symptoms worse In dampness and cold; from weather changes; from the warmth of the bed; in the evening; at night; from touching or rubbing the affected area.

Theridion curassavicum
THERIDION

COMMON NAME Orange spider.
ORIGIN Native to Curaçao and the West Indies.
BACKGROUND This small spider has orange spots on its back. Its bite can cause trembling, cold sweats, and fainting.
PREPARATION The whole, live spider is macerated in alcohol.

REMEDY PROFILE
Sensitivity to noise may be so extreme in people who respond to *Theridion* that it causes pain and vibrations to penetrate through the body. There may be a feeling that time is passing too quickly, and a tendency to be chilly. *Theridion* is generally used for acute sensitivity of the bones, nerves, and spine. The spine tends to be so highly sensitive that the least jarring motion, such as walking, may be unbearable; on sitting, one buttock may be raised off the seat to ease the pressure on the lower spine. There may be accompanying vertigo, dizziness, or motion sickness. *Theridion* may also be used to treat diabetes.
Symptoms better With warmth; with rest; from drinking warm water.
Symptoms worse At night; near noise; if touched; from pressure on the affected area; from travel; jarring movement; from closing the eyes; from bending forward.

SEE ALSO Diabetes, *page 191*; Dizziness, *page 266*

Trinitrum syn. *Nitroglycerinum*

GLONOINUM

COMMON NAMES Nitroglycerine, trinitroglycerine, glyceryl trinitrate.
ORIGIN Chemically prepared.
BACKGROUND An Italian chemist, Ascanio Sobreoro, created nitroglycerine in 1846, and 20 years later the Swedish chemist Alfred Nobel used it to develop dynamite.
PREPARATION Nitroglycerine is dissolved in purified water, diluted, and succussed.

REMEDY PROFILE

Symptoms that are treated with *Glonoinum* focus on the regulation of the circulation between the head and the heart. The remedy is used when an increase in blood supply causes flushes of heat, similar to those experienced during heatstroke, which surge up to the brain in waves, resulting in severe headaches. There is typically a bursting, "full" sensation in the head, with great confusion and a compulsion to hold the head and squeeze it. *Glonoinum* is also used for high blood pressure, particularly in the elderly, for heat exhaustion, and for hot flashes during menopause.
Symptoms better In fresh air.
Symptoms worse With heat, especially that of the sun; from movement such as shaking the head.

Uranium nitricum

URANIUM NIT.

COMMON NAME Uranium nitrate.
ORIGIN Chemically prepared.
BACKGROUND This is a compound of the radioactive metal uranium, which was named in 1789 by Klaproth after the planet Uranus, since the element was first located soon after the planet's discovery.
PREPARATION Uranium nitrate is triturated with lactose sugar.

REMEDY PROFILE

There is no well-defined picture for people who respond best to *Uranium nit.*, although irritability and depression may be evident.

Diabetes, kidney inflammation, high blood pressure, and liver problems can all respond to *Uranium nit.* It has an affinity with the digestive system and may be used for indigestion, bloating, and abdominal gas. Diabetes with water retention and increased urination may also be treated with this remedy.
Symptoms better In open air; with rapid movement; from bathing in cold water.
Symptoms worse With heat; with rest; from sour foods; from wine.

SEE ALSO Diabetes, *page 191*

Urginea maritima var. *rubra*
syn. *Drimia maritima* var. *rubra*

SQUILLA

COMMON NAMES Sea onion, sea squill.
ORIGIN Native to the shores of the Mediterranean region.
BACKGROUND The bulb of this plant is cultivated for the drug industry, since it contains scillarin, which affects the heart. Highly toxic, it has also been used in the manufacture of rat poison.
PREPARATION The fresh bulb is steeped in alcohol.

REMEDY PROFILE

Squilla is most appropriate for people who are irritable, weak, and weary. They tend to sleep badly, and definitely prefer to sit up rather than lie down.

This is a slow-acting remedy, used for conditions that take several days to develop. It can be used for chronic bronchitis in the elderly, or for childhood measles, but its primary use is for chronic respiratory conditions, including bronchitis, pleurisy, coughs, and asthma with panting. *Squilla* is typically prescribed for symptoms such as a dry, loose, short, violent cough that comes from deep in the lungs, sharp pain in the lower left side of the chest, and involuntary passing of urine.
Symptoms better With rest; from sitting up; from coughing up even a small quantity of mucus.
Symptoms worse In the early morning; with movement.

Urtica urens

URTICA URENS

COMMON NAME Annual nettle.
ORIGIN Found wild in temperate regions throughout the world.
BACKGROUND In the 1st century CE the ancient Greek physician Dioscorides advocated this nettle and its relative, *Urtica dioica*, as a treatment for festering wounds, nosebleeds, and delayed menstruation. The plant has a long tradition of use for many ailments in Western herbalism, and is still highly valued today.
PREPARATION The whole flowering plant, including the root, is steeped in alcohol.

REMEDY PROFILE

Appropriately, hives (urticaria) is a key condition treated by *Urtica urens*. It is given for red, burning, stinging skin eruptions that may be swollen or itchy. Symptoms are often aggravated by warmth, bathing, and vigorous exercise. Itching tends to be worse on rising in the morning, perhaps causing a fear of going to bed at night. *Urtica urens* is also used for actual burns or scalds with classic redness and blistering, and for blistering, burning, stinging, red, allergic rashes caused by insect bites, stings, shellfish, and plants.
Symptoms better From rubbing the affected area; lying down.
Symptoms worse With warmth; during a snowfall; from bathing in cold water; at the same time each year; if touched; after childbirth.

SEE ALSO Urticaria (hives), *page 242*

URTICA URENS
(Annual nettle)

Ustilago zeae
USTILAGO

COMMON NAME Corn smut.
ORIGIN Found as a fungus on corn grain, especially in Central and South America.
BACKGROUND The Zuni Indians of New Mexico traditionally used corn smut to hasten labor and prevent uterine bleeding.
PREPARATION The ripe, fresh fungus is macerated in alcohol.

REMEDY PROFILE

This remedy is best suited to people who tend to be irritable and sad. It is used for women's problems such as uterine fibroids, or hemorrhaging that develops following miscarriage or labor. The characteristic symptom picture is of slow, congestive bleeding, with clots that sometimes form long strings.
Symptoms better With rest.
Symptoms worse If touched; with movement; during menopause.

Valeriana officinalis
VALERIANA

COMMON NAME Common valerian.
ORIGIN Native to Europe and northern Asia, and cultivated in central Europe.
BACKGROUND Once known as "all-heal," valerian has been used since the time of ancient Rome for anxiety, insomnia, and high blood pressure. In World War I the tincture was widely used for shell shock.
PREPARATION The fresh root is unearthed and macerated in alcohol.

REMEDY PROFILE

Those with a nervous, irritable, restless, and mentally or emotionally unstable state of mind respond best to *Valeriana*. It is used for an extreme nervous state possibly characterized by hysteria, raving, swearing, and madness, accompanied by a sensation of dreaming or floating. Fluctuating mood swings that alternate between extreme joy and deepest grief are typically linked to this remedy.

Physically, *Valeriana* is associated with neuralgic pains, a rapid pulse, and blood congestion in the head. Pains tend to be darting and tearing, alternating between the upper and lower limbs. The limbs feel painful, heavy, and difficult to move, and may jerk on resting. Headaches tend to develop slowly, in spurts, or suddenly, as if caused by a blow to the head.
Symptoms better Changing position; walking around; from sleep; sweating.
Symptoms worse In the early afternoon; in the late evening; at rest; from standing or sitting still; from excitement; fasting.

Veratrum viride
VERATRUM VIR.

COMMON NAME American white hellebore.
ORIGIN Found throughout northwestern North America.
BACKGROUND Although once used as an herbal remedy by the Iroquois and Cherokee Indians, this highly toxic plant is now little used in herbal medicine.
PREPARATION The fresh root is gathered in autumn and macerated in alcohol.

REMEDY PROFILE
People who respond best to this remedy are often restless, argumentative, and prone to complaining.

Veratrum vir. has a strong affinity with lung conditions such as asthma, pleurisy, and pneumonia. Symptoms appear rapidly, including a strong or slow pulse, high fever, anxiety, and vomiting. There may be a red streak in the center of the tongue.

Another rapid-onset condition for which *Veratrum vir.* is given is intense fever with twitching, especially during sleep, spasms, delirium, chorea (involuntary, random, jerky movements), or even manic behavior or puerperal fever (infection in the genital tract after miscarriage, an abortion, or childbirth). Violent, rapidly appearing headaches may occur, with a bursting, congested sensation in the head, as if it contains too much blood.
Symptoms better From rubbing the affected area; lying with the head held low; from hot, strong coffee.
Symptoms worse With cold; from the heat of the sun; from rising; with movement; lying on the back; after childbirth; if menstruation is suppressed, possibly by jet lag.

Verbascum thapsiforme
VERBASCUM

COMMON NAMES Great mullein, Aaron's rod.
ORIGIN Native to central and southern Europe and western Asia.
BACKGROUND Greek mythology relates that Odysseus used great mullein to protect himself from Circe, and in the Middle Ages it was thought to be magical. Today it is generally used in herbalism for coughs.
PREPARATION The fresh aerial parts in flower, excluding the woody parts, are finely chopped and steeped in alcohol.

REMEDY PROFILE
Verbascum is of most benefit to those who are apathetic, lazy, and easily distracted by the varied thoughts that crowd upon them.

The symptoms treated by *Verbascum* are often associated with painful neuralgic conditions, particularly of the facial area. Typical symptoms include neuralgic pains in the face and teeth, especially on the left side, with severe pain in the cheekbones. Irritation and inflammation of the bladder, ears, or respiratory tract may also be eased by the remedy.

In addition, *Verbascum* is given for painful colds with profuse discharge, watery eyes, and a sensation of the ears having been blocked up. The chest may be congested with phlegm, and the voice may be deep and hoarse. Coughs tend to sound hollow, deep, and hoarse, and occur mainly at night. An intake of breath may cause the coughing to die down.
Symptoms better From rising after sitting; from taking a deep breath.
Symptoms worse For drafts; from changes in temperature; if touched; from talking or reading aloud; from biting hard.

SEE ALSO Neuralgia, *page 268*

Vespa crabro
VESPA

COMMON NAME European hornet.
ORIGIN Native to Europe.
BACKGROUND The female hornet has a severe sting, but it is rarely fatal.
PREPARATION The whole, live insect is steeped in alcohol, diluted, and succussed.

REMEDY PROFILE
VESPA CRABRO (European hornet)

People for whom *Vespa* is best suited are prone to insomnia, often due to anxiety. Their nerves and muscles are often sensitive.

Red, swollen skin complaints and disorders of the female reproductive organs are usually treated with *Vespa*. Typical skin symptoms include sore, stinging boils, raised, itchy bumps and weals, and itchy, lentil-shaped spots. Stinging, burning pains, as if the body is being pierced by something sharp, are another symptom associated with this remedy.

Vespa is also used for mucous membrane problems and complaints associated with menstruation, such as premenstrual depression, pain, and constipation.
Symptoms better From washing the hands in cold water; from bathing the affected area with vinegar.
Symptoms worse In closed, stuffy surroundings; from being near a source of direct heat.

Vetiveria zizianoides
ANANTHERUM

COMMON NAMES Cuscus grass, vetiver.
ORIGIN Native to tropical Asia, and commonly found in India and Sri Lanka.
BACKGROUND In India and Sri Lanka this grass's oil is called "the oil of tranquility," and its heavy, earthy aroma is used to repel flies, cockroaches, bedbugs, and moths.
PREPARATION The dried root is steeped in alcohol, diluted, and succussed.

REMEDY PROFILE
Anantherum is best suited to people who seem overexcited or even drunk. Their behavior may be restless and manic.

The remedy is typically prescribed for skin disorders, and for hard, glandular swellings, especially in the neck. It is used for itchy skin eruptions, notably on the scalp and eyebrows, and particularly if accompanied by herpes or warty growths. *Anantherum* may also be given to ease neuralgic headaches with a sensation of the facial bones being crushed.
Symptoms better A few hours after drinking coffee.
Symptoms worse With movement; immediately after drinking coffee.

Viburnum opulus
VIBURNUM

COMMON NAMES Cramp bark, guelder rose, bark elder, high cranberry.
ORIGIN Grows wild in Europe and eastern North America.
BACKGROUND Native American tribes such as the Meskwaki and the Penobscot used this plant to treat cramps, swollen glands, and mumps.
PREPARATION The fresh, young bark is collected in autumn, chopped finely, and macerated in alcohol.

REMEDY PROFILE
Specifically a women's remedy, *Viburnum* best suits those who feel depressed, dazed, and disoriented, and are unable to decide where they are or what they should do.

The classic symptom picture for this remedy is of uterine problems, including painful menstruation, false labor, pains following labor, threatened abortion, and recurrent miscarriage. Menstrual pain may be so severe that it feels as if breathing and the heartbeat will stop.
Symptoms better In the open air; with rest; from pressure on the affected area; from moving around.
Symptoms worse In the evening; at night; during a snowfall; before menstruation; from fright; from jarring.

Vinca minor
VINCA

COMMON NAME Lesser periwinkle.
ORIGIN Native to Europe.
BACKGROUND Lesser periwinkle was traditionally known as the "flower of death" by Italians, who placed it on the coffins of dead children.
PREPARATION The whole, fresh plant, including the root, is finely chopped and macerated in alcohol.

REMEDY PROFILE
Vinca is most suitable for people who seem sad, weepy, weak, and faint. They may have an empty, hungry sensation, and possibly a feeling that they are going to die.

Skin problems such as eczema are key conditions treated by this remedy. It is used for weeping eczema that is infected with thick, foul-smelling crusts, for itchy, burning skin, for a warm scalp with foul-smelling eruptions and corrosive itching, for cradle cap, and for burning leg ulcers. *Vinca* is also given for excessive menstrual flow that causes great weakness.
Symptoms better From moving in the open air.
Symptoms worse From anger; from walking; from stooping; from swallowing.

Viola tricolor
VIOLA TRI.

COMMON NAMES Heartsease, wild pansy.
ORIGIN Native to Europe, north Africa, and parts of Asia.
BACKGROUND Heartsease is a member of the violet family, long renowned as a "purifier" and used as a treatment for eczema and itching.
PREPARATION The fresh aerial parts in flower are chopped and steeped in alcohol.

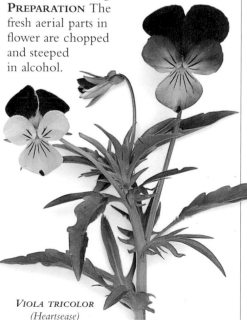

VIOLA TRICOLOR
(Heartsease)

REMEDY PROFILE
Viola tri. is best suited to those who feel discontented and capricious, and to children who are prone to disobedience.

Persistent skin problems are typically treated with *Viola tri.* These include impetigo, rashes, eczema, rosacea, and pustular eruptions. The typical symptom picture is of intolerable itching and burning, especially at night. The skin does not heal easily, and is prone to thick scabs, which may crack and discharge yellow pus or fluid.

Viola tri. is particularly suited to skin symptoms in conjunction with urinary problems. Typical urinary symptoms may include cloudy, foul-smelling urine, frequent, profuse urination, bed-wetting at night, and sharp pains in the urethra.
Symptoms better No specific factors.
Symptoms worse In cold air; in winter; with movement.

SEE ALSO Rosacea, *page 193*

Vipera berus
VIPERA

COMMON NAME European adder, viper.
ORIGIN Widely distributed in Europe and Asia.
BACKGROUND Dark gray with black zigzags on its back, the adder has hollow fangs in the upper jaw for injecting venom.
PREPARATION The fresh venom is triturated with lactose sugar.

REMEDY PROFILE
Vipera is best suited to people with a rather dizzy, even delirious, state of mind. It is also associated with slow-developing children, and people who age prematurely.

Key symptoms associated with *Vipera* include inflammation and swelling of the veins, typically accompanied by faintness and collapse. The remedy is commonly used for recurrent nosebleeds, varicose veins, or phlebitis (inflammation of a vein, often due to a blockage caused by a clot).
Symptoms better From raising the affected limbs.
Symptoms worse With cold; from changes in the weather; if touched; from letting the affected limbs hang down; at the same time each year.

Viscum album
VISCUM ALB.

COMMON NAME Mistletoe.
ORIGIN Native to Europe and northern Asia, and found growing as a parasite on host trees.
BACKGROUND Revered in Nordic and

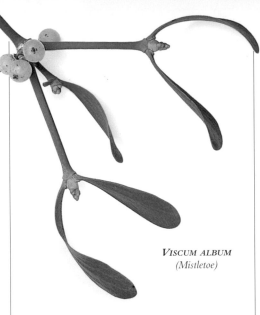

VISCUM ALBUM
(Mistletoe)

Druidic legend, this plant has long been used in herbal medicine and is currently being researched as a treatment for cancer.
PREPARATION The fresh, leafy shoots and berries are harvested in autumn, chopped finely, and macerated in alcohol.

REMEDY PROFILE

Fear and detachment from others is typical in those for whom *Viscum alb.* is most appropriate. They seem to dream constantly, both when awake and asleep, and may talk incoherently. They may be alternately cold and hot.

The classic symptom picture for *Viscum alb.* is of seizures, tremors, or epilepsy, tearing joint and neuralgic pains, and asthma. It is prescribed for generalized tremors, uncontrollable jerking after a fright, seizures, including "absences," petit mal, chorea, and epilepsy that begins as a glow radiating from the head to the feet. Attacks may be accompanied by breathing difficulties or asthma, and followed by persistent dizziness and by twitching of the body that causes insomnia.

Neuralgic pains usually treated with *Viscum alb.* include headaches with a numb, tightening sensation and throbbing in the top of the head, as though the skull is being lifted off the body. Headaches are sometimes accompanied by eye pains, difficulty in opening the eyelids, and crackling noises or deafness in the ears.
Symptoms better No specific factors.
Symptoms worse In winter; in cold, stormy weather; from becoming chilled when hot; with movement.

Vitex agnus-castus
AGNUS CASTUS

COMMON NAMES Agnus castus, chaste tree, monk's pepper, wild lavender.
ORIGIN Native to the Mediterranean region and western Asia.
BACKGROUND As the name "chaste tree" suggests, this plant was once thought to lower the libido. It was often chewed by monks, and in Italy blossoms are still strewn in the path of novices entering a convent.
PREPARATION The dried, ripe berries are macerated in alcohol.

REMEDY PROFILE

People who respond well to this remedy may be anxious about their health, especially their sexual health, and may have a strong presentiment of their own death.

Agnus castus is given chiefly to people with low energy levels, depression, poor sexual vitality, and a low libido. It is helpful for fatigue due to menopause, or caused by alcohol or drug abuse, or following numerous instances of sexual intercourse.

In men the remedy is generally prescribed for sexual conditions such as impotence, premature ejaculation with sexual arousal, or disinterest, particularly in men who formerly had a high libido. In women *Agnus castus* may help when there is a loss of libido, especially during menopause, scant or excessively heavy menstruation, or an enlarged uterus, possibly with a staining vaginal discharge. Postnatal depression and a lack of breast milk following childbirth may also be helped by the remedy.
Symptoms better From scratching or pressing on the affected area.
Symptoms worse From sexual excess; when ejaculating.

SEE ALSO Erectile dysfunction, *page 264*

VITEX AGNUS-CASTUS
(Agnus castus)

Wyethia helenoides
syn. *Alarconia helenoides*
WYETHIA

COMMON NAMES Poison weed, California compass plant.
ORIGIN Native to North America.
BACKGROUND This plant takes its Latin name from N. B. Wyeth, the naturalist who first discovered it in the mountains of North America.
PREPARATION The fresh root is steeped in alcohol, diluted, and succussed.

REMEDY PROFILE

Uneasy, nervous behavior is typical of people who respond best to *Wyethia*. They may expect a calamity to befall them.

The classic symptom picture for *Wyethia* is of hay fever with violent sneezing, dryness, and itching in the ears, palate, and the back of the nose, and a scalding sensation in the mouth. There is often a great urge to rub the palate with the tongue to relieve the itching.
Symptoms better No specific factors.
Symptoms worse In the afternoon; with movement; from exercise that raises a sweat; from eating.

SEE ALSO Allergies, *page 206*

Zingiber officinale
ZINGIBER

COMMON NAME Ginger.
ORIGIN Native to southern Asia and grown throughout the tropics.
BACKGROUND Ginger has played a major medicinal and culinary role in many cultures for millennia, and is highly valued, especially for relieving indigestion and nausea and stimulating the circulation.
PREPARATION The rhizome is dried and stripped of its outer layer, before being macerated in alcohol.

REMEDY PROFILE

People who benefit most from *Zingiber* are cheerful even when in great pain. They are nervous and fidgety, and often restless at night, despite being sleepy.

Digestive disorders are chiefly associated with *Zingiber*. Typical symptoms treated include nausea, vomiting, and colicky pain in the abdomen, with chronic excess mucus production in the intestine. The remedy is also prescribed for asthma that is marked by a total absence of any accompanying anxiety.
Symptoms better No specific factors.
Symptoms worse In cold air; from uncovering the body; with touch; lying down; with movement; from bread; from melons.

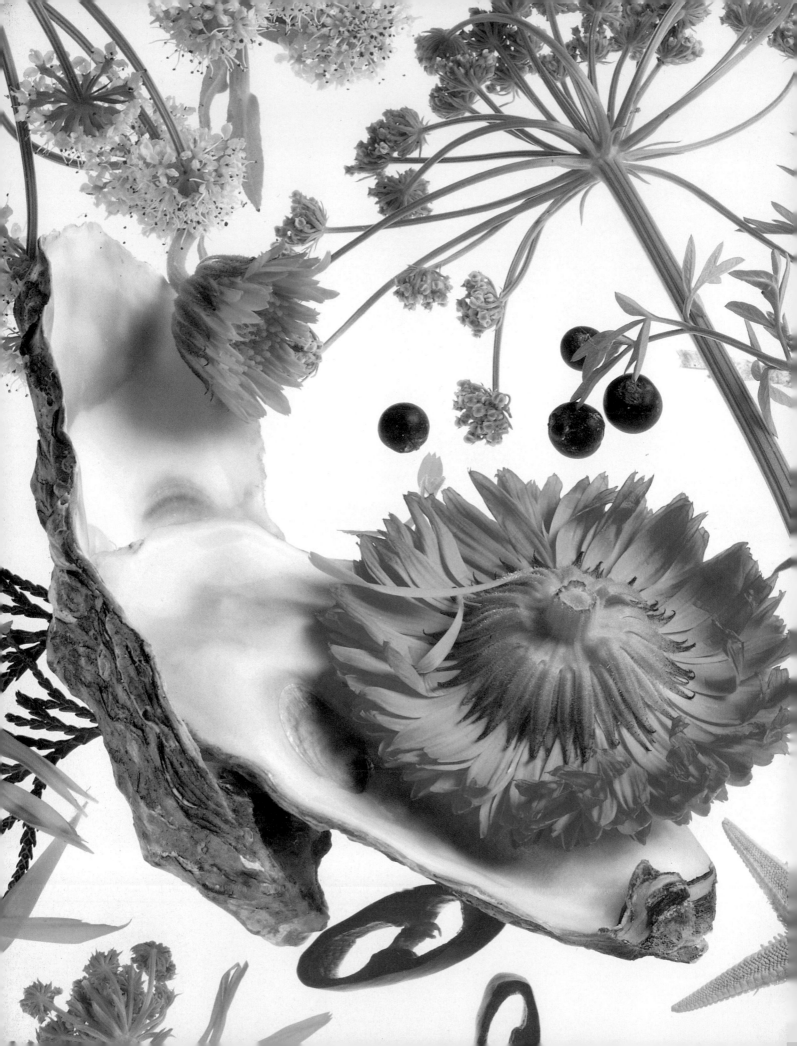

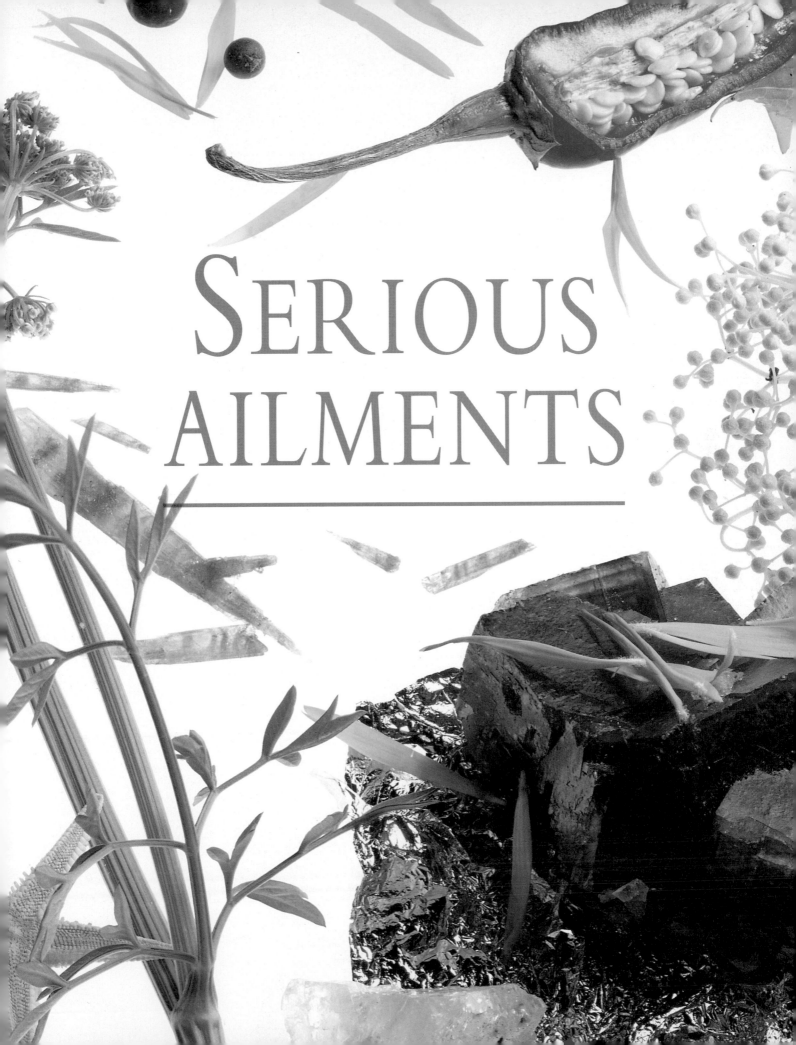

SERIOUS
AILMENTS

CONSULTING A PRACTITIONER

AN INTERVIEW WITH a homeopathic practitioner will be longer than a conventional medical consultation, and is likely to involve a series of follow-up visits several weeks apart, especially if a long-term condition is being treated. This allows the progress of an ailment to be carefully monitored and subtle changes noted. At the initial appointment, a person's current state of health and previous medical history will form the basis of a complete health, personality, and lifestyle profile as the foundation of homeopathic prescription.

AMASSING INFORMATION

Homeopaths believe that a person's state of health reflects the level of their inner vitality at the time, and that good health is defined as freedom from illness combined with general physical and emotional well-being. Homeopaths also consider that certain health problems develop from an acquired or inherited "root"; and that a person has a tendency to become ill in a particular way – his or her susceptibility (*see page 18*). According to homeopathic theory, illness results from imbalances in body systems, which have a great capacity for self-healing. This can be stimulated and nurtured by homeopathic treatment.

Homeopathy presupposes that the human body is always attempting to maintain a healthy balance (*see page 18*) and has a compulsion to flourish. If that balance is threatened – from outside or within – the body tries to reestablish it, and symptoms of an ailment are manifested as it does so. Symptoms develop as the body responds to the stress of illness, and a person's physical and mental resources are temporarily redeployed in order to deal with the illness.

PROFILING PATIENTS

Many factors constitute a whole person, so a wide range of details are required in order to build up a profile of a patient before "constitutional" homeopathic treatment can be prescribed. Despite the individualistic nature of homeopathic assessment and treatment, many people can be grouped according to "type." Types are described in terms of physical attributes as well as mental and emotional traits. People of a particular type very often have the same habits, develop the same likes and dislikes, and may well share a susceptibility to particular ailments.

SEARCHING FOR CLUES

First and foremost, a homeopathic practitioner requires a full description of a patient's symptoms, how they have evolved since onset, and what makes them better or worse. The choice of remedy will ultimately be based on the law of similars, which states that "like cures like" (*see page 18*). A person's symptoms are seen as reliable clues to the most suitable remedy to activate the self-healing powers of the individual's "vital force." Characteristics of bodily functions and functional disturbances are also noted. So, for instance, someone might be prone to indigestion, which manifests itself as heartburn when certain foods are eaten.

Also of interest to a homeopathic practitioner are a person's medical history, including details of pharmaceutical medications, other treatments, and family medical history. This information may reveal significant evidence of both genetic tendency and susceptibility.

DESCRIBING PERSONALITY

A homeopathic practitioner will then ask a person to describe themselves in terms of basic temperament, moods, feelings, and beliefs. This will include temporary psychological factors associated with their physical symptoms, such as irritability or an aversion to sympathy. Of significance are details about any emotional traumas – from deep-seated childhood experiences to events of the recent past, for example, bereavement. Details such as how the weather, seasons, and times of day affect the individual, personal likes and dislikes, and in particular objects of fear, are all important in building up a complete picture of that person.

LOOKING AT LIFESTYLE

Finally, general features of a person's lifestyle are considered. Dietary factors of significance include caffeine, alcohol, and tobacco consumption, food preferences and aversions, and potential sources of irritation or digestive upset. Stress levels are also significant: does the person have a stressful job, time for relaxation and following interests, an adequate amount of exercise, or enough sleep?

COLLATING INFORMATION

Much disparate information is collected during a consultation. Examinations and tests are carried out on physical symptoms as necessary. Observations and measurable conditions have to be integrated with subjective reportage. Practitioners draw on their experiences of similar symptom pictures and personality types, and compare the information they have with that in a homeopathic repertory, which lists symptoms, remedies, and provings.

PRESCRIBING INDIVIDUALLY

Given the highly individualistic nature of homeopathic prescription, two people are unlikely to be prescribed the same remedy, even if their symptoms are identical. For the same reason, they may find that their remedies do not match any of the general profiles of remedies listed for their ailment in popular homeopathic source books.

One remedy may be prescribed consititutionally to address the underlying causes of an ailment, such as bodily imbalances, with another remedy for a specific, acute symptom. Also, one remedy may be substituted for another on a subsequent visit to the practitioner, depending on the patient's progress.

MAXIMIZING EFFECTS

When taking a homeopathic remedy, observe the following "rules" in order to ensure that it has the best chance of working effectively.

◆ Do not eat for 30 minutes before or after taking a homeopathic remedy so that it enters the system on its own.

◆ Avoid strong foods and drinks, such as spicy foods and alcohol, that may affect body systems, or consume them only in moderation. Some, such as coffee, may actually counteract the remedy.

◆ Avoid using strong substances, for example, household cleaning products, that might have a poisoning effect on the body.

◆ Avoid medicinal substances and certain products, such as some essential oils, so that a remedy can get to work on its own. If in doubt, consult your homeopathic practitioner.

◆ Do not touch or handle a remedy; use a clean, dry spoon to drop it into the mouth. If tablets are touched or dropped, they should not be returned to the container.

◆ Store homeopathic remedies safely and properly (*see page 271*). Make sure that the lids of any bottles are securely in place before storage.

ASSESSING A PATIENT

As the basis of homeopathic assessment, a practitioner collects a wealth of information about a patient's physical condition, mental and emotional states, and life in general (*see below*). An individual's unique adaptations to their surroundings and their idiosyncratic ways are accepted and respected for making an individual what he or she is. A person is regarded as the product of his physical and mental well-being or ill-health, genetic inheritance, and daily experience.

BODY

PHYSICAL WELL-BEING
- General symptoms and ailments: onset of symptoms, and what affects them and how.
- Weight, shape, and physical condition.
- Diet: nutritional balance, food preferences and aversions, food intolerances, and any special requirements or dietary deficiencies.
- Energy levels.
- Sleep: amount and quality, effects of sleep deprivation, and dreams.
- Risks to health: smoking, consumption of alcohol and recreational drugs, or dangerous jobs or pastimes.
- Time out: relaxation and leisure activities.
- Knowledge of what to do if ill or injured.

MEDICAL HISTORY
- Personal medical history: past injuries and illnesses, conventional drug prescriptions, and any complementary treatments.
- Family medical history: incidence in family members of conditions such as heart disease, diabetes, mental health problems, or cancer.
- Inherited susceptibilities: allergies or tendency to contract certain illnesses.
- Diet: susceptibility to cholesterol-related illness, obesity, or food intolerances.
- Awareness of symptoms of genetically inherited disease and preventive measures.
- Checkups: self-examination and regular medical tests or screening.

ENVIRONMENT
- Climate: effects of seasonal changes and day-to-day weather patterns.
- Access to and appreciation of fresh air.
- Exposure to sun and awareness of risks.
- Effects of pollution: air, water, and noise.
- Work environment: office ergonomics, noise levels, amount of personal space, and impact of central heating or air-conditioning systems.
- Home environment: particular allergic responses to household products or toiletries, pollen, animals, tobacco smoke, or air pollution.
- Daily routine: stress and other effects of commuting, working in an office in an urban environment, and working long hours.

MIND

PERSONALITY
- Temperament: positive or negative, passive or assertive, relaxed or anxious.
- Self-image and self-worth.
- Emotions: ability to express and control feelings, laugh, and deal with negative emotions.
- Relationships: sensitivity to others, ability to resolve conflict, desire for approval, and sex drive.
- Any feelings of guilt, insecurity, and degree of control over personal destiny.
- Ability to cope under stress.
- Fears.
- Opportunities for creative expression.
- Spirituality, deeply held beliefs, and motivation.

LIFE EVENTS
- Childhood trauma: impact of death or other loss of a parent, or physical or mental abuse.
- Family circumstances: effects of births, marriage, separation, divorce, death, bullying, exams, children leaving home, or caring for disabled or elderly relatives.
- Proximity of family and friends.
- Ability to deal with serious health problems.
- Property: effects of buying and selling homes, moving, or making extensive alterations.
- Work experience: impact of new job, loss of job, being laid off, retirement, job relocation, overwork, or juggling work and family.
- Financial or legal problems.

LIFE MANAGEMENT
- Time management: ability to set realistic goals, plan and organize projects, cope with deadlines, and delegate tasks.
- Success in maintaining a balance between work and play, and between work and family.
- Stress management: opportunities to relax, and ability to control stressful situations and to turn problems into opportunities.
- Work: ability to rationalize workload, deal with physical strains, or improve working environment.
- Routines developed in order to give structure to the working day and home life.
- Financial planning and organization.

NERVOUS SYSTEM

Tʜᴇ ɴᴇʀᴠᴏᴜs sʏsᴛᴇᴍ is the human body's central command center. It receives and evaluates stimuli from inside and outside the body, and issues directives to tissues and organs in response to these stimuli. It consists of the central nervous system and the peripheral nervous system.

HOW THE SYSTEM WORKS

The central nervous system – the brain and spinal cord – receives information from all over the body. This information takes the form of electrical impulses that are transmitted along a nerve network – the peripheral nervous system – which branches off the central nervous system. The brain then sends out instructions to internal organs, muscles, glands, and tissues throughout the body via the peripheral nervous system.

In terms of function, the parts of the nervous system consisting of nerves that control the muscles involved in voluntary actions are known as the somatic nervous system. Nerves concerned with the unconscious control of bodily functions such as digestion, gland secretions, and temperature regulation are part of the autonomic nervous system.

HOW NERVES FUNCTION
A nerve is made up of strings of nerve cells, or neurons, which are the basic units of the nervous system. Some nerves carry instructions from the brain or spinal cord to muscles, glands, or other tissues throughout the body. Others carry information to the brain from sensory receptors, sensory organs such as the eyes and ears, and internal organs. Each nerve cell (*see right*) has parts that receive electrical messages from other nerve cells, and parts that transmit messages to nerve cells or other tissues. The cell bodies of neurons make up the gray matter of the brain and spinal cord, while the long nerve fibers, or axons, make up the white matter of the central nervous system.

All but the smallest nerve fibers are insulated and protected by a fatty substance called myelin, which also helps to conduct nerve impulses along the fibers quickly. Multiple sclerosis is believed to occur because the myelin becomes damaged in some way. The brain and spinal column are protected by delicate membranes called meninges.

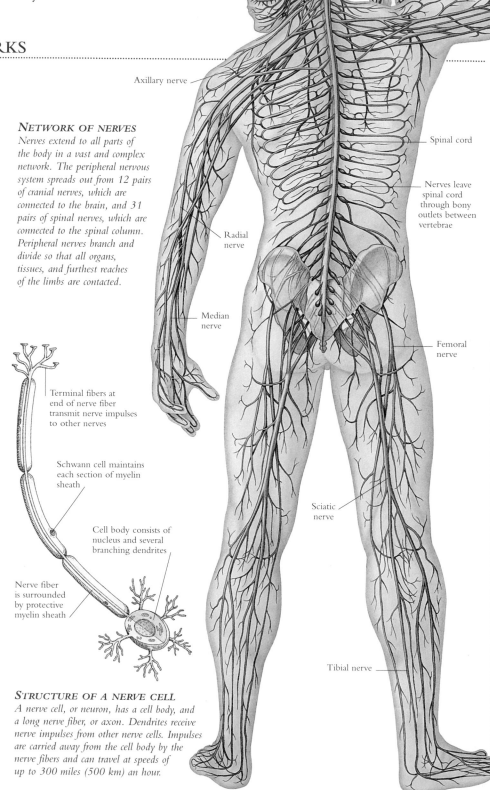

NETWORK OF NERVES
Nerves extend to all parts of the body in a vast and complex network. The peripheral nervous system spreads out from 12 pairs of cranial nerves, which are connected to the brain, and 31 pairs of spinal nerves, which are connected to the spinal column. Peripheral nerves branch and divide so that all organs, tissues, and furthest reaches of the limbs are contacted.

Axillary nerve

Spinal cord

Nerves leave spinal cord through bony outlets between vertebrae

Radial nerve

Median nerve

Femoral nerve

Terminal fibers at end of nerve fiber transmit nerve impulses to other nerves

Schwann cell maintains each section of myelin sheath

Cell body consists of nucleus and several branching dendrites

Nerve fiber is surrounded by protective myelin sheath

Sciatic nerve

Tibial nerve

STRUCTURE OF A NERVE CELL
A nerve cell, or neuron, has a cell body, and a long nerve fiber, or axon. Dendrites receive nerve impulses from other nerve cells. Impulses are carried away from the cell body by the nerve fibers and can travel at speeds of up to 300 miles (500 km) an hour.

MULTIPLE SCLEROSIS

THIS CONDITION OCCURS if the myelin sheaths surrounding nerve fibers are damaged. In temperate regions of the world multiple sclerosis affects one in a thousand people, and more women than men. There may be just a single attack, or repeated attacks that lead to increasing disability. Only in a minority of cases, however, is the condition crippling.

SYMPTOMS

♦ Possible tingling, numbness, or weakness affecting a hand, foot, or a whole side of the body.

♦ Double vision or the misting or blurring of vision.

♦ Possible heaviness, weakness, or constricted feeling in the hands and feet.

♦ Possible strong muscle spasms, constipation, ulceration of the skin, and mood swings.

♦ In more serious cases, possible paralysis and incontinence, which may be associated with fatigue, vertigo, giddiness, clumsiness, muscle weakness, slurred speech, and difficulty in walking.

CAUSES

The causes of multiple sclerosis are unknown. There may be a genetic tendency, but the fact that the disease is five times more common in temperate zones than in the tropics suggests a viral cause. It may be an autoimmune disease, whereby the body's immune system attacks the myelin, gradually leading to damage of the underlying nerve fibers. Sensitivity to toxic metals or to vaccines has also been postulated as a cause.

CONVENTIONAL CARE

Diagnosis is aided by evoked response tests on the eyes (measuring the speed of optic nerve impulses), and magnetic resonance imagery (MRI), which can reveal damage to the white matter of the nervous system. Conventional treatment of multiple sclerosis includes sunflower or evening-primrose oil, interferon (protein produced by the body to fight infection and cultured from human cells or synthesized in the laboratory), and potent drugs such as corticosteroids. An amino acid, phenylalanine, is believed to be beneficial, as well as vitamin B and low doses of antidepressant drugs. Controversy surrounds the use of cannabis to relieve muscle spasms. Physiotherapy may help those affected by multiple sclerosis.

HOMEOPATHIC MEDICINE

Homeopathic treatment is largely constitutional after study of the patient's full history. This includes emotional factors and, especially in the case of multiple sclerosis, any long-suppressed problems from childhood. Homeopathy traditionally attributes this condition to an inherent weakness of the nervous system that is aggravated by trauma, infection, or the effects of toxic metals.

Constitutional prescription will mainly depend on the individual's symptoms (*see page 18*), but some remedies have an affinity with the nervous system. *Argentum nit.* has a direct, qualitative effect on nerves controlling conscious movement; *Causticum* is indicated for the progressive debilitation of the nervous system. *Nat. mur.* is prescribed for problems in the brain and spinal cord that produce tingling, weakness, and eventual numbness in the fingers, hands, and arms. Other constitutional remedies include *Lachesis*, *Phosphorus*, and *Plumbum met.*

Remedies for the relief of specific symptoms include *Phosphorus*, if there is frequent fainting; *Tarentula*, for jerky movements of the hands, feet, and tongue; and *Agaricus*, for weak, shaky movements accompanied by shooting pains.

LIFESTYLE

A diet that is low in animal fats, gluten free, and high in gamma-linoleic acid (found in sunflower seeds and oil) may be beneficial, while caffeine is best avoided. Regular exercise and rest are important. A daily routine might include three rest periods of 10–20 minutes each and fairly vigorous exercise such as weightlifting, which should be built up very gradually.

> ### CAUTION
> ♦ If, despite all treatment, the condition continues to deteriorate, consult a doctor.
> ♦ If a person affected by multiple sclerosis undergoes psychological or physical trauma, homeopathic remedies taken as a preventive measure may preempt an attack.

CASE HISTORY

Christine was a 39-year-old housewife. Eight years before her homeopathic consultation she had noticed that her right foot dragged because of weakness in the leg. Multiple sclerosis was diagnosed six years later, when she began to suffer blurred vision and a frequent urge to urinate. She was taking phenylalanine and vitamin and mineral supplements.

PERSONAL DETAILS
A pleasant, mild-mannered woman on the surface, Christine admitted to anger and a deep sense of injustice. She had a tendency to feel resentful and lose her temper. She lacked confidence, was depressed about her illness deteriorating, and feared the future. Her mother had died when Christine was eight.

FOOD PREFERENCES
Christine had a great desire for coffee and a strong dislike of whiskey. She liked most foods, especially sweet foods, salt, vinegar, and spices, but she disliked fats.

GENERAL DETAILS
Christine felt worse in cold and wet weather, in great heat, and in the late afternoon, but she felt better with warmth. Her symptoms worsened if she was overtired or thought too much about her illness. She woke unrefreshed from sleep.

PRESCRIPTION & FOLLOW-UP
Christine was given a low potency of *Nat. mur.*, and advised to write to her dead mother to unburden her suppressed grief. The remedy was repeated twice in a higher potency, along with advice about rest, exercise, and additional mineral and vitamin supplements, but her condition deteriorated. *Lathyrus* failed to help. Allergy tests proved negative, but her mercury levels were low. A digestive problem was suspected. Herbal and homeopathic remedies improved her bowel function, but the multiple sclerosis worsened. *Phosphorus* failed to help, and Christine was desperate. She was then prescribed *Causticum* on the basis of her oversensitivity to people. Her condition improved immediately. High-potency *Causticum,* with physiotherapy for her abnormal gait, has sustained the improvement.

RESPIRATORY SYSTEM

THE RESPIRATORY SYSTEM runs from the tip of the nose to the smallest air sac deep in each lung. It shares a common passageway with the digestive tract as far as the larynx. The purpose of the respiratory system is to transport oxygen to the lungs, where it is absorbed into the blood. This then carries the oxygen to cells throughout the body, where it is used to produce energy. Carbon dioxide, a by-product of the process, is taken back to the lungs and expelled.

HOW THE SYSTEM WORKS

The breathing process is controlled by the respiratory center of the brain. The purpose of respiration is to obtain oxygen, which is then transported around the body in the blood. It ends up in body cells, where it combines with glucose to produce energy. Carbon dioxide is a by-product of this process and is expelled on breathing out. Breathing is an automatic process: it cannot be stopped voluntarily, although its rate and depth can be controlled. An adult human takes between 13 and 80 breaths a minute, depending on the degree of exertion.

BREATHING IN AND OUT

Air flows in and out of the lungs because the pressure of air in the chest is constantly changing in relation to the pressure of air outside the body. During inhalation the diaphragm contracts and descends while the ribcage rises and expands. The decrease in pressure in the lungs draws air in. The opposite occurs during exhalation as the diaphragm rises and the ribs fall. This increases the pressure in the lungs and air flows out.

RESPIRATORY PROBLEMS

The walls of the airway produce mucus that keeps air moist and warm. The surface of the walls is lined with tiny hairs, which move rather like fields of wheat. They help to move dust and foreign bodies away from the lungs to be coughed up or sneezed out of the airway. If particles are not removed – as in the case of smokers, in whom the hairs become paralyzed by nicotine – they remain in the lung. This encourages viruses and bateria to create infection and excessive amounts of mucus to be produced. Small airways and alveoli (*see right*) may become flooded with mucus, with the result that respiration deteriorates and gas exchange fails. This occurs in pneumonia. Certain irritants may cause spasms of the airway, as in asthma.

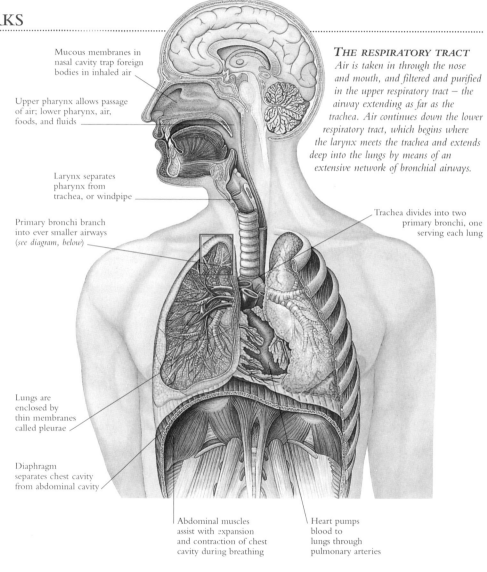

Mucous membranes in nasal cavity trap foreign bodies in inhaled air

Upper pharynx allows passage of air; lower pharynx, air, foods, and fluids

Larynx separates pharynx from trachea, or windpipe

Primary bronchi branch into ever smaller airways (*see diagram, below*)

Lungs are enclosed by thin membranes called pleurae

Diaphragm separates chest cavity from abdominal cavity

Abdominal muscles assist with expansion and contraction of chest cavity during breathing

Heart pumps blood to lungs through pulmonary arteries

THE RESPIRATORY TRACT
Air is taken in through the nose and mouth, and filtered and purified in the upper respiratory tract – the airway extending as far as the trachea. Air continues down the lower respiratory tract, which begins where the larynx meets the trachea and extends deep into the lungs by means of an extensive network of bronchial airways.

Trachea divides into two primary bronchi, one serving each lung

WHERE GASES ARE EXCHANGED
The lungs' branching bronchi feed into tiny respiratory bronchioles and ultimately the alveoli, small balloonlike sacs. Oxygen diffuses through the walls of the alveoli into a network of capillaries, and hence into the bloodstream. Carbon dioxide diffuses from the blood vessels into the alveoli to be exhaled from the lungs.

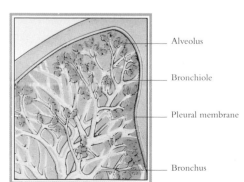

Alveolus

Bronchiole

Pleural membrane

Bronchus

ASTHMA

AN ASTHMA ATTACK occurs when the airways of the lungs become inflamed. This causes contraction of muscles in the walls of the airways and their subsequent narrowing. Asthma affects one in ten children of school age in some industrialized countries, but only three percent of adults. Asthma can be more serious and more difficult to treat in adults.

SYMPTOMS

◆ Breathlessness that is accompanied by a characteristic wheezing.

◆ Tight feeling in the chest.

◆ In severe attacks, possible increased pulse rate and clammy sweats.

◆ Dry cough.

◆ Possible anxiety and fear.

CAUSES

The increase in childhood asthma in the industrialized world during the last two decades of this century has been blamed on increased levels of pollution. A genetic tendency is now thought to be more likely. Asthma is believed to be an allergic reaction to house dust, house-dust mites, pollens, fur, feathers, or tobacco smoke. It can also be induced by drugs, caffeine withdrawal, stress, or exercise. Foods such as dairy products, wheat, nuts, oranges, chocolate, and refined carbohydrates are known triggers. Asthma is also linked to high pollen counts, atmospheric changes, domestic heating systems, and some soft-furnishing materials.

CONVENTIONAL CARE

Asthma sufferers receive treatment plans from doctors or asthma specialists. These include daily checks on the amount of air flowing in and out of the lungs using a peak-flow meter. In acute attacks, bronchodilating drugs are needed to widen the airways. Corticosteroids reduce inflammation. These drugs are taken by means of an inhaler, except in very young children. In serious attacks, hospitalization may be required for oxygen or the use of a powered ventilator to ease breathing. Inhalers used preventively can reduce the impact of irritants.

HOMEOPATHIC MEDICINE

Peak-flow monitoring is necessary, whatever the treatment. Homeopathic treatment of asthma is primarily constitutional. A practitioner will be particularly interested in an individual's food preferences, emotional makeup, and any significant environmental factors. The choice of remedy will largely be determined by symptoms (*see page 18*), but certain remedies have an affinity with the respiratory tract. *Arsen. alb.* is indicated for bronchial constriction and *Antimonium tart.* for bronchial congestion. *Bryonia* is effective for the pain caused by irritation of the pleurae, and *Calc. carb.* for ailments arising out of restrictions in the movement of the ribcage. *Phosphorus* is used for respiratory problems linked with anxiety.

For acute asthma, or to boost the immune system, the tubercular, psoric, or sycotic nosodes (*see page 20*) may be given. Other remedies include *Arsen. alb.*, for attacks in the early hours, with chilliness, restlessness, and a desire for sips of water; *Ipecac.*, when there is persistent nausea; or *Kali. carb.*, for asthma between 2 a.m. and 4 a.m. causing exhaustion. If the trigger is allergy, the effects of allergens can be reduced by isopathic remedies (*see page 21*), for example by taking a remedy made from cats' hair to treat sensitivity to cats.

LIFESTYLE

A pharmacist can advise about eradicating house-dust mites. Placing a child's cuddly toys in a freezer for a few hours every week will kill dust mites. Bedrooms in particular should be kept as dust-free as possible, and carpets and soft furnishings shampooed regularly. All known sources of irritation should be avoided and smoking forbidden in the home. Asthma sufferers are advised to exercise but must learn to control their breathing, especially during an asthma attack.

CAUTION

◆ If an asthma sufferer turns pale or blue, with clammy skin, and is experiencing severe breathing difficulties, call an ambulance.

◆ If an acute attack persists for more than 12 hours, consult a doctor.

◆ If the stated dose of treatment for acute asthma does not bring an attack under control, consult a doctor immediately.

CASE HISTORY

John Carpenter, age three, had a year-long history of recurrent chest infections. Asthma had been diagnosed two months previously. His attacks developed from chesty coughs. He had taken antibiotics, bronchodilators, and corticosteroids, but had not responded to treatment or to the removal of house dust and pollens.

PERSONAL DETAILS
Described by his mother as an easy child but one that liked messiness, John had been a poor sleeper as a baby and had walked early. He tended to cry when disciplined and was highly sensitive. He was very protective of his sister and was a talkative little boy.

FOOD PREFERENCES
John had a very sweet tooth and a slight desire for salt. He enjoyed fatty foods and loved smoked meats.

GENERAL DETAILS
John lived with his parents and sister and attended nursery school five mornings a week. He was part of a happy family, and there appeared to be no major stresses within it.

PRESCRIPTION & FOLLOW-UP
John was prescribed high-potency *Tuberculinum*. Two weeks later, he developed a wheezing cough after a cold. He was given *Tuberculinum* again, which made him better initially, but then he deteriorated. He was then given sodium cromoglycate, a conventional asthma drug, four times daily. He still complained of a dry, tickly cough and was given *Coccus cacti* and encouraged to use salbutamol, a bronchodilator. None of a series of constitutional remedies helped. John was given corticosteroids, the long-term prospect of which concerned his mother. He was then prescribed *Bacillinum* as a preventive measure against colds and the flu, and advised to eliminate refined carbohydrates from his diet and to eat little and often. He developed an acute infection soon after but responded to *Phosphorus* and then *Sulfur*, which had a very marked effect. He now takes an occasional dose of *Sulfur*, but he is largely free of asthma and takes no conventional medication.

TUBERCULOSIS

AN INFECTIOUS, BACTERIAL DISEASE, tuberculosis was once common worldwide and a killer, especially in mid-19th-century Europe, where it was responsible for one-quarter of deaths. This incidence fell until the 1980s but has increased since with the spread of HIV. The disease is now prevalent in Africa, Asia, and countries of the former USSR.

SYMPTOMS

◆ A mild attack of tuberculosis has the same symptoms as a mild case of the flu.

◆ In second-stage tuberculosis, there may be a slight fever, night sweats, fatigue, weight loss, a dry cough that eventually produces pus or bloody sputum, breathlessness, and chest pain.

◆ If the disease progresses further still, it may cause a pleural effusion (fluid between the lining, or pleura, of the lung and that of the chest cavity) or pneumothorax (air between the pleurae).

CAUSES

Tuberculosis is caused by *Mycobacterium tuberculosis*, and is spread in droplets of mucus expelled in coughs and sneezes. If the infection is fought off successfully, a small scar forms in the lung tissue. The person is then immune unless he becomes undernourished or generally ill in the future, in which case tuberculosis may flare up again. Sometimes the primary infection spreads to other parts of the body via the lymphatic system and the bloodstream, a condition known as miliary tuberculosis, which is occasionally fatal. Tuberculosis is most common among the elderly, alcoholics, and people living in economically deprived areas.

CONVENTIONAL CARE

In many industrialized countries preventive measures are taken against tuberculosis in the form of innoculation of all children by the age of 13 with a live strain of the bacterium that causes tuberculosis in cattle. This is too weak to cause the disease in humans, yet it stimulates the immune system. Diagnosis of tuberculosis is by a primary test followed by a chest X ray if the test is positive. The most common treatment is with two drugs – usually isoniazid and rifampicin – taken over a long period. There is concern in some regions of the world that the disease has become resistant to these drugs. Other, shorter treatment regimes are therefore being tried.

HOMEOPATHIC MEDICINE

It is rare for a homeopathic practitioner to treat a tuberculosis patient exclusively. The disease has to be notified to the medical authorities, and will inevitably, and justifiably, be treated conventionally. Homeopathy can, however, play an important supportive role, and if indeed the disease is developing a resistance to conventional drugs, complementary treatment may become important, for example, in boosting the immune system.

The patient's specific symptoms will be the main criteria in determining constitutional prescription (*see page 18*). Certain remedies, however, have an affinity with respiratory ailments. *Arsen. alb.* is indicated for bronchial constriction. *Lycopodium* is associated with infection of the right lung; *Phosphorus* is effective for treating inflammation of the mucous membranes; and *Calc. carb.* is prescribed for gland enlargement.

For acute attacks, remedies include *Bacillinum* for head sweats; *Calc. carb.* if the extremities are cold and clammy, with weakness and apprehension; and *Arsen. alb.* if there is chilliness, exhaustion, anxiety, and a desire for sips of water.

LIFESTYLE

Tuberculosis tends to affect people who are generally run-down and otherwise in poor health. Adequate rest is important, as is a good diet, which should include plenty of potassium-rich foods, raw vegetables, fruits, and protein from legumes and whole grains as well as fish and meat. Plenty of fresh air is beneficial. Bad habits such as smoking, drinking too much alcohol, and taking recreational drugs should be avoided.

CAUTION

◆ If tuberculosis is suspected because of contact with someone who has it, consult a doctor.

◆ If there are symptoms of tuberculous meningitis (stiff neck, severe headache, light intolerance, and confusion and drowsiness leading to coma) see a doctor immediately.

CASE HISTORY

The author has not personally treated a case of tuberculosis. The following is based on a report in French homeopathic literature by Dr. Nebel of Monteau at the beginning of the 20th century.

Charles had suffered from pulmonary tuberculosis for ten years. His father and three siblings had died from it. Clinically, he showed signs of extensive tuberculosis, mainly affecting the left lung, with a cough and copious green sputum, which frequently contained blood.

PERSONAL DETAILS
Charles was very tall and thin, with an emaciated chest. He suffered sleeplessness and weariness. He was extremely depressed and worried about his health, being convinced that he would die.

FOOD PREFERENCES
A lover of acidic foods and fat, particularly meat fat, Charles had been known to eat lard. He also liked smoked meats and salty foods. He had a great thirst, sipping water constantly. His stomach was upset by acidic foods and very cold drinks. He would become very hungry during the night and have to eat something.

GENERAL DETAILS
Charles was often constipated and, although he felt the cold, he experienced night sweats. His symptoms were worse between midnight and 2 A.M. He exuded from his armpits and chest what his doctor described as the smell of tuberculosis.

PRESCRIPTION & FOLLOW-UP
Charles was prescribed *Tuberculinum*, which gave him chest pains. Within a few days, however, his cough and perspiration reduced significantly, although he lost a little more weight. He tried other remedies. After taking *Silica*, his weight dropped further but his general health improved. After taking *Arsen. alb.*, he coughed only slightly in the morning and evening, he produced no sputum, his chest sounded better to his doctor, and he started gaining weight. After ten weeks his appetite was good, and he could walk farther than before without feeling breathless. He felt stronger than he had for years and was hopeful for a complete recovery.

PNEUMONIA

PNEUMONIA IS INFLAMMATION of the lungs, which may be mild if a person is generally healthy, but life-threatening in those who are very young, elderly, immobilized or inactive, alcoholic, or already suffering from respiratory, heart, or kidney disease. Lobar pneumonia affects only one lung; bronchopneumonia affects both lungs.

SYMPTOMS

- Breathlessness even when resting.

- Fever with alternate sweats and chills.

- Cough that produces yellow or green sputum. When the chest is listened to, there may be an absence of breathing sounds, or there may be wheezing or crackling sounds.

CAUSES

Pneumonia occurs when an infection of the upper airway spreads deep into the lung tissue and invades the alveoli. It may develop from a cold virus, but it is usually caused by bacteria, especially pneumococcal bacteria. Other, more obscure sources of infection are carried by mycoplasma and rickettsia (micro-organisms). Pneumonia may be associated with immunodeficiency disorders, in which case unusual fungi or protozoa may be responsible. Pneumocystis pneumonia – common among AIDS sufferers – is an example of this. People taking inflammatory or immuno-suppressive drugs long-term, or who smoke, are more likely to develop pneumonia than those who do not. The disease may also be caused by inhaling liquids or poisonous gases such as chlorine.

CONVENTIONAL CARE

Diagnosis is by examination, chest X ray, blood test, and sputum test, whereby a culture is grown in a laboratory. Patients with lobar pneumonia were once said to heal "by lysis or crisis" within five days. That is to say, the disease came to a head and then abated, or death followed from respiratory failure. Modern drugs enable recovery from pneumonia within about two weeks unless the patient is debilitated or old. In severe cases, oxygen therapy or artificial ventilation may be necessary.

HOMEOPATHIC MEDICINE

In the initial stages of mild, viral pneumonia, treatment by an experienced homeopathic physician may be beneficial.

With recurrent pneumonia, constitutional homeopathic treatment is certainly advisable in addition to conventional treatment. A person's specific symptoms will largely determine constitutional prescription (*see page 18*), but certain remedies have an affinity with the lungs. *Arsen. alb.* is prescribed for bronchial constriction, while *Bacillinum* may be used for those with respiratory problems in whom chronic phlegm may easily give rise to infection, such as the elderly. *Calc. carb.* is effective for complications arising out of restrictions in the movement of the ribcage; and either *Pulsatilla* or *Phosphorus* may be used to treat irritation of the mucous membranes lining the respiratory tract.

In acute cases of pneumonia, *Aconite* may be prescribed if the onset is sudden, particularly in cold, dry weather, and there is chest pain, fever, anxiety, and a fear of dying. *Phosphorus* is given for a cough producing rust-colored sputum, with weakness, trembling, nervousness, and numb extremities, and symptoms that are worse lying on the left side. *Bryonia* is prescribed for chest pain that is worse with the slightest movement but better lying on the affected side.

LIFESTYLE

Plenty of vitamin C, which can also be taken as a preventive measure, and a good deal of rest, preferably sitting up in bed, are beneficial. Since dry air tends to make pneumonia worse, rooms should be humidified. Inhalations of steam or herbs such as echinacea may help. The diet should ideally be low in refined carbohydrates and include plenty of fluids. It is advisable not to smoke. Manipulation by an osteopath or a physiotherapist may help to clear the lungs of sputum.

CAUTION

- If symptoms do not respond to treatment within 24 hours, see a doctor.

- If there is blood in the sputum or chest pain, or if the lips turn blue, consult a doctor immediately.

CASE HISTORY

Fiona, a 38-year-old dental nurse, suffered from whooping cough at the age of six and had a history of recurrent pneumonia. She was also a migraine sufferer. The pneumonia would be heralded by a sudden drop in energy levels, cold sweats and shakiness, constipation, a characteristic cough, and the production of sputum.

PERSONAL DETAILS
Of medium build and slightly plump, Fiona described herself as having a quick temper and being overemotional, crying easily when angry or frustrated. She craved sympathy and reassurance, especially when sick, and hated being alone. She had a high sex drive, which was based more on an emotional than a physical need.

FOOD PREFERENCES
Fiona had a strong craving for sweets, especially before a migraine or attack of pneumonia. Even when she had a fever, she was not thirsty. She had an intolerance of, and an aversion to, anything fatty, although she liked butter and cream. She disliked warm foods and drinks. Rich foods, ice cream, and pork gave her indigestion.

GENERAL DETAILS
Fiona preferred hot weather but disliked being in stuffy rooms, where she craved cool air. She felt worse at the beach and was disturbed by noise. Her energy levels were low, and she had never slept well, even as a child. The pneumonia tended to occur when she was premenstrual.

PRESCRIPTION & FOLLOW-UP
A diet was devised to strengthen Fiona's liver and make her bowels more efficient. This relieved the constipation, and her energy levels rose. She then developed a cold that went into her chest. She was prescribed *Pulsatilla* and advised to take antibiotics, although she chose not to. She recovered from the acute attack within a week. She still had a cough, which responded to *Sticta*, but she still had a lot of phlegm. She was then given *Merc. sol.* and has been healthy ever since. She takes this remedy at the first signs of a cold.

PALPITATIONS

PALPITATIONS IS THE TERM used to describe a general awareness that the heart is beating, or the sensation that it is beating irregularly, or faster, or with more force than it should, given the level of exertion. Not all palpitations indicate a serious condition, but they should be investigated. The heart normally beats at a rate of 70 beats a minute.

SYMPTOMS

◆ Heart feels as though it is beating harder or faster than usual.

◆ Fluttering or thumping in the chest, with an alarming sensation as though the heart has stopped beating.

◆ Possible faintness and breathlessness.

CAUSES

Heartbeat is controlled by the autonomic nervous system. If nerve impulses are disrupted, the heart will continue beating, but at its own, usually slower rate. The most common form of palpitation – usually experienced at rest – is caused by ectopic heartbeats, when a premature beat is followed by an unusually long pause. This feels like a thumping or fluttering in the chest, and is not usually indicative of heart disease. It is caused by stimulants, for example, large amounts of caffeine or heavy smoking. Palpitations with an irregular heartbeat may be symptomatic of heart disease. They may also be caused by an overactive thyroid gland, high fever, food allergy, and certain recreational drugs, such as amphetamines or cocaine. Palpitations may be a side effect of some prescribed drugs, particularly those that regulate blood pressure, or they may be triggered by anxiety.

CONVENTIONAL CARE

Treatment depends on the underlying cause. Investigations may include 24-hour electrocardiograms (ECGs) to explore the level of electrical activity in the heart, and thyroid-function tests to identify gland disorders. Appropriate drug therapy will follow. In extreme cases, a normal heart rhythm may have to be reestablished using cardioversion (electric shocks).

HOMEOPATHIC MEDICINE

In addition to an individual's medical history, a homeopath will consider emotional state, any local aggravating factors, such as the effects of cold air or physical exhaustion, and food preferences.

Prescription of constitutional remedies will be largely determined by specific symptoms (see page 18), but some remedies have an affinity with the heart. *Agaricus* is associated with heart irregularities induced by stimulants. *Apis* is indicated for organic heart disease accompanied by fluid retention. *China* is associated with nervous exhaustion. *Conium* is effective for an incompetent mitral valve, and *Kali. carb.* is indicated if there are associated respiratory problems such as asthma. Other remedies include *Argentum nit., Aurum met., Calc. carb., Lachesis, Nat. mur., Nux vomica, Phosphorus, Sepia,* and *Sulfur.*

Acute attacks are also treated according to specific symptoms. Remedies include *Aconite,* if onset is sudden, especially after shock, with a fear of dying; and *Nux vomica,* if palpitations result from overindulgence, or if there is physical and mental exhaustion with overarousal from doing too much, chilliness, and irritability. *Digitalis* is given for palpitations preceding a feeling as though the heart has stopped, with a fear that the least movement might make it stop again; and *Lachesis* is prescribed for menopausal women who feel faint and anxious, and complain of a constricted feeling in the chest.

LIFESTYLE

Smoking is inadvisable, and those who consume large amounts of caffeine should reduce their intake. The diet should be low in fat and refined carbohydrates, and high in oily fish and vegetarian proteins. A nutritionist can advise about possible food allergy, but it is worth eliminating suspected triggers from the diet, one by one. Plenty of rest and sleep are advisable, as are relaxation techniques or meditation. Time-management techniques can help to reduce stress levels.

CAUTION

◆ If palpitations are accompanied by chest pain, breathing difficulties, dizziness, sweating, or fainting, see a doctor immediately.

◆ If palpitations last for several hours, or recur over several days, consult a doctor.

CASE HISTORY

Clare, a credit controller aged 37, had a two-month history of palpitations. She described thuds in her chest – three a minute or one every two minutes – at any time of day. She had cut out caffeine and increased the amount of oats in her diet, but neither helped. She felt worse under stress. An ECG was normal. She had been referred to a cardiologist and prescribed a beta-blocker, which helped a good deal. She was taking an oral contraceptive and was a nonsmoker.

PERSONAL DETAILS
Clare was a nervous person, concerned about what others were thinking and, in her view, not tough enough. She was easily offended, but bottled up her feelings. She resented what she considered to be bad treatment by her mother-in-law.

FOOD PREFERENCES
Clare liked sweet foods, vinegar, and spices, and especially chocolate and sodas. She disliked herbal teas.

GENERAL DETAILS
Clare was better in the sun and heat. She slept six hours a night and awoke unrefreshed. She complained of a poor memory, a lack of energy since puberty, split ends, brittle nails, cold extremities, and loose bowel movements when she was anxious.

PRESCRIPTION & FOLLOW-UP
On her first visit Clare was given *Staphysagria*, and it was suggested that she write a letter to her mother-in-law airing her grievances, but that she not mail it. She was also advised not to take the contraceptive pill. By her next visit, four weeks later, the cardiologist had confirmed that there was no heart disease. The palpitations were less frequent and less severe, and Clare's energy levels were higher. She was put on mineral supplements and seen a month later. She had not had any palpitations, felt much less stressed, and was sleeping better, although she was restless, and had become insecure and fastidious. She had also developed a craving for fats. After being prescribed *Arsen. alb.,* Clare had no further problems. She now takes no medication other than the contraceptive pill.

STROKE

A CEREBRAL VASCULAR ACCIDENT, or stroke, occurs when the blood supply to part of the brain is interrupted or insufficient. Symptoms vary, depending on which part of the brain is affected. Strokes are quite common, affecting 200 in 100,000 people each year – more men than women – in the industrialized world. Incidence rises sharply with age.

SYMPTOMS

◆ Possible sudden loss of speech or the ability to move.

◆ Sudden heaviness or numbness of the limbs.

◆ Blurred vision.

◆ Confusion, dizziness, and loss of consciousness.

CAUSES

A stroke may result from a thrombosis, an embolism, or a hemorrhage. Cerebral thrombosis may be due to atherosclerosis, when blood vessels are narrowed by fatty deposits. In an embolism, a small blood clot breaks off an artery wall somewhere in the body and lodges in an artery supplying the brain. A hemorrhage occurs when blood leaks out of a weak-walled artery in the brain. Other causes of stroke include atrial fibrillation (irregular heartbeat), damaged heart valves, or heart attack. All three may lead to the formation of clots in the heart. These may travel to the brain, causing an embolism. Strokes are more common in those with diabetes, smokers, women on oral contraceptives, and people with high cholesterol levels.

CONVENTIONAL CARE

One in two first strokes is fatal. Recovery depends upon the severity of the stroke and rehabilitation. Scanning methods can establish the cause of a stroke and the extent of the damage. Thrombolytic drugs may be used to dissolve blood clots, and aspirin and anticoagulants to prevent further clots. Surgery may be needed to remove arterial obstructions. About half of those who survive a stroke recover to a greater or lesser degree. Those with disabilities may require physiotherapy, speech therapy, or occupational therapy.

HOMEOPATHIC MEDICINE

Constitutional treatment from an experienced homeopathic practitioner can play an important complementary role in recuperation after a stroke. The choice of constitutional remedy will be mainly influenced by the stroke victim's specific symptoms (*see page 18*), but remedies that have an affinity with the blood vessels include *Arnica*, which is indicated for shock and a hemorrhagic stroke; *Hyoscyamus*, which is effective for a paralytic stroke that is associated with confused and inappropriate behavior; and *Opium*, for a major stroke with total muscular relaxation and unconsciousness. *Nux vomica* and *Rhus tox.* may also be prescribed constitutionally.

Specific remedies to be taken during a stroke and to aid recovery include *Aconite*, if a patient is panicky and afraid of dying; and *Opium*, if they become unconscious, with a bluish, florid face and heavy, labored breathing. *Arnica* is good immediately after a stroke and *Aurum met.* if there is major depression. *Baryta carb.* is suitable for the very elderly and the physically and mentally weak.

LIFESTYLE

Diet and the management of stress levels are important in stroke prevention and for those who have already suffered a stroke. The diet should be modified in order to reduce the amount of animal fats and proteins consumed – including dairy products – and to increase fiber intake. It is advisable to eat plenty of fruits and fresh vegetables every day, and to lose excess weight and get regular exercise. If the stroke is thrombotic, the herb gingko biloba may improve blood flow. Smoking is inadvisable. Relaxation and meditation are beneficial, especially for those with high blood pressure or who are under stress. Women who have had a stroke, or who have a family history of heart disease, should avoid taking oral contraceptives.

CAUTION

◆ If there are any symptoms of a stroke, see a doctor immediately.
◆ If a stroke victim loses consciousness, place them in a safe position (*see page 270*) and call an ambulance.

CASE HISTORY

Thomas was a 79-year-old former engineer. Nine months before his consultation he had fallen in the bathtub. Three months later, he fell twice more. He had since been complaining of unsteadiness, difficulty in writing, frequent urination, general confusion, and poor short-term memory. His doctor had diagnosed a minor stroke. Thomas's blood pressure was high, and he showed all the signs of a right-sided stroke.

PERSONAL DETAILS
Thomas' character had changed since the stroke. He was by nature a leader and was used to being in control of his life. He was thorough to the point of fastidiousness. He now felt frustrated because he could no longer drive and had had to slow down generally. His wife claimed that he was more attentive to her, but that at times he appeared to look through her. Thomas slept fitfully.

FOOD PREFERENCES
Thomas liked sweets, and salty and acidic foods, but hated pork, milk, and desserts. He claimed that pork and alcohol upset his stomach.

GENERAL DETAILS
Thomas tended to get hot at night and to feel as though there was a lump in his throat preventing him from swallowing. His stomach was tender and sensitive to touch.

PRESCRIPTION & FOLLOW-UP
Thomas was originally prescribed *Anacardium or.* because of his feeling of being detached from reality. This remedy improved his memory, and he felt more himself. His blood pressure came down, and he felt steadier on his feet. He was then given *Baryta mur.* and sent for physiotherapy. This improved his unsteady gait. His blood pressure was normal by now. He looked much better and was getting exercise, although he was still forgetful. Thomas then had a fall, after which he was prescribed *Arnica* followed by another dose of *Baryta mur.* He continued to get better and even his memory started to improve. He is still making a slow and steady recovery, and to date has exhibited no further symptoms of stroke.

1e

CIRCULATORY SYSTEM

DIGESTIVE SYSTEM

THE DIGESTIVE SYSTEM basically consists of a long tube that starts at the mouth and ends at the anus. The aim of the system is to break food down for absorption into the body. Associated digestive organs, such as the liver, process nutrients into substances that can be used for the production of energy and for the building and repair of body tissues, cells, and the constituents of blood – metabolic processes that take digestion a stage further.

DIGESTION & METABOLISM

The human body needs energy to function. That energy comes from food, but only after it has been processed into substances that can be assimilated by various parts of the body. Some nutrients, such as minerals, can be absorbed directly along the way down the digestive tract, but substances such as proteins have to be broken down into smaller molecules.

FOOD PROCESSING

Digestion starts in the mouth, where saliva containing a digestive enzyme called amylase lubricates food as it is chewed. In the stomach proteins and fats are broken down in an acidic environment, and salt, water, and alcohol are absorbed. Beyond the stomach (in the duodenum) acidity is neutralized before food is treated by secretions from associated digestive organs – the liver, gallbladder, and pancreas. Bile from the liver and gallbladder emulsifies fats, and pancreatic enzymes break down proteins, starch, and fats.

USING NUTRIENTS

The liver is, in effect, the chemical factory of the body. Among many important metabolic functions, it stores glucose, vitamins, and minerals produced by food processing but not immediately usable by the body, and facilitates the breakdown of fats, which is vital for the conversion of food into energy. As well as digestive enzymes, the pancreas produces insulin (a hormone) and glycogen (a starch), both of which regulate sugar levels. Diabetes is the result of inadequate insulin production. In the small intestine the breakdown of food is completed. Nutrients are absorbed into the blood, carried to cells, and used in the release of energy. Undigested food is expelled from the anus.

Digestive ailments such as irritable bowel syndrome or ulcerative colitis are believed to result from, among other factors, an unsuitable diet or chemical imbalances in the metabolic process.

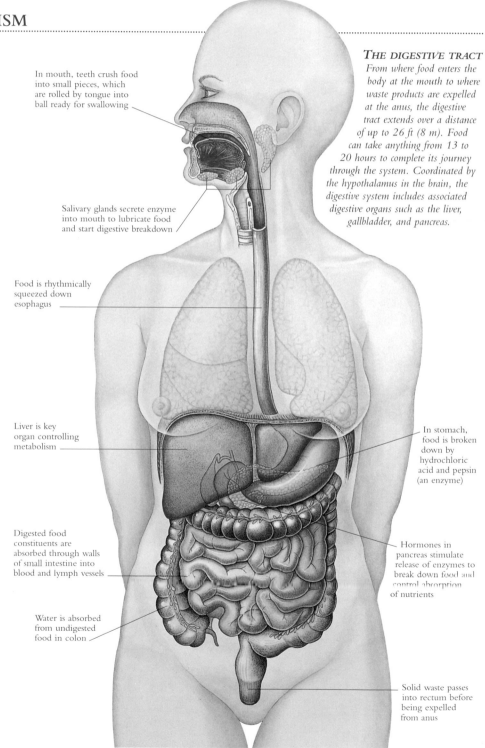

In mouth, teeth crush food into small pieces, which are rolled by tongue into ball ready for swallowing

Salivary glands secrete enzyme into mouth to lubricate food and start digestive breakdown

Food is rhythmically squeezed down esophagus

Liver is key organ controlling metabolism

Digested food constituents are absorbed through walls of small intestine into blood and lymph vessels

Water is absorbed from undigested food in colon

THE DIGESTIVE TRACT
From where food enters the body at the mouth to where waste products are expelled at the anus, the digestive tract extends over a distance of up to 26 ft (8 m). Food can take anything from 13 to 20 hours to complete its journey through the system. Coordinated by the hypothalamus in the brain, the digestive system includes associated digestive organs such as the liver, gallbladder, and pancreas.

In stomach, food is broken down by hydrochloric acid and pepsin (an enzyme)

Hormones in pancreas stimulate release of enzymes to break down food and control absorption of nutrients

Solid waste passes into rectum before being expelled from anus

IRRITABLE BOWEL SYNDROME (IBS)

IRRITABLE BOWEL SYNDROME is the most common intestinal disorder. It afflicts 10–20 percent of adults in parts of the developed world, and twice as many women as men. It often starts in early adulthood and, although distressing, is not life-threatening. Formerly known as irritable colon syndrome or spastic colon, IBS tends to be intermittent.

SYMPTOMS

◆ Alternating constipation and diarrhea.

◆ Cramping pains in the lower abdomen and sometimes the feeling of not having emptied the bowel on passing stools.

◆ Production of copious amounts of flatulence, the passing of which usually brings relief.

CAUSES

There may be several causes of IBS. The basic one is a disturbance in the action of the large intestinal muscle. This may be the result of stress, because of emotional upset or work, or of fear, such as that of serious illness. It may be the result of a low-fiber diet or an intolerance of wheat, corn, dairy products, fruits, tea, coffee, or vegetables. IBS may also be due to an overgrowth of organisms such as *Candida albicans* in the digestive tract, to the excessive use of laxatives, or to spinal maladjustment that affects nerves serving the digestive system.

CONVENTIONAL CARE

IBS is treated with antispasmodic drugs and other painkillers, antidiarrheal drugs, and a high-fiber diet. Counseling may be recommended for those suffering from stress. Diagnosis is made after ruling out the possibility of other ailments with similar symptoms, such as ulcerative colitis or cancer. A physical examination may include the passing of an instrument into the anus and colon – a colonoscopy or sigmoidoscopy – or a barium enema, which outlines the inside of the intestine so it can be seen on X-ray examination.

HOMEOPATHIC MEDICINE

A homeopathic practitioner will take a full medical history, paying particular attention to food preferences and IBS triggers. Constitutional remedies will be determined largely by an individual's symptoms (*see page 18*), but certain remedies have an affinity with the colon. *Argentum nit.* is indicated for irritation of the mucous membranes of the intestine and problems with the control of the gut by the autonomic nervous system. *Cantharis* is associated with inflammation of the whole gastrointestinal tract, especially the lower bowel. *Colocynthis* is also used to treat irritation of the gastrointestinal tract. Constitutional remedies also include *Arsen. alb., Carbo veg., Nux vomica, Pulsatilla, Lycopodium,* and *China.*

Remedies for acute symptoms include *Argentum nit.* for excessive flatulence, constipation alternating with diarrhea, pain in the left, upper abdomen, mucus in the stools, fluttering in the stomach, and great apprehension. *Colocynthis* is prescribed for intense pains that are relieved by bending double or applying pressure to the abdomen, and which are associated with anger. *Cantharis* is particularly suitable for treating women who have burning abdominal pains, cystitis, great thirst, nausea, and vomiting.

LIFESTYLE

Relaxation techniques will help stress-related problems. Fluid intake should be increased, but alcohol consumption reduced. Regular meals and exercise are both essential. If a particular food is believed to aggravate the condition, it should be eliminated from the diet for at least four days, and then reintroduced and symptoms observed. A nutritionist can advise about this and dietary changes that might be beneficial. An osteopath or physiotherapist may be able to help if there is spinal maladjustment.

CAUTION

◆ If symptoms are associated with persistent weight loss, consult a doctor.

◆ If there is fever and blood in the feces, see a doctor within 12 hours.

◆ Symptoms should be investigated promptly in patients over 50 in order to rule out cancer.

CASE HISTORY

Alf was a 42-year-old builder who experienced periods of loose bowel movements and lower-abdominal spasms lasting for a couple of months. This had begun two years before – after the break-up of a relationship. He was taking antispasmodic and antidiarrheal drugs.

PERSONAL DETAILS
Alf was convinced that his symptoms were stress-induced. He would get diarrhea, for example, if he was lonely. He often woke terrified in the middle of the night.

FOOD PREFERENCES
Alf had very few likes and dislikes, and no foods seemed to aggravate his condition. He had a great thirst, mainly for acidic drinks. Lemon juice relieved his symptoms.

FEARS
Alf feared darkness, looking into deep water, being alone, and worried that dogs might attack him. He hated cemeteries and anything connected with death.

GENERAL DETAILS
Alf slept badly and snored loudly. He complained of yeast infections, ear infections, bad breath, dry skin, and fatigue. He was better in company and with warmth. He was incontinent when frightened.

PRESCRIPTION & FOLLOW-UP
Since Alf's condition was related to emotional stress, he was given *Stramonium*. A month later he was much better but still complained of abdominal spasms and colicky pains in the intestines. He was prescribed *Cuprum*. At his next appointment, he revealed that a preference for masturbation had contributed to the failure of his relationship. He was given *Bufo* for this masturbatory tendency. A month later his bowels were much better as a result of the *Cuprum*. He felt that he had come to terms with his sexuality, and he had a new relationship. He rarely suffered pain or diarrhea, but was still not happy on his own. *Stramonium* was repeated. Alf was not seen for eight months, when IBS recurred due to stress. *Stramonium* was again given, since when Alf has been fine.

ULCERATIVE COLITIS

A FAIRLY RARE CONDITION, ulcerative colitis is an inflammatory bowel disease in which the linings of the rectum and colon become progressively more ulcerated. Colitis affects between 40 and 50 people per 100,000 in parts of the developed world and is most common in young and middle-aged adults. Attacks usually occur at intervals.

SYMPTOMS

◆ Abdominal pain on the left side.

◆ Diarrhea, with mucus and blood in the feces.

◆ In severe cases, fever and general malaise.

◆ Possible anemia and, if toxins get into the bloodstream, septicemia.

CAUSES

Although the exact cause of ulcerative colitis is unknown, it is believed that food allergy, infection, autoimmune problems, low levels of digestive enzymes and stomach acid, stress, and some antibiotics aggravate the condition. There may be a genetic tendency. Many sufferers are found to be emotionally stressed, especially if they are frustrated at work or grieving.

CONVENTIONAL CARE

Diagnosis is by means of a barium enema and an endoscopy of the rectum and lower colon. If these are not conclusive, a biopsy, whereby a small piece of the bowel lining is removed, may be performed. Infections can be discounted by analyzing samples of feces. Treatment is with sulfasalazine and its derivatives and possibly corticosteroid drugs. Ulcerative colitis is a potentially serious condition, and surgery may be necessary. In a few cases of persistent colitis, colonic cancer has been known to develop, so regular examinations are advisable.

HOMEOPATHIC MEDICINE

Constitutional assessment is a prerequisite of effective homeopathic treatment. A full medical will include referral for colonic investigation if necessary. Specific symptoms will then be studied, along with any aggravating factors that have been observed, and emotional temperament.

The most important criteria in determining constitutional treatment are the individual's symptoms (*see page 18*). Some remedies have an affinity for the digestive tract, and are particularly effective in treating the symptoms of inflammation of the colon. *Cantharis* is prescribed for inflammation of the lining of the gut and the production of thick, sticky mucus. *Colchicum* is given for colitis with symptoms similar to dysentry. *Colocynthis* is effective for colicky and neuralgic pains induced by irritation of the intestine; and *Merc. corr.* is used for constant straining of the rectum, which is not eased by passing stools. *Arsen. alb.*, *Nux vomica*, and *Sulfur* are other commonly used constitutional remedies.

Remedies for acute flare-ups of colitis include *Merc. corr.*, when there are hot, foul-smelling stools containing blood and mucus, and cutting pains in the abdomen on passing a stool, which are not relieved by emptying the bowel; *Arsen. alb.*, for restlessness, anxiety, burning abdominal pains with vomiting, a frequent desire for sips of warm drinks, and attacks that come on around midnight; and *Phosphorus,* if stools are bloody, and pain is relieved by passing a stool but then the anus feels as though it is gaping.

LIFESTYLE

Changing to a high-fiber diet with few dairy products may reduce the likelihood of further attacks. Other foods and drinks that are best avoided include refined carbohydrates, those containing caffeine, and alcohol. A nutritionist will be able to advise further. Smoking is inadvisable. When consulting a doctor about infections, colitis sufferers should draw attention to their condition, which may be exacerbated by taking antibiotics. Relaxation techniques and meditation are advisable for those leading stressful lives. During a colitis attack, the most suitable foods are those that are easily digested.

CAUTION

◆ If there is persistent weight loss of more than about 1 lb (0.5 kg) a week, consult a doctor.

◆ If there is fever, and blood and mucus in the stools, see a doctor within 12 hours.

CASE HISTORY

David was a 41-year-old stockbroker. Originally diagnosed as having irritable bowel syndrome, his condition had since been identified by a colonoscopy as ulcerative colitis. He believed that an infection picked up while traveling had made his condition worse. He was taking a corticosteroid and a sulfasalazine derivative, before which he had five or six watery bowel movements a day. His anus was raw and sore. He had great flatulence, with some pain, and had to get up in the early morning to empty his bowel.

PERSONAL DETAILS
David's father had died when he was eight, and his mother had relied heavily on him. He felt great relief on going away to university, and did well in his work, although it was his main source of stress. He had lost a daughter at the age of nine months, a victim of crib death. David was not sure he had gotten over this. He described himself as solid, but feared being incapacitated by illness.

FOOD PREFERENCES
David had a fairly sweet tooth. He liked vinegar and spices but avoided them in case they upset him. He believed that milk and cheese upset his bowel. He loved tea and had not smoked for 12 years.

GENERAL DETAILS
David felt better in dry heat and worse in humid conditions. He slept well and awoke refreshed but had to get up immediately.

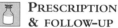

PRESCRIPTION & FOLLOW-UP
David was treated with *Sulfur*, after which his condition improved, with fewer and firmer bowel movements. The corticosteroid dosage was reduced, and David was able to sleep in later in the mornings. About this time he had dreams concerning his job and family, but he continued to improve, reducing his conventional drugs. He was then prescribed the nosode of measles (*see page 20*) since he had suffered a bad attack as a child. This remedy worked to good effect, so the potency was increased. David's progress continued and he reduced his drugs further. When last seen, he was on a maintenance dose of mesalazine, and continued to improve.

DIABETES

THE MOST COMMON FORM of diabetes, diabetes mellitus, occurs if the pancreas secretes insufficient insulin or none at all. This prevents the glucose needed for energy production being taken from the blood, so that blood-sugar levels rise. Insulin-dependent diabetes affects the young, while late-onset diabetes afflicts those in middle or old age.

SYMPTOMS

◆ Frequent and copious urination.

◆ Continuous thirst.

◆ Tiredness and apathy as a result of reduced energy production.

◆ Possible loss of weight.

◆ Possible cramps, blurred vision, faintness, breathlessness, erectile dysfunction, menstrual problems, and lowering of resistance to infection.

CAUSES

There is a genetic tendency to develop diabetes. In young people it is believed to result from a viral infection, although it may be due to autoimmune problems. It usually strikes between the ages of 10 and 15, although it can affect those aged up to 35. In older people the main factor is obesity. It is thought that not enough insulin is produced for a body that is overweight, or that, with age, the body becomes resistant to the effects of insulin.

Diabetes often comes to light during illnesses such as pancreatitis or after an infection, while taking drugs such as diuretics, or during pregnancy. Chromium deficiency may also be a factor. The cells of the pancreas are destroyed as diabetes progresses, so that insulin production stops almost completely. In the absence of regular injections of insulin, a diabetes sufferer will become hyperglycemic (too much glucose in the blood).

CONVENTIONAL CARE

People with insulin-dependent diabetes require insulin injections and a balanced diet that regulates carbohydrate intake. Glucose levels in the blood or urine are monitored carefully; high levels indicate that glucose is not being absorbed. Late-onset diabetes may be controlled mainly by means of a balanced diet, although drugs may be necessary to stimulate the production of insulin. It is important, especially for those taking drugs, to eat at regular intervals to prevent hypoglycemia (too little glucose in the blood).

HOMEOPATHIC MEDICINE

Constitutional homeopathic treatment for diabetes is recommended in support of conventional measures, and is compatible with them. Prescription depends upon specific symptoms (*see page 18*), but certain remedies have an affinity with the metabolic system. *Phosphoric ac.* is effective when emotional stress has played a part in the onset of diabetes. *Silica* is prescribed for diabetes that has arisen from infection; while *Tarentula* is used for diabetes linked to anxiety or grief. *Argentum nit.*, *Lycopodium*, *Phosphorus*, *Plumbum met.*, *Theridion*, and *Uranium nit.* are other constitutional remedies often used in the treatment of diabetes.

Remedies for acute symptoms include *Phosphoric ac.*, when diabetes is worse because of nervous exhaustion; *Uranium nit.* for digestive upset, great weight loss, weakness, and incontinence; *Argentum nit.*, when the usual symptoms of diabetes are accompanied by swollen ankles and there is apprehension; and *Silica*, when the person complains of cold, sweaty, smelly feet, and a lack of stamina.

LIFESTYLE

Carbohydrate intake should be carefully monitored, and the diet should include plenty of pulses and legumes as long as they do not upset the bowel. A nutritionist can advise about vitamin and mineral supplements. The loss of excess weight, stress-management techniques, and regular exercise will all help diabetes sufferers. Smoking is inadvisable.

CAUTION

◆ If a person with diabetes and taking insulin develops a sudden loss of energy, hunger, perspiration, dizziness, weakness, headache, irritability, slurred speech, or pins and needles, or is unsteady (hypoglycemia), administer sugar or glucose immediately and call a doctor. If the person loses consciousness, place them in a safe position (*see page 270*) and call an ambulance.

◆ If, despite treatment, there is increased urine production, great thirst, and loss of energy (hyperglycemia), see a doctor within two days.

CASE HISTORY

Sam was a 61-year-old, retired policeman, working part-time as a van driver. He had been diagnosed two years before his consultation with diabetes mellitus, revealed by a routine urine sample. He had responded fairly well to a diabetic diet, but still had high blood-sugar levels. He complained of anxiety, poor memory and concentration, anger, confusion, a lack of purpose in his life, depression, and tiredness.

PERSONAL DETAILS
Sam went to the UK in his thirties, having been born in India and having lived in Africa. He was used to responsibility and pleased with his achievements but felt that he was burnt out. He now wanted to put himself first, but he feared poverty. He felt his wife was not his equal intellectually, and they argued a lot. Sam was tidy but not fastidious.

FOOD PREFERENCES
Sam had a sweet tooth and liked spicy foods. He was often very thirsty since his blood-sugar levels had been brought under control, and he passed large quantities of urine.

GENERAL DETAILS
As well as mental tension, Sam had tension in the back of his skull. He had lower-back pain that was worse under stress, and he suffered sudden losses of energy. He preferred warm, damp weather.

PRESCRIPTION & FOLLOW-UP
Sam was advised to eat unrefined carbohydrate snacks little and often, and to avoid caffeine and alcohol. He felt better because of this, but still had sugar in his urine. He was prescribed *Nux vomica*, which aggravated him initially, then made him feel better. He soon became irritable and depressed, however. The remedy was repeated twice, after which he had more energy and felt less irritable. *China* was tried because of Sam's history of malaria while in Africa, but to little effect. *Sulfuric ac.* seemed to help him most, especially with the restlessness and irritation that he experienced on exposure to pollution while driving. When last seen, Sam had detected no sugar in his urine for several months.

SKIN & BONES

THE SKIN AND BONES are important components of the body's basic support systems. The skin keeps the internal parts within the body and protects them from the environment, while the skeletal system, among other functions, provides a strong, mobile framework that enables the body to move and protects internal organs.

THE BODY'S SUPPORT SYSTEMS

The skin is the body's outermost boundary and, in effect, its largest organ, accounting for 16 percent of total body weight. It is shed and renewed at a rate of 1 oz (25 g) a month. The skin protects the body by waterproofing it, reacting to sunlight, regulating temperature, and providing a barrier to invading organisms. It also supplies the brain with a range of sensory information. Skin problems often result from regulatory imbalances (acne rosacea and psoriasis) or allergy (eczema).

The skeleton is an extensive framework of bones, attached to which are skeletal muscles. Together they coordinate the body's movements. Individual bones move against each other by means of joints. The skeleton also provides support and protection for some of the body's most important organs, such as the brain, spinal cord, heart, and lungs. Diseases of the skeleton often result from degeneration of joints (osteoarthritis) or autoimmune problems (rheumatoid arthritis).

SYSTEM OF JOINTS
A joint is where two bones meet. There are different types of joint throughout the body, depending on their location. Most joints are mobile (see diagram, below). They are versatile and lubricated so that bone surfaces slide over each other easily, facilitating body movement. Other joints are less moveable, or fixed, and their main function is to provide support for the body.

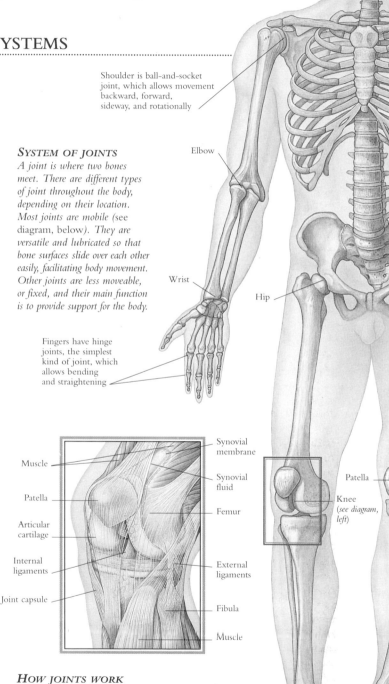

Shoulder is ball-and-socket joint, which allows movement backward, forward, sideway, and rotationally

Elbow

Wrist

Hip

Fingers have hinge joints, the simplest kind of joint, which allows bending and straightening

Femur

Patella

Knee (*see diagram, left*)

Fibula

Ankle

Toe joints

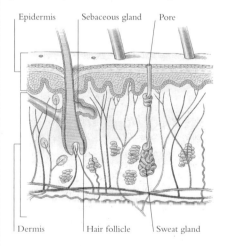

Epidermis — Sebaceous gland — Pore

Dermis — Hair follicle — Sweat gland

STRUCTURE OF SKIN
The skin has two main layers. The epidermis consists of flat, dead, or dying cells, which waterproof the skin and protect it from infection. These surface cells are continuously shed and replaced from below. The underlying dermis is where cells are created. Here there are blood vessels, nerves, muscles, sensory cells, sweat glands, sebaceous glands, and hair follicles.

Muscle

Patella

Articular cartilage

Internal ligaments

Joint capsule

Synovial membrane

Synovial fluid

Femur

External ligaments

Fibula

Muscle

HOW JOINTS WORK
Joints such as the knee – the largest joint in the body – are mobile joints. Their bone surfaces are covered with smooth cartilage to reduce friction during movement. Each mobile joint lies within a capsule lined with a membrane that secretes a lubricating fluid – the synovial fluid. Mobile joints are surrounded by ligaments that support them and prevent too much movement.

ROSACEA

ROSACEA, OR ACNE ROSACEA, resembles mild adolescent acne in some respects, but its main feature is flushing of the skin. It is most common among middle-aged women. In serious cases in elderly men it may lead to a bulbous swelling of the nose called rhinophyma. Rosacea tends to last between five and ten years before disappearing.

SYMPTOMS

◆ Flushed cheeks and nose, possibly induced by drinking hot drinks or alcohol, eating spicy foods, or entering a warm room.

◆ Possible permanent redness of the skin and small, pus-filled pimples that are similar to mild acne.

CAUSES

The causes of rosacea are largely unknown, but oral contraceptive drugs and corticosteroid ointments prescribed for other skin conditions, such as eczema, may precipitate it. Stress may exacerbate the condition. In women rosacea often strikes during or after menopause, when the condition is most probably linked to hormonal changes affecting the sebaceous glands in the skin.

CONVENTIONAL CARE

The usual treatment for rosacea is a long course of tetracyclines. These are very effective in suppressing the small, pus-filled pimples, but they do not tend to make much difference to the underlying red discoloration. Being antibiotics, they may harm the bacterial flora of the intestine, necessitating the subsequent use of acidophilic supplements.

HOMEOPATHIC MEDICINE

A homeopathic practitioner will take a full medical history, paying particular attention to the onset and progression of rosacea and its possible triggers, followed by an examination of affected areas.

Many remedies are suitable for the constitutional treatment of symptoms of rosacea (*see page 18*), but prescription will depend upon the individual. Among the remedies often chosen are *Carbo veg.*, for when blood stagnates in capillaries, resulting in poor oxygen supply to facial tissue; and *Lachesis* for hemorrhaging that allows infection to set in. *Psorinum* is prescribed for problems of the sebaceous glands; and *Rhus tox.* is given for infection such as that forming boils.

Homeopathic remedies prescribed for acute symptoms include *Belladonna*, for the early stages of rosacea, when the face is red, dry, and burning hot; and *Arsen. alb.*, when the skin is flaky and scaly, there is restlessness, and the condition is better with warmth generally as well as applying warm compresses to the affected areas. *Viola tri.* may be prescribed if rosacea is mainly concentrated on the chin, and the urine smells like cats' urine; while *Silica* is given if the main problem is pustules that remain for long periods of time. *Calc. phos.* is prescribed for rosacea that is found mainly on the nose and is accompanied by many pimples; and *Kali. brom.* is given when the forehead and cheeks in particular are flushed, and there are itchy pustules.

LIFESTYLE

Specifically, if rosacea is associated with vaginal discharge and general fatigue in women, a yeast- and sugar-free diet accompanied by acidophilic supplements is advisable. Naturopaths – those who promote health and natural healing by means of diet, exercise, and complementary care – believe that rosacea develops as a result of both stress and an inappropriate diet, especially one that is high in animal protein and fat, refined carbohydrates, and dairy products. Following a mainly fish and vegetarian diet for one month may be beneficial. Alcohol and coffee are best avoided. If stress is an aggravating factor, relaxation techniques, yoga, meditation, or t'ai chi may help on a daily basis. Any emotional problems should be solved, with the help of a counselor if necessary. Local applications of calendula solution or tea-tree oil may alleviate the condition (10 drops calendula mother tincture to 2 pints/1.25 liters cooled, boiled water, or 2 drops tea-tree oil).

> ### CAUTION
> ◆ If the nose is swelling, consult a doctor.
> ◆ If an acnelike rash develops while taking steroids, either orally or in an ointment, consult a doctor to discuss discontinuation.

CASE HISTORY

William was a 57-year-old retired blacksmith. He came to the consultation with a ten-year history of rosacea. It had started with small spots above the eyebrows but had progressed to boils and redness of the whole face. He had been prescribed an antibiotic, oxytetracycline, which upset his bowels, and then another form of tetracycline to be applied (as a solution) to the affected areas.

PERSONAL DETAILS
As well as a red face and several small boils on his nose, William had a coated tongue, a slightly swollen upper lip, and a strong body odor. He described himself as superstitious and a perfectionist. He became depressed easily and worried constantly about his health.

FOOD PREFERENCES
William had a huge appetite, even needing to eat in the middle of the night, but he never put on any weight. He liked beer and acidic foods, but not meat. He had a great thirst, but his skin condition was exacerbated by drinking coffee.

GENERAL DETAILS
William felt the cold greatly and wore a lot of clothes even in summer. He hated winter and loved hot, sunny weather. Despite this, he had a tendency to feel very hot in bed and did not like becoming overheated by physical exertion.

PRESCRIPTION & FOLLOW-UP
William was prescribed *Sulfur*, which helped the rosacea initially. The condition deteriorated, however, if he stopped using tetracycline. He was then given *Psorinum* in increasing potencies over a period of about 18 months, and this produced a remarkable improvement in his condition. He was able to stop applying tetracycline, and eventually to take *Psorinum* on the rare occasion only if he felt the rosacea might be about to flare up again. Interestingly, William had also suffered from irritable bowel syndrome for about 40 years, and this condition also improved for taking *Psorinum*. When last heard of, William had been completely clear of symptoms of rosacea for four years.

SEVERE ECZEMA

LOCAL INFLAMMATION OF THE SKIN, or eczema, may be accompanied by itching, blistering, and oozing, may be associated with an allergic reaction, but the cause is often unknown. Childhood eczema, which usually occurs in the flexures behind a knee or in the bend of an elbow, usually clears up by the time the child reaches puberty.

SYMPTOMS

◆ Red, itchy, and scaly skin.

◆ Inflamed areas, possibly with small, red pimples that weep or bleed if scratched.

◆ Possible blistering of skin.

◆ Possible cracked and painful skin.

◆ Possible issue of pus if broken skin becomes infected.

CAUSES

Atopic eczema occurs in people with a genetic tendency to develop allergies. Contact eczema – or contact dermatitis (some forms of eczema are also known as dermatitis) – is caused by touching items to which the body is sensitive, such as fabric, metal, or plants. Seborrheic dermatitis may be inherited but is not linked to allergy. Of unknown cause, it produces flakiness and itchiness on the face, scalp, and other hairy areas, and may be worse with stress. Detergent dermatitis afflicts those using cleaning products. Varicose eczema tends to be associated with inefficient circulation in the legs, although the precise cause is unknown.

CONVENTIONAL CARE

With atopic eczema, eliminating certain foods or food additives from the diet may identify an allergy. With contact eczema, patch tests are useful. Antihistamine drugs can reduce irritation, while antibiotics are prescribed for infection. Corticosteroid ointments inhibit inflammation, but they should be used only when the risk of infection or irritation is so severe that it prevents sleep, thus increasing stress and exacerbating the eczema. Moisturizing ointments may be beneficial.

HOMEOPATHIC MEDICINE

A full medical history of the condition, any family history of allergy, and possible triggers will be studied by a homeopath. A person's psychological makeup, food preferences, and environmental factors will also be investigated.

Constitutional remedies will be largely determined by an individual's symptoms (*see page 18*). *Calc. sulf.* is indicated for skin eruptions that easily become infected; while *Dulcamara* is effective for thickening of the epidermis. *Graphites* is associated with sticky fluid exuded from inflamed patches that dry out to become rough and hard; and *Rhus tox.* is also prescribed for infected skin. Other remedies commonly prescribed are *Arsen. alb.*, *Baryta mur.*, *Calc. carb.*, *Hepar sulf.*, and *Sulfur*.

Local remedies prescribed for acute conditions include *Psorinum*, if the skin is broken and very sensitive, and the slightest scratch becomes infected, forming a green crust that burns and itches, then cracks and bleeds. *Oleander* is given for skin that is very dry, sensitive, and itchy so that the slightest friction results in soreness, and scratching causes the skin to bleed and weep. *Mezereum* is prescribed for itchy, thick scabs, beneath which there is pus, and which are worse with warm baths. *Cicuta* is used for eczema that is worse on the face and hands, feels hot to the touch, and may include pustules.

LIFESTYLE

Rubber gloves should be worn for most household tasks, with cotton gloves inside them if there is sensitivity to rubber. As well as known irritants, substances and situations best avoided include colored sanitary paper, antiperspirants, false nails, dehumidified air, and rapid temperature changes. The skin may benefit from lukewarm oatmeal herbal baths and cold milk compresses, but it should always be dried thoroughly. Clothes should be rinsed well after washing. The diet should ideally include plenty of fish and vegetables, while quantities of animal protein, fats, refined carbohydrates, and dairy products should all be reduced.

CAUTION

◆ If eczema deteriorates markedly, and especially if the skin is broken, inflamed, and appears to be infected, consult a doctor within 48 hours.

CASE HISTORY

Five-year-old Alex had experienced eczema for two years. The inflammation was widespread, and although it came and went on most parts of the body, it was constantly on his forehead. His arms and legs were worst affected, with some scarring. He was on hydrocortisone, and had been prescribed antibiotics for skin infections on two occasions. The eczema worsened when Alex was ill.

PERSONAL DETAILS
Alex was born in Hong Kong. His eczema started about the time that his baby brother was born. The family then moved to the UK, the father changed careers, and the family moved again before life settled down. His mother described Alex as lively, excitable, loving, and nonaggressive. He was good with his hands and liked taking things apart. He loved attention and was sometimes jealous of his younger brother.

FOOD PREFERENCES
Alex loved most foods, especially fatty and sweet ones, and those with strong flavors, which was unusual for a child of his age.

GENERAL DETAILS
Alex tended to grab everything and put it in his mouth, behavior characteristic of a child younger than he was. His itching was worse from bathing, or if he was overheated or overexcited. The itching was also worse at night, and Alex had many a sleepless night as a result of his condition. His skin was always dry, and bled if he scratched it.

PRESCRIPTION & FOLLOW-UP
When first seen, Alex's skin was slightly infected. He was given *Silica* for the infection, and his mother was advised to bathe Alex's skin with a solution of calendula and hypericum, and apply calendula ointment. Alex's eczema symptoms and general picture indicated *Sulfur*, and he was prescribed a variety of potencies of this remedy over the next eight months. By the end of that time, his condition was much improved, and he hardly needed to take the *Sulfur* at all. He was finally discharged, having been totally weaned off his conventional drug treatment.

PSORIASIS

THIS FAIRLY COMMON SKIN DISEASE consists of inflamed areas that are often covered by silvery scales. A chronic condition that flares up at intervals, psoriasis can cover a large area, including the face, and can be very disfiguring. It affects about two percent of the population in North America and Europe, but is less common in other regions.

SYMPTOMS

- Unsightly patches of flaky skin that can occur anywhere on the body, possibly with itching.
- Patches are slightly raised and deep pink, often overlain with silvery scales.
- Possible pitting of the nails.
- Possible inflammation of the joints.

CAUSES

There may be a genetic tendency. The basic problem with psoriasis is that new skin cells form more quickly than usual, causing accumulations of living cells. These create thickened patches of skin covered with dead, flaking cells. The condition varies in severity and may be triggered by infection, particularly that caused by the streptococcal bacteria, by drugs such as chloroquine used in the treatment of rheumatic pain and malaria. Stress or injury may also trigger psoriasis.

CONVENTIONAL CARE

In mild cases, light therapy can help up to 75 percent of those afflicted. It may be combined with a psoralen, a substance that makes skin more sensitive to light. Exposure times should be increased only gradually, and soothing, moisturizing ointments should be applied. Moderate cases of psoriasis are treated with dithranol or coaltar ointments, and corticosteroids. Severe cases may be treated with vitamin-A derivatives or cytotoxic drugs such as methotrexate, which retards cell division. This may cause serious side effects such as abnormal bleeding or a decreased resistance to infection. Nonsteroidal anti-inflammatory drugs may be used to treat psoriasis, but they may cause digestive problems, even stomach ulcers.

HOMEOPATHIC MEDICINE

A full medical history is obtained and, if there is doubt about the diagnosis, skin scrapings are taken. In treating psoriasis, great emphasis is placed on an individual's psychological makeup, in particular factors that might have triggered the condition, such as stress or emotional upset. Environmental factors and food preferences are also significant.

The most important criteria in determining constitutional prescription are the person's individual symptoms (*see page 18*). Some remedies in particular are associated with the treatment of psoriasis, however. *Arsen. alb.* is indicated for dry, rough, and scaly skin; and *Lycopodium* is effective for dry skin and raw areas in the flexures. *Sepia* is prescribed for the thick crusts that form on the elbows; while *Staphysagria* is used to treat skin conditions that are affected by irritability of the nervous system.

Specific remedies for local problems include *Sulfur*, for dry, red, scaly, itchy patches that are worse after a bath; *Graphites*, if the skin behind the ears is affected; *Petroleum*, when the skin is extremely dry, and psoriasis is worse in winter, with deep, bloody cracks, especially on the hands, fingertips, genitals, and elbows; and *Phytolacca*, when there are lesions with a purple coloration.

LIFESTYLE

Reducing stress by means of relaxation techniques, meditation, t'ai chi, or yoga, and nutritional therapies can help this condition enormously, as can a diet that includes plenty of fish and vegetarian sources of protein rather than meat and dairy products. Refined carbohydrates should be eliminated, along with caffeine, alcohol, and tobacco. It is advisable to lose excess weight, and make sure that the bowel functions well, taking extra fiber if necessary, and plenty of water. It may be worth using marine oils, such as cod-liver oil, for cooking, and avoiding foods containing yeast.

CAUTION

- If symptoms show no improvement after two weeks of homeopathic remedies and lifestyle changes, see a doctor.

CASE HISTORY

Kate, 22, had been affected by psoriasis since she was six. It had worsened in the last year following the breakup of a relationship. She was taking corticosteroids and applying a vitamin-D-based ointment. Her skin was inflamed and itchy. The condition was worse if Kate was tired, and often coincided with attacks of tonsilitis.

PERSONAL DETAILS
Kate believed herself to be ambitious, but she lacked confidence. She felt as though the psoriasis had eaten away every part of her body.

FOOD PREFERENCES
Kate had a great thirst and liked very cold drinks. She would drink ice-cold milk, which was sometimes vomited as soon as it was warmed in the stomach. She loved salt, acidic and spicy foods, and ice cream. She disliked fruits, warm foods and drinks, and coffee.

FEARS
Kate had fears of failure, of letting down her parents and her friends, of living alone, and of thunderstorms.

GENERAL DETAILS
Kate was better in the sun, but disliked great heat. She felt faint if she put her hands in cold water. She was aware of falling pressure before thunderstorms, and sometimes suffered headaches. She disliked mornings and evenings, and was better after catnapping, eating, and massage.

PRESCRIPTION & FOLLOW-UP
Kate was given *Phosphorus,* and her skin condition started to improve. She began to take life more easily, and sleep more. In fact, she felt that the *Phosphorus* relaxed her so much that all she wanted to do was sleep. Over 12 months she weaned herself off the corticosteroids and reduced the application of cream to once a week. She no longer suffered from recurrent sore throats. Kate's psoriasis returned after a year, when she had a cancer scare and started to work in Boston, with the stress of commuting. She was again prescribed *Phosphorus* and the psoriasis settled down. It still flares up if Kate is stressed, but *Phosphorus* is usually effective.

OSTEOARTHRITIS

OSTEOARTHRITIS IS A DEGENERATIVE DISEASE of the joints that breaks down cartilage, causing restriction of movement and sometimes pain. It has been estimated that in some parts of the developed world up to 90 percent of people over 40 have osteoarthritis in one or more joints. Severe osteoarthritis affects three times as many women as men.

SYMPTOMS

- Stiffness and pain in the affected joints.

- Possible swelling of the joints, most commonly weight-bearing joints such as those in the hips, knees, and spine.

- Weakness and loss of bulk in the muscles surrounding the affected joints if they are not used regularly.

- Possible deformation of affected joints.

CAUSES

The degeneration of cartilage covering the ends of bones occurs with age or as a result of injury or overuse. The bone ends touch, causing them to thicken and thus restrict joint movement. This results in inflammation. There may also be outgrowths on a bone called osteophytes, which increase the pain and stiffness, and may press on blood vessels and nerves. The early onset of osteoarthritis may be the result of a congenital joint deformity.

CONVENTIONAL CARE

Diagnosis is usually possible following examination, but can be confirmed by an X ray. Conventional treatment is largely symptomatic, using painkillers and non-steroidal, anti-inflammatory drugs. Steroids are sometimes injected into the joint. If a joint is badly worn, it may need replacing surgically with an artificial joint. Hip-replacement operations, for example, have a high success rate but need to be repeated after 20 to 30 years. If replacement is not an option, the joint may be fused to prevent pain.

HOMEOPATHIC MEDICINE

Homeopathic treatment of osteoarthritis is mostly localized, depending on the joint affected, the nature of the pain, and other symptoms. Constitutional treatment may be required if there is a genetic tendency. Emotional or environmental factors will be less significant than in other serious ailments since osteoarthritis is a mechanical failure, although stress makes any symptoms less bearable. The choice of constitutional remedy will depend upon an individual's symptoms (*see page 18*), but remedies commonly used include *Apis*, which is prescribed for inflammation of synovial membranes and overproduction of synovial fluid; and *Silica*, which is given for the destruction of bone and enlarged bursae (fluid-filled pads that cushion pressure points near a joint). *Calc. carb.* is indicated for osteoarthritis associated with growths on the bone; and *Causticum* is prescribed for inflammation of the joints leading to deformity. Other constitutional remedies used include *Kali. carb.*, *Lycopodium*, *Merc. sol.*, *Nat. mur.*, *Pulsatilla*, *Sepia*, and *Sulfur*.

Remedies given for acute symptoms include *Aconite*, for shooting pains in a joint accompanied by numbness and tingling; and *Belladonna*, for joints that become red, swollen, and shiny quickly, and are unbearably painful if jarred. *Bryonia* is prescribed for joints that are red, swollen, and hot, with the least movement causing agonizing pain; and *Ledum* is given for joints that feel cold, are swollen, make cracking noises on moving, and are better with cold compresses.

LIFESTYLE

A diet that is high in alkaline-forming foods and low in acid-forming ones is beneficial. This means more fish and vegetarian protein and less caffeine, sugar, citrus fruits, wheat, and dairy products. Losing excess weight will relieve pressure on the joints. Smoking is inadvisable. Exercise such as cycling or walking is beneficial; well-cushioned shoes should be worn. Sleeping on a firm bed and rest or catnaps during the day are also helpful. Yoga may relieve stress and warm compresses may help to alleviate pain. Dependency on tranquilizers, painkillers, or sleeping pills should be avoided.

CAUTION

- If the pain suddenly becomes more severe, or additional joints become affected, consult a doctor within a week.

CASE HISTORY

Doris, 60, had suffered from osteoarthritis for six years. It had started in the right wrist, then developed in the left. An X ray had revealed bone changes in the thumb joint. Doris was not aware of any precipitative factors. She was unable to take nonsteroidal, anti-inflammatory drugs because they upset her stomach.

PERSONAL DETAILS
Doris had been a dental nurse before getting married and having three children, the eldest of whom had died in a car accident. Doris was generally happy and contented, although she often felt restless and worried constantly about her other two children, even though they had long since left the family home. She had a great interest in the arts and practiced meditation.

FOOD PREFERENCES
Doris had a desire for mayonnaise, milk, coffee, and wine. She disliked pineapple, vinegar, coconut, and some fish.

GENERAL DETAILS
Doris hated cold, damp weather, which made her condition worse. Her joints would seize up during sleep and when at rest, were painful when they were first moved, then better with continuous motion. Doris also had a red-tipped tongue.

PRESCRIPTION & FOLLOW-UP
First of all, Doris was put on an alkaline diet for arthritis but to no avail. There was a family history of allergy and respiratory problems, so she was given *Tuberculinum* on a weekly basis, and *Rhus tox.* three times daily for the arthritis. On this regime there was a slow improvement, but Doris then developed phlegm and sinusitis. As the phlegm continued, her wrist pain diminished until she could unscrew the lid of a jar, a task that she had been unable to do for years. She continued to take *Tuberculinum* until the phlegm cleared up. She was not seen for a couple of years, when pain recurred in her right thumb. She was prescribed *Rhus tox.* again, which was effective. When Doris was seen nine years later for another complaint, she reported that her joints were fine.

RHEUMATOID ARTHRITIS

RHEUMATOID ARTHRITIS IS AN AUTOIMMUNE DISEASE, in which the body's immune system attacks the joints. There is a juvenile form, but the disease usually starts in early adulthood or middle age. This form of arthritis affects about two percent of the world's population, and afflicts more women then men.

SYMPTOMS

◆ Mild fever, muscle aches and pains, loss of appetite, and weight loss may precede the main symptoms.

◆ Pain and stiffness – mainly in the small joints of the hands and feet, but also in the wrists, neck, ankles, and knees – that may start suddenly and are worse in the morning and with rest.

◆ Possible exacerbation of symptoms during menstruation.

◆ Possible rheumatoid nodules beneath the skin.

◆ Possible association with Raynaud's disease or anemia.

◆ Possible deformation of joints, fluid-filled swelling around joints, and inflammation of the tendon sheaths.

CAUSES

It is not known why the immune system should start to attack the joints. There may be a genetic tendency; some people with a certain tissue type may be prone to rheumatoid arthritis. The result is that the linings of joint capsules become inflamed. The inflammation spreads to other parts of the joint and even the bones themselves. The process may be triggered by infection, environmental pollutants, stress, or taking certain drugs.

CONVENTIONAL CARE

Diagnosis is confirmed by X ray and a blood test that can identify a "rheumatoid factor." Conventional treatment focuses on reducing inflammation with non-steroidal, anti-inflammatory drugs and penicillamine or sulfasalazine injections. Failing these, immunosuppressant drugs such as steroids or azathioprine will retard the autoimmune response. Physiotherapy can relieve muscle spasms and stiffness, and splints help to reduce pain in the hands and wrists. Replacement surgery may be necessary if a joint has been damaged.

HOMEOPATHIC MEDICINE

Homeopathy considers rheumatoid arthritis to be a complex condition. A genetic tendency may be addressed by antimiasmatic treatment (*see page 20*). Diet and lifestyle will be studied closely, as will stress or psychological factors as potential triggers of the disease. The choice of remedy will largely be determined by individual symptoms (*see page 18*). *Aurum met.* is indicated for destruction of the bone; and *Bryonia* is used for inflammation and the overproduction of synovial fluid. *Calc. phos.* affects the maintenance of bones, and is given if they are soft, thin, and brittle. *Causticum* is prescribed for inflammation of the joints leading to deformity. *Iodum*, *Kali. bich.*, *Lycopodium*, and *Medorrhinum* are also commonly used.

Local remedies include *Rhus tox.*, when there is pain on waking and in cold, damp conditions; and *Colchicum*, for hot, stiff joints, and pain that moves from joint to joint and is agonizing at night or if touched. *Iodum* is used for joints that feel tight and pain that is worse at night, when the bones are also affected; and *Spigelia*, for tearing pain near the joints as if a knife were scraping along the bones.

LIFESTYLE

A high-alkaline diet is beneficial, as are evening-primrose oil, antioxidants, green-lipped-mussel extract, brazil nuts, and the wearing of a copper bracelet. Regular but moderate exercise that does not exert pressure on weight-bearing joints is advisable. Swimming is ideal, preferably in a heated pool. Catnaps, or periods of rest with the eyes closed, are beneficial.

CAUTION

◆ If a joint becomes deformed, see a doctor.

◆ If there are breathing difficulties or chest pains, see a doctor immediately.

◆ If the eyes are dry and there are lumps in the neck, under the arms, or in the groin, see a doctor as soon as possible.

CASE HISTORY

Penelope, a 54-year-old former dental nurse, had developed arthritis gradually in her feet, especially the toes and ankles, four years before her consultation. A few months before she was seen, it had spread to her fingers, an alarming development since Penelope was a piano player. She had been prescribed anti-inflammatory drugs, but they had made her nauseous. She had tried acupuncture and Bryonia, *which had helped slightly.*

PERSONAL DETAILS

Penelope was a pleasant, intelligent woman, who liked the arts and reading. Her main fear was of feathers. She described herself as emotionally closed, and disliked sympathy, which made her feel sorry for herself. She had a happy marriage, but her mother had lived in Penelope's home for 30 years after her husband's death. Having become ill about five years previously, her mother had moved into a nursing home a few months before Penelope's homeopathic consultation.

FOOD PREFERENCES

There were no particular foods that Penelope strongly liked or disliked, although she did prefer salty rather than sweet foods.

GENERAL DETAILS

Penelope was worse on first moving in the morning, but did not appear to be affected by any particular weather conditions.

PRESCRIPTION & FOLLOW-UP

The deterioration of Penelope's health seemed to be closely linked to events in her mother's life. Penelope had not grieved properly for her father, however, and this increased the emotional impact of her mother's experiences and took its toll on Penelope's immune system. She was prescribed *Nat. mur.* in a high potency and *Rhus tox* specifically for her joints. One month on, she had stopped taking anti-inflammatories, and felt better from having dealt with the loss of her father. Her joint pain had reduced to such an extent that she was teaching the piano again. Two years later she reported only the slightest twinges of pain, which responded to *Rhus. tox.*

REPRODUCTIVE SYSTEMS

THE URGE TO PROCREATE is one of the most basic instincts driving human beings. Reproduction involves the fertilization of an egg from the ovary of the female by a sperm from the male, and the development of a fetus to term. Contraception has facilitated greater control over childbearing than ever before. In parallel the science of assisted reproduction has developed as couples delay having children until their fertility may have begun to decline.

HOW THE SYSTEMS WORK

Reproduction depends on the efficient functioning of both the female and male systems. This is impaired by physiological problems such as blockages, which are either congenital or the result of infection or scarring and which may give rise to infertility; growths such as fibroids; and malformation such as an enlarged prostate gland. The reproductive process may also be interrupted by hormonal imbalances.

FEMALE REPRODUTION

The vagina receives sperm from the penis of the male during sexual intercourse. The sperm pass through the opening of the cervix into the uterus on their way to find an egg that has been expelled from an ovary. A fertilized egg travels down the fallopian tube and, after many cell divisions, embeds itself in the wall of the uterus. For the first eight weeks of its development it is called an embryo; thereafter, it is a fetus.

If no fertilization occurs, the lining of the uterus, or endometrium, is shed during menstruation. This occurs about every 28 days. The menstrual cycle is under the control of hormones produced by the pituitary gland in the brain.

MALE REPRODUCTION

Male sex cells, or sperm, are produced in the testes. These are outside the body so that the sperm are kept cool. From the testes sperm travel up a narrow tube, the vas deferens, in which they are joined by secretions from the seminal vesicles and the prostate gland to create semen. During sexual intercourse semen is ejaculated into the vagina of the female. Erectile tissue in the penis expands as a result of increased blood flow during sexual arousal, allowing the insertion of the erect penis into the vagina during intercourse and the emission of semen. Once in the vagina, sperm "swim" by means of long, whiplike tails. Each sperm head contains genetic material.

FEMALE REPRODUCTION
An egg shed by an ovary is swept up by the pronglike ends of the fallopian tube. A fertilized egg will pass down into the uterus and embed itself in the lining. The uterus expands greatly to accommodate a developing fetus.

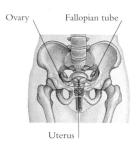

LOCATION OF SYSTEM
The female reproductive system lies inside the pelvic cavity, surrounded and protected by the pelvic bones. This space is wider than in the male to accommodate the enlarging uterus in pregnancy.

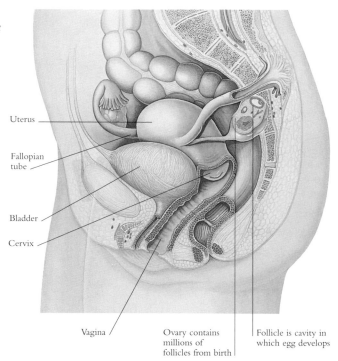

Uterus

Fallopian tube

Bladder

Cervix

Vagina

Ovary contains millions of follicles from birth

Follicle is cavity in which egg develops

MALE REPRODUCTION
During sexual intercourse sperm are propelled by means of muscle contractions from the testes along the vas deferens to the ejaculatory duct. At ejaculation, semen is propelled along the urethra and out of the penis.

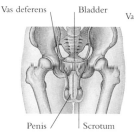

Vas deferens   Bladder

Penis   Scrotum

LOCATION OF SYSTEM
The male reproductive organs are not within the pelvic cavity. In fact, they lie outside the body altogether – in the scrotum.

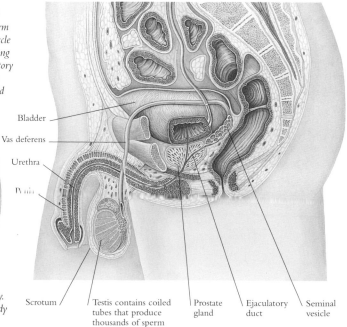

Bladder

Vas deferens

Urethra

Penis

Scrotum

Testis contains coiled tubes that produce thousands of sperm

Prostate gland

Ejaculatory duct

Seminal vesicle

FIBROIDS

FIBROIDS ARE BENIGN (noncancerous) tumors in the uterus. In the developed world they occur in about 20 percent of women over 30, mainly between 35 and 45. A fibroid may grow steadily in the wall of the uterus, or project into the uterine cavity, in which case it will be attached to the wall by a stalk. Fibroids may shrink after menopause.

SYMPTOMS

◆ Possibly no symptoms at all if a fibroid is very small.

◆ Possible heavy or lengthy menstrual periods that may cause anemia if a fibroid is large.

◆ Symptoms of cystitis if a large fibroid presses on the bladder.

◆ Backache or constipation if a large fibroid presses on the bowel.

◆ Possible difficulty in conceiving, miscarriage, pain during pregnancy, or problems during labor if there is a large fibroid in the uterine cavity.

◆ Severe pain if a fibroid stalk becomes twisted, cutting off its blood supply.

CAUSES

Fibroids are growths in smooth muscle and connective tissue. It is believed that they grow in response to estrogen stimulation or as an abnormal response to normal levels of estrogen. They can be caused by taking oral contraceptives, and tend to enlarge during pregnancy. As a result of the decrease in estrogen levels during menopause, fibroids often shrink and eventually disappear.

CONVENTIONAL CARE

Small, symptom-free fibroids are often discovered during routine gynecological examinations or ultrasound scanning. Small fibroids do not require treatment, but they are usually monitored. The conventional treatment for fibroids that cause pain involves the removal of the fibroid (myomectomy), or – especially if there is heavy bleeding – the removal of the uterus (hysterectomy).

HOMEOPATHIC MEDICINE

Homeopathic treatment aims to correct imbalances in estrogen levels or the body's extraordinary response to normal estrogen levels. A constitutional approach will address the interaction between the ovaries and the pituitary gland. The choice of remedy will depend on an individual's particular symptoms (*see page 18*). *Calc. carb.* is used for the treatment of growths on stalks that project from the uterine wall. For problems that may be associated with fibroids, *Lachesis* is indicated when the circulation of blood in the uterus leads to bleeding into surrounding muscle. *Phosphorous* is used for the overdevelopment of muscle, and *Sepia* is associated with inflammation of the uterus and prolapse (displacement of the uterus).

Remedies may be prescribed specifically in an attempt to shrink a fibroid. These include *Calc. iod.*, when fibroids are small and there is a profuse, yellow vaginal discharge; and *Fraxinus,* when the uterus is swollen and accompanied by an urge to bear down, and there are painful cramps and a watery, brown vaginal discharge during menstruation. *Silica* is used when menstrual periods are heavy, possibly with intermittent bleeding, and the body feels ice cold; and *Aurum mur.* is often prescribed for a swollen, painful uterus with spasmodic vaginal contractions.

LIFESTYLE

A diet that is high in fish and vegetarian sources of protein and raw vegetables, and low in meat, dairy products, refined carbohydrates, caffeine, and alcohol is advisable, especially if the fibroids are associated with heavy bleeding. Half-an-hour's moderate exercise a day, with care not to overexert, is recommended. There is some evidence that progesterones extracted from Mexican yams and applied to the skin as a cream may counteract the effects of estrogen and therefore shrink the fibroids. This product is not always readily available over the counter, however.

> ### CAUTION
>
> ◆ If there is severe pain in the lower abdomen, see a doctor immediately.
>
> ◆ If a fibroid is causing abdominal swelling comparable with that in the twelfth week of pregnancy, and the person is not approaching menopause, removal may be necessary.

CASE HISTORY

Natasha, 35, went to the UK from the former USSR ten years previously with her husband, an international banker. She had two children. Before her consultation a plum-sized fibroid had been revealed by a checkup following a pap smear. Natasha complained of heavy periods with a black discharge two days before the onset of menstruation.

PERSONAL DETAILS
Natasha was an anxious person who worried about her health and that of her children, death, the future, and being deserted by her husband. She was dissatisfied, restless, fastidious, and always rushing. She dreamed of being in quicksand or drowning. She would awake in panic at around 1 A.M.

FOOD PREFERENCES
A stomach problem diagnosed as a hiatus hernia made Natasha vomit at night. She loved sweet, salty, fatty, and acidic foods, but at times completely lost her appetite. Milk, coffee, spicy foods, chocolate, and too much fat upset her digestion.

GENERAL DETAILS
Natasha felt the cold greatly and loved hot weather. She liked to place hot compresses on her stomach during menstruation. She was worse from exertion and between midnight and 2 A.M., and hated tobacco smoke.

PRESCRIPTION & FOLLOW-UP
Natasha was given *Arsen. alb.*, and within a few days felt more relaxed. Her period was a week early, with the discharge as before, but it was less heavy than usual. She was then put on a diet low in refined carbohydrates and free of caffeine. This made her feel weak but generally better. Her next period occurred at the right time, with no discharge, but it was still heavy. Within the next couple of months, normal menstruation was restored with the prescription of *Solidago*. Two months later at a checkup, Natasha's gynecologist reported that the fibroid had reduced to the size of a small bean. After two years, Natasha developed benign breast lumps, which were treated effectively with *Sulfur*. Following a subsequent gynecological checkup, the fibroid was reported to have disappeared.

CANDIDIASIS

CANDIDIASIS, THRUSH, OR YEAST INFECTION is caused by *Candida albicans*, a fungus that lives in warm, moist conditions and thrives if the immune system is at a low ebb. Candidiasis mainly affects the vagina, in up to 50 percent of women in the developed world, even if there are no symptoms. It may also affect the mouth, digestive tract, and skin.

SYMPTOMS

♦ Thick, white discharge from the vagina, possibly with itching and discomfort on passing urine. In men, candidiasis causes inflammation of the head of the penis.

♦ Yellowish-white, raised patches on the lining of the mouth. If the digestive tract is affected, symptoms include indigestion, nausea, bloating, flatulence, diarrhea, constipation, and itching of the anus.

♦ In babies, inflamed type of diaper rash.

♦ Other symptoms associated with candidiasis include a skin rash, aches and pains, recurrent sore throat, dizziness, fatigue, blurred vision, and headache.

CAUSES

Candida albicans is normally present in the vagina and often in the mouth, but is kept under control by bacteria. Some drugs, such as antibiotics, interfere with this. Candidiasis may flare up if the immune system is compromised, as in AIDS, or if there are metabolic problems, such as diabetes. Oral contraceptives and immuno-suppressive and progestogen drugs also encourage it to proliferate. Local factors may affect its growth (*see* Lifestyle).

CONVENTIONAL CARE

Candida albicans can be identified in the mouth or genitals from swabs, but there is as yet no definitive test for the digestive tract. It is treated with antifungal drugs. These come as pessaries for the vagina or as creams for applying to the vulva or penis. There are oral drops for the mouth.

HOMEOPATHIC MEDICINE

Homeopathy is most effective in treating candidiasis in the genitals. A practitioner will study the reason for the proliferation of the bacteria. Choice of constitutional remedy will depend on individual symptoms (*see page 18*), and especially the characteristics of the vaginal discharge. *Arsen. alb.* is prescribed for a burning, offensive-smelling discharge associated with inflammation; and *Graphites* for a profuse, thin, white discharge associated with inflammation. *Medorrhinum* is given for a fishy-smelling discharge that feels as if it is stripping the skin off the vagina; while *Merc. sol.* is indicated for vaginal inflammation and bleeding along with a greenish discharge, and for inflammation of the penis. *Nitric ac.* is used to treat blisters and ulcers on the genitals.

Remedies include *Lycopodium*, for an irritating vaginal discharge that is worse after menstruation, with itching and thickening of the vulval skin from scratching; and *Carbo veg.*, for an offensive-smelling, itchy, greenish, burning discharge that is worse with heat, and on cracking of the vulva. *Kreosotum* is prescribed for an offensive, sour-smelling discharge that stains underwear, with soreness and burning in the vagina; and *Nux vomica*, for an offensive-smelling discharge, especially during pregnancy, that is worse with heat and is associated with frequent urination.

LIFESTYLE

Drugs known to aggravate the condition should be avoided. *Candida albicans* thrives on sugar, so the diet should be low in refined carbohydrates and, if allergy to fungal products is suspected, free of yeasts and molds. Acidophilic supplements encourage the growth of intestinal organisms to keep *Candida albicans* in check; garlic inhibits its growth. Regular exercise without overexertion is good.

Both sexual partners should be treated. Adequate lubrication during intercourse is advisable, using a lubricant if necessary, and condoms will prevent the spread of infection. The vagina may benefit from an acidic douche or the application of live yogurt; an infected penis may be treated with calendula ointment. Perfumed toiletries are best avoided.

CAUTION

♦ If discharge does not respond to treatment or lifestyle changes, and especially if it is green and irritating, see a doctor within five days.

♦ If a diaper rash becomes uncomfortable, red, and raw, consult a doctor within 48 hours.

CASE HISTORY

Thirty-year-old Sophie had suffered from vaginal candidiasis for eight months. She was also prone to eczema and hives (urticaria). The candidiasis had been brought on by taking oral contraceptives but improved with treatment using antifungal drugs, although it usually recurred at the end of a menstrual period.

PERSONAL DETAILS

Sophie described herself as a worrier. She did not dwell on the past, but felt angry that she was unable to find a part-time job that fitted in with looking after her son. She was ambitious and wanted to be a high achiever, but she tended to be untidy and disorganized.

FOOD PREFERENCES

Sophie had a large appetite, although she did not put on weight. She loved sweet foods, the fat on meat, spicy foods, and alcohol. Alcohol tended to upset her digestion, however. She disliked meat, eggs, olives, and chicken.

GENERAL DETAILS

Sophie's condition was worse after bathing and in bed at night. She slept throughout the night but woke feeling unrefreshed. She disliked heat and felt better in cold weather. She often experienced a fall in her level of energy at about 11 A.M. or if she had to stand for any length of time.

PRESCRIPTION & FOLLOW–UP

Based on her symptoms, particularly the itching, Sophie was prescribed *Sulfur*. She was also advised to cut down on refined carbohydrates, to take acidophilic supplements and garlic, and to practice relaxation techniques, meditation, yoga, or t'ai chi. After a couple of months of treatment, the candidiasis disappeared completely, and she felt better. She resolved the conflict regarding her work and the care of her son by taking a job two days a week and finding an excellent babysitter to look after him. Two years later Sophie had another child and was not bothered by candidiasis either during the pregnancy or after the birth. She has kept to a diet that is low in refined carbohydrates but has needed no further treatment.

BREAST PROBLEMS

THE MAIN PROBLEMS affecting the breasts are inflammation (mastitis), breast lumps, and discharges from the nipples. Lumps occur mainly between the ages of 30 and 50, and 80 percent are benign. They should all be investigated promptly by a doctor, however. Regular self-examination and breast awareness are important for all women.

SYMPTOMS

◆ Inflammation: possibly with tender glands under the arms, mild fever (mastitis), cysts (fluid-filled growths or swellings), or boils in the areola (brown areas surrounding the nipples).

◆ Benign lump (fibroadenosis): possible premenstrual tenderness in the breasts.

◆ Abscess: increasingly tender breast and hard, red, and painful spot, possibly accompanied by mild fever and tender glands under the arms.

◆ Tumor: a milky discharge (in women who are not pregnant or lactating) or a dark red discharge from the nipple, possibly accompanied by an unusual retraction of the nipple or an outbreak of eczema around the nipple.

CAUSES

Inflammation of the breast may be caused by a blocked milk duct, or bacteria entering a cracked nipple during lactation, or by infection from an abscess or from elsewhere in the body. Most benign lumps are hormonal in origin.

CONVENTIONAL CARE

Mastitis and abscesses are usually treated with painkillers and antibiotics. An abscess may be surgically incised. Ultrasound, mammography, or biopsy are used to investigate lumps. Biopsy involves either the removal of the lump or the aspiration of fluid in order to identify cancerous cells. Discharge from the nipples may be investigated using the methods above or, in order to indentify infection, by culturing a sample. Hormone levels are also measured.

HOMEOPATHIC MEDICINE

A physical examination and investigative tests will be carried out, and details taken of a woman's gynecological and obstetric history. A homeopath will also study precipitative factors affecting her general health – especially hormonal balances –

in an attempt to identify the underlying causes of breast problems. The choice of constitutional remedy will depend upon individual symptoms (see page 18). Silica is effective for abscesses; while Sulfur may be used to treat infection that has entered through cracked nipples, causing mastitis. Calc. phos. is prescribed for painful breast lumps and swelling; and Conium is used to treat hard tumors. Calc. carb. and Pulsatilla are indicated for lumps or inflammation that occur premenstrually or are linked to hormonal imbalances. Other remedies include Arnica, Causticum, and Lachesis for nipple pain; and Graphites for eczema and cracked, blistered nipples.

Local remedies include Belladonna, if an abscess or mastitis is developing and the breast is red, heavy, throbbing, and painful with the slightest movement; and Bryonia, if a breast is hard and painful with the slightest movement. Conium is given for a breast lump causing discomfort that is better with firm pressure, or for a cyst; and Phytolacca is prescribed for cysts that are tender before and during menstruation.

LIFESTYLE

Regular self-examination of the breasts is very important. It should be done at the same time every month, first standing in front of a mirror to observe any visual changes to the breasts or nipples, then lying down to feel any lumps, thickening, or tenderness in the breasts or armpits. Breast-feeding women with mastitis should bathe the affected breast in hot water, then breast-feed with the baby positioned lower than the affected area of the breast so as to drain the area of milk. A fish- and vegetable-rich diet with no caffeine is advisable for women affected by breast lumps.

CASE HISTORY

Catherine, a 43-year-old former teacher, first started having mild mastitis after a kidney infection. She was prescribed the contraceptive pill, which helped. She also felt better when pregnant. After a couple of miscarriages, however, the mastitis got worse. She was given vitamin B_6 and a hormone regulator, which made the condition worse. Catherine had an irregular menstrual cycle.

PERSONAL DETAILS
Catherine appeared to be easy going, but inside she was a great worrier, and very anxious about what others thought about her. A highly sensitive woman, she was deeply moved by sad stories. At times she felt that she would go insane with pain and discomfort.

FOOD PREFERENCES
Catherine had a craving for boiled eggs, especially when she was premenstrual or pregnant. She also had a desire to eat indigestible items, such as chalk, coal, and pencils, and had a sweet tooth.

GENERAL DETAILS
Catherine felt the cold very easily, but tended to sweat profusely in bed, particularly on the back of her head so that the pillow would become damp. Her feet were often so hot that she had to stick them out of the bed during the night. She felt worse in cold, northeasterly winds, and better when the weather was warm and dry.

PRESCRIPTION & FOLLOW-UP
Catherine was prescribed a variety of homeopathic remedies, including Conium, Lachesis, and Phytolacca, and advised about dietary changes, but nothing brought more than temporary relief. When she was given Calc. carb., however, the mastitis symptoms disappeared completely. After that she had the occasional dose of Calc. carb., but remained largely free of pain and discomfort. During menopause Catherine developed the first symptoms of mastitis that she had experienced in five years. She again responded well to Calc. carb., needing just two or three doses during menopause. She has remained symptom-free ever since.

PROSTATE PROBLEMS

DISORDERS OF THE PROSTATE GLAND rarely occur in men under 30. Enlargement of the prostate, and the consequent pressure on the bladder and urethra, commonly occur among men over 45. Prostatitis, or inflammation of the prostate, usually affects those in their thirties and forties, while prostate cancer generally affects men over 60.

SYMPTOMS

◆ Enlarged prostate: difficulty in starting a stream of urine, weak urine flow, and the need to urinate during the night. In later stages, possible incontinence due to overflow from the bladder and frequency of urination. In severe cases, possible obstruction of urine flow associated with distension of the abdomen.

◆ Prostatitis: pain when passing urine, increased frequency of urination, possible fever, discharge from the penis associated with pain in the colon and lower abdomen, and blood in the urine.

◆ Cancer: symptoms resemble those of an enlarged prostate, but there may be none at all. Possible pain from secondary cancers. If cancer has spread locally, possible urinary obstruction or pelvic pain.

CAUSES

The precise cause of prostate enlargement with age is unknown, although it may be due to an excess of a testosterone-type hormone or to a nutritional deficiency. Prostatitis is caused by a urinary infection, possibly following the use of a catheter or excessive sexual activity. The causes of cancer are unknown (see page 208).

CONVENTIONAL CARE

Prostate enlargement and prostatitis are diagnosed by examination, ultrasound scanning, urinanalysis, and blood tests to check kidney function. Strength of urine flow may be measured. Cancer is detected by examination, scanning, or biopsy. Treatment for an enlarged prostate includes alpha-blockers, which relax smooth muscle thus increasing urinary flow, and testerone-inhibiting drugs, or surgical removal. Prostatitis is treated with antibiotics, and cancer by the conventional methods (see page 208).

HOMEOPATHIC MEDICINE

Treatment is constitutional for all prostate problems, especially if they result from a hormonal imbalance. The choice of remedy will depend upon an individual's symptoms (see page 18). Apis is indicated for an enlarged prostate with urine retention. Baryta carb. is prescribed for enlargement and hardening of the prostate. Conium is often effective for an enlarged prostate accompanied by a discharge of prostatic fluid; and Thuja is used to treat chronic enlargement of the prostate and inflammation associated with infection. Other constitutional remedies commonly used to treat prostate problems include Calc. carb., Lycopodium, Nux vomica, Pulsatilla, and Sulfur.

Remedies for the specific symptoms of an enlarged prostate include Sabal, if urination is difficult or if there are spasms of the bladder or urethra; Baryta carb., when there is a frequent urge to urinate, a slow stream of urine, and impotence; Iodum, when there are shrunken testicles, impotence, and the prostate feels hard; and Argentum nit., for prostate problems associated with erectile dysfunction. For symptoms of prostatitis, Sabal is given if the prostate is enlarged and the area around the gland feels cold; Chimaphila, if prostatic fluid is leaking from the penis and there is urine retention; Selenium, when urine dribbles from the penis and there is impotence; and Capsicum for burning pains in the prostate.

LIFESTYLE

An enlarged prostate may benefit from 15 ml (1 tbsp) of lecithin as instructed, a zinc supplement, and evening-primrose oil. The diet should include plenty of oily fish, but no caffeine, alcohol, or refined sugar. Constipation is to be avoided. Sabal is available in a herbal form called palmetto which is good for prostatitis, as is 10–15 ml (2–3 tsp) cold, pressed linseed oil taken twice a day.

> ### CAUTION
> ◆ If there is a dragging feeling between the legs, difficulty in passing urine, and blood in the urine, or if there is acute urine retention (a few drops may be passed) causing abdominal discomfort, see a doctor as soon as possible.

CASE HISTORY

George was 74 and had a seven-year history of an enlarged prostate. It caused him to urinate every couple of hours, and he had to get up at least three times a night. Following a biopsy, he had been assured that there was no cancer. He had been generally healthy all his life, apart from having a tubercular lymph node removed when he was in his twenties.

PERSONAL DETAILS
This rather shy, apprehensive man was something of a perfectionist. Extremely ambitious, George had progressed to become chairman of one company he worked for and, when seen, had his own consultancy business – for relaxation, he claimed. He found the prospect of addressing large groups of people daunting, but performed well once he had begun.

FOOD PREFERENCES
George disliked extremes of heat and cold. Apart from his prostate problem, he was in extremely good health for his age. He experienced a lot of flatulence, and eating even small amounts of food made him feel full.

GENERAL DETAILS
George had a very sweet tooth and enjoyed alcohol. He liked his foods warm, and hated cold foods or drinks. Oysters, onions, and brassicas such as cabbage upset his digestion.

PRESCRIPTION & FOLLOW-UP
George was prescribed *Phosphorus* as a constitutional remedy and an herbal form of *Sabal* for his symptoms. This treatment reduced his urination at night slightly for a couple of months, after which the frequency increased to what it had been before. He was then prescribed *Lycopodium*, and his condition began to improve generally. He was getting up only once a night – considered to be normal at his age – and his sexual function also improved. George experienced a setback following minor surgery, but again responded well to *Lycopodium*. He continues to get up just once a night, and does not suffer from frequency of urination at all during the day. He takes the occasional dose of *Sabal* if he feels his condition might start to deteriorate.

INFERTILITY

INFERTILITY IS SAID TO EXIST if a couple has been having regular sexual intercourse without the use of contraceptives for more than a year and the woman has not become pregnant. About one in seven couples in the developed world have infertility problems; 30 percent because of the male, 30 percent because of the female, and 40 percent due to both.

SYMPTOMS

◆ Inability to conceive a child despite having regular sexual intercourse without the use of contraceptives.

CAUSES

Male infertility is usually due to a low sperm count, which may be the result of physiological problems, taking drugs, or environmental factors; malformed sperm; or the inability of sperm to reach the egg. It may also be caused by problems in the testicles or vas deferens, often the result of sexually transmitted disease; or malformation of the testes due to an endocrine (glandular) disorder. Erectile dysfuntion or ejaculatory problems may also result in infertility, and this situation may be aggravated by stress, overwork, tiredness, or psychological problems.

The most common cause of female infertility is failure to produce eggs. This may be the result of a hormonal disorder, stress, problems with the ovaries such as cysts, damaged fallopian tubes caused by pelvic inflammatory disease, or uterine abnormalities such as fibroids. The cervical mucus may be too stringy for sperm to get through, or it may contain antibodies that kill sperm. Rarely, defective chromosomes are responsible.

CONVENTIONAL CARE

The full medical history of each partner is studied, physical examinations made, and any sexual problems discussed. Semen analysis and a biopsy of the testes can identify a low sperm count. A postcoital semen test can reveal whether the cervical mucus is deterring the sperm. A temperature chart kept by the woman will reveal if and when ovulation occurs. Hormone levels will be checked and X rays taken. A laparoscopy can explore the fallopian tubes and ovaries.

Artificial insemination can solve the problem of defective sperm. Hormone treatment can be given to either sex, and surgery can repair certain damage to the female reproductive organs. In vitro fertilization is an option for some couples.

HOMEOPATHIC MEDICINE

Provided there are no physiological problems, constitutional treatment will try to rectify imbalances in the body systems controlling reproduction. Remedies are determined largely by an individual's symptoms (*see page 18*). In men, *Aurum met.* is indicated for childhood atrophy of the testes or painful, swollen testicles; and *Causticum* for infertility associated with testicular pain or blood in the spermatic fluid. In women, *Nat. carb.* is prescribed for the nonretention of semen; and *Sepia* when infertility results from a hormonal imbalance and an aversion to sexual intercourse. Although not strictly an infertility problem, *Sabina* is effective for recurrent miscarriage in early pregnancy.

Specific local remedies for men include *Agnus castus*, for erectile dysfunction and a lack of energy; *Conium*, for erectile dysfunction, with cramps and cold legs; and *Lycopodium*, when there is increased sexual desire, but intercourse is spoiled by the anticipation of the failure to conceive. *Conium* is prescribed for women when infertility is associated with breast tenderness and suppressed sexual desire; and *Lycopodium* when there is lower-abdominal tenderness and vaginal dryness.

LIFESTYLE

It is advisable to reduce intake of alcohol and caffeine, and desirable to eat organic foods and those that are high in zinc, such as whole grains and nuts. Drugs such as anabolic steroids and tobacco should be avoided. Overexertion is inadvisable, while relaxation techniques, meditation, and stress-reduction methods are all beneficial. Men should not wear tight-fitting trousers and, if they have a low sperm count, should abstain from sexual intercourse in the week before the woman ovulates. There is some evidence to suggest that adopting the missionary position during intercourse, with the woman remaining still for 20 minutes afterward, will increase the chances of conception. Women are advised not to use vaginal douches, and to substitute egg white for commercial gel lubricants.

CASE HISTORY

Bob and Alice had two children, the first by a difficult forceps delivery and the second delivered normally after some homeopathic treatment. Alice, 35, had then had two miscarriages, since when she had been unable to conceive. Her periods were irregular, and tests showed that she was not ovulating. Bob, 42, had been diagnosed as having a low sperm count and poor mobility of sperm.

PERSONAL DETAILS
The couple had been happily married for 15 years. Alice had been upset by her doctor and hospital staff during the birth of her first child, and she also had problems with her stepmother (her father had remarried after his wife died when Alice was six). Bob was a taciturn, overweight man, who possibly only attended the consultation at his wife's request.

FOOD PREFERENCES
Both had a sweet tooth and ate a lot of refined carbohydrates. Bob drank a lot of coffee. He had a large appetite and felt better after eating. He liked eggs but not fats.

GENERAL DETAILS
Bob felt the cold easily, but sweated at night. Alice also felt the cold. She was worse with emotional stress and in the evening, but revived after midnight. She felt better after hot baths, eating, and massage.

PRESCRIPTION & FOLLOW-UP
Bob and Alice were put on a diet low in refined carbohydrates and caffeine, and given vitamin and mineral supplements. Bob was prescribed *Calc. carb.*, and Alice *Staphysagria*. Alice was advised to write, but not send, letters to the medical staff and her stepmother expressing her feelings. On her return a month later, she reported that Bob had lost 14 lb (6 kg) in weight and felt healthier. Alice felt emotionally relieved but somewhat detached from reality. She stayed on the diet and was given *Anacardium*. One month later Alice became pregnant and was given *Pulsatilla* for morning sickness. She was treated homeopathically to stabilize the pregnancy and relieve symptoms during the next few months before giving birth to a boy.

IMMUNE SYSTEM

T HE IMMUNE SYSTEM is the collective name given to various mechanisms that enable the body to defend itself against invasion by infection-carrying agents such as bacteria, viruses, fungi, and foreign proteins. The skin, certain glands, and the lymphatic system are all part of the immune system.

HOW THE SYSTEM WORKS

Any invading organism trying to enter the body must break down the defensive barriers erected by the immune system. It will probably pass through an area of broken skin or enter the respiratory and digestive tract via the mouth or nose. There are glands along these routes that produce protective enzymes or natural antibiotic secretions, but if an organism does break through into body tissue, the immune system relies heavily on the lymphatic system.

THE LYMPHATIC SYSTEM

This body system consists of lymph vessels that carry lymph from the tissue spaces between cells all over the body to lymph glands, or nodes. Lymph is a clear fluid that derives from plasma in blood from which proteins and other nutrients have been removed. Lymph drains from the bloodstream into capillaries and then into the lymph vessels. The flow of lymph is controlled by muscle contractions and valves. Invading organisms are trapped in lymph glands dotted throughout the lymphatic system. Here they are attacked by scavenging white blood cells called macrophages. Lymph glands also produce lymphocytes, another form of white blood cell. Some lymphocytes (B-cells) produce antibodies that attack antigens on the surface of an invading organism (*see page 206*); other lymphocytes (T-cells) destroy invading organisms directly.

Lymphocytes have the ability to remember invaders that they have come across before, and so respond quickly if the body is invaded again. On the other hand, the immune system can fail to detect invaders, or it can overreact – by developing allergies – or react abnormally to the body's own tissues, as in auto-immune diseases such as rheumatoid arthritis (*see page 197*). Alternatively, it may fail to recognize that its own cells have begun to function abnormally, hence the development of cancer.

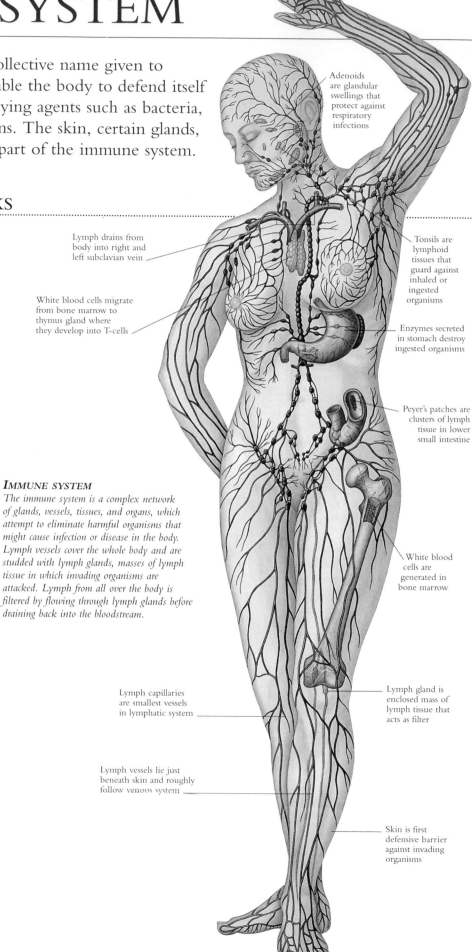

Lymph drains from body into right and left subclavian vein

White blood cells migrate from bone marrow to thymus gland where they develop into T-cells

Adenoids are glandular swellings that protect against respiratory infections

Tonsils are lymphoid tissues that guard against inhaled or ingested organisms

Enzymes secreted in stomach destroy ingested organisms

Peyer's patches are clusters of lymph tissue in lower small intestine

White blood cells are generated in bone marrow

Lymph gland is enclosed mass of lymph tissue that acts as filter

Skin is first defensive barrier against invading organisms

Lymph vessels lie just beneath skin and roughly follow venous system

Lymph capillaries are smallest vessels in lymphatic system

IMMUNE SYSTEM

The immune system is a complex network of glands, vessels, tissues, and organs, which attempt to eliminate harmful organisms that might cause infection or disease in the body. Lymph vessels cover the whole body and are studded with lymph glands, masses of lymph tissue in which invading organisms are attacked. Lymph from all over the body is filtered by flowing through lymph glands before draining back into the bloodstream.

CHRONIC FATIGUE SYNDROME (CFS)

ALSO KNOWN AS myalgic encephalomyelitis (ME), postviral syndrome, and yuppie flu, CFS has only recently been recognized as a condition in conventional medical circles, its symptoms mimicking many other illnesses. It has been described as a physical illness brought on by stress. Three times more women than men are affected in the developed world.

SYMPTOMS

◆ Identifiable fatigue that is present for 50 percent of the time and for at least six months, severely affecting physical and mental functioning.

◆ Muscular pain, weight fluctuation, and sleep disturbance.

◆ Possible abnormal temperature regulation, recurrent sore throat, swelling of the lymph glands, and depression.

CAUSES

CFS often follows a viral infection of the upper respiratory or digestive tract. It is not known why some people do not recover fully. It may be due to malfunctions of the immune or metabolic system, stress, overwork, the overuse of antibiotics, dysfunctional production of the hormone melatonin, the effects on neurotransmitters in the brain of chemicals leaking out of the digestive tract, pollution or toxicity, or even geopathic stress (disruptions in radiation emitted by the Earth).

CONVENTIONAL CARE

There is no single diagnostic test for CFS, and the nature of the condition makes it very difficult to conduct conventional research. A detailed medical history is required, together with a physical examination that concentrates on the body's neurological system. There is no conventional treatment as such. Anti-depressant drugs may be prescribed for sleep disturbances, but lifestyle guidelines form the basis of conventional care.

HOMEOPATHIC MEDICINE

As a result of the large range of physical and mental symptoms possible, CFS is treated constitutionally. Psychological and environmental factors are studied in particular, together with the person's dietary history. The choice of remedy is determined largely by an individual's symptoms (see page 18). Phosphoric ac. is prescribed for weakness in the spinal cord and associated nerves; Nat. mur. is effective for fatigue – affecting the knees, ankles, and dorsal spine in particular – caused by mental exertion. Calc. carb. is used to treat fatigue, particularly of the thigh muscles, caused by walking; and Arsen. alb. is given for fatigue, especially of the chest muscles, caused by walking.

Remedies for localized, specific symptoms include Belladonna, when there are swollen glands in the neck and groin, muscular and joint pains, aches and burning pains all over the body, and a constant sore throat; and Causticum, when there is permanent chilliness, stiffness and pain in the joints and muscles, and weakness after the slightest exertion. Kali carb. may be given for swollen glands in the neck and groin, joint pains, numbness in the throat, panic attacks, and permanent chilliness; Carbo veg. for aches and burning pains all over the body, confusion, bloating and great flatulence, and faintness in the morning; and China for bloating, anxiety, sleeplessness, and a feeling of weakness after the slightest exertion.

LIFESTYLE

The key to recovery from CFS is rest. In planning a strategy for recuperation, it is helpful to imagine the energy of the body as if it were being supplied from checking and savings bank accounts. CFS occurs if the savings account has been seriously depleted over a lengthy period. In order to recover, the savings account needs reimbursing from the checking account. What this means in practical terms is that any activity should leave in reserve 25 percent of the energy normally used when 100 percent is what can be achieved without tiring. So, if someone can walk 100 yards without getting tired, they should only walk 75 yards. A diet that is low in refined carbohydrates, with vitamin and mineral supplements, is beneficial. Recreational drug-taking and smoking are inadvisable, and alcohol intake should be reduced.

ALLERGIES

AN ALLERGY IS DEFINED as a condition that is caused by an inappropriate or exaggerated reaction by the body's immune system. Harmless substances are misidentified by it as potentially dangerous, so the immune response is to form antibodies. These attack the perceived irritants – or allergens – on the surface of the offending substance. The reaction between antibodies and allergens stimulates the release of substances within the body, such as histamine, which cause a variety of irritating symptoms.

SYMPTOMS

◆ Rash or itchy swelling on the skin.

◆ Hay fever: irritation of mucous membranes in the sinuses, causing sneezing and the production of watery phlegm.

◆ Asthma: possible spasms and narrowing of the airways.

◆ Inflamed and possibly watering eyes.

◆ Possible nausea, vomiting, and diarrhea.

◆ In severe cases of type I allergy (*see right*), there is a danger of anaphylactic shock, which is an extreme nervous reaction that includes breathing difficulties, a drop in blood pressure, swelling of the tongue or throat, pain in the abdomen, and diarrhea.

ANTIBODIES AT WORK

REACTING TO ALLERGENS
When under threat from harmful substances – or antigens – the body produces antibodies that attach themselves to special immune cells (mast cells) and can destroy invading particles. An allergic reaction occurs when large numbers of antibodies are activated in response to harmless, misidentified substances called allergens. This triggers the release of histamine, causing unpleasant side effects.

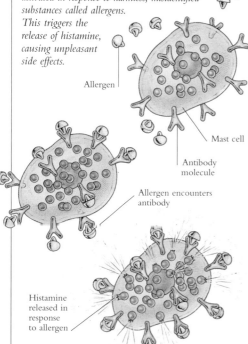

Allergen

Mast cell

Antibody molecule

Allergen encounters antibody

Histamine released in response to allergen

CAUSES

Conventionally, allergies are described in terms of four categories of hypersensitivity reaction. Type I is the most common of the four, and is known as anaphylactic or immediate hypersensitivity. It includes allergies to pollens, animal dander, house dust, house-dust mites, some drugs, yeast, insect venom, and certain foods, especially milk, eggs, shellfish, nuts, and some fruits. These allergens stimulate the body to produce a specific kind of antibody called immunoglobulin E (IgE), which coats cells in the skin, sinuses, lungs, and stomach. When a further exposure to the allergen occurs, the immunoglobulin antibodies become attached to cells in body tissues called mast cells. In response, these cells release chemicals, mainly histamine, which cause allergic reactions. Asthma, hay fever, hives (urticaria), anaphylactic shock, some forms of eczema, and food allergy are type I allergies.

Types II, III, and IV are all much less common than type I. In the case of type II, antibodies bind themselves to antigens on cell surfaces, resulting in the damage to and destruction of cells, as in certain autoimmune disorders. With type III allergies, antibodies combine with antigens to form particles called immune complexes. These travel around the body in the bloodstream and can lodge anywhere, stimulating the immune system further. This mechanism is responsible for reactions to immunization and allergic alveolitis (inflammation of the alveolar walls in the lungs). Type IV is known as delayed hypersensitivity. T-cells (white blood cells) combine with antigens and release chemicals called lymphokines, which cause inflammation. These chemicals are responsible for measles rashes and contact dermatitis.

Another possible cause of allergy considered in complementary medical circles is leaky gut syndrome, whereby cells in the lining of the bowel are not as adherent as they should be. Parts of proteins may pass into the bloodstream, triggering antibody production. Leakage may occur from birth, or be caused by infection or by taking certain drugs.

CONVENTIONAL CARE

Allergies are investigated by means of skin-testing. A small amount of the suspected allergen is pin-pricked under the skin, or placed beneath a patch resembling a bandage, and the reaction monitored. Blood tests can measure the reactions of antibodies and allergens that have been highlighted by dyes. Elimination and challenge, whereby a suspected irritant is removed from the diet or the surroundings for a while and then reintroduced, is another method of allergy identification.

Once an allergen has been identified, the effects of the antibody-antigen reaction can be relieved, using mainly antihistamine drugs. These block the effects of histamine, thus preventing allergic symptoms from developing. Other drugs include sodium chromoglycate, used mainly to treat asthma, and corticosteroids. Allergic skin reactions can be treated with ointments containing corticosteroids. Drugs may be combined with vitamin supplements, reflexology, hypnotherapy, and desensitization, the last of which involves the gradual introduction of the source of irritation in order to increase a person's level of tolerance until they no longer have an allergic reaction.

HOMEOPATHIC MEDICINE

Where there is only one allergy (a fixed allergy), homeopathic treatment is similar to conventional treatment. Constitutional

---

CAUTION

◆ If a person goes into anaphylactic shock, that is, they collapse with pale, cold, and clammy skin, anxiety, nausea, thirst, faintness, or difficulty in breathing, call an ambulance.

◆ If someone who is known to suffer from asthma develops pale, cold, and clammy skin, anxiety, and labored breathing, or their breathing rate exceeds 40 breaths a minute, call an ambulance.

◆ If an asthma sufferer does not respond to any treatment within 12 hours, see a doctor. If their condition appears to be deteriorating rapidly, consult a doctor immediately.

treatment is used to correct imbalances in the body, and to discourage the immune system from overreacting. Such treatment is even more beneficial when there is not a fixed allergy but a cyclic allergy situation. This is when, even though the sources of irritation are removed from the diet, the body develops oversensitivity to something else. In this case, it is necessary to investigate the malfunctioning of the immune system, which may be due to an inherited weakness or body imbalances.

The choice of constitutional remedy will largely be determined by an individual's symptoms (*see page 18*). *Apis* is indicated for allergic swelling of the face, eyelids, lips, or mouth. *Arsen. alb.* is prescribed for allergic reactions associated with the nose such as allergic rhinitis and hay fever. *Calc. carb.* is used to treat allergic reactions of the skin and mucous membranes, while *Carcinosin* is indicated when there are multiple allergies. Other constitutional remedies often used include *Nat. carb.*, *Nat. mur.*, *Nux vomica*, *Pulsatilla*, *Sulfur*, and *Tuberculinum*.

Acute symptoms can be treated with a number of other remedies, such as *Allium cepa*, for hay fever with profuse watering of the eyes and phlegm that irritates and inflames the nostrils and upper lip; and *Arundo*, when there is great itchiness around the nostrils and palate, with sneezing, pain in the bridge of the nose, and copious saliva. *Wyethia* is prescribed for great itchiness in the nose and palate, which the person constantly rubs with the tongue; and *Arum triph.* is effective for cracked lips and hoarseness.

LIFESTYLE

Allergies, like many conditions, tend to become worse if a person is run-down, stressed, overtired, has a poor diet, or does not get adequate exercise. If a food allergy is suspected, the potential irritant should be eliminated from the diet for four days, then reintroduced within 12 days and any changes of symptoms noted. This is a method worth trying for a number of foods, one at a time, until the culprit is isolated. If household products are believed to be the cause of an allergic reaction, the affected person should walk in the open air for an hour, then return home and sniff any strong-smelling products. If a substance provokes excessive sneezing, it is probably the cause of the allergic reaction and should be removed from the home.

CASE HISTORIES

Vera, a 59-year-old housewife, had developed allergic rhinitis when camping in Maine, at age 30. She had what appeared to be cold symptoms that lasted for three months. She then developed prolonged sneezing attacks, during which she felt dreadful. She was allergy-tested and found to be allergic to mold. Desensitization relieved the condition until a recurrence during renovations on Vera's house. She was diagnosed as allergic to grass. All conventional medication upset her, and her condition deteriorated. Symptoms were profuse, watery phlegm, with sneezing and a frontal headache. When first seen, Vera's attacks occurred every four days.

PERSONAL DETAILS
A placid, happy person, Vera had a tendency to be overcritical. During attacks, however, she was tearful, had difficulty speaking, and hated being fussed over. She sighed a lot. She was oversensitive and finicky.

FOOD PREFERENCES
Vera tended to be thirsty rather than hungry, and she liked acidic foods, the fat from meat, and brandy. She liked to drink water little and often, but ice-cold water made her sick.

GENERAL DETAILS
Vera felt the cold very easily, but if she had a headache she liked to put her head out of a window. She loved hot, dry weather and being in bed, and loathed damp weather and autumn.

PRESCRIPTION & FOLLOW-UP
Vera was put on a detoxification program, which had little effect on her condition. She felt that dampness exacerbated her problems. *Nat. sulf.* was prescribed twice a day in damp weather, and *Arsen. alb.* in different potencies for the allergic symptoms. At first Vera lost weight, the rhinitis attacks became less frequent, and a long-standing burning sensation in her feet disappeared. Over the next few months, the attacks diminished even further and, a year on from her initial consultation, the occasional attack was much less severe. A year later she did have a bad attack, but recovered well until a bout of the flu another 12 months later. After she recovered from this the rhinitis cleared up completely, and she was able to stop all medication, including homeopathic remedies.

Jodie was a 40-year-old schoolteacher who had experienced migraines since childhood. They had improved once she identified chocolate, red wine, and citrus fruits as triggers. She also had allergic rhinitis, with heavy and painful sinuses, a dry nose, one-sided headaches, a stiff neck, watery phlegm, and an itchy palate. The rhinitis was triggered by fumes, flowers, house-dust mites, cold wind, and hot air.

PERSONAL DETAILS
Jodie had left a poor American farming community to go to college. She was unattached, but this suited her because her career was important to her. She disliked being overweight, and felt she could achieve more. She was open and sensitive, and liked people to make a fuss of her and reassure her. If overworked, she became apathetic and indifferent.

FOOD PREFERENCES
Jodie liked to drink very cold water and milk. She liked ice cream, fish, and salty, spicy, and acidic foods, but she disliked fruits, and warm foods and drinks, especially coffee.

FEARS
Jodie described many fears, including old age, snakes, heights, and thunderstorms.

GENERAL DETAILS
Jodie felt worse in hot weather, and experienced headaches before thunderstorms. She felt better after eating, with sleep, and a massage. She thought she should have more energy.

PRESCRIPTION & FOLLOW-UP
Jodie was prescribed *Belladonna,* and then had no migraines for a month, although the rhinitis was worse. She was put on a diet to balance her blood-sugar levels, and given antioxidants and chromium and zinc supplements. After feeling ill initially, her energy levels rose, although she still had sinus-related headaches and an occasional migraine. She was given three doses of *Phosphorus*. A month later her sinuses had improved, she was migraine-free, and her energy levels were normal. A fitness regime improved her health further. Now Jodie has an occasional migraine only if she is overworked.

CANCER

CANCER IS A BY-PRODUCT of the growth and repair processes within the body whereby 500 billion new cells are formed each day. Inevitably, some of them are defective, and their growth may become out of control. Defective cells are usually destroyed by the immune system, but if this does not occur, a rapidly dividing colony of cells becomes a tumor that may grow and spread into adjacent body tissue. Cancer may affect major organs, bones, glands, skin, or muscles. Symptoms vary from site to site.

SYMPTOMS

◆ Lumps or changes in the color or other features of the skin.

◆ Symptoms of obstruction in the digestive tract, or hoarseness.

◆ Bleeding from orifices such as the mouth or anus.

◆ Severe, recurrent, or constant headaches.

◆ Ulcers or sores that do not heal.

◆ Changes in bowel habits.

◆ Changes in the breasts.

◆ Painful, numb, or tingling nerves.

◆ Rapid, unexplained weight loss.

CAUSES

The exact causes of cancer are unknown. Most experts agree that probably at least two factors, such as genetic tendency and diet, or pollution and infection, combine to create a disturbance within a cell. Chromosomes may be damaged before birth, as a result of inherited or acquired defects of the immune system, or by radiation, viruses, tobacco smoke, carcinogenic substances such as asbestos, a lack of antioxidants such as vitamins A, C, E, and selenium, other dietary deficiencies, or aging. Complementary medical practitioners believe that other factors are significant too, such as food intolerance, carcinogens in food – for example preservatives, other additives, and pesticide traces – and psychological factors, particularly suppressed emotional shock or great stress. It has also been postulated that some people are more than usually sensitive to geopathic stress (natural radiation emitted by the Earth) or emissions from buildings or power cables.

CONVENTIONAL CARE

Cancer can be detected by cytology tests such as pap smears, X rays, imaging techniques such as mammograms, and chemical markers in the blood, for example, prostate specific antigen, which can identify otherwise undetectable prostate cancer. Often, however, diagnosis of cancer follows the appearance of symptoms and is confirmed by a biopsy.

In most cases, treatment involves radiotherapy, chemotherapy, or surgery, or a combination of these. Radiotherapy uses radiation to reduce and destroy tumors and cancer cells that have spread beyond the original tumor or traveled to other parts of the body (metastasis). Chemotherapy has the same aim but uses anticancer drugs. Surgery removes the primary tumor. The principal aim of conventional methods is to suppress the rate of growth of the cancer. They are more effective with cancers in certain parts of the body than in others.

HOMEOPATHIC MEDICINE

Most homeopathic practitioners would agree that a combination of homeopathic and conventional techniques, along with dietary and other lifestyle changes, is the best program of treatment. The ability of a cancerous growth to destroy the surrounding healthy tissue has to be dealt with quickly, and conventional medicine can do this. Homeopathy, on the other hand, attempts to address the underlying causes. As with other chronic ailments, this takes the form of constitutional assessment. Of particular interest is the psychological makeup of a person, especially signs of severe emotional stress that might have impaired immunity. Constitutional remedies will be largely

HOW CANCER DEVELOPS

ABNORMAL CELL DIVISION
All cells multiply by dividing into two. This is usually controlled so that just the right amount of cell division occurs to replace dead or damaged cells. This process sometimes proceeds at an abnormally fast rate, however, creating a tumor. As it grows, cells force their way into neighboring tissues or organs. Rogue cells from a tumor in the skin, for example, can then travel via the lymphatic system to other parts of the body, where secondaries may form.

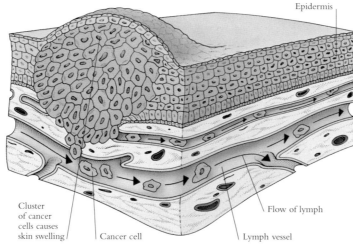

Epidermis
Cluster of cancer cells causes skin swelling
Cancer cell
Flow of lymph
Lymph vessel

CAUTION

Although many of these symptoms may not necessarily be indicative of cancer, it is wise to consult a doctor about any of the following:

◆ Persistent lump or thickening anywhere on the skin or in a testicle or breast.
◆ Unexplained swelling of a limb.
◆ Enlargement, bleeding, irritation or other change in the appearance of a mole.
◆ Severe recurrent headaches.
◆ Difficulty in swallowing.
◆ Hoarseness that lasts for more than a month.

◆ Difficulty in passing urine.
◆ Unexplained weight loss of more than about 1 lb (0.5 kg) a week.
◆ Unusual bleeding from the mouth, nipples, anus, or genitals, or the coughing up of blood.
◆ Bleeding from the vagina between menstrual periods and altered bleeding during them.
◆ Persistent indigestion.
◆ Abdominal pain or change in bowel habits unrelated to dietary changes.
◆ Sores that do not heal.

determined by an individual's symptoms (*see page 18*), but *Arsen. alb.* is often indicated for cancers with burning pain and in any location. *Bromium*, on the other hand, is effective for breast cancer in particular. *Carbo an.* is used to treat cancers of the breast, stomach, uterus, and glands in the later stages, while *Nitric ac.* is associated with cancer of the breast, uterus, vagina, and rectum. Other constitutional remedies often used to treat cancer are *Conium, Lycopodium, Hydrastis, Phosphorus,* and *Silica*. Those associated with cancer in particular organs include *Phosphorus, Calcium, Fluoric ac., Conium,* and *Hecla* for bones; *Crotalus* and *Kali. mur.* for connective tissue; and *Carbo an., Conium,* and *Aurum mur.* for glands.

OTHER TREATMENTS

It is generally acknowledged that dietary excess or deficiency may predispose an individual to the formation of cancer. Controversy surrounds the use of dietary treatment for the disease, but it can play a supportive role. Most therapies have their origins in the Gerson treatment based on an initially vegan, then lactovegetarian diet, along with fruit and vegetable juices and coffee enemas to detoxify the liver.

Many nutritional therapies include high doses of antioxidants to counteract cellular damage inflicted by free radicals in the bloodstream. These are absorbed from the environment as well as foods. Other complementary therapies use combinations of herbs or substances such as extractions of mistletoe and shark cartilage, but many await further trials.

LIFESTYLE

The diet should include plenty of unrefined carbohydrates and fresh fruits and vegetables, but few animal fats or animal proteins. Nutritional supplements prescribed by a doctor may safely be accompanied by over-the-counter antioxidants, and are advisable during radiotherapy or chemotherapy. Adequate physical exercise is desirable, although symptoms may restrict choice.

Emotional or other psychological problems need to be tackled. Meditation, prayer, and relaxation may help to establish a positive outlook and strengthen the will to live. Visualization techniques can be used to encourage the destruction of the cancer by treatment, and to focus on a fully functioning immune system.

CASE HISTORIES

Clarissa, 69, had had her left breast removed eight years previously, followed by the right breast and associated lymph glands two years after that. One year before her consultation, an X ray had revealed secondary cancers in the ribs, lungs, and scar tissue. Chemotherapy eliminated the skin cancer, but Clarissa did not respond well to the treatment. She recovered but developed back pain due to secondaries in the spine. Chemotherapy was again unsuitable for Clarissa, who was then given steroids and sent home to die.

PERSONAL DETAILS
Of Jewish origin, Clarissa had fled Nazi Germany in 1933. She was tense, with a quick temper. She felt a great need for fresh air and lacked strength. She believed her role was to keep her family happy, but had argued with her daughter and son-in-law over religion. Each breast operation followed a driving test, which she failed as a result of anxiety.

FOOD PREFERENCES
Clarissa had put herself on a vegan diet for the cancer and because she hated meat. Her appetite was not good. She craved ice cream and disliked warm foods. She liked salad vegetables, whole-wheat bread, and oats, but disliked legumes and beans.

GENERAL DETAILS
Clarissa felt the cold but loved the open air. She preferred wet, humid weather. She was sensitive to light and noise, disliked mental exertion, and felt sick if she became nervous.

PRESCRIPTION & FOLLOW-UP
It was decided to detoxify Clarissa with a variation of the Gerson diet. Her drugs were gradually reduced to low dosages, and she was then given *Silica*. Within three months she was stronger and off the steroids. The levels of red and white cells in her blood were improving, although she still had back pain, for which *Chelidonium* was prescribed. She could soon climb stairs easily as her energy levels rose. She was then given injections of bamboo to strengthen her back. Over the next two years her energy levels and appetite continued to improve. She was seen once a year until she died, at age 86. The cause of death was unknown.

Sheila was a 41-year-old personnel manager. She had been diagnosed nine months before her consultation with a malignant melanoma on her left breast. The growth was removed, followed by another. She was worried about a melanoma on her right foot, and she also complained of a recurrent sore throat, premenstrual problems, and joint pain. On examination, she had tenderness in the left breast and lower abdomen, and a melanoma on the left foot.

PERSONAL DETAILS
Sheila had been insecure as a child despite a supportive family. She had a successful career, but her first husband had been violent. She was now remarried, but her husband had had a mild heart attack, and Sheila was angry that her new-found happiness was threatened. She was open, vital, friendly, and enthusiastic. Despite appearing confident, she needed reassurance. She was businesslike, competent, and thrived on the stress of a high-powered job.

FOOD PREFERENCES
Sheila had a good appetite. She craved sweet foods, especially before menstruation. She liked salt, the fat on meat, and acidic and spicy foods, but not vegetables. She had begun to modify her diet.

GENERAL DETAILS
Sheila felt worse after a bath and from being overheated, which made her skin itch. She was better after walking in the open air. Talking sometimes exhausted her.

PRESCRIPTION & FOLLOW-UP
Sheila was prescribed *Sulfur* and advised to reduce her workload and take beta-carotene and vitamin C. She also went on a variation of the Gerson diet. Within six months she felt a lot better, her menstrual periods had improved, and the joint pain she had experienced had gone. The melanomas on her feet were noninvasive and surgery was not required. Sheila was also suffering from irritable bowel syndrome. Nutritional supplements helped, but symptoms returned if Sheila's work became too stressful. A year later, the *Sulfur* was repeated because of further menstrual problems, but five years later Sheila has had no further melanomas.

MIND & EMOTIONS

A GREAT DEAL IS ALREADY KNOWN about the location of certain mental functions in different areas of the brain. There remain many gaps in this knowledge, however, especially concerning the nature of the emotions and consciousness, and the links between brain activity and psychiatric illness. The workings of the body, mental functions, and the expression of emotions are believed to be closely linked by a part of the brain known as the limbic system.

HOW THE LIMBIC SYSTEM WORKS

The limbic system lies in the midbrain area. The word "limbic" means "border" or "boundary," and the limbic system forms the border between the higher, more complex, mental processes and emotional facilities of the cerebral cortex – the folded gray matter in the outer brain – and less complex centers of the brain, such as the hypothalamus, which control automatic body functions. Unlike less complex parts of the brain, where information received (*see page 178*) undergoes only rudimentary filtering, in higher areas of the brain information from the peripheral nervous system is subjected to elaborate perception processes involving memory, decision-making, and other thought processes.

The limbic system plays a role in the expression of instinctive responses relating to survival, emotions and the effects of mood on behavior, and the activities of what are known as neurotransmitters – a sort of chemical messenger. Some of these are mood enhancers, and a deficiency may contribute to depression.

COMPLEX INTERACTIONS

The highly complex nature of interactions that take place in the brain, together with consciousness, higher emotions, and spiritual feelings, produce unique and complex patterns of behavior. The expression of grief, for example, differs greatly from individual to individual. It is therefore difficult to draw a line between balance and imbalance on mental or emotional levels. In addition, mental health is determined largely by what is acceptable or tolerable either to an individual or to the society in which they live. Many mental and emotional problems, such as phobias, are rooted in childhood experiences and are affected by illnesses and stress. In tackling and solving mental and emotional problems, a person often has to recognize and come to terms with factors that make him what he is.

LOCATION OF THE LIMBIC SYSTEM
The limbic system forms a boundary between the cortical and midbrain areas such as the thalamus and mamillary bodies.

COMPONENTS OF THE LIMBIC SYSTEM
The various parts of this circular-shaped system are extremely important in the expression of human basic instincts, drives, and emotions. The links between the limbic system and sensory structures help to explain why a sense of smell can evoke a memory or emotion.

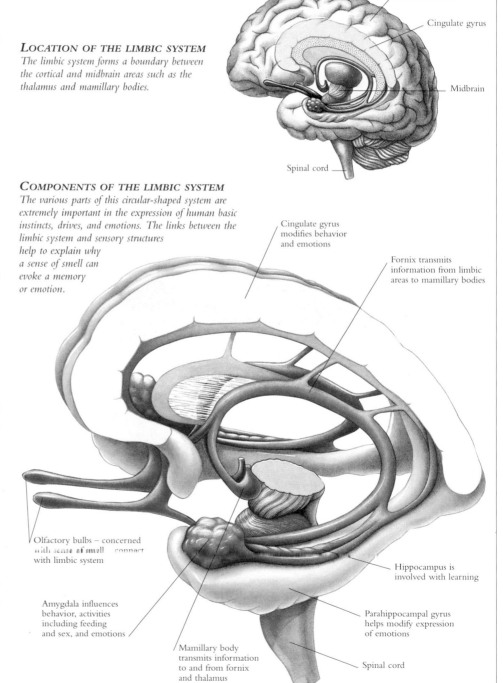

Cerebral cortex

Cingulate gyrus

Midbrain

Spinal cord

Cingulate gyrus modifies behavior and emotions

Fornix transmits information from limbic areas to mamillary bodies

Olfactory bulbs – concerned with sense of smell connect with limbic system

Amygdala influences behavior, activities including feeding and sex, and emotions

Mamillary body transmits information to and from fornix and thalamus

Hippocampus is involved with learning

Parahippocampal gyrus helps modify expression of emotions

Spinal cord

PHOBIAS

A PHOBIA IS A FEAR so disabling that it affects a person's ability to cope with everyday life. Minor phobias are extremely common, but most people learn either to keep them in check or to overcome their fears. Someone who is seriously phobic will be overtaken by an intense, irrational fear when confronted by the object of their phobia.

SYMPTOMS

- Intense anxiety, even a panic attack, when faced with the object of the phobia.
- Possible depression.
- Possible obsessive–compulsive behavior in order to avoid the perceived harmful effects of the feared object.
- Possible attempt to relieve the anxiety by consuming alcohol or drugs.

CAUSES

A phobia may be the result of a personal past experience that was extremely unpleasant, or it may be "inherited," from a parent for example. It may be a fear that has been transferred from another object or set of circumstances, or dredged up from the collective unconscious – a term that is used to describe the collective memory of the human species. Occasionally, phobias can be due to organic disease such as epilepsy or to a brain tumor.

There are various types of phobia. These include a fear of animals such as dogs, mice, spiders, or snakes, or a fear of situations, such as enclosed spaces (claustrophobia), or open or public places (agoraphobia). Social phobias involve a dread of being in public, and anxiety about being observed by other people. They may lead ultimately to an inability to speak or perform in public, to eat out in a restaurant, or even, in severe cases, to use any public facilities at all.

CONVENTIONAL CARE

If, on examination, no organic cause of a phobia is found, antianxiety drugs such as tranquilizers may be prescribed. More commonly, antidepressant drugs are given, especially the "new" selective serotonin reuptake inhibitors (SSRIs) such as Prozac. These drugs are often combined with some form of behavioral therapy. This may involve desensitization techniques, whereby the person is increasingly exposed to the object of fear while, at the same time, being instructed in relaxation techniques.

HOMEOPATHIC MEDICINE

Just as a person's psychological state provides clues about remedies for physical conditions, with a condition such as phobia it is often the accompanying physical symptoms that indicate a specific constitutional remedy (*see page 18*). *Argentum nit.* is prescribed for multiple phobias associated with anxiety neuroses that originate in previous experiences. *Calc. carb.* may be used to treat fears of heights and open spaces; while *Calc. phos.* is often prescribed for phobias centered around school. *Phosphorus* is used for fears that develop into phobias when the sufferer spends too much time alone. Other consitutional remedies include *Aurum met.*, *Graphites*, *Ignatia*, *Lycopodium*, *Nat. carb.*, *Psorinum*, *Sepia*, and *Stramonium*.

Remedies given for specific symptoms include *Borax*, for fear of heights associated with a sensation of falling; *Sulfur*, when a fear of heights is associated with great giddiness; and *Gelsemium*, for a fear of appearing in public associated with weak limbs. *Anacardium or.* is used to treat the sensation of having a plug in the stomach, especially in performers; and *Aconite* is given for a fear of dying with palpitations.

LIFESTYLE

Particularly in the case of claustrophobia, agoraphobia, and some animal phobias, if the motivation is strong enough, it may be possible to desensitize oneself by very gradual exposure to the object of fear. It is advisable at the same time to learn simple breathing or relaxation techniques, or practice yoga, meditation, or t'ai chi. Breathing techniques are able to defuse anxiety when it threatens to overwhelm. Drugs and alcohol should not be used in an attempt to suppress fear since this may lead to dependence.

CAUTION
- If a person is feeling suicidal, contact their doctor or a counseling service immediately.
- If simple fear is greatly interfering with daily activities, consult a doctor.

CASE HISTORY

Maria, 24, was phobic about having contracted AIDS. She was unable to touch anything for fear of passing it to others and suffering unbearable guilt as a result. Maria's fears had been exacerbated after she terminated a pregnancy, causing her to feel extremely guilty.

PERSONAL DETAILS
Maria had been the victim of bullying at school. She had left college because of depression and agoraphobia. She was sensitive, lacked confidence, and felt detached from herself. She would decide on a course of action, but would then doubt that she could see it through. She had received psychiatric help.

FOOD PREFERENCES
Maria craved sweet foods, vinegar, and fat, particularly the fat on meat. She hated licorice, and avocados and bananas upset her digestion. She felt as though there was a plug at the end of her gullet.

GENERAL DETAILS
Maria felt generally ill after studying or emotional stress. She disliked drafts and the open air – particularly if it was cold – and was sensitive to strong smells. She felt worse in the morning and evening, but better after eating and hot baths. She was prone to eczema on her wrists, and had lost more than 20 lb (9 kg) in weight over nine months.

PRESCRIPTION & FOLLOW-UP
Maria was given *Anacardium or.* and advised to write about the abortion to release her suppressed feelings. One month later she felt better and was less depressed. She was better able to make decisions, except before menstruation. She was given *Alumina* to take premenstrually. Soon after Maria went into dramatic decline, having learned that the father of the baby she had lost might move into the area. She felt angry, guilty, and hurt. *Anarcardium or.* was repeated and, with behavioral therapy, she was able to overcome her phobia. It recurred briefly, but over the next few months, with *Lac. can.* for fatigue and headaches that she had developed and repeat doses of *Anacardium or.*, Maria's phobia was fully overcome.

DEPRESSION

MEDICALLY SPEAKING, depression is more than the sadness many people feel periodically. It combines despondency, hopelessness, apathy, and a lack of well-being, and can persist for some time. There may be physical symptoms. In parts of the developed world one person in 25 feels depressed enough at some point in their life to seek professional help.

SYMPTOMS

♦ Slow thinking, inability to concentrate, indecision, general lack of interest, and recurrent thoughts about death.

♦ Increase or decrease in appetite or weight, slowing down of movement, and loss of energy.

CAUSES

Depression may have an obvious external cause, such as the death of a loved one. It may follow a viral infection, childbirth, or be caused by chemical imbalances in the body. These may occur naturally, for example, due to an underactive thyroid gland, or result from taking prescribed drugs, such as the contraceptive pill or sleeping pills, or from drug or alcohol addiction. Periods of depression may alternate with impulsive, energetic behavior – a condition known as manic depression. There is an affliction called seasonal affective disorder (SAD), whereby people become depressed in winter, possibly due to insufficient sunlight.

More often, however, depression is a spiritual problem, involving a negative attitude to life that leads to feelings of fear, anger, guilt, and frustration, possibly accompanied by a sense of persecution, loneliness, and hopelessness. Severely depressed people may become suicidal or experience delusions. Long-term depression may result from childhood trauma such as the death of a parent.

CONVENTIONAL CARE

Mild depression may be treated with antidepressant drugs, sometimes together with psychotherapy or psychoanalysis. Severe depression is still treated with electroconvulsive therapy (ECT), but only after all other methods have failed.

HOMEOPATHIC MEDICINE

Most homeopathic practitioners treat depression constitutionally. Remedies are determined largely by an individual's symptoms (see page 18). It may be the case that if emotional problems are alleviated, physical problems come to the fore (see page 19). *Aurum met.* is associated with the kind of despair that might lead to suicide; while *Causticum* is indicated for a feeling of loss of control. *China* is prescribed for low spirits following menstruation or associated with neuralgic pain; and *Lachesis* is given for premenstrual or menopausal depression. *Nat. mur.* is used for depression associated with the suppression of grief. Other remedies prescribed constitutionally include *Arsen. alb.*, *Calc. carb.*, *Graphites*, *Lycopodium*, *Nat. carb.*, *Platina*, *Pulsatilla*, *Sepia*, *Sulfur*, and *Thuja*.

Specific remedies include *Ignatia*, when depression results from bereavement or the breakup of a relationship; or *Cadmium sul.*, after a viral illness such as infectious mononucleosis that produces a lack of energy. *Nux vomica* is used when there is great irritability, extreme chilliness, and extreme criticism of others; while *Aconite* is often given for the sudden onset of depression following a fright or shock, and which is linked with a fear of death.

LIFESTYLE

If minor depression is brought on by overwork or stress, time-management techniques will provide for the prioritization of tasks and time out for relaxation and the pursuit of interests. A sense of isolation can be reduced by taking up an interest that involves meeting new people. Those often confined to the home should arrange to go out frequently. Mild depression can be helped by dietary changes, especially the elimination of caffeine and the inclusion of vitamin and mineral supplements. Some prescribed drugs may have depressive side effects. It might be worth consulting a doctor with a view to changing the prescription.

CAUTION

♦ If symptoms of depression last for more than a month, consult a doctor.

♦ If a depressed person is talking about suicide, alert their doctor or a counseling service.

CASE HISTORY

Rosa, a 30-year-old Argentinian, had been depressed for about a year. The depression had started after she gave birth, but she attributed it initially to an exhausting house move six months before. She was tearful, anxious, and fearful that she might kill her children. She felt physically and mentally exhausted, was too depressed to answer the telephone, and felt she would never recover. She was taking antidepressant drugs.

PERSONAL DETAILS
At the age of 19, Rosa had married an Englishman and moved to England. She described herself as a very organized perfectionist. She was sensitive to those close to her to the extent of having prophetic dreams about them, particularly her children.

FOOD PREFERENCES
Rosa was often very thirsty and loved cold fruit juices and milk, ice cream, and salty and spicy foods. She disliked fruits, warm foods and drinks, coffee, onions, and tomatoes.

GENERAL DETAILS
Rosa could sleep only lying on the right side. She felt faint if she put her hands in cold water and suffered indigestion and constipation. She had headaches before thunderstorms. She improved after catnaps and a massage.

PRESCRIPTION & FOLLOW-UP
On the basis of her digestive problems and irrational fears, Rosa was given *Argentum nit.* Her digestion and energy levels improved, but she developed headaches, for which she was given *Bryonia.* She was put on a lactovegetarian diet and advised to have physiotherapy for muscle spasms in her neck. She stopped taking the antidepressants, but felt weepy and irritable. Over a few months she took doses of *Pulsatilla*, *Ammonium carb.*, *Coffea*, and *Phosphorus*, the last of which made her feel much better. On visiting Argentina she felt extremely well, but a significant decline on her return revealed great homesickness. *Phosphorus* revived her, and she took a part-time job. A car accident and two stress-related illnesses set her back, but again she responded to *Phosphorus* and is on the whole no longer depressed.

GRIEF

GRIEF IS A PERFECTLY NATURAL REACTION to the loss of a loved one, an animal, a job, a house, or anything in which a great amount of emotion has been invested. The grieving process has definite stages through which most individuals must pass in order to come to terms with their loss and resolve the situation satisfactorily.

SYMPTOMS OF STAGES

◆ Initial sense of unreality or numbness.

◆ Refusal to believe that the loss has occurred, with hallucinations of a loved one or the feeling that they are present. This can last for up to three months.

◆ Series of complex emotions such as guilt (for example, for not spending more time with the lost person) and anger (for example, with God for taking the person or with the doctors for not doing enough to save the deceased's life), leading to despair and depression, possibly associated with bowel upsets, mental disorders, and even a susceptibility to suicide.

◆ State of depression with a tendency to increase the use of drugs or alcohol, sleeping problems, general feelings of a lack of well-being, agitation, and tearfulness. Eventually, life becomes bearable, and even enjoyable, but the whole process may take up to two years or more. There is some evidence that the death of a partner may increase the chance of death in the bereaved.

CONVENTIONAL CARE

Treatment of long-term depression may require the involvement of a psychiatrist, in conjunction with antidepressant drugs, psychotherapy, and counseling. Help may also be obtained from a variety of support groups and religious organizations.

HOMEOPATHIC MEDICINE

Homeopathic remedies can help at each stage of the grieving process. If a person does not appear to be recovering, however, constitutional treatment may be necessary, the remedy depending on individual symptoms (*see page 18*). *Aurum met.* is indicated for those who are grieving over the loss of a loved one or the failure of a business. *Causticum* is given for chronic, long-term grief and feelings akin to grief that are triggered by childbirth; *Ignatia* is used to treat the initial impact of grief; and *Phosphoric ac.* is used in the treatment of grief associated with great exhaustion.

Staphysagria is indicated for suppressed grief that is linked to embarrassment or humiliation. Other remedies prescribed constitutionally include *Lachesis*, *Nat. mur.*, and *Phosphorus*.

Remedies specifically for the early stages of grief include *Arnica*, when the grieving person wants to be left alone, insists they are all right, rejects physical comfort, and displays the reactions of a person in shock; *Aconite*, if there is great fear and the person is on the verge of collapse, having witnessed a violent death for example; and *Opium*, when the bereaved is literally numb with grief, and is very frightened by the death of their loved one. In the later stages of grief, *Nux vomica* is indicated when there is great anger and criticism of others, and *Pulsatilla* is prescribed for tearfulness at the slightest provocation, insomnia, and recurrent colds accompanied by yellow or green phlegm.

LIFESTYLE

The most important thing for a grieving person to do is to express their emotions. If they have difficulty talking about their problems, they should write down their thoughts, paint a picture, or use some other form of expression. Bottling up emotions may lead to chronic depression or lowered resistance to physical illnesses. Relaxation techniques or massage may also be of great benefit.

It is also important that someone who is grieving is kind to and patient with themselves. They may believe that life will never be the same again, but time does heal, and their anguish will lessen. If progress through the grieving process is slow, however, talking to a counselor who has received specific training in dealing with grief, such as those working for support groups, is advisable.

CAUTION

◆ If grief lasts for more than 18 months, seek professional help.

◆ If a depressed person is talking about suicide, alert their doctor or a counseling service.

CASE HISTORY

Celia was 54 and was seen after her daughter had drowned while on vacation in Italy. Celia was distraught. She described feeling terrified on waking at the realization that her daughter was dead, and feared that she was losing her sanity. She had received a lot of support from her church and did not want to take conventional drugs.

PERSONAL DETAILS
It was impossible to assess Celia at first due to her appalling grief. Normally, she would not be seen to cry, would bottle up her feelings, and be reluctant to confide in others. She hated fuss, but became irritated if not shown any attention. Celia felt that she had to be strong for others in times of crisis. Her greatest fear was of her home being burglarized.

FOOD PREFERENCES
Celia craved salty and acidic foods, and liked starchy foods, but nothing slimy, such as shellfish. She disliked rich foods, meats, and coffee.

GENERAL DETAILS
Celia felt better in the open air on cool days, but was exhausted by heat. She was worse if her eyes got tired, and was sensitive to noise.

PRESCRIPTION & FOLLOW-UP
Celia was treated with *Phosphoric ac.* A month later, she was still feeling guilty about her daughter's death and was given *Nat. mur.* This relieved the guilt, but Celia missed her daughter terribly. She tried several Bach remedies and gradually improved until the anniversary of the death, when she developed cystitis. For this she was given *Pulsatilla*. Over several years she was treated homeopathically for a variety of ailments, including high blood pressure caused by the stress of caring for her granddaughter. *Nat. mur.* and relaxation therapy helped, but she also had to take hypotensive drugs. She was generally well until her son committed suicide 12 years after his sister's death. Celia sank into deep despair, angry that her family had been made to suffer so much. She was prescribed *Ignatia* and then *Nat. mur.* over four months, and was able to work through her anger and the depression that followed.

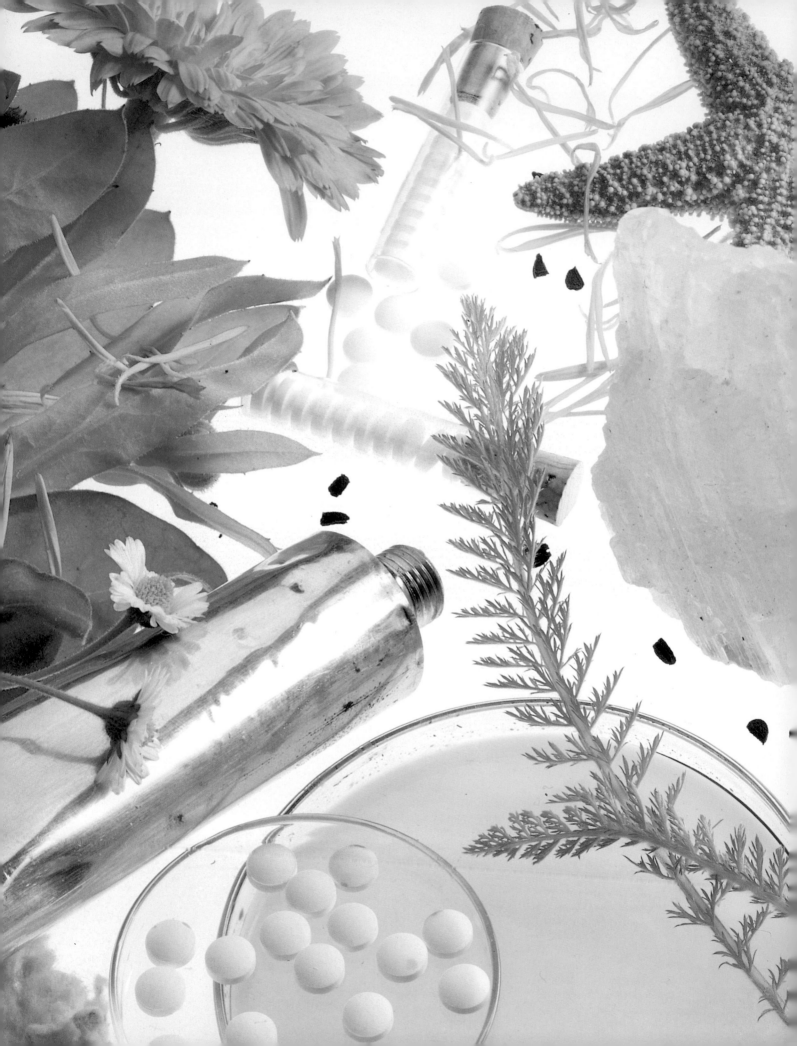

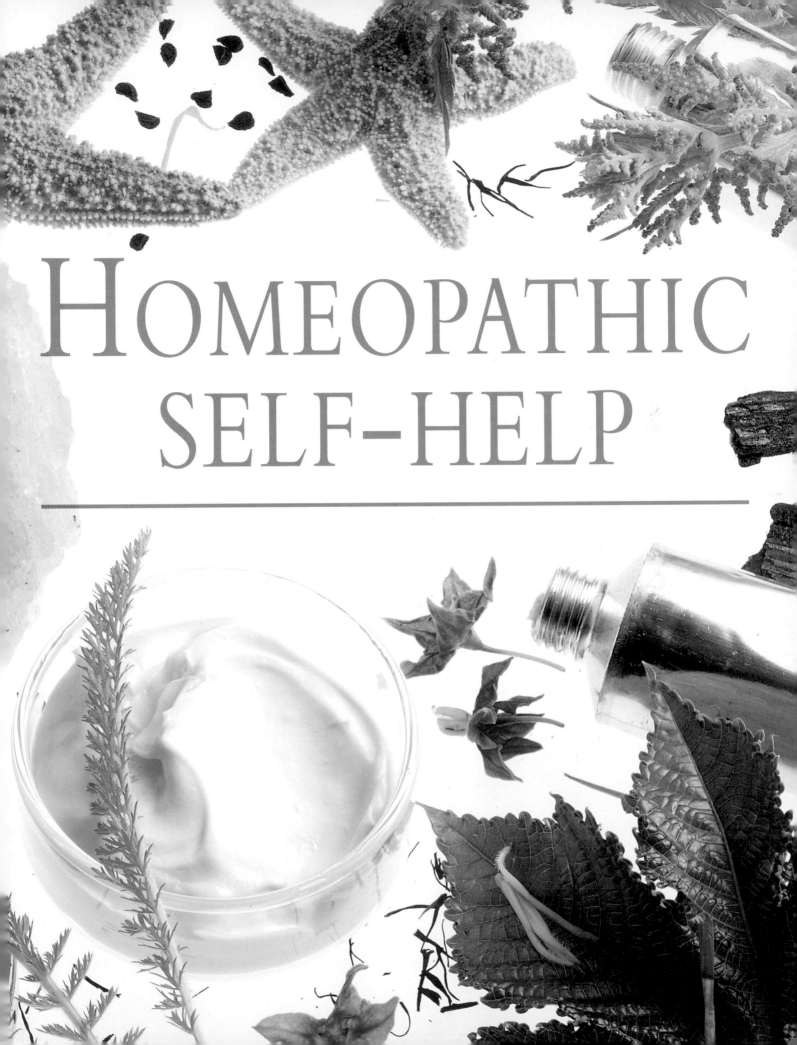

HOMEOPATHIC
SELF-HELP

CHOOSING A REMEDY

HOMEOPATHIC REMEDIES can be used effectively and safely by lay people to treat many minor ailments and injuries. Careful observation enables a person to select a remedy to match their symptoms. While not necessarily providing an instant cure, a homeopathic remedy is believed to encourage the body's self-healing mechanisms and nurture a sense of well-being, good energy levels, and a resistance to ill-health. A remedy can be helped to work by adopting a lifestyle that will promote good health and a positive outlook.

CONDUCTING SELF-PRESCRIPTION

A person must first decide whether or not it is safe to self-prescribe. Some symptoms (see Warning symptoms, *page 9*) may be indicative of a serious ailment and require the immediate attention of a conventional doctor. If pharmaceutical drugs are already being taken, it may be necessary to consult a doctor before considering additional medication. Babies and small children, pregnant women, the elderly, and those with chronic medical conditions need careful consideration in terms of self-help treatment (*see* Safety issues, *page 9*).

IDENTIFYING SYMPTOMS

A diagnostic picture needs to be compiled in order to self-prescribe. A person must describe the characteristics of his or her symptoms (*see right*) or, if prescribing for someone else, make a note of what can be seen or heard, and what is reported by the patient. Some symptoms may be associated with other manifestations of an ailment, or with a particular state of mind. A fever may develop after a person becomes wet and chilled, for example; a headache may follow a head injury; or diarrhea may be linked with anxiety.

BUILDING SYMPTOM PICTURES

Armed with a "symptom picture," a person can proceed to the homeopathic directory (*see pages 218–69*) in which symptom descriptions can be compared and suitable remedies identified. Some symptoms are common to several ailments. A sore throat may be indicative of a cold, the flu, or laryngitis. It may be necessary, therefore, to study the symptom pictures of several ailments, comparing the accompanying physical symptoms and psychological symptoms listed. The remedy lists in the self-help section that follows are not exhaustive, but are common examples of homeopathic treatment for minor ailments. It is not necessary to exhibit all the symptoms listed, nor to match all the better or worse factors, for a remedy to be suitable. One can be chosen on the basis of the main symptoms, the likely cause, and onset characteristics.

DIAGNOSTIC CHECKLIST

WHAT ARE YOUR MOST OBVIOUS PHYSICAL SYMPTOMS?	**Examples**: pain, soreness, inflammation, skin eruption, itching, bleeding, nausea, vomiting, diarrhea, sore throat, cough, fever, fainting, dizziness, headache.
ARE MAIN SYMPTOMS ACCOMPANIED BY LESS ACUTE SYMPTOMS?	**Examples**: perspiration, chilliness, great thirst, desire for or aversion to certain foods, loss of appetite, sensitivity to touch, weak limbs, coated tongue, swollen glands.
WHAT ARE THE CHARACTERISTICS OF YOUR SYMPTOMS?	**Examples**: location in the body, sudden or gradual onset, constant or intermittent occurrence, frequency of recurrence.
DO YOU HAVE ANY PSYCHOLOGICAL SYMPTOMS?	**Examples**: restlessness, irritability, anger, anxiety, tearfulness, self-pity, emotional oversensitivity, indifference, desire to be alone, irrational fears, desire for sympathy.
ARE YOU AWARE OF ANY OBVIOUS CAUSE OF THE SYMPTOMS?	**Examples**: injury, viral infection, bacterial infection, exposure to extremes of temperature or strong wind, stress, anxiety, grief, overwork.
DO YOUR SYMPTOMS GET BETTER OR WORSE IN CERTAIN CONDITONS?	**Examples**: warmth or cold, fresh air, application of hot or cold compresses, sitting or standing, lying in a particular way, physical or mental exertion, emotional stress.

TYPES OF REMEDY

Lactose tablets are the most common form of homeopathic remedy, although sucrose tablets are available for those who are lactose-intolerant. Dissolved under the tongue, a remedy enters the bloodstream directly. Remedies come in different forms (*see below, left*), and choice depends upon personal preference or aptitude for taking medication (*see* Administering remedies, *page 271*). Homeopathic mother tinctures can be diluted to make soothing solutions (*see page 271*), and ointments and creams can be applied directly. Biochemic tissue salts are minerals that are taken individually or in combination to treat common ailments. They can be used on their own or with other homeopathic remedies.

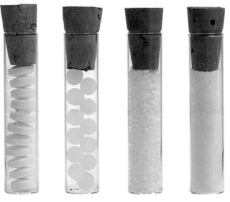

FORMS OF HOMEOPATHIC REMEDY
Homeopathic remedies are available in different potencies (see page 28) and a variety of forms; from left to right, tablets, pilules, granules, and powder.

PROMOTING RECOVERY

It is best to take only one homeopathic remedy at a time. Repeating the dosage relies on being able to assess whether or not a remedy has worked and symptoms have improved. It is also advisable to follow certain guidelines (*see page 176*). All remedies are best combined with good nutrition, a low-stress environment, exercise, and emotional and intellectual states that promote balanced body systems.

HELPING REMEDIES TO WORK

A homeopathic remedy helps the body to heal itself. This self-healing can be encouraged, and future health and well-being promoted, by a series of measures put in place along with the treatment (*see below*). The importance of a good, balanced diet and adequate exercise is obvious, but many other aspects of a person's life, such as how they combine work and play, whether or not they have a network of family and friends, and their general outlook on life, can help or hinder healing.

COMPLEMENTARY LIFESTYLE GUIDE

EATING FOR HEALTH
◆ Obtain protein from vegetarian sources rather than meat and dairy products.
◆ Eat foods that are rich in vitamins and minerals or take supplements.
◆ Cut down on refined carbohydrates, salt, animal fats, sugar, yeast, and processed foods.
◆ Drink plenty of fluids.
◆ Reduce consumption of caffeine and alcohol.
◆ Eat regular meals.
◆ Lose weight if necessary.
◆ Consult a dietician about specific needs.
◆ Include plenty of fiber in the diet.
◆ Use healthy cooking methods, for example broiling rather than frying.

KEEPING IN SHAPE
◆ Learn breathing techniques to maximize the benefits of exercise.
◆ Include exercise in a daily routine, for example climb stairs rather than take an elevator.
◆ Plan a weekly exercise program.
◆ Aim to improve energy levels, brain-power, and mood.
◆ Choose activities for specific purposes such as muscle coordination, strength, and endurance, cardiovascular endurance, or flexibility.
◆ Always warm up before exercising and stretch out afterward.
◆ Use exercise as a means of getting time to yourself, or meeting people, or as a challenge.

IMPROVING SURROUNDINGS
◆ Prohibit smoking at home and at work.
◆ Reduce the risk of allergies by keeping the home dust-free.
◆ Use environmentally friendly household products rather than strong, chemical-based substances that are potentially irritating.
◆ Avoid using heavily perfumed toiletries and skin-care products.
◆ Avoid polluted or noisy environments.
◆ Humidify or dehumidify rooms as necessary.
◆ Make rooms draft-free but with adequate ventilation.
◆ Wear natural fibers.
◆ Create an area that is conducive to relaxation.

TREATMENTS FOR THE BODY
◆ Breathing and relaxation techniques: for relief of pain and stress-related symptoms.
◆ Touch therapies: pressure or massage for relaxation, relief of ailments, and promotion of health (for example, aromatherapy, reflexology).
◆ Manipulation: for disorders of the spine, joints, and muscles, and for body alignment (for example, physiotherapy, osteopathy).
◆ Physical reeducation: for tension release, body alignment, and improved posture and flexibility (for example, Hellerwork, Alexander technique).
◆ Movement therapies: for increased vitality and promotion of self-healing (for example, t'ai chi, yoga, dance movement therapy).

MANAGING STRESS
◆ Allow for periods of rest during the day and get enough sleep at night.
◆ Include periods of relaxation and exercise in a daily routine.
◆ Prioritize and organize tasks.
◆ Delegate, and learn to say "no" to extra work.
◆ Eat properly and regularly and get plenty of fresh air.
◆ Make time for leisure activites and socializing with family and friends.
◆ Take a vacation.
◆ Cultivate a positive attitude to all things.
◆ Face up to problems rather than putting them off.

TREATMENTS FOR THE MIND
◆ Breathing and relaxation techniques: for managing stress and treating mental conditions including phobias, insomnia, and depression.
◆ Meditation: focusing on feelings of inner peace and fulfillment rather than on thought processes for relief of stress and promotion of well-being.
◆ Psychotherapy and counseling: talking to a skilled listener as a treatment for mental and emotional disorders.
◆ Hypnotherapy: use of a trancelike state of consciousness to influence physical and mental conditions, for example, desensitizing pain.
◆ Creative therapies: use of sounds, music, or art to treat mental and emotional disorders.

NERVOUS SYSTEM

THE NERVOUS SYSTEM is a huge and immensely complex structure (*see page 178*), with the brain as the control center. The brain contains up to 14 billion nerve cells and weighs about 3 lb (1.5 kg).

It receives stimuli from inside and outside the body, processes the information received, and then sends instructions in response to that information via the rest of the nervous system to various parts of the

DISORDER	SPECIFIC AILMENT	PHYSICAL SYMPTOMS
HEADACHE A constant headache may be indicative of a serious ailment, but most headaches are due to anxiety, stress, physical tension, fatigue, stimulants, allergy, eyestrain, or low blood sugar. Pain results from strain on the head or neck muscles or congestion (too much blood) in the blood vessels supplying them. **SELF-HELP** If pain is related to the neck, see a physiotherapist. **CAUTION** If a headache follows a head injury or drowsiness, intolerance of light, or vomiting exists, call an ambulance. If there is a temperature of more than 100°F (38°C) with light intolerance, or a headache behind one eye with blurred vision, see a doctor within two hours. If a headache has lasted for several days, with nausea and vomiting, see a doctor within 12 hours.	HEADACHE THAT COMES ON SUDDENLY	◆ Pain may feel like a tight band around the head ◆ Head may feel full and heavy as though the brain is being pushed out through the forehead ◆ Possible pulsating pain in the head and teeth ◆ Possible hot, bursting pain that is worse on the left side
	HEADACHE CAUSED BY DRINKING TOO MUCH ALCOHOL	◆ Head may feel as though it has been beaten ◆ Dizziness ◆ Possible pain in the back of the head as though the skull is going to burst ◆ Possible violent, jerking pain or dull, shooting pain in the left side of the brain
MIGRAINE An intermittent, severe headache may be a migraine, which usually occurs on one side of the head, and is associated with nausea, vomiting, blurred vision or other visual disturbances such as zigzags, intolerance of light, and sometimes tingling or numb arms. Symptoms are caused by the alternate constriction and swelling of arteries supplying the brain. Stress, low blood sugar, and food allergy are common triggers. Migraines affect women more than men, especially premenstrually. **SELF-HELP** Avoid stress and learn relaxation techniques (*see page 217*). Consult a dietician, or eliminate trigger foods such as chocolate, citrus fruits, and cheese from the diet for about four weeks. Reintroduce them and observe any changes in symptoms. If you smoke, stop. If you feel a migraine coming on, splash your face with cold water and lie down quietly for an hour. **CAUTION** Follow the same cautionary advice as for a headache (*see above*).	HEADACHE THAT IS WORSE ON THE RIGHT SIDE OF THE HEAD	◆ Pain on the right side of the head ◆ Sensation of the temples being screwed into each other ◆ Pain made worse by concentration ◆ Possible dizziness
	THROBBING, BLINDING HEADACHE	◆ Headache preceded by numbness and tingling in the lips, nose, and tongue ◆ Head feels stuffy, possibly with dizziness, and as though the brain is being hit by tiny hammers ◆ Pain over the eyes and on top of the head
	HEADACHE WITH TEARFULNESS	◆ Head feels as though it is about to burst ◆ Pain starts in the right temple ◆ Possible weeping of the right eye ◆ Bruised sensation in the forehead
SCIATICA This term describes pain that is transmitted along the sciatic nerve, which is the principal nerve in the leg and is connected to nerves in the pelvis and spine. Sciatica is usually felt in the buttock and thigh on one side, although sometimes it extends down the leg, and may affect both sides. It is caused by pressure on the nerve as a result of a prolapsed vertebral disk, the degeneration of a disk from osteoarthritis (*see page 196*), or an unusual autoimmune disease known as ankylosing spondylitis. Sciatic pain is exacerbated by bending, sneezing, or coughing. **SELF-HELP** Osteopathy, physiotherapy, or acupuncture may relieve the condition. Rest the back well by lying flat on a fairly hard mattress with a firm pad 2–3 in (5–7 cm) thick beneath the head. Try placing a hot-water bottle on the affected area. Learn how to lift and carry heavy objects correctly. Swimming may be beneficial.	SCIATICA THAT IS WORSE WHEN SITTING	◆ Difficulty straightening the affected leg because of contractions of the hamstring ◆ Hip pain as though the tendons are too short ◆ Tearing pain along the front of the thigh ◆ Lopsided walking style
	SCIATICA THAT IS WORSE IN COLD, DAMP WEATHER	◆ Shooting pain down the right leg to the foot ◆ Possible numbness and weakness in the leg ◆ Muscles are contracted ◆ Cramplike pain in the hip
	SCIATICA THAT IS RELIEVED BY HEAT AND MOVEMENT	◆ Tearing pain ◆ Numbness and tingling in the leg ◆ Pain extends down the back of the affected leg when passing stools ◆ Cramp in the calf

body. As a result of the complexity of the nervous system, nerve cells are vulnerable to damage and have little capacity for self-repair. Disorders of the brain and nervous system range from slight nerve twinges to traumatic events such as a stroke (*see page 187*). Serious ailments require immediate conventional treatment, but there is a role for homeopathy's mind-and-body approach, especially during recuperation. Homeopathic treatment follows exploration of imbalances within the body and analysis of constitutional type (*see page 176*). The prescribed remedies treat the nervous system by calming the mind, thereby encouraging healing processes, as well as by addressing specific symptoms.

PSYCHOLOGICAL SYMPTOMS	SYMPTOMS BETTER	SYMPTOMS WORSE	REMEDY & DOSAGE
◆ Apprehension ◆ Fear of the future and of death ◆ Fear of crowds ◆ Restlessness and impatience ◆ Feeling of despair	◆ In fresh air ◆ With warmth ◆ With rest ◆ From perspiring	◆ In stuffy rooms ◆ With cold and in drafts ◆ From a shock or fright ◆ From light or noise	**Aconite** (*see page 32*) 30c every 10–15 minutes up to 6 doses
◆ Mental dullness ◆ Extreme irritability ◆ Harsh criticism of others	◆ With warmth ◆ From applying firm pressure to the head ◆ Washing the hair or applying cold compresses to the head ◆ From being alone in the evening	◆ In cold, dry, or windy weather ◆ Between 3 A.M. and 4 A.M. ◆ From taking stimulants ◆ From eating ◆ With physical or mental exertion ◆ Near noise	**Nux vomica** (*see page 63*) 6c every 10–15 minutes up to 6 doses
◆ Lack of confidence ◆ Apprehension ◆ Memory appears to be failing ◆ Lack of concentration ◆ Sudden outbursts of anger	◆ From loosening tight clothing ◆ With movement ◆ In cool air ◆ From hot foods and drinks ◆ At night	◆ From wearing tight clothing ◆ From overeating ◆ In stuffy rooms ◆ Between 4 A.M. and 8 A.M. and 4 P.M. and 8 P.M.	**Lycopodium** (*see page 59*) 6c every 15 minutes up to 10 doses after first signs
◆ Rejection of sympathy ◆ Desire to be left alone ◆ Symptoms associated with grief ◆ Tendency to dwell on unpleasant memories	◆ In fresh air ◆ From applying cold compresses to the head ◆ From fasting ◆ Lying down	◆ With warmth ◆ With movement ◆ In stuffy rooms ◆ From grief	**Nat. mur.** (*see page 92*) 6c every 15 minutes up to 10 doses after first signs
◆ Tearfulness at the least provocation ◆ Timidity ◆ Desire for sympathy and reassurance	◆ In cold, fresh, open air ◆ With gentle movement ◆ From crying	◆ With warmth ◆ From rich or fatty foods ◆ In the evening ◆ During menstruation	**Pulsatilla** (*see page 61*) 6c every 15 minutes up to 10 doses after first signs
◆ Melancholia ◆ Apprehension ◆ Desire to cry but inability to do so ◆ Discontentment	◆ In the open air ◆ With rapid movement ◆ From walking bent over ◆ Lying down ◆ With sleep	◆ From walking around ◆ Between 2 A.M. and 4 A.M. ◆ In the evening ◆ When sitting down	**Ammonium mur.** (*see page 123*) 6c hourly up to 10 doses, or half-hourly if acute
◆ Irritability ◆ Symptoms associated with anger, especially if suppressed ◆ Frequent embarrassment ◆ Anguish but no desire to talk	◆ From applying firm pressure to the affected area ◆ From bending down ◆ With heat ◆ With rest or gentle movement	◆ In cold, wet weather ◆ From emotional stress ◆ Lying on the pain-free side ◆ At night	**Colocynthis** (*see page 52*) 6c hourly up to 10 doses, or half-hourly if acute
◆ Great restlessness ◆ Apprehension at night to the extent of having to get up ◆ Anxiety, depression, hopelessness, and tearfulness	◆ With heat ◆ With continuous movement ◆ From rubbing the affected area ◆ From stretching the limbs	◆ With rest ◆ On moving for the first time after rest ◆ In cold and dampness ◆ After midnight	**Rhus tox.** (*see page 162*) 6c hourly up to 10 doses, or half-hourly if acute

THE EYES

THE EYES SUPPLY THE BRAIN with information from the outside world – along with the other sensory organs (the ears, nose, tongue, and skin) – and are complex, delicate mechanisms. The cornea and lens in each eye focus incoming rays of light, forming an image on the retina, a membrane covering the back of the inside of the eye. Millions of extremely sensitive nerve cells in the retina convert the image

DISORDER	SPECIFIC AILMENT	PHYSICAL SYMPTOMS
EYESTRAIN Eye strain can be caused by overwork or by working in poor light. Stress, especially following an emotional upset, can weaken the eye muscles and cause eyestrain. The condition may manifest itself as a tightness around the eyes, or as difficulty in focusing on long-distance objects after focusing on near ones. **SELF-HELP** Apply dry, cold compresses to the eyes or bathe them with a euphrasia solution (*see Conjunctivitis below*). Rest the eyes by placing the palms lightly against closed eyes, thus relaxing them, for a couple of minutes.	EYES ACHE ON MOVEMENT	◆ Dull, aching pain in the eyes when looking up, down, or sideways
	BURNING EYES	◆ Eyes burn and feel strained after a prolonged period of studying or reading ◆ Eyes feel hot and are red ◆ Possible headache
CONJUNCTIVITIS Inflammation of the conjunctiva results from infection (yellow discharge) or allergy (whites of the eyes are red and gritty). **SELF-HELP** Bathe the eyes with euphrasia solution (2 drops mother tincture added to a saltwater eyebath – 1 tsp/5 ml salt to 5 fl oz/150 ml boiled, cooled water). Rest the eyes, do not share a towel, and wash your hands after touching the eyes.	SWOLLEN EYELIDS WITH BURNING DISCHARGE	◆ Eyes water continuously, which irritates the skin on the cheeks beneath them ◆ Eyelids are swollen and burning ◆ Frequent need to blink ◆ Little blisters may form inside the eyelids ◆ Bland nasal discharge
STIES A sty is a small, pus-filled boil that forms at the base of an eyelash. It is caused by an infection and usually clears up by itself within about seven days, but it can be aggravated by tiredness. For recurrent sties, constitutional treatment (*see page 176*) is advisable. **SELF-HELP** Rest the eyes. Avoid touching the eyes, especially with dirty hands, and never squeeze a sty. If a sty persists, try hot-spoon bathing: wrap cotton batting around the handle of a wooden spoon, dip it into very hot water, then place the cotton batting against the sty. Repeat several times.	INFLAMED EYES WITH ITCHY EYELIDS	◆ Eyes are red and swollen ◆ Eyelids itch ◆ Small boils on the eyelids develop heads of pus
	INFLAMED AND PAINFUL EYES	◆ Eyes are red, swollen, and painful ◆ Small boils on the eyelids develop heads of pus
TWITCHING EYELIDS The eyelids may twitch when there is no other bodily twitching or trembling. This usually indicates tiredness or tension. **SELF-HELP** Increase the amount of sleep you get and take naps if necessary. Learn relaxation or meditation techniques	TWITCHING WITH ANXIETY ABOUT HEALTH	◆ Spasmodic twitching of the eyelids ◆ Difficulty in reading because type seems to "swim" on the page ◆ Possible itching and burning of the eyelids
WATERING EYES Watering eyes are common in cold winds and drafts. If constant, this condition may be due to blocked tear ducts as a result of infection or injury to the bridge or sides of the nose. **SELF-HELP** Massage the sides of the nose to clear the tear ducts. **CAUTION** If discharge contains pus or if there is tenderness at the sides of the nose, see a doctor within 24 hours.	WATERING CAUSED BY INFECTION OF TEAR DUCT	◆ Eyes water because of mild but persistent infection of the tear ducts, which the body seems unable to overcome ◆ Lack of physical stamina

into suitable messages for transmission along the optic nerve to the brain. The front of the eye is protected by another membrane – the conjunctiva. The eyes are continuously bombarded with atmospheric particles, such as spores, bacteria, viruses, chemicals, and air pollutants, which may give rise to irritation or infection. Complaints in the eyes may be exacerbated by fluctuations in temperature, stress, and fatigue, all of which weaken the ability of the body's immune system to fight infection. Homeopathic self-help remedies are particularly suitable for soothing tired, irritated, or infected eyes. Regular, standard eye tests are essential for maintaining healthy eyes and monitoring degeneration with age.

PSYCHOLOGICAL SYMPTOMS	SYMPTOMS BETTER	SYMPTOMS WORSE	REMEDY & DOSAGE
◆ Aversion to sympathy and consolation ◆ Symptoms possibly associated with stress, particularly after the loss of a loved one	◆ In fresh air ◆ From fasting ◆ From applying cold compresses to the affected eye	◆ In cold, thundery weather ◆ In drafts or hot sun ◆ At the beach ◆ From physical or mental exertion ◆ From emotional stress	**Nat. mur.** (see page 92) 6c 4 times daily up to 7 days
◆ Depression ◆ Lack of personal satisfaction ◆ Criticism of others ◆ Anxiety	◆ With movement ◆ With warmth ◆ From gently massaging the eyes	◆ In cold, damp weather ◆ With rest ◆ Lying down ◆ From drinking alcohol	**Ruta** (see page 163) 6c 4 times daily up to 7 days
◆ None, apart from irritability due to discomfort of symptoms ◆ Aversion to answering questions ◆ Tendency to wake with a start	◆ When the eyes are closed ◆ From coffee	◆ In the evening ◆ Indoors ◆ With warmth ◆ In light ◆ In warm, windy weather	**Euphrasia** (see page 142) 6c hourly up to 10 doses
◆ Depression ◆ Self-pity ◆ Tearfulness	◆ From applying cold compresses to the affected area	◆ From rich, fatty foods ◆ From hormonal changes such as those associated with puberty or pregnancy	**Pulsatilla** (see page 61) 6c hourly up to 10 doses
◆ Feelings of resentment or anger, especially concerning a loved one	◆ From resting the eyes ◆ From applying cold compresses to the affected area	◆ When the sty is touched ◆ From the suppression of emotions, especially following an argument	**Staphysagria** (see page 54) 6c hourly up to 10 doses
◆ Possible tension brought on by anxiety about health ◆ Tendency to exaggerate small problems, even to the extent of fearing death ◆ Extreme excitability at night	◆ Lying down ◆ With sleep	◆ Before thunderstorms ◆ From sexual intercourse	**Agaricus** (see page 33) 6c every 4 hours up to 6 doses
◆ Lack of confidence ◆ Lack of mental stamina	◆ With warmth ◆ From applying warm compresses to the eyes ◆ In summer	◆ In cold air and drafts ◆ In damp conditions ◆ From applying gentle pressure to the eyes ◆ From mental exertion	**Silica** (see page 97) 6c 4 times daily up to 7 days

THE EARS

THE EARS ARE INTRICATE SENSORY ORGANS that provide details to the brain about the body's external experiences, as well as controlling balance. An ear has an outer, a middle, and an inner section, the first two being responsible for the collection and relaying of sound waves, while the third interprets them. The external folds of the ear lead into the ear canal, at the end of which is a membrane – the eardrum –

DISORDER	SPECIFIC AILMENT	PHYSICAL SYMPTOMS
EARACHE Earache can result from a buildup of wax in the ear or an infection of the outer, inner, or middle ear – after a cold, for example. It can worsen as a result of barotrauma (pressure damage) after flying, or if there is mucus in the eustachian tube (*see below*). Earache may also occur as a result of infection in the outer ear following ear piercing. The body's natural mechanisms for fighting infection may be impeded if the ears are exposed to extremes of temperature. **SELF-HELP** Hold a covered hot-water bottle against the affected ear. **CAUTION** If earache is associated with fever or discharge, see a doctor immediately. Consult a doctor about all types of earache in children.	EARACHE WITH SHARP PAIN	◆ Acute, throbbing pain ◆ Extreme sensitivity to touch
	THROBBING EARACHE WITH REDNESS	◆ Bright red ear ◆ Throbbing pain ◆ High fever ◆ Dry mouth and throat ◆ Wide, staring eyes
	FEELING OF PRESSURE BEHIND THE EARDRUM	◆ Pain resulting from pressure behind the eardrum pushing it out slightly
BLOCKAGE OF THE EUSTACHIAN TUBE The eustachian tube may become blocked by mucus resulting from an infection of the upper respiratory tract, a middle ear or adenoid infection, or tonsillitis; by swollen adenoids (which cover the opening to the eustachian tube at the back of the nose); or because of barotrauma after flying. **SELF-HELP** To dislodge mucus, inhale three drops of lemon juice up each nostril three times a day for five days, using a dropper. Do not do this if you are prone to nosebleeds. **CAUTION** If there is no improvement after seven days, consult a doctor within 48 hours.	EUSTACHIAN TUBE BLOCKAGE WITH CONSTRICTING FEELING IN THE THROAT	◆ Glands in the throat may be swollen and hard ◆ Painful, constricting feeling in the throat
	EUSTACHIAN TUBE BLOCKAGE WITH COUGHING UP OF PHLEGM	◆ Deafness caused by the swelling of the eustachian tube ◆ Cracking noise in the ear on blowing the nose or swallowing ◆ Runny nose and coughing up of mucus from the back of the throat
TINNITUS Tinnitus is a persistent noise in the ears, commonly ringing or roaring. It may result from the presence of a foreign body in the ear canal, barotrauma after flying, or taking certain drugs, especially aspirin. It may be brought on by the flu or aging, and is an occupational hazard for those employed in noisy workplaces. The condition may be accompanied by deafness and giddiness, tenderness as a result of pressure on the nerves at the base of the skull, or a headache. **SELF-HELP** Place two drops of pure almond oil in each ear once a week. Reduce the stress that may be generated by this disorder by means of relaxation techniques (*see page 217*). Tinnitus may be exacerbated by neck problems, in which case consult an osteopath or physiotherapist. **CAUTION** If you cannot identify the cause of noise or discomfort in the ears, consult a doctor within 48 hours.	ROARING IN THE EARS WITH DIFFICULTY IN HEARING	◆ Possible deafness or muffled hearing and giddiness and nausea ◆ Noises in the ear heard as music or the buzzing of insects
	TINNITUS WITH BLOCKED FEELING IN THE EARS	◆ Singing or hissing noise resembling the sound of an aeolian harp ◆ Ears feel blocked and tingly ◆ Hearing is impaired
	BUZZING IN THE EARS WITH DIZZINESS	◆ Buzzing, especially in the left ear, sometimes accompanied by deafness and dizziness ◆ Deafness accompanied by a severe headache and violent noise in the ears ◆ Possible tenderness in the cervical or dorsal spine and pain in the head

which vibrates according to variations in air pressure caused by sound waves. Beyond the eardrum is the middle ear, where a series of small bones transforms vibrations so that they can pass through the liquid in the inner ear. From here, information is transmitted along the auditory nerve to the brain. The eustachian tube links the middle ear to the back of the nose and maintains the same air pressure on either side of the eardrum. The ears are susceptible to invasion by particles and microorganisms and are easily damaged, so any pain or other kind of discomfort should be investigated promptly. Homeopathic remedies can be of particular help in treating ailments linked to mucus resulting from respiratory infections.

PSYCHOLOGICAL SYMPTOMS	SYMPTOMS BETTER	SYMPTOMS WORSE	REMEDY & DOSAGE
◆ Extreme irritability and anger ◆ Emotional sensitivity ◆ Great sensitivity to even the slightest jarring of the body	◆ With warmth ◆ From applying warm compresses to the head ◆ When the head is warmly wrapped	◆ In cold air and drafts ◆ From undressing when chilled ◆ When the ear is touched ◆ Lying on the affected side	**Hepar sulf.** (see page 84) 6c half-hourly until you see a doctor
◆ Restlessness and agitation that may be accompanied by hallucinations or violent outbursts ◆ Sensitivity to heat, light, noise, or touch	◆ When standing or sitting upright ◆ From applying cold compresses to the forehead	◆ When the head is chilled ◆ With movement, jarring, near noise, in light, or from pressure ◆ Lying on the right side ◆ At night	**Belladonna** (see page 39) 30c half-hourly until you see a doctor
◆ Tearfulness and self-pity ◆ Desire for company ◆ In small children, constant desire for cuddling	◆ With gentle movement ◆ In fresh air ◆ In cool, dry conditions	◆ In hot, stuffy conditions ◆ In the evening ◆ Lying on the left side ◆ From prolonged standing	**Pulsatilla** (see page 61) 6c hourly up to 10 doses
◆ Restlessness and great excitability ◆ Desire to keep constantly busy ◆ Obsessive checking to make sure things have not been forgotten	◆ In cold conditions ◆ From emotional stress	◆ With heat ◆ At night ◆ With rest	**Iodum** (see page 86) 6c 4 times daily up to 7 days
◆ Irritability ◆ Anger ◆ Discontent	◆ From cold drinks ◆ From gently rubbing the ear	◆ In fresh air ◆ In drafts ◆ Lying down at night ◆ In damp conditions	**Kali. mur.** (see page 150) 6c 4 times daily up to 7 days
◆ None, apart from irritability or depression caused by discomfort of symptoms	◆ From applying heat, especially dry heat, to the ear	◆ When the ear is touched ◆ With movement ◆ At night ◆ In cold air	**Salicylic ac.** (see page 120) 6c 3 times daily up to 14 days
◆ Irritability, anxiety, intolerance, and mood swings ◆ Possible hallucinations	◆ In the open air	◆ After breakfast ◆ From bathing	**Carbon sulf.** (see page 134) 6c 3 times daily up to 14 days
◆ Nervousness ◆ Nominal aphasia (difficulty in naming objects) ◆ Great anguish and fits of anxiety, despair, and melancholia	◆ From applying pressure to the ear ◆ From yawning ◆ When bending forward	◆ At precise, regular intervals ◆ With cold ◆ Between 10 A.M. and 11 A.M. ◆ If touched ◆ With movement	**China sulf.** (see page 136) 6c 3 times daily up to 14 days

RESPIRATORY SYSTEM

WITH EVERY BREATH THAT WE TAKE, spores, viruses, bacteria, and microscopic particles of dust, smoke, and chemical pollutants enter the body. The nose moistens, warms, and filters air before it is drawn into the airway and lungs (*see page 180*). The respiratory system is therefore highly susceptible to the effects of atmospheric irritants. If the immune system is strong, it is able to ward off all but the most virulent infections.

DISORDER	SPECIFIC AILMENT	PHYSICAL SYMPTOMS
HAY FEVER & ALLERGIC RHINITIS Seasonal airborne irritants such as grass, tree, and flower pollens cause the allergic reaction that is called hay fever. Mucous membranes lining the nose and eyes are principally affected, but the ears, throat, and lungs may also become irritated. Symptoms include repeated sneezing, a runny nose, watering eyes, and itching of the eyes, nose, palate, and throat. Allergic rhinitis, or perennial rhinitis, is the name given to similar symptoms that occur all year round and are caused by other irritants, including dust mites and animal dander. **SELF-HELP** Avoid all known irritants. If symptoms are severe, try using air filters or ionizers in the home. Wear sunglasses and a hat when outdoors to shade your face. Eat lots of fresh, raw fruits and vegetables. Blow the nose gently; hard blowing may burst pollen grains in the nose and increase irritation. Rub a small dab of petroleum jelly inside each nostril a few times a day to prevent the nose from becoming dry and sore. Take combination H tissue salts (*see page 216*).	HAY FEVER WITH BURNING MUCUS	◆ Streaming, burning mucus that may start in the left nostril and move to the right, and that makes the nostrils and upper lip sore ◆ Pain in the forehead ◆ Larynx feels as if it has hooks sticking in it ◆ Eyes stream with a bland discharge
	HAY FEVER WITH CONSTANT DESIRE TO SNEEZE	◆ Thick, honey-colored mucus follows three or four days of continuous, violent sneezing that brings no relief ◆ Nostrils are sore, red, and painful ◆ Burning throat and irritating cough
	HAY FEVER IN WHICH MAINLY THE EYES ARE AFFECTED	◆ Eyes are swollen and sensitive to bright light ◆ Thick, burning discharge from the eyes that irritates the skin on the cheeks beneath ◆ Bland mucus from the nose ◆ Mucus drips down the back of the throat
COLDS Colds are caused by viral infections of the respiratory tract. Early symptoms include a sore throat, watery mucus, and sneezing. As a cold runs its course, the mucus thickens and may become yellow in color. Colds are usually self-limiting, but a neglected cold may develop into a chest infection such as bronchitis (*see page 228*), or infection may spread to the ears (*see page 222*), sinuses (*see page 226*), throat (*see page 226*), or larynx (*see page 228*). Vulnerability to infection is increased by overwork and exhaustion, emotional stress – especially after a shock or a scare – and anxiety. **SELF-HELP** Rest and drink plenty of fluids, especially hot water mixed with fresh lemon juice and a little honey. Eat plenty of fresh fruits and vegetables, and get some fresh air. Take combination Q tissue salts (*see page 216*). **CAUTION** If there is pain in the throat, larynx, chest, sinuses, or ears, consult a doctor.	COLD THAT COMES ON SLOWLY	◆ Mouth feels hot ◆ Throat is inflamed ◆ Mild fever ◆ Nose may bleed
	COLD WITH IRRITABILITY	◆ Chilliness ◆ Runny nose by day, blocked nose by night ◆ Watering eyes and sneezing ◆ Headache ◆ Sore throat
	EARLY STAGES OF A COLD WITH SNEEZING	◆ Violent sneezing and thin mucus resembling the white of a raw egg ◆ Possible blocked nose ◆ Possible cold sores
THE FLU There are many different strains of flu virus, and the whole body is usually affected. Symptoms include fever, muscular aches and pains, a headache, a sore throat, and a cough. Children, the elderly, smokers, and people with chronic diseases are the most likely to be seriously affected by the flu. **SELF-HELP** Rest and drink frequently, especially hot water mixed with fresh lemon juice and a little honey. Eat plenty of fresh fruits and vegetables, and take combination Q tissue salts (*see page 216*). Get some fresh air once the acute stage has passed. **CAUTION** If fever persists for four days, see a doctor.	THE FLU WITH WEAKNESS	◆ Chills running up and down the spine ◆ Shakiness and trembling, mainly in the legs ◆ Bursting headache that is eased by urinating ◆ Fever with lack of thirst and fatigue ◆ Sore throat
	THE FLU WITH HIGH FEVER	◆ High fever that comes on suddenly ◆ Flushed face ◆ Bright red, sore throat ◆ Wide, staring eyes

Colds, coughs, and the flu strike easily when the immune system is weak, making the body vulnerable. Variations in the efficiency of the immune system explain why only some of the people exposed to a cold actually catch it. The immune system may be impaired by poor diet, overindulgence, exposure to cold or windy weather, or being chilled or overheated.

In addition, the body's defenses are weakened by overwork, exhaustion, anxiety, and stress. A weak system also increases the possibility of allergic reactions to atmospheric particles. Homeopathy addresses imbalances in the immune system rather than fighting infection. Allergies may require constitutional homeopathic treatment (*see page 176*).

PSYCHOLOGICAL SYMPTOMS	SYMPTOMS BETTER	SYMPTOMS WORSE	REMEDY & DOSAGE
• None, apart from irritability caused by discomfort of symptoms	• In cool rooms • In fresh air • From bathing • With movement	• In warm rooms • In cold or damp weather • From warm foods and drinks	**Allium cepa** (*see page 34*) 6c as required up to 10 doses
• Restlessness • Anxiety and worry • Possible hyperactivity in children	• In the open air • From eating • With rest	• From sneezing • With warmth • In dry weather	**Arsen. iod.** (*see page 126*) 6c as required up to 10 doses
• None, apart from irritability caused by discomfort of symptoms	• Lying down in a darkened room • From coffee	• With warmth • In warm, windy weather • In bright light • Indoors • In the evening	**Euphrasia** (*see page 142*) 6c as required up to 10 doses
• Fear of losing touch with friends • Talkativeness • Excitability	• From applying cold compresses to the forehead • With gentle exercise • From lying down	• From jarring and touch • Lying on the right side • In fresh air and sun • Between 4 A.M. and 6 A.M. • When overheated but not perspiring	**Ferrum phos.** (*see page 82*) 6c every 2 hours up to 4 doses
• Irritability • Harsh criticism of others	• With warmth • With sleep • From applying firm pressure and warm compresses to the nose • In the evening	• In dry, cold wind • In public places • Between 3 A.M. and 4 A.M. • From emotional stress • From spicy foods or stimulants	**Nux vomica** (*see page 63*) 6c every 2 hours up to 4 doses
• Desire to be left alone • Aversion to sympathy	• In fresh air • From fasting • From applying cold compresses to the sinuses	• Around 10 A.M. • In cold, thundery weather • From physical or mental exertion • In drafts, salt air, or hot sun • Near noise, talking, or music	**Nat. mur.** (*see page 92*) 6c every 2 hours up to 4 doses
• Apprehension and worry about upcoming events • Brain feels dull and drowsy	• In fresh air • From urinating • From applying hot compresses to the back of the head and top of the neck	• In the sun • In humid conditions • From emotional stress • In the early morning and late at night	**Gelsemium** (*see page 144*) 6c every 2 hours up to 10 doses
• Confusion and delirium • Horrible visions • Violent outbursts	• When standing or sitting up • In warm rooms	• With jarring and movement • Near noise and in light • In hot sun • Lying on the right side • At night	**Belladonna** (*see page 39*) 30c every 2 hours up to 10 doses

DISORDER	SPECIFIC AILMENT	PHYSICAL SYMPTOMS
MUCUS (PHLEGM) This is the intermittent discharge of runny or viscous fluid, or mucus, from the nose, which may alternate with a stuffy, blocked-up feeling. Phlegm may be a symptom of an infection, such as a cold or the flu (*see page 224*), or sinusitis (*see below*). Alternatively, phlegm may be part of an allergic reaction to a number of things, including pollen or dust (*see Hay fever, page 224*), cigarette smoke, chemical pollution, gas or oil heaters, central heating or air-conditioning systems, certain drugs, or cold and dampness. These may irritate the mucous membranes, which stimulates mucus production in an attempt to lubricate the membranes and remove the irritation. A cough (*see page 228*) may develop if phlegm drips down the back of the throat. **SELF-HELP** Drink plenty of fluids. Avoid eating dairy products, bread, and potatoes – which may increase mucus production – for a couple of weeks and make a note of any changes to symptoms. Take combination Q tissue salts (*see page 216*).	THICK, WHITE MUCUS	◆ Thick, white mucus in the second stage of a cold after the inital inflammation of mucous membranes has subsided ◆ Mucus flows down the nose or the back of the throat
	MUCUS RESEMBLING THE WHITE OF A RAW EGG	◆ Watery mucus may be so profuse that is it necessary to hold a handkerchief below the nose ◆ Loss of smell and taste
	MUCUS WITH CONSTANTLY RUNNY NOSE	◆ Nose runs constantly with need to blow it all the time ◆ Mucus is yellow or green, watery, and burning
	MUCUS WITH EXTREME SENSITIVITY TO STRONG SMELLS	◆ Crusts and cracks inside the nostrils that make blowing the nose painful ◆ Nose may bleed ◆ Heightened sense of smell may make even the scent of flowers unbearable
SINUSITIS The sinuses are air-filled cavities in the bones around the nose. Sinusitis is inflammation of the mucous membranes lining the sinuses due to infection or allergy. The cavities may fill up with mucus, creating pressure that in turn causes pain. Symptoms include a blocked nose, general malaise, possibly a headache over one or both eyes, and tender cheeks with pain resembling toothache. The condition is aggravated by stress. **SELF-HELP** Take care when blowing your nose: blow one nostril at a time. Humidify all rooms, and inhale steam. Rest, drink plenty of fluids, and take combination Q tissue salts (*see page 216*). Avoid eating dairy products, bread, and potatoes. If you smoke, stop. Do not use decongestants repeatedly. **CAUTION** If symptoms persist beyond 48 hours, consult a doctor. If you are in severe pain, see a doctor within 12 hours.	SINUSITIS WITH STRINGY MUCUS	◆ Stringy, stretchy, greenish yellow mucus ◆ Nose feels blocked, with loss of smell ◆ Mucus drips down the back of the throat ◆ Violent sneezing
	SINUSITIS ACCOMPANIED BY TEARFULNESS	◆ Pain above the eyes, in the right cheekbone, or on the right side of the face generally ◆ Yellow mucus ◆ Nose feels blocked
	SINUSITIS WITH FACIAL TENDERNESS	◆ Facial bones are tender, even to the slightest touch ◆ Excessive yellow mucus and sneezing ◆ Chilliness
SORE THROAT A relatively mild irritation or a more serious infection, such as laryngitis (*see page 228*), may produce a sore throat. Soreness may affect the whole throat, or areas such as the larynx, tonsils, adenoids, pharynx, or vocal chords. Symptoms include a dry mouth and throat, discomfort on swallowing, an unpleasant taste in the mouth, bad breath, fatigue, and fever. They may be made worse by cold and dampness, overusing the voice, smoking, food allergy, being run down, or emotional stress. **SELF-HELP** Take garlic preparations. Drink plenty of fluids. Gargle with a solution of calendula and hypericum (*see page 271*). **CAUTION** If symptoms lasts for more than one week, or if loss of voice persists, see a doctor. If there is high fever, children should see a doctor within 12 hours, adults within 48 hours. If the tonsils are inflamed and accompanied by fever, see a doctor within 12 hours.	ACUTE, PAINFUL SORE THROAT	◆ Throat looks red and feels dry, rough, constricted, burning, and tingly ◆ Extreme thirst, usually for warm drinks, but at infrequent intervals ◆ Skin is dry and hot
	RAW, BURNING SORE THROAT	◆ Very painful throat with thick saliva and hoarse voice ◆ Possible cold sores or hives (urticaria) ◆ Desire for cold drinks
	SORENESS EXTENDING TO THE NECK AND EARS	◆ Unpleasant taste in the mouth ◆ Pain on swallowing ◆ Body feels alternately hot and cold due to fever ◆ Exhaustion, weakness, and shakiness ◆ Head is heavy and feels as though it is bound

PSYCHOLOGICAL SYMPTOMS	SYMPTOMS BETTER	SYMPTOMS WORSE	REMEDY & DOSAGE
• Dogmatism • Depression	• From cold drinks • From a massage • From letting the hair down, literally	• In fresh air • In cold air and drafts • From fatty foods • During menstruation	**Kali. mur.** (see page 150) 6c 4 times daily up to 14 days
• Desire to be left alone • Dislike of sympathy	• With rest • In fresh air • From perspiring • From applying pressure to tender areas	• In sun and heat • Before menstruation • In damp conditions • With physical exertion	**Nat. mur.** (see page 92) 6c 4 times daily up to 14 days
• Depression • Irritability • Poor memory	• From applying pressure to the sinuses • In dry weather • From keeping the head warm	• After dinner • From inhaling cold air • From drug abuse	**Hydrastis** (see page 147) 6c 4 times daily up to 14 days
• Melancholia • Tendency to weep while listening to music • Timidity and indecisiveness • Poor short-term memory	• With sleep	• From cold or sweet foods, or seafood • During menstruation • On the left side of the face	**Graphites** (see page 83) 6c 4 times daily up to 14 days
• Dogmatism • Depression	• From applying warm compresses to the sinuses • From undressing when chilled	• From drinking beer • In the morning • In hot weather	**Kali. bich.** (see page 87) 6c every 2 hours up to 2 days
• Self-pity and tearfulness • Desire for sympathy and reassurance	• From crying and sympathy • With the hands above the head • With gentle exercise and fresh air • From cold drinks and applying cold compresses to the sinuses	• In stuffy rooms • In sun, heat, and extremes of temperature • From rich, fatty foods • Lying on the painful side	**Pulsatilla** (see page 61) 6c every 2 hours up to 2 days
• Irritability • Emotional sensitivity	• When sitting in warm surroundings • When the head is wrapped up	• In drafts • With touch • From undressing when chilled	**Hepar sulf.** (see page 84) 6c every 2 hours up to 2 days
• Extreme anxiety, even to the extent of fearing death, caused by sudden onset and severity of symptoms	• With movement • With warmth • In the open air if not too cold	• In cold, windy weather • In warm rooms • On exposure to tobacco smoke • In the evening and at night • With music	**Aconite** (see page 32) 30c every 2 hours up to 10 doses
• Tendency to argue • Harsh criticism of others	• In fresh air • With exercise • From stimulants • With warmth around the throat • When bending forward	• At night • In cold, damp weather • With rest	**Dulcamara** (see page 62) 6c every 12 hours up to 10 doses
• Depression • Irritability	• In fresh air • From drinking alcohol • From perspiring	• Early in the morning and late at night • In sun, fog, and dampness • Before thunderstorms	**Gelsemium** (see page 144) 6c every 2 hours up to 10 doses

DISORDER	SPECIFIC AILMENT	PHYSICAL SYMPTOMS
LARYNGITIS Laryngitis is hoarseness or loss of voice caused by inflammation of the larynx as a result of an allergy or infection. It may also be caused by continuous coughing, breathing through the mouth rather than the nose, exposure to cold, dry, winds, inhaling toxic fumes, heavy smoking, drinking too much alcohol, or vomiting. If you are inherently susceptible to throat conditions (*see page 20*), a scare or emotional shock may cause inflammation. Laryngitis can also be triggered by overuse of the voice, and is an occupational hazard for teachers, singers, and street vendors. **SELF-HELP** Do not smoke or drink alcohol, and avoid hot, smoky rooms. Rest the voice and increase your fluid intake. Gargle with a solution of calendula and hypericum (*see page 271*) every four hours. If you sing, and loss of voice is a persistent problem, your voice may need retraining. Recurrent laryngitis may be the result of poor posture: The Alexander technique (*see page 217*) may be helpful. **CAUTION** If there is no improvement within a week to ten days, or if loss of voice persists, consult a doctor.	LARYNGITIS WITH HIGH FEVER	◆ Hoarseness or loss of voice ◆ Sudden onset of high temperature ◆ Larynx very sensitive to touch and inhaled air
	LARYNGITIS WITH DRY, TICKLY COUGH	◆ Throat feels dry and sore ◆ Talking may be painful ◆ Desire for cold drinks, which may be vomited when warmed in the stomach
	DRY, RAW THROAT AND VIOLENT COUGH	◆ Copious mucus drips down the back of the throat and makes talking difficult ◆ Cough may be violent enough to cause leakage of urine ◆ Loss of voice that is usually painful
COUGHS A cough is the body's attempt to expel an irritant from the respiratory tract. The lungs build up a pressure of air that is released suddenly in an attempt to dispose of the cause of irritation. A cough either produces mucus or it is dry. Irritation of the lining of the airway may be caused by mucus dripping down the back of the throat, smoking, or atmospheric particles. Coughing can also be triggered by a shock or scare. **SELF-HELP** Humidify all rooms. If you smoke, stop. Avoid dusty, smoky places and going out in cold, damp weather. Rest and drink a lot, especially hot water with fresh lemon juice and a little honey. If you are producing copious phlegm, avoid dairy products and starchy foods, which may increase mucus production. Try homeopathic or herbal over-the-counter cough mixtures. **CAUTION** If a cough is accompanied by breathing difficulties, fever, or chest pain, see a doctor. If it results from inhaling dust or fumes, and does not improve within two days, see a doctor.	DRY, IRRITATING COUGH THAT COMES ON SUDDENLY	◆ Dry, hollow-sounding, croaky cough ◆ Great thirst ◆ Possible rapid rise in temperature
	COUGH WITH CHEST PAIN	◆ Bursting headache, aggravated by even the slightest cough, possibly with fever ◆ Extreme thirst, usually for warm drinks, but at infrequent intervals ◆ Whole body feels dehydrated
	COUGH WITH THICK, GREEN MUCUS	◆ Thick, green, bitter-tasting mucus is coughed up, leaving an unpleasant taste in the mouth ◆ Poor appetite ◆ Tongue has a white coating ◆ Green, bland mucus may issue from the nose ◆ Little or no thirst
BRONCHITIS Bronchitis is inflammation of the bronchi – the airways connecting the windpipe to the lungs (*see page 180*) – resulting in a cough (*see above*) that produces a lot of mucus. Other symptoms include fever, breathing difficulties, and wheezing. Bronchitis usually develops from a viral infection such as a cold or the flu, and is aggravated by atmospheric pollution, and by cold or damp air. **SELF-HELP** If you smoke, stop; avoid smoky atmospheres. Try inhaling steam. If you have a bad attack, stay in bed for two or three days with a hot-water bottle placed on your chest, and plenty of hot drinks. Avoid eating refined carbohydrates. **CAUTION** If symptoms persist, see a doctor. If temperature rises above 102°F (39°C), if the mucus has blood in it, or if there are breathing difficulties, see a doctor within two hours.	BRONCHITIS THAT COMES ON SUDDENLY AFTER EXPOSURE TO COLD, DRY AIR	◆ Sudden onset of symptoms ◆ Dry, staccato cough ◆ High fever ◆ Chilliness
	BRONCHITIS WITH DESIRE FOR ICE WATER	◆ Tight, dry, tickly cough ◆ Frequent desire to drink iced water ◆ Pale, anxious appearance
	BRONCHITIS WITH PAINFUL COUGH	◆ Dry, stabbing, painful cough ◆ Headache that gets worse from coughing ◆ Chest pain that is relieved by supporting the elbows on the back of a chair ◆ Great thirst

PSYCHOLOGICAL SYMPTOMS	SYMPTOMS BETTER	SYMPTOMS WORSE	REMEDY & DOSAGE
• Anxiety, even to the extent of fearing death, caused by sudden onset of symptoms • Restlessness	• In fresh air • With movement • With warmth	• In warm rooms • On exposure to tobacco smoke • From music • In the evening and at night	**Aconite** (*see page 32*) 30c every 4 hours up to 10 doses
• Strong desire for company and sympathy • Irrational fears, for example, of darkness or thunderstorms	• With sleep • From a massage • In fresh air • From drinking	• From talking and laughing • From hot foods and drinks • Lying on the left or the painful side • Between sunset and midnight	**Phosphorus** (*see page 94*) 6c 4 times daily up to 7 days
• Depression • Extreme sensitivity to the suffering of others	• In warm, humid weather • From cold drinks • With gentle movement	• In the morning • From sweet foods • From coffee	**Causticum** (*see page 79*) 6c 4 times daily up to 7 days
• Extreme anxiety, even to the extent of fearing death	• In fresh air • With movement • With warmth	• In warm rooms • On exposure to tobacco smoke or pollen • In the evening and at night • In cold, hot, or windy weather	**Aconite** (*see page 32*) 30c every 4 hours up to 10 doses
• Irritability • Desire to be at home even if already there • Reluctance to move or speak • Stress about financial problems	• In cool conditions • From applying firm, cool pressure to the head and chest	• With movement and if touched • In bright light • Near noise • In the morning and around 9 P.M. and 3 A.M.	**Bryonia** (*see page 42*) 30c every 4 hours up to 10 doses
• Tearfulness • Self-pity • In young children, constant desire for cuddling	• In fresh air • From a good cry • From applying cold compresses to the chest	• In the evening • In warm, stuffy rooms	**Pulsatilla** (*see page 61*) 30c every 4 hours up to 10 doses
• Restlessness • Anxiety, even to the extent of fearing death	• In fresh air • With rest • From warm perspiration	• In cold, dry wind • With shock • At night	**Aconite** (*see page 32*) 30c every 4 hours up to 10 doses
• Anxiety and fear, especially during thunderstorms • Excitability • Great desire for reassurance	• Lying on the right side • From cold foods and drinks • From massaging the chest	• With touch • From warm foods • In the evening • In windy or cold weather • During thunderstorms	**Phosphorus** (*see page 94*) 6c every 4 hours up to 2 days
• Extreme irritability • Desire to be left alone • Delirium and desire to be at home even if already there	• Lying on the painful side • From applying pressure to the chest • With rest and quiet • In cool, open air	• When sitting up or stooping • With movement or if touched • From coughing, breathing, becoming hot, or eating • With stress	**Bryonia** (*see page 42*) 30c every 4 hours up to 2 days

CIRCULATORY SYSTEM

THE CIRCULATORY SYSTEM transports blood around the body (*see page 184*), supplying body tissues with oxygen and nutrients. Circulatory disorders may arise if the heart is not capable of pumping properly, or if blood flow is disrupted because arteries become clogged or less elastic, with the result that the heart has to work harder in order to circulate the blood. Arteries very often become less efficient with age.

DISORDER	SPECIFIC AILMENT	PHYSICAL SYMPTOMS
CHILBLAINS (SENSITIVITY TO COLD) This condition is most common on the hands and feet, and when superficial blood vessels contract excessively because of an extreme sensitivity to cold. The skin becomes pale and numb, then red, swollen, and itchy. Eventually the skin may break. **SELF-HELP** Keep the hands and feet as warm and dry as possible, especially during cold, damp weather. Apply calendula ointment. Do not scratch the affected area. Regular exercise will improve circulation, as will "windmilling" the arms.	BURNING, ITCHY SKIN	♦ Skin in affected areas is red, prickly, and swollen ♦ Intolerable itching ♦ Burning pain in affected areas
	SENSITIVITY TO COLD WITH SWOLLEN VEINS	♦ Burning, throbbing pain in affected areas ♦ Bluish inflammation ♦ Biting, itching sensation if affected areas are scratched
CRAMPS A cramp is an acute pain that occurs when muscles go into spasm as a result of a shortage of oxygen or a buildup of lactic acid. Poor circulation reduces oxygen supply to the muscles, and may occur after prolonged sitting or standing, lying awkwardly, if the arteries narrow suddenly on being chilled, during pregnancy, or because of salt deficiency after vomiting or excessive perspiration. A buildup of lactic acid occurs after strenuous or unaccustomed exercise. **SELF-HELP** If cramps are worse at night, raise the foot of your bed by about 4 in (10 cm). As a cramp comes on, stretch the muscles and massage them to increase the blood supply.	SEVERE CRAMPS IN THE LEGS OR FEET	♦ Muscle twitching leading to violent muscle spasms in the toes, ankles, soles of the feet, and legs ♦ Ankles are painfully heavy ♦ Knees bend involuntarily when walking
	CRAMPS FROM MUSCLE FATIGUE	♦ Pain resembling bruising brought on by overexertion ♦ Limbs feel as if they have been beaten ♦ Heaviness in limbs
VARICOSE VEINS When the valves inside the veins start to fail, blood pools form, a condition known as varicose veins. They show up as twisted, purple lines, mainly affecting the legs, and may be hereditary, or the result of thrombosis (blood clot), obesity, or pregnancy. **SELF-HELP** Stand as little as possible and wear support hose. Sit with the feet raised above the level of the hips. **CAUTION** If the condition persists for three weeks, see a doctor. If a vein bursts and bleeds, bandage the leg tightly and keep it raised. See a doctor within two hours if the bleeding continues.	VARICOSE VEINS WITH A SORE, BRUISED FEELING	♦ Veins are inflamed, possibly with a burning feeling ♦ Veins are sore, swollen, and lumpy, and feel bruised and tender to the touch ♦ Veins may bleed
	VARICOSE VEINS THAT ARE WORSE WHEN SITTING WITH THE LEGS HANGING DOWN	♦ Veins feel full ♦ Chilliness ♦ Veins smart and sting
RESTLESS LEGS This condition may be partly hereditary and partly nervous in origin, and is most common among the elderly and those who smoke, or if the leg muscles are overexerted and fatigued. It has been linked to diabetes, vitamin B deficiency, excess caffeine, drug withdrawal, and food allergies. Symptoms are tickling, burning, or prickling sensations that are mainly in the lower legs and cause involuntary twitching or jerking. **SELF-HELP** Use a hot-water bottle in bed or wear warm socks. Cut out caffeine and eat plenty of fresh vegetables and fruits. Check for a food allergy if symptoms persist.	RESTLESS LEGS THAT ARE BETTER WITH CONTINUOUS MOVEMENT	♦ Tickling feeling, like ants moving around beneath the skin ♦ Burning, prickling sensations in the legs ♦ Legs feel wooden and dead
	FEET THAT ARE RESTLESS EVEN AT NIGHT	♦ Trembling, twitching feet and restless legs, even when asleep ♦ Restlessness that makes sleep difficult

The circulation of blood is regulated by the autonomic nervous system (*see page 178*), and as such may be adversely affected by stress. As well as homeopathic self-help remedies for specific ailments, constitutional treatment (*see page 176*) may improve the body's general metabolic function, reduce stress, and maintain the health of other organs, for example, the liver, on which the functioning of the heart depends. Circulatory disorders, especially heart disease, benefit most from a complete health program that, as well as homeopathic treatment, includes key dietary practices, an adequate amount of appropriate exercise and relaxation, and a lifestyle that avoids smoking, stress, overwork, and excesses of any kind.

PSYCHOLOGICAL SYMPTOMS	SYMPTOMS BETTER	SYMPTOMS WORSE	REMEDY & DOSAGE
◆ Great anxiety based on fear that symptoms are a harbinger of more serious disease	◆ With slow movement ◆ When warm in bed	◆ With cold and dampness ◆ In cold weather ◆ Before thunderstorms	**Agaricus** (*see page 33*) 6c half-hourly up to 6 doses
◆ Possible tearfulness caused by discomfort of symptoms ◆ Desire for sympathy	◆ With the hands above the head ◆ With gentle exercise ◆ In cold, fresh air	◆ With heat ◆ In extremes of temperature ◆ In the evening and at night	**Pulsatilla** (*see page 61*) 6c half-hourly up to 6 doses
◆ Tendency to shriek shrilly ◆ Violent tearfulness ◆ Fearfulness	◆ From applying firm pressure to the affected area ◆ From cold drinks ◆ From perspiring	◆ With movement ◆ From applying light pressure to the affected area ◆ During sexual intercourse	**Cuprum met.** (*see page 80*) 6c 4 times daily up to 14 days
◆ Fear of being touched ◆ Nervousness about pain ◆ Great sensitivity to noise	◆ On starting to move ◆ In clear, cold weather ◆ When lying down	◆ With heat ◆ From applying light pressure to the affected area ◆ With prolonged movement	**Arnica** (*see page 37*) 6c 4 times daily up to 14 days
◆ Irritability ◆ Anxiety at night ◆ Lack of desire to work or study	◆ With rest ◆ From lying down quietly ◆ In winter	◆ From injury ◆ With movement or jarring ◆ From applying pressure to the affected area ◆ In warm, humid weather	**Hamamelis** (*see page 145*) 30c twice daily up to 7 days
◆ Timidity and submissiveness ◆ Tearfulness ◆ Desire for reassurance and consolation	◆ In cold, fresh air ◆ From applying cold compresses to the affected areas ◆ When standing upright ◆ Lying on the back	◆ With warmth ◆ In the evening ◆ During pregnancy	**Pulsatilla** (*see page 61*) 30c twice daily up to 7 days
◆ Mental restlessness ◆ Inability to concentrate	◆ With continuous movement ◆ With heat ◆ From holding the legs	◆ With rest ◆ On starting to move ◆ In cold, damp weather	**Rhus tox.** (*see page 162*) 6c 4 times daily up to 14 days
◆ Mental hyperactivity ◆ Intolerance of noise	◆ With movement ◆ From applying firm pressure to the affected area ◆ From massaging the legs	◆ From being exhausted ◆ Near noise ◆ If touched ◆ From being overheated	**Zinc. met.** (*see page 101*) 6c 4 times daily up to 14 days

THE MOUTH

DIGESTION BEGINS IN THE MOUTH, where the digestive enzyme amylase, found in saliva, begins to break down carbohydrates. The teeth crush and chew food to break it up into smaller pieces, and the muscular tongue mixes it with lubricating saliva and rolls it into a ball ready for swallowing. When food enters the mouth, it stimulates taste buds on the tongue. These send signals along nerves to taste centers

DISORDER	SPECIFIC AILMENT	PHYSICAL SYMPTOMS
## TOOTHACHE Often an indication of tooth decay, a toothache may also be a symptom of an infection such as gum disease, an abscess (a pus-filled sac surrounding the root of a tooth), or sinusitis (*see page 226*). The pain may be sharp and shooting or dull and throbbing; it may be continuous, come in waves, or occur only when a decayed tooth comes into contact with sweet foods, or very hot or very cold foods. **SELF-HELP** Rub oil of cloves onto the affected tooth and surrounding gums except when taking a homeopathic remedy, in which case the oil may act as an antidote. **CAUTION** If a toothache is accompanied by fever and swelling of the gums or face, or if a tooth feels loose, see a dentist within 12 hours. If a tooth is sensitive to hot or cold, and to sweet foods and drinks, or if there is pain on biting, see a dentist within 48 hours.	TOOTHACHE WITH SEVERE, SHOOTING PAIN	◆ Oversensitivity to agonizing pain that causes restlessness and thrashing around ◆ Pain makes sleeping difficult ◆ Jerking, tearing pain
	TOOTHACHE WITH UNBEARABLE PAIN	◆ Agonizing pain ◆ Swollen, red cheek on the same side of the face as a decayed tooth ◆ In young children, symptoms may be associated with teething
	TOOTHACHE WITH THROBBING PAIN	◆ Gums and cheeks are swollen and hot and painful to the touch ◆ Shooting pains extend to the ear ◆ Waves of pain that increase in severity to become excruciating before subsiding
## GINGIVITIS This condition causes the gums to bleed and become darker in color, swollen, and infected. Gingivitis usually occurs because of poor toothbrushing, but it may be a side effect of taking drugs, or be due to a vitamin deficiency, a serious blood disorder, or the immune system being weakened by stress. **SELF-HELP** Use a solution of calendula and hypericum (*see page 271*) as a mouthwash. **CAUTION** If the condition does not improve after three days, see a dentist.	BLEEDING GUMS WITH HALITOSIS	◆ Gums are tender, spongy, and bleed easily ◆ Excessive production of saliva, which dribbles onto the pillow during sleep ◆ Teeth may feel loose
	SWOLLEN, BLEEDING GUMS WITH CANKER SORES	◆ Taste of pus in the mouth ◆ Teeth are very sensitive to heat and cold ◆ Possible canker sores or cold sores
## HALITOSIS Halitosis, or bad breath, can be caused by tooth decay, smoking, gingivitis (*see above*), indigestion (*see page 234*), tonsillitis, sinusitis (*see page 226*), or fasting. To test whether your breath smells, breathe into the cupped palms of your hands and inhale. **SELF-HELP** Avoid foods and drinks that leave a strong odor behind or cause indigestion. If you smoke, stop. Visit your dentist regularly and practice good oral hygiene.	HALITOSIS ASSOCIATED WITH TOOTH DECAY AND GINGIVITIS	◆ Breath and sweat smell offensive ◆ Excessive production of saliva, which dribbles onto the pillow during sleep ◆ Tongue is yellow and thickly coated
## CANKER SORES Canker sores are ulcerated spots that can occur anywhere inside the mouth, and result from careless toothbrushing, biting the mouth, eating hot foods, an allergy, being run down, or stress. **SELF-HELP** Avoid spicy, sweet, or acidic foods. If you smoke, stop. Rinse the mouth with a warm saline solution (1 tsp/5 ml salt to 5 fl oz/150 ml boiled, cooled water) several times a day. **CAUTION** If sores have not healed in three weeks, see a doctor.	BURNING CANKER SORES	◆ Mouth feels dry ◆ Stinging, burning soreness in ulcerated areas ◆ Metallic or bitter taste in the mouth ◆ Tongue is clean, dry, and red

in the brain, which in turn activate digestive secretions. Bacteria naturally present in the mouth feed on sugary food particles and combine with saliva to form plaque – a sticky coating on the teeth and gums. If unchecked, plaque eventually erodes tooth enamel. Problems with teeth and gums are common in developed countries, where the diet is rich in sugar.

Many mouth problems can be prevented by regular dental checkups, good oral hygiene, and a diet that includes fibrous, chewy, nonsugary foods that stimulate the production of saliva, which contains infection-fighting white blood cells. Homeopathic treatment includes soothing mouthwashes as well as standard remedies that depend on specific symptoms.

PSYCHOLOGICAL SYMPTOMS	SYMPTOMS BETTER	SYMPTOMS WORSE	REMEDY & DOSAGE
◆ Great sensitivity to pain ◆ Inability to relax ◆ Hyperactive mind	◆ With ice-cold water in the mouth ◆ Lying down ◆ With sleep	◆ With heat ◆ From hot foods ◆ Near noise	**Coffea** (*see page 50*) 6c 4 times daily up to 14 days
◆ Irritability ◆ Irascibility ◆ Desire to be left alone and not be bothered by anything	◆ From sympathy ◆ In young children, from being carried around ◆ With cold applications, for example, ice on the tooth	◆ At night ◆ From being angry ◆ From warm foods and drinks ◆ In cold air	**Chamomilla** (*see page 46*) 6c 4 times daily up to 14 days
◆ Possible violent outbursts, if the condition is severe and accompanied by fever	◆ With rest ◆ From leaning the head against something ◆ From bending backward	◆ With touch ◆ From jarring ◆ At night ◆ In fresh air	**Belladonna** (*see page 39*) 30c every 5 minutes up to 10 doses
◆ Mental dullness ◆ Hesitant speech ◆ Slow comprehension ◆ Lack of willpower or motivation	◆ With rest ◆ When warmly dressed ◆ In the morning	◆ In extremes of temperature ◆ From perspiring at night ◆ From stress ◆ In drafts	**Merc. sol.** (*see page 85*) 6c every 4 hours up to 3 days
◆ Desire to be left alone ◆ Aversion to sympathy and consolation	◆ In fresh air ◆ From fasting ◆ From rubbing the affected area	◆ From physical or mental exertion ◆ From emotional stress ◆ With warmth ◆ In hot sun ◆ Near noise or from jarring	**Nat. mur.** (*see page 92*) 6c every 4 hours up to 3 days
◆ Desire to be left alone ◆ Aversion to sympathy and consolation	◆ With rest ◆ When warmly dressed ◆ From rubbing the gums	◆ With cold and extremes of temperature ◆ From perspiring at night ◆ From stress	**Merc. sol.** (*see page 85*) 6c 3 times daily up to 7 days
◆ Restlessness ◆ Anxiety	◆ From a warm mouthwash ◆ From applying warm compresses to the face ◆ Lying with the head higher than the body	◆ From cold foods and drinks ◆ In cold, dry, windy weather ◆ Between midnight and 2 A.M. ◆ From stress ◆ From being run down	**Arsen. alb.** (*see page 68*) 6c 4 times daily up to 5 days

DIGESTIVE SYSTEM

DIGESTION IS A COMPLEX process that starts with the chewing of food in the mouth and ends with the passing of waste from the rectum (*see page 188*). A healthy, efficient digestive system is essential for both physical and mental well-being, but it can be upset by many factors. Some can be controlled, such as diet and, to a certain extent, emotional stress or allergy, and some cannot, like infection or inherited problems.

DISORDER	SPECIFIC AILMENT	PHYSICAL SYMPTOMS
INDIGESTION Indigestion is a blanket term for a number of symptoms that include excessive burping, a stomachache, and heartburn (*see below*). It may be caused by the defective production or flow of digestive enzymes, fluids, or hormones, or by something more serious, such as a peptic ulcer. Alternatively, it may result simply from eating too much, or eating the kinds of food that the digestive system finds difficult to process. Indigestion tends to worsen with stress and with age. **SELF-HELP** Practice some form of relaxation or meditation before you eat. Do not rush your meal, and relax for at least 30 minutes after eating. Avoid coffee, tea, alcohol, sodas, smoking, and eating late at night. Avoid foods that may cause problems, such as citrus fruits, tomatoes, onions, beans, nuts, spices, bread, pork, and rich, fatty foods. Cut down on unrefined carbohydrates. **CAUTION** If you experience serious pain radiating toward the back, with or without vomiting, see a doctor within two hours. If you vomit blood, consult a doctor immediately.	INDIGESTION WITH EXCESSIVE FLATULENCE	◆ Digestion seems to have slowed down ◆ Pain when eating even the plainest food ◆ Burning feeling in the stomach extending through to the back ◆ Craving for salty, acidic, or sweet foods and coffee, and aversion to meat or milk
	INDIGESTION WITH PAINFUL RETCHING	◆ Heartburn 30 minutes after eating, with a putrid taste in the mouth ◆ Craving for fatty, acidic, or spicy foods and alcohol, even though they upset the digestion
	INDIGESTION WITH NAUSEA AND/OR VOMITING	◆ Indigestion two hours after eating, and especially in the evening ◆ Pounding heart ◆ Unpleasant taste in the mouth ◆ Feeling of pressure under the breastbone ◆ Possible headache around the eyes
HEARTBURN Heartburn is a common form of indigestion consisting of a burning pain in the stomach or the esophagus and the chest. It tends to worsen with age, and may be associated with a hiatal hernia (protrusion of the stomach through the opening in the diaphragm into the esophagus). It is exacerbated by stress, and by eating certain foods (*see Indigestion, above*). Eating too quickly, or eating too much, and swallowing air also aggravate the condition. Heartburn is very common during pregnancy, when digestive efficiency is impaired. **SELF-HELP** Try relaxation or meditation before you eat. Eat calmly, and relax for 30 minutes afterward. Avoid eating late, and do not eat foods that you know upset you. If you smoke, stop. **CAUTION** If you have serious pain radiating toward the back, see a doctor within two hours. If you vomit blood, consult a doctor immediately.	HEARTBURN WITH DESIRE FOR ICE-COLD WATER	◆ Burning sensation in the chest ◆ Craving for ice-cold water that may be vomited as soon as it is warmed in the stomach ◆ Constant hunger ◆ Wakefulness and night hunger but eating produces no weight gain ◆ Desire for salt, ice cream, chocolate, fish, and cool drinks, and aversion to oysters, eggs, and meat
	HEARTBURN WITH CRAVING FOR SWEETS	◆ Burning sensation associated with hunger and weakness due to low blood-sugar levels (hypoglycemia) ◆ Strong craving for sweet, spicy, and fatty foods
HICCUPS Hiccups are caused by spasms of the diaphragm that produce a rush of air into the lungs. This, in turn, causes the vocal chords to snap shut with a click. The spasms are caused by irritation of the diaphragm as a result of too much air in the stomach, laughing, being tickled, or emotional stress. **SELF-HELP** Traditional cures include holding the breath, breathing rapidly, breathing into a paper bag, having someone give you a shock, or squirting lemon juice down the back of the throat. Water with a little glucose may help infants.	HICCUPS WITH BURPING	◆ Hiccups an hour or two after eating a very rich meal ◆ Possible retching
	HICCUPS ASSOCIATED WITH EMOTIONAL STRESS	◆ Hiccups after eating, drinking, or smoking

Dietary discretion – what a person chooses to eat – and eating habits have an obvious impact on digestion. Some foods are difficult to digest, and routines such as eating late may also cause problems. Minor ailments, such as indigestion, lend themselves to homeopathic self-help, especially if combined with dietary controls. Homeopathic remedies are concerned with improving the condition of the digestive tract, by adjusting the number of beneficial bacteria; reducing irritation caused by some foods; improving waste elimination; and maintaining other organs involved in the digestive process, such as the liver. Some ailments, such as hemorrhoids, may need constitutional treatment (*see page 176*), especially if they recur.

PSYCHOLOGICAL SYMPTOMS	SYMPTOMS BETTER	SYMPTOMS WORSE	REMEDY & DOSAGE
◆ Lack of mental energy ◆ Lack of interest in life ◆ Intransigence	◆ From burping ◆ In cold, fresh air	◆ From overeating ◆ From rich, fatty foods ◆ From eating too late in the day ◆ Lying down ◆ In the evening ◆ In warm, wet weather	**Carbo veg.** (*see page 44*) 30c every 10–15 minutes up to 7 doses
◆ Irritability ◆ Agitation resulting from stress and lack of sleep ◆ Criticism of others	◆ With warmth ◆ With sleep ◆ From applying firm pressure to the stomach ◆ In the evening ◆ From being alone	◆ With touch ◆ From fatty, acidic, or spicy foods or alcohol ◆ From stress ◆ With lack of sleep ◆ In cold, windy weather	**Nux vomica** (*see page 63*) 6c every 10–15 minutes up to 7 doses
◆ Tearfulness at the slightest provocation ◆ Depression ◆ Self-pity ◆ Desire for sympathy	◆ With gentle exercise ◆ From crying	◆ From rich, fatty foods ◆ From emotional stress ◆ With hormonal changes due to menstruation or pregnancy ◆ In the evening and at night ◆ In hot, stuffy conditions	**Pulsatilla** (*see page 61*) 6c every 10–15 minutes up to 7 doses
◆ Anxiety about health ◆ Irrational fear of the dark, being alone, death, and thunderstorms	◆ From cold foods and water ◆ With sleep ◆ From a general body massage	◆ Lying on the back ◆ From stress ◆ From warm foods	**Phosphorus** (*see page 94*) 6c every 10–15 minutes up to 7 doses if acute
◆ Laziness and lack of mental energy ◆ Melancholia ◆ Hypochondria ◆ Tendency to daydream ◆ Indecision	◆ In the open air ◆ From applying warm compresses to the stomach and lower chest ◆ From warm drinks	◆ From bathing ◆ From becoming overheated, especially in a warm room or in bed at night ◆ When standing up	**Sulfur** (*see page 99*) 6c every 10–15 minutes up to 7 doses if acute
◆ Irritability ◆ Fussiness ◆ Lack of mental energy ◆ Exhaustion from lack of sleep ◆ Harsh criticism	◆ From hot drinks ◆ From loosening clothing	◆ From the pressure of clothing ◆ From overindulgence ◆ From food, drink, or drugs	**Nux vomica** (*see page 63*) 6c every 15 minutes up to 6 doses
◆ Moodiness ◆ Extreme sensitivity ◆ Lack of mental energy ◆ Guilt ◆ Sensitivity to noise	◆ From swallowing ◆ From eating ◆ Lying on the back	◆ From emotional stress ◆ From smoking, eating, or drinking when upset	**Ignatia** (*see page 57*) 6c every 15 minutes up to 6 doses

DISORDER	SPECIFIC AILMENT	PHYSICAL SYMPTOMS
NAUSEA & VOMITING Nausea, or the feeling of a need to vomit, is not necessarily followed by vomiting, the involuntary expulsion of the contents of the stomach, but the causes of the two are the same. Nausea and vomiting may be symptoms of digestive disorders caused by eating fatty foods, drinking too much alcohol, food poisoning, or infections such as gastroenteritis (*see below*). Stress, migraines, or the hormonal changes associated with menstruation or pregnancy (*see page 262*) may also trigger these conditions. Nausea and vomiting may also indicate more serious ailments, many of which are digestive disorders, such as a peptic ulcer (erosion of areas of the digestive tract by acidic gastric juices) or cancer of the stomach, but some of which are connected to the brain and nervous system. Self-help treatments are not appropriate in these cases. **SELF-HELP** Drink small amounts of cooled, boiled water frequently and avoid solid foods. If you smoke, stop. **CAUTION** If vomiting persists for more than 48 hours, or is accompanied by fever, see a doctor within two hours. If there is severe abdominal pain or blood in the vomit, seek medical help immediately. If you think you may have vomited prescribed drugs, consult a doctor.	CONSTANT NAUSEA	◆ Constant nausea that is not relieved by vomiting ◆ Vomit may include green mucus ◆ Possible headaches, perspiration, and diarrhea ◆ Spasmodic abdominal pain
	VOMITING WITH GREAT THIRST	◆ Craving for ice-cold drinks, which are then vomited when warmed in the stomach ◆ Burning pain in the pit of the stomach with retching and vomiting
	NAUSEA AND VOMITING WITH TEARFULNESS	◆ Nausea and vomiting may be accompanied by mucus dripping down the back of the throat
	NAUSEA AND VOMITING WITH IRRITABILITY	◆ Vomiting two to three hours after eating ◆ Painful retching ◆ Sensation resembling a hangover ◆ Tendency to wake up around 4 A.M. for a couple of hours
GASTROENTERITIS (GASTRIC FLU) This inflammation of the digestive tract is usually caused by a virus transmitted directly from person to person or via contaminated food and water. Symptoms of gastroenteritis vary in severity but usually pass within 48 hours. At worst, there is nausea, vomiting, diarrhea, abdominal pain, fever, and exhaustion. Infants and the elderly are most at risk because of the danger of dehydration. **SELF-HELP** Rest and drink plenty of fluids, preferably salted, cooled, boiled water (1 tsp/5 ml salt and 8 tsp/40 ml sugar to approximately 2 pints/1 liter water), to prevent dehydration. Avoid drinking milk and eating any solid food until the stomach settles. Be meticulous about personal hygiene. **CAUTION** If symptoms persist for more than 48 hours, or if there is blood in the feces or a fever, see a doctor within two hours. If symptoms are accompanied by severe abdominal pain that lasts for more than an hour, consult a doctor immediately.	VOMITING AND DIARRHEA AT THE SAME TIME	◆ Vomiting with burning pain in the abdomen ◆ Diarrhea that causes soreness of the anus and stinging in the rectum ◆ Craving for cold drinks that may be vomited as soon as they are warmed in the stomach ◆ Chilliness
	GASTROENTERITIS WITH SEVERE ABDOMINAL CRAMPS	◆ Colicky pains that are better when the body is bent double ◆ Possible diarrhea ◆ Pain relieved by passing gas
	GASTROENTERITIS WITH DIFFERENT TYPES OF STOOL	◆ Rumbling, gurgling stomach ◆ Pressure under the breastbone after meals ◆ No two stools are alike in texture or color ◆ Possible vomiting
BLOATING & FLATULENCE Bloating and flatulence – a feeling of fullness in the stomach associated with burping or the passing of air out through the anus – may be due to constipation (*see page 238*) or intestinal dysbios (an overgrowth of bacteria or fungi in the intestine). The condition may be worse prior to menstruation, and is aggravated by anxiety, food intolerance, or swallowing air. **SELF-HELP** Avoid eating legumes, onions, cabbage, and nuts, and use cumin, aniseed, or ginger in your cooking.	BLOATING AFTER EATING ONLY SMALL AMOUNTS OF FOOD	◆ Hunger, but bloated feeling after only small quantities of food have been eaten ◆ Difficulty in passing stools without straining ◆ Main discomfort is on the right side of the abdomen, and is not relieved by passing gas
	BLOATING AND FLATULENCE RELIEVED BY BURPING	◆ All foods produce flatulence ◆ Burning sensation in the stomach ◆ Craving for salty, acidic, and sweet foods and coffee, and an aversion to meat and milk

PSYCHOLOGICAL SYMPTOMS	SYMPTOMS BETTER	SYMPTOMS WORSE	REMEDY & DOSAGE
◆ None marked, but possible tendency to be very hard to please	◆ In the open air ◆ With rest	◆ In a moving car or when looking at moving objects ◆ With movement ◆ Lying down	**Ipecac.** (*see page 45*) 6c hourly up to 10 doses (mild); 6c every 15 minutes up to 10 doses (acute)
◆ Fear and anxiety ◆ Great concern for others or complete indifference, even toward loved ones	◆ With sleep ◆ From a massage and relaxation ◆ Lying on the right side	◆ From physical or mental exertion ◆ From hot foods and drinks ◆ Between sunset and midnight ◆ When the hands are held in cold water	**Phosphorus** (*see page 94*) 6c hourly up to 10 doses (mild); 6c every 15 minutes up to 10 doses (acute)
◆ Tearfulness ◆ Self-pity ◆ Great need for sympathy ◆ Depression	◆ From crying and sympathy ◆ With gentle exercise ◆ In fresh air ◆ From cold drinks ◆ With the hands above the head	◆ From rich, fatty foods ◆ In hot, stuffy rooms ◆ In the sun ◆ In the evening and at night	**Pulsatilla** (*see page 61*) 6c hourly up to 10 doses (mild); 6c every 15 minutes up to 10 doses (acute)
◆ Irritability ◆ Harsh criticism of others ◆ Overactive brain when awake during the night	◆ With warmth ◆ With sleep ◆ From applying firm pressure to the abdomen	◆ From overindulgence ◆ With cold ◆ Near noise ◆ From stress	**Nux vomica** (*see page 63*) 6c every 15 minutes up to 10 doses
◆ Restlessness, fear, and anxiety ◆ Despair about recovery ◆ Irritability	◆ With warmth ◆ From hot drinks	◆ At the sight and smell of food ◆ Between midnight and 2 A.M. ◆ From cold drinks ◆ From alcohol	**Arsen. alb.** (*see page 68*) 6c hourly up to 10 doses
◆ Irritability and extreme sensitivity ◆ Possible suppressed anger and indignation at real or imagined ill-treatment	◆ Lying on one side with the knees pulled up to the chest ◆ With warmth ◆ From sleep ◆ From coffee	◆ From eating or drinking ◆ In cold, damp weather ◆ Around 4 P.M.	**Colocynthis** (*see page 52*) 6c hourly up to 10 doses
◆ Depression and self-pity ◆ Tearfulness and great desire for sympathy and consolation	◆ From crying and sympathy ◆ In fresh air ◆ From cold drinks	◆ In hot, stuffy rooms ◆ In the evening and at night ◆ From rich, fatty foods ◆ From stress	**Pulsatilla** (*see page 61*) 6c hourly up to 10 doses
◆ Melancholia ◆ Apprehension ◆ Poor memory	◆ From hot foods and drinks ◆ After midnight ◆ In cool conditions	◆ From wearing tight clothing ◆ From overeating ◆ Between 4 P.M. and 8 P.M. ◆ In stuffy rooms	**Lycopodium** (*see page 59*) 6c half-hourly up to 10 doses
◆ Lethargy, sluggishness, and indifference ◆ Irritability with mood swings	◆ From burping ◆ In fresh air ◆ With cold	◆ From overeating ◆ From rich, fatty foods ◆ From eating too late in the day ◆ In the evening ◆ Lying down	**Carbo veg.** (*see page 44*) 6c half-hourly up to 10 doses

DISORDER	SPECIFIC AILMENT	PHYSICAL SYMPTOMS

DIARRHEA

Diarrhea is the frequent passing of watery or loose stools as a result of the failure of the large intestine to absorb water from undigested material. This may be the result of dietary or digestive problems, such as eating too many prunes or legumes, a lack of vitamin B or folic acid, too much vitamin D, food intolerance, parasites, or gastroenteritis (*see page 236*). Diarrhea may indicate a more serious condition, such as irritable bowel syndrome (*see page 189*), or be a reaction to certain drugs, anxiety, or stress.

SELF-HELP Drink plenty of boiled, cooled water with a little honey in it, ice water, or barley water to avoid dehydration. Progress to arrowroot, tapioca, semolina, or slippery elm food, then thin soups. A supplement of acidophilus, or eating live yogurt, is advisable if diarrhea follows taking certain drugs such as antibiotics. Avoid analgesics and vitamin E supplements.

CAUTION If diarrhea continues for more than 48 hours, or if there is blood in the feces, see a doctor within two hours. Recurrent diarrhea may require constitutional homeopathic treatment (*see page 176*).

DIARRHEA CAUSED BY FOOD INTOLERANCE
- Yellowish green stools accompanied by severe flatulence
- Painful urination
- Tip of the tongue is red

DIARRHEA CAUSED BY NERVOUS EXCITEMENT
- Diarrhea followed by severe flatulence
- Stools may be greenish in color
- Flatulence not relieved by burping
- Craving for salty, sweet, and cold foods

DIARRHEA AFTER SHOCK
- Green, watery diarrhea resembling chopped spinach
- Possible nausea and perspiration
- Possible colicky pains or lack of pain

DIARRHEA AFTER COLD FOODS AND DRINKS
- Stools are scanty, odorless, and brown
- Stools burn the skin around the anus

CONSTIPATION

Constipation is the difficult and/or infrequent passing of stools. It is commonly caused by a diet that includes too little fiber, but it can also result from a lack of exercise, stress, poor bowel training, taking certain drugs, and thyroid or liver problems. Chronic constipation may be due to the recurrent use of laxatives or drinking too much coffee or alcohol, and is viewed in homeopathy as a constitutional problem (*see page 176*).

SELF-HELP Try eating plenty of raw vegetables before resorting to laxatives based on substances such as senna, which, over a long period, may irritate the lining of the gut. Increase the amount of exercise you get.

CAUTION If a marked change in bowel function is accompanied by a weight loss of more than 1 lb (0.5 kg) in a week, see a doctor within 48 hours. If there is any bleeding from the anus or blood in the stools, see a doctor within 12 hours. If no stools have been passed for several days despite self-help measures, especially if there is pain in the abdomen, see a doctor as soon as possible.

DRY, HARD STOOLS AND DRY MUCOUS MEMBRANES
- Stools are large, dry, hard, and look burned
- Headache and congested feeling
- Bloated abdomen
- Burning in the rectum after passing a stool
- Great thirst
- All mucous membranes are dry

CONSTIPATION WITH STRONG URGE TO PASS STOOLS
- Cramps and spasms in the anus resulting in a great urgency to pass a stool, but with increasing difficulty in doing so
- Great thirst

CONSTIPATION WITH DIFFICULTY IN PASSING EVEN SOFT STOOLS
- No desire to open the bowels until the rectum is completely distended
- Difficulty in passing stools
- Stools may be soft and claylike or covered in mucus
- Sensation of a stool having been coughed up and caught beneath the left rib cage

HEMORRHOIDS

Hemorrhoids, or piles, are swollen veins in the lower rectum and around the anus, often due to constipation (*see above*), but also associated with hormonal problems, pregnancy, childbirth, the overuse of laxatives, and sitting on hard surfaces.

SELF-HELP Try peony ointment or hamamelis suppositories. Include more fiber in your diet to avoid constipation.

CAUTION If there is bleeding from the anus, do not assume that it is due to hemorrhoids until other possible causes have been ruled out. If bleeding persists, see a doctor within 12 hours.

HEMORRHOIDS RESEMBLING A BUNCH OF GRAPES
- Itchy inflammation of the veins
- Sore, bruised feeling in the anus
- Hemorrhoids may bleed
- Hemorrhoids feel strained and rigid
- Great thirst

INTERNAL HEMORRHOIDS WITH SPLINTER-LIKE PAIN
- Internal hemorrhoids associated with constipation
- Dry, splinterlike sensation in the rectum
- Lumpy stools that cause stitching pain
- Hot, dry, itchy anus

PSYCHOLOGICAL SYMPTOMS	SYMPTOMS BETTER	SYMPTOMS WORSE	REMEDY & DOSAGE
◆ Irritability caused by discomfort of symptoms ◆ Anxiety about whether gas or stools will be passed	◆ With cold ◆ In fresh air ◆ From fasting	◆ In hot weather ◆ After eating or drinking ◆ Early in the morning	**Aloe** (*see page 35*) 6c hourly up to 10 doses
◆ Apprehension	◆ In fresh air ◆ With cold	◆ With warmth ◆ From sweet foods ◆ At night	**Argentum nit.** (*see page 74*) 6c half-hourly up to 10 doses
◆ Great fear of death, even to the extent of predicting the time of death	◆ From passing stools	◆ On exposure to cold wind ◆ From overeating in summer	**Aconite** (*see page 32*) 30c half-hourly up to 10 doses
◆ Fear, particularly of having an incurable illness ◆ Restlessness ◆ Wakefulness between midnight and about 2 A.M.	◆ From frequent, small sips of warm drinks	◆ From cold drinks, ice cream or popsicles, and overripe fruits	**Arsen. alb.** (*see page 68*) 6c half-hourly up to 10 doses
◆ Irritability	◆ From applying pressure to the head and abdomen ◆ With cold ◆ From being left alone and keeping quiet	◆ From overeating ◆ From rich, fatty foods ◆ From eating too late in the day	**Bryonia** (*see page 42*) 30c every 2 hours up to 10 doses
◆ Anger and irritability ◆ Extreme sensitivity to noise, touch, and pressure	◆ With heat ◆ With sleep ◆ In the evening	◆ From too much mental stimulation ◆ If touched and from pressure ◆ Near noise ◆ Early in the morning	**Nux vomica** (*see page 63*) 6c every 2 hours up to 10 doses
◆ Sense of urgency internally despite outward appearance of slowing down ◆ Feeling of foreboding ◆ Possible confusion ◆ Possible sense of unreality	◆ From stretching the body backward ◆ From standing up	◆ In cold weather ◆ From wine, vinegar, pepper, salt, and starchy foods	**Alumina** (*see page 72*) 6c every 2 hours up to 10 doses
◆ None, apart from irritability caused by discomfort of symptoms	◆ With rest	◆ With warmth ◆ From pressure on the affected area ◆ With movement	**Hamamelis** (*see page 145*) 6c 4 times daily up to 5 days
◆ Depression ◆ Irritability ◆ Difficulty in concentrating ◆ Confusion upon waking	◆ If the hemorrhoids bleed ◆ From kneeling ◆ In cool, open air	◆ In the morning ◆ From passing a stool ◆ From standing	**Aesculus** (*see page 121*) 6c 4 times daily up to 5 days

THE SKIN

THE SKIN ACCOUNTS FOR 16 PERCENT of the total weight of the human body and as such may be described as its largest organ. Stretched out flat it would cover between 15 and 20 square feet (2 and 2.6 square meters). It protects the internal organs of the body from environmental impact and injury, and acts as a sensory organ, regulating body temperature and metabolism, for example, the control of bodily

DISORDER	SPECIFIC AILMENT	PHYSICAL SYMPTOMS
## MILD ACNE The term acne includes common blemishes such as blackheads (comedones), whiteheads (milia), and yellowheads (pustules). Acne is associated with high hormone levels, for example, during puberty, which increase the production of sebum, the skin's oily secretion, leading to clogged pores. If pores become infected, acne forms. Acne may be exacerbated by taking certain drugs or stress. If there is a firm swelling beneath the skin, treat as for boils (see below). **SELF-HELP** Sunlight in moderation and fresh air are beneficial. Avoid refined carbohydrates, chocolate, cheese, nuts, citrus soda drinks, and processed foods. Wash affected areas thoroughly twice a day. Do not scrub the skin, since this spreads infection, or pick acne and risk scarring. Use commercial preparations sparingly. **CAUTION** If there is scarring or large, fluid-filled cysts, treat as for rosacea (see page 193). If cysts persist for 14 days, or are causing distress, see a doctor.	ITCHY ACNE ON THE FACE AND SHOULDERS	◆ Itchy acne including blackheads and yellowheads with depressed centers ◆ Tendency for scarring if the acne is scratched ◆ Fidgety feet and hands
	PAINFUL, PUS-FILLED PIMPLES	◆ Yellowheads that are extremely painful to the touch
	ACNE ASSOCIATED WITH HORMONAL IMBALANCE, ESPECIALLY IN ADOLESCENT GIRLS	◆ Acne occurs during puberty ◆ Associated with delayed or scant menstruation in adolescent girls ◆ Acne is worse from eating rich, fatty foods
## MILD ECZEMA Mild eczema is common, especially in children. The skin is inflamed and itchy, possibly with small pimples and scaly patches. If scratched, the skin may bleed. Eczema is commonly found in the flexures, such as the bend of an elbow, and on the face, but it can occur anywhere. It may be an allergic reaction to a variety of chemical irritants, plants, food, or metals, or it may be hereditary. Eczema may be exacerbated by stress, hormonal changes, or dietary factors. **SELF-HELP** Avoid known irritants. Use moisturizing ointments, preferably paraffin-based, to keep the skin soft. Use emulsifying ointments rather than soap for washing. Wear cotton next to the skin. Avoid potentially irritating foods, such as dairy products, one at a time for a month, and see if the condition improves. **CAUTION** If the skin produces a watery discharge, or becomes infected, creating a yellow discharge, or if irritation causes sleeplessness, treat as for severe eczema (see page 194).	ECZEMA WITH RESTLESSNESS	◆ Skin is dry and burning, but is aggravated by the application of cold compresses ◆ Inability to sit still ◆ Sleeplessness, especially after midnight
	DRY ECZEMA	◆ Skin is rough, red, and itchy ◆ Possible diarrhea, especially early in the morning ◆ Desire for salty, fatty, spicy, or sweet foods
	ECZEMA THAT IS WORST BEHIND THE EARS	◆ Skin is rough, dry, and may be cracked ◆ Eruptions are worst behind the ears and possibly on the palms of the hands ◆ Face feels dry, as if covered by a cobweb
## BOILS A boil is a firm swelling (nodule) beneath the skin caused by the infection of a hair follicle. Thick, white or yellow pus accumulates and comes to a head. Boils may be associated with illness, fatigue, stress, or being run-down. Recurrent boils may be due to an infection or they may be a symptom of diabetes. **SELF-HELP** Bathe a boil with a solution of hypericum and calendula (see page 271). Never squeeze a boil, and if it bursts, let it drain naturally. Avoid handling food after dealing with boils. **CAUTION** If boils recur, are accompanied by fever or severe pain, or do not heal within a week, consult a doctor.	EARLY STAGES OF BOIL FORMATION	◆ Possible sudden onset of symptoms ◆ Boil is round and hard ◆ Skin around the boil is dry, inflamed, painful, and throbbing ◆ Possible fever
	LATER STAGES OF BOIL WHEN PUS HAS FORMED	◆ Boil has a head of pus that is on the point of bursting ◆ Boil is sensitive to the slightest touch

fluids and elimination of waste. The skin contains blood vessels, lymph vessels, and nerve endings that perform its sensory function, glands that manufacture sebum to keep the skin supple and waterproof, and follicles that produce hair and nails. Homeopathic practitioners tend to regard skin complaints as an outer manifestation of what is going on within the body, and look for underlying causes of skin eruptions. Stress, poor diet, and allergies, as well as infections may all cause outbreaks. Skin conditions may be aggravated by factors such as lack of exercise; eating sugary foods, refined carbohydrates, or other foods; caffeine and alcohol; constipation; the use of cosmetics; and contact irritants in the environment.

Psychological symptoms	Symptoms better	Symptoms worse	Remedy & dosage
• Restlessness • Nervousness • Suspicion • Feeling of helplessness	• From physical or mental exertion • In cold weather	• From hormonal changes such as those associated with puberty or menstruation • From emotional stress	**Kali. brom.** (see page 149) 6c 3 times daily up to 14 days
• Great irritability • Petulance • Tendency to lash out if the pimples are touched	• With heat • In damp weather • From eating	• When the pimples are touched, even lightly • With cold • Lying on the affected areas	**Hepar sulf.** (see page 84) 6c 3 times daily up to 14 days
• Tearfulness • Self-pity • Desire for sympathy	• From crying • In the open air • From applying cold compresses to the affected areas	• From rich, fatty foods • In warm, stuffy rooms • From hormonal changes such as those associated with puberty, menstruation, or pregnancy	**Pulsatilla** (see page 61) 6c 3 times daily up to 14 days
• Possible anxiety • Restlessness • Desire for reassurance	• With warmth • From applying warm compresses to the affected areas • From walking around	• With cold • Between midnight and 2 A.M. • From physical or mental exertion • From drinking milk	**Arsen. alb.** (see page 68) 6c 4 times daily up to 7 days
• Anxiety • Lack of mental energy • Harsh criticism of others but tolerance of one's own failings	• In fresh air • With cold • From perspiring	• From washing • From becoming overheated • Early in the morning	**Sulfur** (see page 99) 6c 4 times daily up to 7 days
• Timidity • Indecisiveness • Possible anxiety and depression • Emotionalism	• With sleep • When wrapped up warmly • In fresh air	• From cold or sweet foods, or seafood • From hormonal changes associated with menstruation • In cold conditions • From scratching the skin	**Graphites** (see page 83) 6c 4 times daily up to 7 days
• None, unless multiple boils are accompanied by fever, in which case there may be delirium and hallucinations	• From applying pressure to the affected area • At night • With warmth	• From applying cold compresses to the affected area • In drafts • If touched	**Belladonna** (see page 39) 30c hourly up to 10 doses
• Possible extreme bad temper • Desire not to be touched, physically or emotionally	• With warmth • From applying warm compresses to the affected area • In damp weather	• In cold air and drafts • From even the lightest touch • Lying on the affected area	**Hepar sulf.** (see page 84) 6c hourly up to 10 doses

DISORDER	SPECIFIC AILMENT	PHYSICAL SYMPTOMS
HIVES (URTICARIA) This condition consists of raised red patches – sometimes with paler centers – which itch intensely. It may be caused by a food allergy, certain drugs, bites or stings, or heat, cold, or sunlight. Hives may also be a symptom of stress or leaky gut syndrome (*see* Allergy, page 206). **SELF-HELP** Take a cool shower or place a covered ice pack on the affected area. Urtica ointment may relieve itchiness. **CAUTION** If the eyes, lips, or throat swell dramatically, call an ambulance, and take *Apis 30c* every minute until help arrives.	HIVES WITH SWELLING ON THE LIPS AND EYELIDS	◆ Skin on the lips and eyelids is red, swollen, and burning ◆ Throat may be swollen
	HIVES WITH VIOLENTLY ITCHY BLOTCHES	◆ Burning sensation, especially on the hands ◆ Itchy, red, or pale, slightly raised blotches ◆ Stinging blemishes on the skin
COLD SORES Cold sores are blisters on and around the mouth caused by a virus. They are triggered by being run-down or by hot, cold, or windy weather. Accompanying symptoms include canker sores, inflamed gums, a furry tongue, and mild fever. **SELF-HELP** Avoid peanuts, chocolate, seeds, and cereal grains.	SORES ON THE LIPS AND AROUND THE MOUTH	◆ Mouth feels dry ◆ Lips are swollen and burning, with pearl-like blisters ◆ Blisters weep before becoming crusty ◆ As blisters dry up they may develop into deep, painful cracks
WARTS A wart is caused by a virus that causes cells to multiply rapidly, forming a raised lump. Warts on the feet (verrucas) tend to grow inward as a result of the pressure placed on them. **SELF-HELP** Cover a wart, but not the surrounding skin, with a fabric bandage. Drip thuja mother tincture onto it twice daily. Over-the-counter treatments can be used with homeopathic ones except on facial warts. Keep treatments away from the eyes. **CAUTION** If the condition does not improve, and especially if a wart changes size or color, or if it itches or bleeds, consult a doctor.	SOFT, FLESHY, CAULIFLOWER-SHAPED WARTS	◆ Warts are found anywhere on the body, but especially on the back of the hand ◆ Warts ooze or bleed easily ◆ Restless sleep
	WARTS MAINLY NEAR THE NAILS	◆ Warts appear on the fingers, near or even under the nails ◆ Possible warts on the face and eyelids ◆ Verrucas may be painful
DANDRUFF Dandruff is characterized by a flaking scalp, which is sometimes itchy and red. It may be caused by seborrheic dermatitis, a form of eczema (*see* page 240). More rarely, it may be symptomatic of psoriasis (*see* page 195) or a fungal infection. **SELF-HELP** Reduce your intake of refined carbohydrates and animal fats. If the whole scalp itches, place a cold compress soaked in olive oil on the head overnight; wash off with a pure soap shampoo. If all else fails, use a shampoo containing selenium, but follow instructions carefully. Apply calendula ointment to itchy areas around the hairline.	DANDRUFF WITH UNBEARABLE ITCHING AT NIGHT	◆ Scalp is dry, flaky, and very hot ◆ Scalp is unbearably itchy at night ◆ Round, bare patches of scalp show through the hair
	DANDRUFF WITH SKIN THAT BURNS WHEN SCRATCHED	◆ Thick dandruff ◆ Scratching, particularly at night, causes the skin to burn ◆ Scalp becomes drier from washing the hair
HAIR LOSS Old hair is lost as new hair grows. Growth may slow sometimes so that hair is lost faster than it is replaced. Thinning often occurs with age, especially in men, and may be hereditary. Hair loss may be associated with thyroid problems, anemia, vitamin or mineral deficiency, stress or shock, or certain drugs. **SELF-HELP** Avoid processes such as dying or perming, and do not wash or condition the hair too frequently. Let the hair dry naturally. Scalp massage may help. Eat plenty of protein. **CAUTION** If the condition does not improve, or if there is no explanation for sudden hair loss, consult a doctor.	PREMATURE BALDING OR GRAYING	◆ Great loss of hair or graying of hair at a younger age than would normally be expected ◆ Hair loss possibly associated with eczema on the scalp
	HAIR LOSS DUE TO HORMONAL CHANGES	◆ Greater loss of hair than usual following childbirth or during menopause ◆ Possible chronic headaches

Psychological symptoms	Symptoms better	Symptoms worse	Remedy & dosage
◆ Irritability and nervousness ◆ Clumsiness and a tendency to drop things	◆ From undressing ◆ From cool baths ◆ In cold air	◆ With heat ◆ In the late afternoon ◆ With sleep ◆ If touched ◆ In stuffy rooms	**Apis** (see page 104) 30c hourly up to 10 doses
◆ None, apart from irritability due to discomfort of symptoms	◆ Lying down ◆ From gently massaging the affected area	◆ If touched ◆ In cold, damp air ◆ In water and snow ◆ From scratching the skin	**Urtica urens** (see page 170) 6c hourly up to 10 doses
◆ Depression ◆ Desire to be left alone ◆ Aversion to consolation	◆ In fresh air ◆ From fasting	◆ At around 10 A.M. ◆ In cold, thundery weather ◆ With warmth ◆ In hot sun, salt air, or drafts ◆ Near noise, music, or talking ◆ From jarring ◆ From physical or mental exertion	**Nat. mur.** (see page 92) 6c 4 times daily up to 5 days
◆ Great sensitivity and vulnerability ◆ Disturbing dreams	◆ From covering the affected area ◆ With warmth	◆ From scratching or picking the wart ◆ In cold, damp living conditions ◆ After immunizations	**Thuja** (see page 64) 6c twice daily up to 3 weeks
◆ Pessimism and depression ◆ Intense sympathy for people in distress or for animals ◆ Emotionalism	◆ In damp conditions ◆ With warmth ◆ From cold drinks	◆ In cold air ◆ From sweet foods ◆ From coffee ◆ From emotional stress	**Causticum** (see page 79) 6c twice daily up to 3 weeks
◆ Restlessness and anxiety, especially on waking in the middle of the night	◆ With warmth on the head ◆ From covering the head ◆ From walking around	◆ With cold ◆ From vegetables ◆ From drinking milk	**Arsen. alb.** (see page 68) 6c 3 times daily up to 14 days
◆ Lack of mental energy ◆ Lack of willpower ◆ Harsh criticism of others but tolerance of one's own failings	◆ With cold ◆ From perspiring ◆ In fresh air	◆ With warmth ◆ From washing ◆ Early in the morning	**Sulfur** (see page 99) 6c 3 times daily up to 14 days
◆ Lack of self-confidence ◆ Cowardice ◆ Anger	◆ With relaxation or convalescence ◆ From warm drinks	◆ From stress ◆ After childbirth	**Lycopodium** (see page 59) 6c twice daily up to 4 weeks
◆ Tearfulness ◆ Irritability ◆ Indifference to loved ones ◆ Aversion to sexual intercourse	◆ From applying hot compresses to the head ◆ From bathing in cold water ◆ With vigorous exercise	◆ Before menstruation ◆ During pregnancy, after childbirth, or following a miscarriage ◆ During menopause	**Sepia** (see page 112) 6c twice daily up to 4 weeks

EMOTIONAL PROBLEMS

HOMEOPATHY IS WELL SUITED to the treatment of emotional problems. As a holistic form of medicine, it examines all aspects of an individual – physical, intellectual, and spiritual – and a practitioner does not separate these elements when prescribing treatment. Homeopathic practitioners do not delineate where one ends and the other begins. The investigation of a person's experience on a number of

DISORDER	SPECIFIC AILMENT	PHYSICAL SYMPTOMS
INSOMNIA Insomnia describes a persistent pattern of intermittent sleep that leaves the sufferer feeling tired and unrefreshed. It may occur simply because the bedroom is too hot or airless, or because of having to get up during the night to urinate. It is more likely to be the result of being ill or in pain – to which extreme sensitivity may develop – or of disturbed sleep patterns and exhaustion caused by regular sleep deprivation. Insomnia can also be caused by excessive caffeine or alcohol, food allergies, overexcitement, stress, shock, anxiety (*see below*), or depression (*see page 212*). **SELF-HELP** Increase the amount of exercise you get during the day, and avoid eating late in the evening. Stop work or any other activity an hour before bedtime. Drink a relaxing herbal tea or hot milk, take a warm bath, and read something light and entertaining. With all the homeopathic remedies suggested, take the dose for ten consecutive nights (unless normal sleeping patterns are restored), and repeat the dose if you wake up during the night and cannot get back to sleep. **CAUTION** If there is no improvement within three weeks, consult a doctor.	INSOMNIA WITH INABILITY TO RELAX	◆ Sudden onset of insomnia ◆ Sleep occurs eventually but is fitful ◆ Oversensitivity to light, smell, noise, and touch ◆ Headache resembling a nail being driven into the head
	INSOMNIA WITH IRRITABILITY	◆ Wakefulness between 3 A.M. and 4 A.M., then more settled sleep just before it is time to get up ◆ Craving for stimulants, especially coffee during the day and alcohol in the evening ◆ Constipation with ineffectual urging
	INSOMNIA WITH GREAT FEAR	◆ Sudden onset of insomnia ◆ Fitful sleep associated with acute pain caused by injury, surgery, or exposure to biting wind ◆ Numbness in the limbs
	INSOMNIA WITH FEAR OF NEVER SLEEPING AGAIN	◆ Continuous yawning but inability to get to sleep ◆ Lump in the throat
IRRITABILITY & ANGER These emotions are often a response to events that are perceived to be physically or psychologically threatening. They can be brought on by overindulgence, overwork, or exhaustion, or they may be associated with digestive ailments and, in men, premature ejaculation or impotence. Such feelings may lead to depression. Physical manifestations include an increased pulse rate, fluttering feelings in the stomach, and tense muscles. **SELF-HELP** Increase the amount of exercise you get, and practice relaxation techniques or meditation, or movement therapy such as t'ai chi (*see page 217*). Assertiveness training may help to overcome feelings of insecurity.	IRRITABILITY WITH EXTREMELY CRITICAL ATTITUDE	◆ Sensitivity to the cold ◆ Desire for alcohol and fatty or spicy foods
	ANGER WITH INSECURITY	◆ Craving for sweet foods ◆ Feeling hungry but feeling full after only a few bites
ANXIETY Anxiety, or worry, consists of both an emotional and a physical imbalance, and tends to be provoked by overwork, stress, fear, or insecurity. It may be accompanied by an increased pulse rate, clammy skin, irregular sleep patterns, and appetite disturbance. **SELF-HELP** Avoid stressful situations and caffeine. Practice relaxation techniques or meditation (*see page 217*). **CAUTION** If you are feeling very anxious, with no obvious cause, see a doctor. If anxiety is accompanied by serious chest pains, call an ambulance.	ANXIETY WITH RESTLESSNESS	◆ Physical restlessness ◆ Chilliness ◆ Exhaustion ◆ Possible craving for fatty foods ◆ Possible burning pains ◆ Desire for small sips of fluid
	ANXIETY RELIEVED BY REASSURANCE	◆ Strong craving for cold drinks and ice cream ◆ Burning feeling in the hands and up the back, particularly between the shoulder blades ◆ Palpitations

levels is helpful in dealing with ailments that reveal both a physical and a mental imbalance. Many emotional problems have their origins in stressful situations, exhaustion and overwork, dietary overindulgence or allergies, or fears and insecurities. By focusing on the response of the vital force of the body (*see page 18*) to external problems, homeopathy can stimulate a person's ability to cope with and modify those problems, at least in the short term. Homeopathic treatment for emotional problems is best combined in the long term with dietary changes, regular exercise, relaxation techniques or movement therapies, and stress management in order to maximize the benefits of treatment.

PSYCHOLOGICAL SYMPTOMS	SYMPTOMS BETTER	SYMPTOMS WORSE	REMEDY & DOSAGE
• Overactive mind • Variety of emotions that are often brought on by news received	• With warmth • Lying down • From sucking ice	• From taking sleeping pills • From strong smells • Near noise • In fresh air • In cold conditions	**Coffea** (*see page 50*) 30c hourly before bed for 10 nights
• Possible nightmares • Irritability and oversensitivity • Harsh criticism of others	• Lying on either side • When sitting • With warmth • In the evening	• Lying on the back • From overeating, especially spicy foods • In cold, windy weather • Near noise	**Nux vomica** (*see page 63*) 30c hourly before bed for 10 nights
• Nervousness and restlessness • Great fear of death, even to the extent of predicting the time of death • Possible nightmares	• In fresh air • From warm perspiration	• In warm rooms • On exposure to tobacco smoke • From loud music	**Aconite** (*see page 32*) 30c hourly before bed for 10 nights
• Growing apprehension about going to bed • Rapid changes of mood • Possible nightmares	• From eating • From urinating • From walking around	• In fresh air • With cold • From coffee or alcohol	**Ignatia** (*see page 57*) 30c hourly before bed for 10 nights
• Anger that comes on quickly • Awkwardness and intractability • Harsh criticism of others	• With warmth • With sleep • In the evening	• With cold • Near noise • From overeating • Around 4 A.M.	**Nux vomica** (*see page 63*) 6c half-hourly up to 10 doses
• Lack of self-confidence • Cowardice • Anger, possibly with violent outbursts at infrequent intervals	• From sympathy • In cool conditions • From hot foods and drinks • After midnight	• In stuffy rooms • From wearing tight clothing • From overeating • Between 4 P.M. and 8 P.M.	**Lycopodium** (*see page 59*) 6c half-hourly up to 10 doses
• Mental restlessness • Great insecurity • Anguish and preoccupation with death that are worse from being alone • Fastidiousness masking anxiety	• With warmth • From warm foods and drinks • From being in company	• With cold • Between midnight and 2 A.M. • From physical or mental exertion	**Arsen. alb.** (*see page 68*) 6c every 2 hours up to 10 doses if acute
• Great nervousness • Great sensitivity, affection, and sympathy toward others • Fear and anxiety, especially in the dark and during thunderstorms	• From eating • With sleep, even catnaps • From a general massage	• Lying on the back or side • From stress • Before and during thunderstorms • From warm foods	**Phosphorus** (*see page 94*) 6c every 2 hours up to 10 doses if acute

CHILDREN'S HEALTH

BABYHOOD LASTS FROM BIRTH to one year old, a period of extremely rapid growth. The birth weight of a baby can double within six months and triple within a year. By one year, most babies can stand.

Childhood as a stage of human development extends roughly from one to twelve years old. During this period the immune system flexes its muscles, so to speak, in readiness for puberty and adulthood.

DISORDER	SPECIFIC AILMENT	PHYSICAL SYMPTOMS
COLIC Colic is believed to be spasm of the intestines that causes a baby to scream, pull up its legs, and turn red. Colic occurs at about three months of age, usually in the evening, and for several hours. It may be aggravated by the mother's tension or her diet (if she is breast-feeding), or by the baby gulping milk or swallowing air. **SELF-HELP** If breast-feeding, avoiding foods such as citrus fruits, strong spices, caffeine, legumes, and cows' milk products may be helpful. If bottle-feeding, enlarge the nipple hole. **CAUTION** If the baby vomits or has diarrhea, see a doctor within 12 hours. If the baby is pale and limp, call an ambulance.	COLIC WITH KNEES PULLED UP TO THE CHEST	◆ Knees pulled up to the chest in response to sharp stomach pains ◆ Great distress
	COLIC WITH CRYING RELIEVED BY WARMTH	◆ Bloated abdomen ◆ Sudden onset of intense or shooting pains in the stomach that come in waves due to flatulence ◆ Pains are not relieved by burping ◆ Great distress
DIAPER RASH A baby's buttocks, genitals, and even thighs may become red and sore from contact with soiled diapers. This is caused by irritating chemicals released from urine and feces, or in the detergent used to wash nondisposable diapers. The rash may develop into candidiasis as a secondary infection, especially if a baby or breast-feeding mother is taking antibiotics. **SELF-HELP** Wash the baby's bottom with a solution of calendula and hypericum, dry well, and apply calendula cream. Change the baby's diaper frequently. **CAUTION** If the condition does not improve, consult a doctor.	DRY RASH ON A BABY WITH SENSITIVE SKIN	◆ Skin is generally dry and sensitive ◆ Skin in the diaper area is dry, red, scaly, and irritated ◆ Desire to scratch as soon as a diaper is removed
	INTENSELY ITCHY RASH WITH BLISTERS	◆ Redness and blisters in the diaper area ◆ Extremely itchy skin ◆ Desire to scratch as soon as a diaper is removed
TEETHING Teething describes the discomfort that may arise during the eruption from the gums of a baby's milk teeth. This usually starts at the age of about six months and continues until approximately the end of the child's third year. Symptoms include sore gums, irritability, and an upset stomach. **SELF-HELP** Combination R tissue salts (see page 216) may be given throughout the teething period. **CAUTION** If there is a high fever (see page 248) do not assume that it is a symptom of the teething, and consult a doctor.	TEETHING WITH IRRITABILITY AND ANGER	◆ Acutely inflamed gums that are sore when touched ◆ Diarrhea ◆ One cheek appears hot and red while the other is pale
	TEETHING WITH SUDDEN PAIN AND FLUSHED FACE	◆ Face is hot and flushed ◆ Staring eyes ◆ Mouth is hot and dry ◆ Gums are painful and inflamed
TEMPER TANTRUMS A young child has outbursts of anger, shouting, and crying when thwarted. The causes may be emotional tension within the family, a lack of parental affection, or inconsistent disciplining by parents, which may produce insecurity in a child. Tantrums are exacerbated by teething, allergies, or digestive ailments. **SELF-HELP** Discipline a child consistently, and avoid arguments. Give the child plenty of attention except during a tantrum, when unacceptable behavior is best ignored. Distract the child from the undesirable behavior. **CAUTION** If problems persist, ask a doctor about family therapy.	TEMPER TANTRUMS IN A CHILD WITH PINWORMS	◆ Itching of the rectum and anus (tiny, white pinworms may be detected on clear tape placed across the anus first thing in the morning) ◆ Teeth grinding during sleep
	CHILD IS IMPOSSIBLE TO PLEASE	◆ One cheek may be red if the child is teething ◆ Stools may be green, watery, and smell like rotten eggs ◆ Possible convulsive symptoms in extreme cases, with child going into spasms of rage

Illnesses contracted in childhood help provide the body with the resistance to, and ultimately immunity against, many diseases in later life. Parents often prefer to treat their children with gentle, natural products to reduce the risk of side effects, resorting to conventional drugs only when a child's immune system is unable to cope with extremely serious ailments. Unless there is a congenital, genetic disability, a child's immune system should respond well to homeopathic treatment. In most cases, a child's vital force (see page 18) will enable him or her to deal with many common threats to childhood health. Homeopathic remedies are easily administered to children (see page 216), and can help them bounce back to health quickly and efficiently.

PSYCHOLOGICAL SYMPTOMS	SYMPTOMS BETTER	SYMPTOMS WORSE	REMEDY & DOSAGE
◆ Irritability ◆ Anger	◆ From applying firm pressure to the stomach ◆ With warmth ◆ With sleep ◆ From releasing gas	◆ Around 4 P.M. ◆ In cold drafts ◆ If the mother is stressed ◆ From being fed	**Colocynthis** (see page 52) 6c every 5 minutes up to 10 doses
◆ Irritability and restlessness ◆ Nervous appearance	◆ With warmth ◆ From warm baths ◆ From applying light pressure to the stomach	◆ In cold air ◆ At night ◆ If touched ◆ Lying on the right side	**Mag. phos.** (see page 90) 6c every 5 minutes up to 10 doses
◆ Irritability ◆ Dislike of being put to bed	◆ In fresh air ◆ When warm and dry	◆ From wearing too much clothing ◆ From being washed ◆ From being too warm	**Sulfur** (see page 99) 6c 4 times daily up to 5 days
◆ Great restlessness ◆ Agitation	◆ From changing position ◆ When warm and dry	◆ From being undressed ◆ From getting wet ◆ In drafts	**Rhus tox.** (see page 162) 6c 4 times daily up to 5 days
◆ Great restlessness ◆ Anger ◆ Great sensitivity to pain	◆ From being carried ◆ From applying cold compresses to the face	◆ When angry ◆ With heat ◆ In fresh air ◆ At night, from 9 P.M. onward	**Chamomilla** (see page 46) 30c half-hourly up to 10 doses, or more often if acute
◆ Restlessness ◆ Tendency to lash out	◆ With warmth ◆ From resting in bed	◆ With jarring and movement ◆ From light and noise ◆ From applying pressure to the gums ◆ Lying down and at night	**Belladonna** (see page 39) 30c half-hourly up to 10 doses, or more often if acute
◆ Irritability, anger, and aggression ◆ Rejection of all attempts to please	◆ Lying on the stomach ◆ From being carried over a parent's shoulder	◆ If touched ◆ From being looked at ◆ During a full moon ◆ In the presence of strangers	**Cina** (see page 38) 30c daily up to 7 days
◆ Extreme irritability ◆ Great sensitivity to pain ◆ Dislike of being talked to or touched	◆ From being carried ◆ From perspiring ◆ In mild weather	◆ When teething ◆ At night ◆ After breakfast ◆ From being talked to ◆ If touched	**Chamomilla** (see page 46) 30c daily up to 7 days

DISORDER	SPECIFIC AILMENT	PHYSICAL SYMPTOMS
SLEEPLESSNESS Newborn babies need about 16 hours of sleep, 2-year-olds 12 hours, 6-year-olds 10 hours, and 12-year-olds 9 hours. Sleeplessness in babies may arise from being hot or cold, hunger, a dirty diaper, teething (*see page 246*), colic (*see page 246*), or too much stimulation. In older children it may be caused by being hot or cold, irregular bedtimes, caffeine in canned sodas, food allergies, noise, stress, or anxiety. Nightmares may result from watching television or videos. **SELF-HELP** Keep a baby's or young child's room at 64–68°F (16–20°C). Establish a bedtime routine: bath, last feeding, then bed, at the same time every day; avoid overstimulation. If a child wakes frequently during the night and becomes overtired, bring bedtime forward by 15 minutes every 3 nights until the child sleeps through. Maintain this bedtime, and then gradually put it back by 15-minute intervals. Look for the underlying causes of sleeplessness. Do not punish a child by sending him or her to a bedroom, which will acquire bad associations. **CAUTION** If the problem persists, consult a doctor.	ANGER AND IRRITABILITY THAT PREVENTS SLEEP	◆ Eyes are half-open when asleep ◆ Moaning during sleep ◆ Legs are wide apart when asleep
	SLEEPLESSNESS AFTER SHOCK	◆ Possible dizziness, numbness, flushing, and fainting ◆ Wakefulness any time between midnight and 4 A.M. ◆ Possible feeling of paralysis anywhere in the body
	EARLY WAKING	◆ Wakefulness in the early morning with a desire to play ◆ Possible association with teething or pain ◆ Overtiredness
BED-WETTING (NOCTURNAL ENURESIS) By the end of their second year, most children have a degree of bladder control. Daytime control is usually achieved between 18 months and 3 years of age: nighttime control may take another year. About 10 percent of 4- to 5-year-olds wet the bed regularly. Primary bed-wetting means a child has never been dry at night. This may be due to immaturity of the nervous system or to psychological reasons – for example, a child's diapers may not have been changed often enough so that he or she did not learn what it felt like to be dry. Secondary bed-wetting means a child was dry for a time but then starts to wet the bed again – because of emotional stress, for example. **SELF-HELP** With primary bed-wetting, encourage a child of 7 or over to take control, by changing soiled sheets, for example. **CAUTION** If there is a burning sensation on urinating with secondary bed-wetting, see a doctor within 48 hours.	BED-WETTING WHILE DREAMING	◆ Urination while dreaming ◆ Urination in first stage of sleep as a habit ◆ Symptoms especially associated with children who feel the cold easily
	BED-WETTING SOON AFTER FALLING ASLEEP	◆ Urination soon after falling asleep ◆ Possible association with coughing fits
	BED-WETTING DURING DEEP SLEEP	◆ Reluctance to go to sleep unless soothed ◆ Deep sleep prevents child from waking in time to get to a toilet ◆ Urination during dreams and in the early part of the night
FEVER A rise in body temperature above 98°F (37°C) usually indicates that the body is fighting an infection. In young children, however, before the temperature regulation mechanism has matured, temperature may rise simply because the child is overheated. Other symptoms of fever include restlessness and hot skin. **SELF-HELP** Remove the child's clothes and sponge him or her all over with tepid water. Open the windows or use a fan to cool the air. Provide plenty of fluids. If the child's temperature rises above 102°F (39°C), or if there is a history of febrile convulsions (seizures induced by high fever), give children's acetaminophen. **CAUTION** If the child suffers a febrile convulsion – abnormal breathing and limb movements, rolling eyes, and a loss of consciousness – try to lower the child's temperature and consult a doctor. If the child is unconscious for more than five minutes, call an ambulance. If fever is accompanied by symptoms of meningitis (inflammation of the membranes around the brain) – severe headache, nausea and vomiting, abnormal drowsiness, oversensitivity to light, a stiff neck, and a rash that does not fade when pressure is applied – call an ambulance.	SUDDEN RISE IN TEMPERATURE AFTER EXPOSURE TO COLD	◆ Sudden onset of fever ◆ Pale face ◆ Great thirst ◆ Shivering, especially after exposure to cold, dry wind, even though temperature is raised
	SUDDEN RISE IN TEMPERATURE WITH BURNING, HOT SKIN	◆ Sudden onset of violent fever, with pounding pulse ◆ Skin is dry and hot ◆ Face is flushed ◆ Staring eyes
	FEVER WITH EXHAUSTION	◆ Body feels cold but skin is hot and dry ◆ Thirst for small sips of water ◆ Exhaustion ◆ Burning pains in the limbs ◆ Cold sweats

PSYCHOLOGICAL SYMPTOMS	SYMPTOMS BETTER	SYMPTOMS WORSE	REMEDY & DOSAGE
• Anger • Refusal to be calmed unless carried around	• From being carried • In warm, wet weather • From not eating snacks before bedtime	• From being overheated • In cold, windy weather • From burping • At night, from 9 P.M. onward	**Chamomilla** (*see page 46*) 30c half-hourly from 1 hour before bedtime up to 10 doses
• Fear of death on waking from sleep • Anxiety • Restlessness	• With rest • From being in quiet surroundings • With reassurance	• From a shock or scare • On exposure to cold, dry winds • At night	**Aconite** (*see page 32*) 30c half-hourly from 1 hour before bedtime up to 10 doses
• Extreme excitability • Agitation and nervous tension	• With warmth • Lying down	• From too much excitement • From sleeping in a draft • Near noise • With cold • From strong smells	**Coffea** (*see page 50*) 30c half-hourly from 1 hour before bedtime up to 10 doses
• Possible nightmares • Indolence • Displeasure	• From catnaps	• Lying on the right side • With movement • Lying on a full bladder • If touched	**Equisetum** (*see page 142*) 6c once before bed up to 14 nights
• Excitability • Great sensitivity	• In warm, damp weather • From being in a warm bed	• In cold, dry weather • Between 3 A.M. and 4 A.M. • From physical or mental exertion	**Causticum** (*see page 79*) 6c once before bed up to 14 nights
• Excitability • Restlessness • Irritability • Peevishness	• With warmth • From being cuddled • With movement	• When teething • With cold • Lying down • If touched	**Kreosotum** (*see page 151*) 6c once before bed up to 14 nights
• Restlessness • Tearfulness	• In fresh air • From sleeping	• In warm rooms • On exposure to tobacco smoke • Around midnight	**Aconite** (*see page 32*) 30c hourly up to 10 doses
• Delirium with unusual noises and jerky movements	• When standing or sitting upright • With warmth	• With jarring and movement • With light and noise • From applying pressure to painful areas • Lying on the right side • At night	**Belladonna** (*see page 39*) 30c hourly up to 10 doses
• Restlessness • Anxiety • Stupor or delirium	• Head is better with cold, but heat helps extremities • In the open air • From applying warm, dry compresses all over the body	• Between midnight and 2 A.M. • From physical exertion • From cold drinks and foods	**Arsen. alb.** (*see page 68*) 6c hourly up to 10 doses

DISORDER	SPECIFIC AILMENT	PHYSICAL SYMPTOMS
GLUE EAR Recurrent infections may result in overactivity of the mucous membrane lining the middle ear. This results in a buildup of sticky fluid and the poor transmission of sounds, hence reduced hearing. Glue ear may also be caused by allergies. The insertion of a grommet (a small tube passed through the eardrum) may be necessary to drain the fluid. **SELF-HELP** If symptoms persist, investigate the possibility of an allergy to food or atmospheric irritants. If a child has phlegm, eliminate dairy products from the diet, but only for one month. **CAUTION** If deafness persists, see a doctor within a month.	GLUE EAR WITH SWOLLEN NECK GLANDS	◆ Possible discharge of mucus from the ear ◆ Pain or congested feeling in the ear ◆ Swollen neck glands ◆ Head sweats ◆ Possible association with exposure to drafts
	GLUE EAR WITH THICK, STRINGY MUCUS	◆ Mucus drips down the back of the throat from the sinuses ◆ Pain or congested feeling in the ear ◆ Dull ache or boring pain in the bridge of the nose ◆ Tendency to produce mucus
TONSILLITIS The tonsils are two sacs of lymphatic tissue at the back of the throat that form part of the body's immune system (*see page 204*). They often become infected, especially during childhood. Symptoms include a sore or painful throat, fever, and general malaise. The tonsils look bright red at first, then become covered with a slimy, whitish coating. The glands in the neck may become enlarged. **SELF-HELP** Encourage the child to rest, drink plenty of fluids, and take garlic preparations. Apply alternate hot and cold compresses around the neck. Gargling with sage tea may soothe the soreness or pain in the throat. **CAUTION** If symptoms persist for more than 48 hours, see a doctor. If temperature rises above 102°F (39°C), see a doctor within 12 hours.	TONSILLITIS WITH RED FACE, HIGH FEVER, AND DELIRIUM	◆ Throat is sore and tender and neck feels stiff ◆ Right tonsil is often affected the worst ◆ Spasms of pain in the throat on moving ◆ High fever, red face, and dilated pupils ◆ Tongue has a strawberry-like appearance
	TONSILLITIS WITH SENSATION OF A FISH BONE STUCK IN THE THROAT	◆ Stabbing pain in the throat ◆ Unpleasant-smelling breath ◆ Hoarseness or loss of voice ◆ Yellow mucus is coughed up ◆ Tenderness and swelling of the neck glands ◆ Chilliness
	TONSILLITIS WITH DRIBBLING OF SALIVA ONTO THE PILLOW	◆ Throat is dark red, sore, and swollen ◆ Copious saliva that burns when swallowed ◆ Tongue feels swollen and has a yellow coating ◆ Unpleasant-smelling breath ◆ Copious, offensive-smelling perspiration
CROUP Resulting from an infection of the larynx, epiglottis, or trachea, or from an obstruction of the airway, croup causes a sudden narrowing of the larynx, which produces hoarseness, wheezing, stridor (grunting while breathing), and a distinctive, barking cough. **SELF-HELP** Humidify the bedroom or, during a coughing fit, stay with the child in a bathroom with the hot water running. **CAUTION** If there is fever, call a doctor within two hours. If stridor is acute with no sign of infection and there are breathing difficulties, call an ambulance.	CROUP THAT COMES ON SUDDENLY	◆ Sudden coughing and breathlessness ◆ Cough is hollow-sounding and resembles barking ◆ Possible great thirst
	PERSISTENT CROUP	◆ Dry, hoarse, barking cough ◆ Constant desire for sips of fluid or total lack of thirst ◆ Cough may become rattly, with retching and vomiting
WHOOPING COUGH This highly infectious, bacterial illness is serious in young children, and is occasionally fatal in babies. The incubation period is 1–2 weeks. A child is most infectious during the first week, and may remain infectious for up to three weeks. A fever is followed by spasmodic coughing characterized by a whooping noise. Complications include pneumonia and brain damage. **CAUTION** If you suspect that a child has contracted whooping cough, see a doctor within 48 hours. Antibiotics can minimize severity, but follow up with an acidophilic supplement, such as live yogurt, to reestablish beneficial intestinal bacteria. If a child turns blue during coughing, see a doctor within two hours.	WHOOPING COUGH WITH VOMITING	◆ Throat is dry and tickly ◆ Cough is so violent that the child vomits and can barely catch his or her breath between bouts ◆ Child clutches the stomach in pain from coughing ◆ Chilliness
	WHOOPING COUGH THAT IS WORSE AFTER MIDNIGHT	◆ Dry, hacking cough that starts around 3 A.M. ◆ Chilliness ◆ Exhaustion ◆ Eyelids are puffy, especially the upper eyelids

PSYCHOLOGICAL SYMPTOMS	SYMPTOMS BETTER	SYMPTOMS WORSE	REMEDY & DOSAGE
• Anxiety and insecurity • Many fears, including concern about death and dying • Possible nightmares	• When slightly constipated • Lying on the affected side • In dry weather	• From physical or mental exertion • Between 2 A.M. and 3 A.M. • In cold, raw wind	**Calc. carb.** (*see page 77*) 6c 3 times daily up to 14 days
• Irritability • Despondency	• With warmth • With movement • From vomiting	• In the morning • In hot weather • In spring	**Kali. bich.** (*see page 87*) 6c 3 times daily up to 14 days
• Possible delirium with hallucinations of fantastic shapes or scary things	• When standing or sitting upright • With warmth • From resting in bed	• If the head becomes chilled • With slight jarring or movement • In light and near noise • At night	**Belladonna** (*see page 39*) 30c every 2 hours up to 10 doses
• Touchiness and extreme sensitivity • Unreasonableness and tendency to lash out	• From eating • With warmth • When the neck is warmly wrapped	• In cold air and drafts • From undressing • From touching the throat • Lying on the affected side	**Hepar sulf.** (*see page 84*) 6c every 2 hours up to 10 doses
• Irritability and emotionalism • Shyness and tendency to be withdrawn • Great sensitivity to emotions	• With rest • When warmly dressed	• In extremes of temperature • From perspiring • At night • Lying on the right side	**Merc. sol.** (*see page 85*) 6c every 2 hours up to 10 doses
• Great fear caused by sudden onset and nature of symptoms • Restlessness in bed	• In fresh air • With humidity • From warm perspiration	• On exposure to cold, dry winds • On exposure to tobacco smoke • At night	**Aconite** (*see page 32*) 30c right away, then half an hour later if child is awake
• Great irritability • Extreme sensitivity • Anger that causes lashing out	• With warmth • With humidity • In damp weather	• In cold air and drafts • From undressing • If touched • At night	**Hepar sulf.** (*see page 84*) 6c hourly up to 3 doses, or alternate with *Spongia 6c*
• Restlessness • Suspicion • Anxiety • Anger that develops easily	• From applying pressure to the chest • In the open air • From walking • When sitting up in bed • From keeping quiet	• After midnight • Lying on the left side • With warmth • From talking and laughing	**Drosera** (*see page 141*) 6c once after every coughing bout up to 2 days
• Dislike of being alone • Fear of the dark and ghosts • Anxiety • Irritability • Jumpiness	• With warmth • When sitting with the elbows on the knees • In the open air	• In cold and drafts • Between 2 A.M. and 3 A.M. • From physical or mental exertion	**Kali. carb.** (*see page 88*) 6c once after every coughing bout up to 2 days

DISORDER	SPECIFIC AILMENT	PHYSICAL SYMPTOMS
CHICKEN POX This highly infectious, viral disease is spread in droplets of mucus expelled in coughs and sneezes from an infected child or an adult with shingles. Incubation is 13–17 days. Symptoms are a slight fever for 24 hours, followed by the eruption of a rash and a worsening of the fever. Clusters of small, red, itchy spots evolve into fluid-filled blisters, which heal in 6–10 days. A child is infectious from just before the onset of fever until all the spots heal. Scratched spots may become infected and leave pockmarks. Most children recover completely, but the virus may lie dormant and be triggered in adulthood as shingles. **SELF-HELP** To soothe the rash, rub in honey or vitamin E cream on unbroken skin, dab on baking soda solution (1 tsp/5 ml soda to 1 cup/150 ml water), or have an oatmeal herbal bath. **CAUTION** If you suspect that your child has chicken pox, see a doctor within 24 hours. If the temperature is still high two days after the rash appears, or if the child seems very ill and chesty, see a doctor within two hours because of a risk of pneumonia.	FIRST STAGE OF CHICKEN POX	◆ Sudden rise in temperature ◆ Hot, flushed face, with cold extremities (fingers, hands, toes, and feet) ◆ Possible staring eyes ◆ Sensitivity to noise and light
	CHICKEN POX WITH RESTLESSNESS	◆ Extremely itchy rash ◆ Fever ◆ Restlessness ◆ Headache that develops from a stiff neck
	CHICKEN POX WITH LACK OF THIRST DURING FEVER	◆ Lack of thirst despite high temperature ◆ Typical rash ◆ Thick, bland, yellow discharge from the nose ◆ Chilliness but a desire for fresh air
MEASLES A highly infectious, viral disease, measles is spread in droplets of mucus expelled in coughs and sneezes. The incubation period is about ten days, after which the first symptoms develop – an inflamed throat, runny nose, dry cough, red and watering eyes, and fever. After 3–4 days dark red spots appear, which may join to form blotches. A child is infectious from the first symptoms until five days after the rash develops. Complications include acute middle-ear infection, bronchitis (*see page 228*), encephalitis (inflammation of the brain), and febrile convulsions. **SELF-HELP** Give the child plenty of water and a light diet until the runny nose and the cough clear up. Treat as for fever (*see page 248*). Bathe the eyes with a saline solution (1 tsp/5 ml salt to 1 cup/150 ml boiled, cooled water). **CAUTION** If fever persists, or if the child feels ill after the rash begins to fade or has an earache, see a doctor within 12 hours.	FIRST STAGE OF MEASLES WITH LACK OF THIRST DURING FEVER	◆ Lack of thirst despite high temperature ◆ Great sensitivity to light ◆ Dry cough at night with mucus coughed up in the morning that turns thick and green by day ◆ Nausea, vomiting, or diarrhea ◆ Tiny, raised white spots in the mouth
	SECOND STAGE OF MEASLES WITH DRY, HACKING COUGH	◆ Rash appears slowly ◆ Fever ◆ Great but infrequent thirst ◆ Dry, hacking cough ◆ Headache that is worse from coughing
	SECOND STAGE OF MEASLES WITH A RASH THAT IS SLOW TO DISAPPEAR	◆ Rash disappears very slowly ◆ Spots turn purple ◆ Increased appetite ◆ Great desire for sweet foods
MUMPS A viral infection of certain salivary glands (the parotids in front of the ear and the submandibulars in the lower jaw), mumps is spread by droplets of mucus expelled in coughs and sneezes. The incubation period is 2–3 weeks and a child may be infectious for a week before the symptoms appear. These include fever, headache, and pain in front of the ears as the glands become swollen. The swelling subsides within ten days, during which time a child is still infectious. Complications may include meningitis or inflammation of the pancreas, ovaries, or testes. Rarely, the effect of this disorder on the reproductive organs results in sterility. **SELF-HELP** Avoid acidic drinks, such as citrus fruit juices, since these will stimulate the salivary glands, causing pain. **CAUTION** If there is a severe headache, great sensitivity to light, confusion, drowsiness, or any other symptoms of meningitis, see a doctor within two hours. If the testicles or ovaries are painful, see a doctor within 12 hours.	MUMPS WITH SUDDEN ONSET OF FEVER AND FLUSHED FACE	◆ Sudden rise in temperature ◆ Hot, flushed face ◆ Parotid gland on the right side is worse affected ◆ Wide, staring eyes
	MUMPS WITH PAIN IN THE EARS ON SWALLOWING	◆ Pain on swallowing that extends from the throat to the ears ◆ Submandibular glands are swollen and as hard as stones ◆ Restlessness and a desire to move, but movement makes the symptoms worse
	MUMPS WITH PERSPIRATION AND DRIBBLING WHEN ASLEEP	◆ Glands on the right are affected the worst ◆ Offensive-smelling and unpleasant-tasting saliva that dribbles onto the pillow during sleep ◆ Offensive-smelling, copious perspiration ◆ Tongue is swollen, with teeth imprints

PSYCHOLOGICAL SYMPTOMS	SYMPTOMS BETTER	SYMPTOMS WORSE	REMEDY & DOSAGE
• Possible hallucinations and delirium	• Lying on the front • From bending backward • In a darkened room • From being lightly covered	• In sunlight • From jarring • From stooping • Lying with the head lower than the body • With heat	**Belladonna** (see page 39) 30c every 2 hours up to 10 doses
• Great restlessness	• From changing position • With continuous movement • With warmth • In dry air • From applying hot compresses, especially to the head	• With rest and when first moving • In cold and wet conditions • In drafts, even if only small areas of the body are exposed	**Rhus tox.** (see page 162) 6c every 2 hours up to 10 doses
• Tearfulness and a tendency to cling to an adult • Self-pity • Great desire for attention and comfort	• In the open air • From applying cold compresses to the itchy areas • With gentle movement	• In hot rooms • With warmth • At twilight and in the early evening	**Pulsatilla** (see page 61) 6c every 2 hours up to 10 doses
• Great tearfulness and misery • Desire for plenty of sympathy	• From crying and sympathy • With the hands above the head • With gentle movement • In fresh air • From applying cold compresses to the rash	• With heat • In extremes of temperature • Lying on the painful side • In the evening and at night	**Pulsatilla** (see page 61) 6c every 2 hours up to 10 doses
• Great irritability • Reluctance to be moved	• With rest • In cool air • From applying cold compresses to the rash	• Near noise and in bright light • In the morning and around 9 P.M. and 3 A.M. • With the slightest movement	**Bryonia** (see page 42) 30c every 4 hours up to 10 doses
• Irritability • Anxiety	• In the open air • From applying warm compresses to the rash	• From having a bath • From becoming overheated • From physical or mental exertion	**Sulfur** (see page 99) 6c every 4 hours up to 10 doses
• Possible hallucinations and delirium	• Lying on the front • From applying pressure to the affected glands	• In sunlight • From jarring • When stooping • Lying with the head lower than the body • With heat	**Belladonna** (see page 39) 30c every 4 hours up to 10 doses
• Tearfulness at night • Indifference • Confusion when sitting up	• From cold drinks • With rest • With warmth	• From getting out of bed • From walking around • From swallowing	**Phytolacca** (see page 159) 6c every 4 hours up to 10 doses
• Irritability and emotionalism, or shyness and introversion • Great emotional sensitivity	• With rest • When warmly dressed • In the morning	• From extremes of temperature • From perspiring • At night • Lying on the right side	**Merc. sol.** (see page 85) 6c every 4 hours up to 10 doses

HEALTH IN ADOLESCENCE

ADOLESCENCE DESCRIBES THE TRANSITION from childhood to adulthood, and is ushered in by hormonal changes that occur at about 10 or 11 years of age in girls and a year or so later in boys. Height and weight are gained during adolescence, but more significant is the progression to sexual maturity. In boys, this takes the form of an enlargement of the genitals and the larynx, and the appearance of body hair; in girls it

DISORDER	SPECIFIC AILMENT	PHYSICAL SYMPTOMS
GLANDULAR FEVER (INFECTIOUS MONONUCLEOSIS) This viral infection is spread by personal contact. It starts like the flu, with a fever, sore throat, headache, and general aches and pains. Within a day or two the lymph glands, especially those in the throat, become swollen and painful and the tonsils enlarged and dirty-looking. There may be a rash, and – in rare cases – jaundice. Although symptoms usually wear off in two or three weeks, full recovery may take longer and lethargy may last for months. Stress, such as that generated by intense studying for exams or the breakup of a relationship, may increase susceptibility to infectious mononucleosis. **SELF-HELP** Rest in bed until acute symptoms abate, after which avoid strenuous exercise and do only 75 percent of what you are capable of doing, both physically and mentally, until recovery is complete. **CAUTION** See a doctor for a blood test to confirm the diagnosis.	INFECTIOUS MONONUCLEOSIS WITH ENLARGED TONSILS AND ULCERS	◆ Tonsils are swollen and purple, with weeping ulcers, and swallowing is difficult ◆ Tongue is cracked and parched, and teeth have a brown coating ◆ Great physical exhaustion ◆ Possible headache and muscular pain
	INFECTIOUS MONONUCLEOSIS WITH OFFENSIVE PERSPIRATION	◆ Throat is dark red, sore, and swollen ◆ Saliva burns the throat on swallowing ◆ Tongue feels swollen and is yellow-coated with teeth imprints ◆ Offensive-smelling breath ◆ Copious, smelly perspiration
	INFECTIOUS MONONUCLEOSIS WITH PAIN ON SWALLOWING FOOD AND HOT DRINKS	◆ Tonsils are dark red ◆ Shooting pain up to the ears on swallowing ◆ Swallowing food and hot drinks is especially painful
BODY ODOR Sweat glands in the groin and underarms become functional at about 15 or 16 in girls and a year or two later in boys. Most anxiety about body odor occurs as a result of the unfamiliar smell rather than an excess of perspiration. The odor becomes offensive when bacteria breed in the stale sweat. Perspiration may be increased by stress and during menstruation in girls. **SELF-HELP** Wash thoroughly every day using alkaline soap, which will discourage the proliferation of bacteria. **CAUTION** If symptoms persist, consult a doctor.	BODY ODOR IN OVERWEIGHT PEOPLE WHO FEEL THE COLD EASILY	◆ Perspiration smells sour ◆ Perspiration on the back of the head during sleep that wets the pillow ◆ Profuse perspiration in the morning ◆ Profuse perspiration for only moderate exertion
	BODY ODOR FROM PERSPIRING IN HOT AND COLD CONDITIONS	◆ Copious, unpleasant-smelling perspiration ◆ Perspiration occurs in both hot and cold conditions ◆ Possible large amounts of saliva
EXAM NERVES This describes a state of extreme anxiety about taking exams that almost amounts to a phobia (*see page 211*). Psychological symptoms include a feeling of panic and an inability to concentrate. Physical symptoms include diarrhea, nausea, vomiting, and headaches. The condition may be exacerbated by other problems, for example, difficulty in studying at home or pressure to achieve high marks. Constitutional homeopathic treatment (*see page 176*) may be required. **SELF-HELP** Time management is the key to controlling anxiety. Start studying well in advance; draw up a timetable that divides subjects into manageable units and covers all topics adequately; and always include time out. Also, make sure that you get enough rest. Remedies should be taken on the day of the exam but also for some days before whenever symptoms appear. **CAUTION** If sysmptoms persist, consult a doctor.	EXAM NERVES WITH DIARRHEA	◆ Diarrhea and possibly nausea and vomiting before an exam ◆ Watery stools ◆ Diarrhea accompanied by copious gas ◆ Diarrhea immediately after eating or drinking
	EXAM NERVES WITH INABILITY TO REMEMBER ANYTHING	◆ Sensation of a plug or lump somewhere, usually in the throat or rectum ◆ Sensation of a weight pressing down on the shoulders ◆ Possible worsening of eczema in sufferers
	EXAM NERVES WITH WEAK, WOBBLY LEGS	◆ Limbs feel weak and wobbly ◆ Possible aches and pains resembling the onset of the flu

involves the development of breasts and body hair, and the onset of menstrual periods. Emotionally and intellectually, adolescence is a time of great change as a teenager veers between dependence and independence, and peers very often become more important role models than parents. Many of the disorders encountered during adolescence result from the great hormonal changes that take place at this stage of life. Ailments may be exacerbated by emotional, academic, and peer-group pressures, and may require long-term, constitutional homeopathic treatment in some cases (*see page 176*). Homeopathic remedies and other self-help measures can help address bodily imbalances in the short term.

PSYCHOLOGICAL SYMPTOMS	SYMPTOMS BETTER	SYMPTOMS WORSE	REMEDY & DOSAGE
◆ Mental dullness and apparent stupidity ◆ Confusion ◆ Great anxiety or depression, with constant sighing	◆ From hot drinks ◆ Lying on the right side	◆ From sitting up ◆ At the sight of food ◆ With movement	**Ailanthus** (*see page 122*) 6c every 4 hours up to 10 doses
◆ Irritability and emotionalism or shyness and introversion ◆ Great emotional sensitivity	◆ With rest ◆ When warmly dressed ◆ In the morning	◆ In extremes of temperature ◆ From perspiring ◆ At night ◆ Lying on the right side	**Merc. sol.** (*see page 85*) 6c every 4 hours up to 10 doses
◆ Restlessness ◆ Indifference to life ◆ Fear of dying	◆ Lying on the stomach ◆ With rest ◆ With warmth	◆ From getting out of bed ◆ With movement ◆ From swallowing ◆ From hot foods and drinks ◆ During the hours of darkness	**Phytolacca** (*see page 159*) 6c every 4 hours up to 10 doses
◆ Depression ◆ Apprehension ◆ Forgetfulness ◆ Concern about appearing insane to others	◆ In dry weather ◆ In the morning ◆ After breakfast	◆ With cold ◆ From mainly physical but also mental exertion ◆ From stress ◆ From drinking milk	**Calc. carb.** (*see page 77*) 6c hourly up to 10 doses
◆ Irritability and emotionalism ◆ Shyness and introversion ◆ Great emotional sensitivity	◆ With rest ◆ When warmly dressed ◆ In the morning	◆ In extremes of temperature ◆ From perspiring ◆ At night ◆ Lying on the right side	**Merc. sol.** (*see page 85*) 6c hourly up to 10 doses
◆ Fear of failure ◆ Lack of self-confidence ◆ Self-doubt that undermines concentration	◆ In cold air ◆ From washing the face in cold water ◆ From sitting ◆ From burping	◆ From eating sugar ◆ From eating cold foods ◆ In crowds	**Argentum nit.** (*see page 74*) 6c hourly up to 10 doses before an exam
◆ Lack of self-confidence ◆ Internal conflict that undermines concentration and the retention of information	◆ From eating ◆ With heat ◆ From hot baths	◆ From emotional stress ◆ In the evening up until midnight ◆ From mental exertion	**Anacardium occ.** (*see page 124*) 6c hourly up to 10 doses before an exam
◆ Fear of having to perform that resembles stage fright ◆ Virtual paralysis with fear when thinking about an exam despite great efforts to study	◆ From urinating ◆ From perspiring ◆ With the eyes closed	◆ From emotional stress ◆ In humid weather ◆ From smoking tobacco	**Gelsemium** (*see page 144*) 6c hourly up to 10 doses before an exam

WOMEN'S HEALTH

THE AVERAGE WOMAN ovulates about 400 times between puberty and menopause, usually at intervals of around 28 days. If an egg is fertilized, pregnancy follows; if not, the lining of the uterus is shed during menstruation. The functioning of the female reproductive system (*see page 198*) is controlled by the pituitary gland, which in turn takes its orders from the hypothalamus in the brain. A variety of

DISORDER	SPECIFIC AILMENT	PHYSICAL SYMPTOMS
PREMENSTRUAL SYNDROME (PMS) THIS affects 75 percent of women to some degree over several days preceeding a menstrual period, and includes physiological and psychological symptoms. Many women continue to lead more or less normal lives despite feeling glum and irritable, but in ten percent of cases symptoms are seriously debilitating. Physical symptoms include tender, swollen breasts and abdomen, fluid retention, and minor period-type pains. PMS may be exacerbated by hormonal or nutritional imbalance, stress, overwork, allergies, and psychological factors such as depression. **SELF-HELP** Avoid salty or fatty foods, junk foods, sugar, tea, coffee, and alcohol. Eat regular, small, protein-rich snacks, but reduce meat intake. Get 30 minutes of outdoor exercise daily and practice relaxation techniques (*see page 217*) or meditation. If you smoke, stop. Pace yourself in order to avoid stress. **CAUTION** If symptoms persist, consult a doctor.	PMS WITH APATHY, IRRITABILITY, AND TEARFULNESS	◆ Greasy skin, possibly with acne ◆ Craving for salty or sweet foods ◆ Weariness, especially in the morning ◆ Sensation of the uterus falling out ◆ Possible sinus problems, sore throat, and flashes
	PMS WITH SWOLLEN, TENDER BREASTS	◆ Fluid retention that exacerbates any weight problem ◆ Swollen, tender breasts and painful joints ◆ Lack of energy ◆ Possible vaginal discharge or a yeast infection
	PMS WITH SELF-PITY	◆ Craving for sweet foods ◆ Bloated stomach ◆ Swollen face, especially upper eyelids ◆ Headaches, nausea, and dizziness ◆ Yellowish vaginal discharge
PAINFUL PERIODS (DYSMENORRHEA) Discomfort is common during the first few days of a menstrual period. Symptoms include a dull ache in the lower back or abdomen, or severe abdominal cramps. Pain may be exacerbated by stress, but may improve after childbirth or once a woman reaches her thirties. Sudden pain after years of pain-free periods may indicate pelvic infection, endometriosis (formation of cysts in the pelvic cavity from bleeding fragments of uterus lining), or fibroids (*see page 199*). The use of intrauterine devices or coming off the contraceptive pill can also result in painful menstruation. **SELF-HELP** Eat plenty of raw fruits and vegetables. Get plenty of exercise and lose weight if you need to. Between periods take an occasional short, cold bath; during the week before a period take a long, hot bath every other night. A physiotherapist or osteopath may be able to relieve associated back pain. **CAUTION** If periods are consistently more painful, see a doctor.	ABDOMINAL PAIN WITH DEPRESSION AND SELF-PITY	◆ Uterine cramps causing nausea or vomiting ◆ Tenderness in the abdomen ◆ Tearing pain in the lower abdomen ◆ Possible migraines or diarrhea ◆ Blood flow includes clots or is very scant
	ABDOMINAL PAIN WITH IRRITABILITY, TEARFULNESS, AND INDIFFERENCE	◆ Sharp, piercing pain in the lower abdomen ◆ Sensation of the uterus falling out ◆ Cramps possibly accompanied by a migraine, acne, weakness, perspiration, and fainting
	ABDOMINAL PAIN SOOTHED BY HEAT AND PRESSURE	◆ Colicky, spasmodic pain ◆ Blood flow includes clots ◆ Dark, stringy, and tarlike blood flow ◆ Period starts ahead of schedule
ABSENT PERIODS (AMENORRHEA) The absence of periods may be permanent or temporary. If periods have not started by the age of 16 (primary amenorrhea), the cause is delayed puberty. If menstruation is established but periods suddenly stop (secondary amenorrhea), this may be due to anorexia or great weight loss, or excessive exercise (especially if the diet is vegetarian). Amenorrhea can also be caused by stress, travel (particularly long-haul flights), shock, emotional stress, or coming off the contraceptive pill. Rarely, it is due to displacement of the uterus, for example, if it is tilted backward. Periods may also be delayed after childbirth. **CAUTION** If menstrual periods have been absent for more than nine months, consult a doctor.	PERIODS STOP ABRUPTLY AFTER A SHOCK	◆ Feeling of heaviness and aching pain in the ovaries ◆ Sharp, shooting pain in the uterus ◆ Abdomen is inflated and sensitive ◆ Vagina is hot, dry, and sensitive
	PERIODS STOP AFTER EMOTIONAL STRESS	◆ Possibly no symptoms specifically related to the reproductive organs ◆ Possible lump in the throat ◆ Possible headache resembling a nail being driven into the head

disturbances and imbalances in the body may modify the brain's influence over the pituitary gland, thus upsetting hormone levels, which many women believe are responsible for their psychological as well as physiological problems. A holistic view of the workings of the female body is well suited to the application of homeopathic principles, and there is much anecdotal evidence of homeopathy's success in treating women's complaints. Homeopathic remedies can provide an attractive alternative to conventional treatments such as hormone replacement therapy (HRT) – which may have unpleasant side effects – and are particularly suitable for the treament of recurring ailments associated with the reproductive cycle.

PSYCHOLOGICAL SYMPTOMS	SYMPTOMS BETTER	SYMPTOMS WORSE	REMEDY & DOSAGE
• Irritability and tearfulness • Difficulty in concentrating • Desire to get away from it all • Fits of anger and screaming • Reduction in sex drive	• From eating • With sleep • With vigorous exercise • With heat	• In cold • On exposure to tobacco smoke • From mental exertion • In the early morning and early evening	**Sepia** (see page 112) 30c twice daily up to 3 days, starting 1 day before PMS due
• Irritability and tearfulness • Depression • Indifference • Difficulty in concentrating	• In the morning • When slightly constipated	• In drafts • In cold, damp, windy weather • From overexertion • Between 2 A.M. and 3 A.M.	**Calc. carb**. (see page 77) 30c twice daily up to 3 days, starting 1 day before PMS due
• Self-pity and depression • Sudden tearfulness for no apparent reason • Apprehension about the future • Anxiety in crowded places	• From crying • From sympathy • With exercise • In fresh air • From cold drinks	• With warmth • In the sun • From rich, fatty foods • In the evening and at night	**Pulsatilla** (see page 61) 30c twice daily up to 3 days, starting 1 day before PMS due
• Self-pity and great tearfulness at the slightest provocation • Desire for comfort and reassurance • Depression	• From crying and sympathy • With the hands above the head • With gentle exercise • In fresh air • From cold drinks	• With heat • In extremes of temperature • From rich, fatty foods • Lying on the painful area • In the evening and at night	**Pulsatilla** (see page 61) 30c hourly up to 10 doses
• Irritability and tearfulness • Desire to be left alone • Indifference to loved ones	• Lying on the right side with knees pulled up to the chest • From eating, sleeping, exercise • From applying hot compresses to the abdomen	• With cold • On exposure to tobacco smoke • From mental exertion • In the early morning and between 4 P.M. and 6 P.M.	**Sepia** (see page 112) 30c hourly up to 10 doses
• Irritability, anxiety, and extreme sensitivity • Fixation about pain • Possible fear of thunderstorms and of darkness	• With warmth • From hot baths • From applying pressure to the abdomen • When bending double	• In cold air and drafts • From being uncovered • At night • From being exhausted • With movement	**Mag. phos.** (see page 90) 30c hourly up to 10 doses
• Great fear and anxiety • Nervousness and panic in fear of death, even to the extent of predicting the time of death	• In fresh air • With rest • From warm perspiration • From bending double	• In warm rooms • On exposure to tobacco smoke • In the evening and at night • In dry, cold wind	**Aconite** (see page 32) 30c twice daily up to 14 days
• Suppression of emotions with fear of showing feelings at inappropriate times • Mood swings between laughter and tearfulness • Possible hysteria	• From eating • From urinating • With heat	• In fresh air and cold conditions • From wearing too much clothing • From coffee and alcohol • From strong smells • On exposure to tobacco smoke	**Ignatia** (see page 57) 30c twice daily up to 14 days

DISORDER	SPECIFIC AILMENT	PHYSICAL SYMPTOMS
HEAVY PERIODS (MENORRHAGIA) Heavy periods are defined as those with profuse bleeding, or flooding, which quickly soaks through any sanitary protection and may include large clots of blood, or bleeding that continues for more than seven days. Such periods may be due to pelvic infection, hormonal imbalance, fibroids (*see page 199*), endometriosis (formation of cysts in the pelvic cavity from bleeding fragments of uterus lining), stress, overwork, or approaching menopause (*see below*). The use of intrauterine devices can also increase menstrual blood flow. **SELF-HELP** Reduce your intake of tea, coffee, alcohol, milk, and dairy products, and eat plenty of raw vegetables. Get 30 minutes of moderate exercise every day but avoid overexertion. **CAUTION** If your menstrual cycle is regular but the flow is heavier than usual or exhibits some other change, consult a doctor. If you have had sexual intercourse regularly and a period is late and heavier than usual, see a doctor within 12 hours.	HEAVY PERIODS IN OVERWEIGHT WOMEN	◆ Fluid retention that exacerbates a weight problem ◆ Possible backache, perspiration, and clumsiness ◆ Blood is bright red ◆ Possible abdominal cramps ◆ Periods are irregular
	HEAVY PERIODS WITH APATHY AND INDIFFERENCE	◆ Severe abdominal cramps ◆ Itchy vaginal discharge ◆ Sweating during menstruation ◆ Visual disturbances, such as spots or flashes ◆ Periods are irregular
	HEAVY PERIODS WITH NERVOUS EXCITEMENT	◆ Blood flow includes dark clots ◆ Intermittent bleeding ◆ Abdominal cramps ◆ Headache, dizziness, and fainting ◆ Very pale face
MENOPAUSE Menopause is the cessation of menstruation that occurs in women between the ages of 45 and 55. It should not be considered an ailment but rather a fact of physical and emotional life that some women adjust to better than others. Symptoms occur as a result of diminishing hormone production by the ovaries, and include hot flashes, vaginal dryness, aches and pains, dizziness, loss of appetite, weariness, chilliness, and palpitations. Psychological symptoms include tearfulness, irritability, anxiety, nervousness, depression, and insomnia. Menopausal symptoms may be exacerbated by stress. Counterbalancing the reduction in hormone production is the basis of conventional treatment – hormone replacement therapy (HRT). Homeopathy does not view menopause simply in terms of hormones, but adopts a more holistic approach to body imbalances that may have existed for a long time. Constitutional treatment (*see page 176*) may be required. **SELF-HELP** Avoid tea, coffee, alcohol, and spicy foods, and eat little and often. Cotton underwear, lightweight clothes, and cool showers or baths will reduce the impact of hot flashes. Get moderate exercise and practice deep breathing (*see page 217*) or yoga. Ease vaginal dryness with calendula ointment, and increase lubrication during sexual intercourse with a vaginal lubricant. **CAUTION** If there is any bleeding six months beyond the last period, or prolonged spotting between periods, consult a doctor.	INABILITY TO COPE DURING MENOPAUSE	◆ Headache that is worse on the left side ◆ Perspiration on the face and back of the neck during sleep ◆ Craving for sweet foods ◆ Swollen finger joints
	MENOPAUSE WITH HOT FLASHES, PERSPIRATION, AND FAINTING	◆ Sensation of a kettle boiling inside the body, which is relieved by perspiring ◆ Headache that is worse on the left side ◆ Dizziness and fainting ◆ Hot flashes on the face ◆ Constricted feeling in the throat and abdomen
	LOSS OF LIBIDO DURING MENOPAUSE	◆ Heavy, irregular periods leading into menopause ◆ Possible candidiasis ◆ Vaginal dryness causing pain during sexual intercourse
	MENOPAUSE WITH HOT FLASHES IN WARM CONDITIONS	◆ Hot flashes if in a hot room or a room full of people ◆ Tendency to put on weight easily ◆ Headaches and migraines that are worse on the left side ◆ Craving for sweet foods
BREAST PAIN General tenderness in the breast is common before a period. Localized pain may be due to an abscess or a lump. Abscesses may develop from mastitis (*see page 201*), while lumps may be caused by fibroadenosis (thickening of breast tissue), benign growths, or cancer. **SELF-HELP** If breast-feeding, bathe the breast in hot water. If breast pain has other causes, reduce intake of animal fats, tea, and caffeine, and substitute oily fish for meat and dairy products. **CAUTION** If you are breast-feeding and have breast pain, especially if it is accompanied by a fever, see a doctor within 24 hours. If the nipple or breast changes, or if a hard, tender area develops, see a doctor immediately.	BREAST IS TENDER EVEN WHEN LIGHTLY TOUCHED	◆ Breast is tender to the slightest touch ◆ Breast is swollen ◆ Stitchlike pain in the nipple ◆ Desire to press the breast hard with the hands ◆ Legs feel heavy ◆ Possible reduction in sex drive
	BREAST IS HARD AND INFLAMED	◆ Breast is hard and inflamed, and feels as though there might be an abscess forming ◆ Discomfort on the slightest movement ◆ Possible bursting headache ◆ Great but infrequent thirst ◆ Possible constipation

PSYCHOLOGICAL SYMPTOMS	SYMPTOMS BETTER	SYMPTOMS WORSE	REMEDY & DOSAGE
• Confusion and difficulty in concentrating • Anxiety about symptoms having been noticed by others • Fear of insanity	• In the morning • When slightly constipated	• In drafts • In cold, damp, windy weather • With exercise • Between 2 A.M. and 3 A.M. • From stress and overexertion	**Calc. carb.** (*see page 77*) 30c 3 times daily up to 14 days
• Tearfulness and irritability • Indifference even to loved ones • General apathy	• From eating and with sleep • From exercise • From applying hot compresses to the lower abdomen	• With cold • On exposure to tobacco smoke • From mental exertion or stress • In the early morning and evening	**Sepia** (*see page 112*) 30c 3 times daily up to 14 days
• Irritability • Extreme sensitivity • Fear of domesticated animals • Mood swings and depression	• From applying firm pressure to the abdomen • From loosening clothing • When bending double • Lying down	• If touched and with jarring • Near noise • In cold drafts • From mental exertion • At night	**China** (*see page 49*) 30c 3 times daily up to 14 days
• Feeling of being unable to cope • Confusion • Anxiety about symptoms having been noticed by others • Claustrophobia	• In dry weather • After breakfast • From rubbing the affected joints	• In cold, raw air • From cold baths • From physical or mental exertion • From the pressure of clothing • From sexual intercourse	**Calc. carb.** (*see page 77*) 30c twice daily up to 7 days
• Poor memory • Difficulty in concentrating • Extreme excitability with great talkativeness • Confusion	• In the open air • From cold drinks • From loosening clothing • From eating	• On waking • In the summer and in the sun • From swallowing liquids • From the pressure of clothing • From hot drinks or alcohol	**Lachesis** (*see page 109*) 30c twice daily up to 7 days
• Irritability • Tearfulness • Apathy and indifference • Difficulty in concentrating	• With sleep • From cold baths • From strenuous walking in the open air • From being warm in bed	• With cold • From sexual intercourse • In the early morning and evening • Before thunderstorms	**Sepia** (*see page 112*) 30c twice daily up to 7 days
• Poor memory • Depression • Irritability	• In the open air • From perspiring • From gentle walking	• From hot baths • From physical or mental overexertion • From becoming hot in bed • From drinking alcohol	**Sulfur** (*see page 99*) 30c twice daily up to 7 days
• Depression • Confusion • Mental dullness and fatigue • Anxiety, hysteria, or sadness associated with grief	• From fasting • From expressing emotion • With the arms hanging down	• Lying down • From turning over in bed • In cold	**Conium** (*see page 51*) 6c every 4 hours up to 5 days
• Irritability • Desire to be alone • Great concern about financial problems	• In cool air • From applying firm, cold pressure to the breast	• With the slightest movement • In the morning and around 9 P.M. and 3 A.M. • In cold, dry, windy weather	**Bryonia** (*see page 42*) 6c every 4 hours up to 5 days

DISORDER	SPECIFIC AILMENT	PHYSICAL SYMPTOMS
CYSTITIS This term is used generally to describe increased frequency of urination with pain, but cystitis proper is inflammation of the bladder due to infection from the bowel. It may be accompanied by fever and a burning sensation when urinating. Cystitis mainly affects women; the female urethra is short and easily invaded by germs. The condition may be exacerbated by stress, antibiotics, contraceptives, poor diet, food allergies, poor personal hygiene, panty hose or underwear, and sexual intercourse. **SELF-HELP** Increase the alkalinity of the urine by drinking 10 fl oz (300 ml) of cold water or barley water every 20 minutes. Avoid tea, coffee, and alcohol. Cystitis may be aggravated by some foods, such as asparagus, beets, citrus fruits, strawberries, milk, ice cream, spicy foods, and junk foods. Never suppress the urge to urinate, and be scrupulous about personal hygiene. Avoid using tampons, douches, and perfumed bath products. Use lubrication during sexual intercourse. Urinate after intercourse. **CAUTION** If there is pain in the kidneys or blood in the urine, or if an attack lasts for more than 48 hours, see a doctor.	CYSTITIS WITH CUTTING, BURNING PAINS	◆ Burning, cutting pains in the lower abdomen ◆ Constant urge to urinate and a sensation as though the bladder cannot be emptied properly ◆ Only small amounts of urine are passed ◆ Aching in the small of the back
	CYSTITIS WITH IRRITABILITY	◆ Only small amounts of urine are passed despite frequent urging ◆ Chilliness
	CYSTITIS WITH A FEELING OF RESENTMENT	◆ Sensation of a drop of urine constantly trickling through the urethra ◆ Possible association with surgery to the urinary tract or other vaginal invasion, including sexual intercourse
VAGINAL YEAST INFECTIONS Sometimes called thrush, these infections are caused by a fungus, *Candida albicans*. Symptoms include itchiness or soreness of the vagina and vulva, discharge, and frequent urination. Acidifying, infection-fighting bacteria that occur naturally in the vagina can be destroyed by antibiotics, contraceptives, vaginal deodorants, and medicated douches. Infections are aggravated by stress, overwork, hormonal imbalance, pregnancy, and wearing tight clothes. **SELF-HELP** Avoid all potential irritants. Use lubrication and condoms during sexual intercourse. Allow air to reach the vagina as often as possible. Wear cotton underwear and avoid panty hose. Avoid sugar and yeast. Follow antibiotics with an acidophilic supplement (such as live yogurt). Douche the vagina three times a day with 5 oz (150 g) natural live yogurt diluted in 3 pints (1.5 liters) of boiled, cooled water or a weak solution of fresh lemon juice or vinegar (1 tbsp/15 ml) and water (10 fl oz/ 300 ml). Acidifying preparations are available over the counter. **CAUTION** If symptoms persist, consult a doctor.	YEAST INFECTION WITH ITCHING IN THE VULVA THAT IS WORSE BEFORE MENSTRUATION	◆ Itching of the vagina and vulva that is worse after urination and before menstruation ◆ Possible vaginal warts ◆ Possible chronic headache or increased appetite
	YEAST INFECTION WITH DISCHARGE THAT IS WORSE AFTER SEXUAL INTERCOURSE	◆ Itching of the vagina and vulva ◆ White, offensive-smelling discharge that is worse after sexual intercourse ◆ Soreness and burning in the vagina ◆ Possible ulceration of the labia
	YEAST INFECTION WITH ITCHING IN THE RECTUM	◆ Itching in the rectum and around the anus ◆ Offensive-smelling, yellow or white vaginal discharge ◆ Vaginal pain during sexual intercourse ◆ Alternating constipation and diarrhea ◆ Flatulence
VAGINISMUS This is an unusual condition in which the muscles surrounding the entrance of the vagina go into spasm. This makes sexual intercourse, medical examination of the vagina, or the use of tampons painful or even impossible. The spasms may be accompanied by arching of the back and straightening and drawing together of the legs. Vaginismus usually occurs in women who are anxious about penetration of the vagina as a result of a previous medical condition or examination, trauma such as sexual abuse, or psychological factors such as fear or guilt associated with sexual intercourse. **SELF-HELP** Practice relaxation techniques (*see page 217*), meditation, or yoga before any vaginal invasion. **CAUTION** If symptoms persist, consult a doctor for referral to a gynecologist or a psychotherapist.	EXTREME SENSITIVITY OF THE VAGINA AND THE VULVA	◆ Great sensitivity of the vagina and vulva ◆ Increased sexual desire despite symptoms ◆ Possible retention of urine ◆ Constipation that is accompanied by colicky abdominal pains
	VAGINISMUS AFTER MEDICAL EXAMINATION	◆ Extreme sensitivity of the vagina and vulva ◆ Possible irritation of the bladder
	VAGINISMUS SECONDARY TO GRIEF	◆ Vaginismus is spasmodic and erratic ◆ Itching of the vulva that extends into the vagina ◆ Possible association with a lump in the throat

PSYCHOLOGICAL SYMPTOMS	SYMPTOMS BETTER	SYMPTOMS WORSE	REMEDY & DOSAGE
• Anger or extreme irritability • Possible fear of mirrors and other reflective surfaces	• With warmth • From a gentle massage • At night and in the morning	• With movement • From drinking coffee or cold water • In the afternoon	**Cantharis** (*see page 105*) 30c half-hourly up to 10 doses
• Irritability • Great criticism of others • Desire to be left alone	• With warmth • With sleep • From applying pressure to the bladder • From washing • In the evening	• In cold, windy weather • Near noise • From eating, especially spicy foods • From taking stimulants • Between 3 A.M. and 4 A.M.	**Nux vomica** (*see page 63*) 6c half-hourly up to 10 doses
• Resentment • Anger	• With warmth • From a good night's sleep	• From applying pressure to the bladder • From not drinking enough fluids	**Staphysagria** (*see page 54*) 30c half-hourly up to 10 doses
• Anxiety, especially that brought on by overwork and stress • Depression	• In the morning • When slightly constipated	• Before and after menstruation • From applying heat to the vulva • During pregnancy • In cold, damp, windy weather • From physical or mental exertion	**Calc. carb.** (*see page 77*) 6c 6 times daily up to 5 days
• Tearfulness • Irritability • Indifference toward loved ones • Aversion to sexual intercourse	• From eating • With sleep • From exercise • From applying heat to the vulva	• In cold • On exposure to tobacco smoke • From being overtired • Between 2 A.M. and 3 A.M., and in the early morning and evening	**Sepia** (*see page 112*) 6c 6 times daily up to 5 days
• Stress • Stubbornness and irritability • Anxiety and hypochondria	• In fresh air • With dry warmth • From walking	• From prolonged standing • From wearing too much clothing • In cold and damp • From washing • For being too warm in bed	**Sulfur** (*see page 99*) 6c 6 times daily up to 5 days
• Selfishness and self-indulgence • Loss of memory and slow perception • Tendency to malinger	• From massaging the vagina • From applying firm pressure to the muscles at the tops of the thighs • From stretching the legs	• From exertion • From being in company • With excitement	**Plumbum met.** (*see page 96*) 30c twice daily up to 5 days
• Resentment and suppressed anger	• With warmth • With rest • From applying firm pressure to the muscles at the tops of the thighs	• From emotional stress or arguing • From sexual excess or masturbation • From operative investigation	**Staphysagria** (*see page 54*) 30c twice daily up to 5 days
• Association with grief, introspection, and the suppression of emotions	• From changing position • With warmth • From urinating	• From emotional stress • With consolation • From the slightest touch	**Ignatia** (*see page 57*) 30c twice daily up to 5 days

DISORDER	SPECIFIC AILMENT	PHYSICAL SYMPTOMS
MORNING SICKNESS Nausea and vomiting are fairly common during pregnancy, especially a first pregnancy. It is thought that changing hormone levels during pregnancy activate the vomiting center in the brain. Women often experience nausea and vomiting during the second and third months of pregnancy, although not necessarily only in the mornings. Symptoms usually wear off by about 14 to 16 weeks, although a few women vomit excessively (hyperemesis), which can cause dehydration and chemical imbalances in the body. This condition may, in the worst cases, require hospitalization. **SELF-HELP** Eat small, frequent meals and avoid fatty foods. If there is sickness immediately upon waking, eat a dry cracker before getting out of bed. The use of fresh ginger in cooking may also help. An acupressure band, available from pharmacies, worn around the wrist may also be effective. Get plenty of rest. **CAUTION** If you are vomiting after most meals, consult a doctor.	NAUSEA WITH A THICKLY COATED TONGUE	◆ Nausea that is worse in the morning ◆ Vomiting of small amounts of food with mucus ◆ Retching spasms ◆ Dry mouth and thickly coated tongue ◆ Craving for fresh, fatty, spicy, or acidic foods and aversion to bread, meat, coffee, and tobacco
	NAUSEA THAT IS WORSE IN THE EVENING	◆ Nausea that is worse during the early evening but wears off during the night ◆ Dry mouth but lack of thirst ◆ Digestion is upset by rich, fatty foods ◆ Pressure under the breastbone after meals ◆ Craving for sweet foods
	CONSTANT NAUSEA WITH A CLEAN TONGUE	◆ Vomiting of all foods and drinks ◆ Nausea is not relieved by vomiting ◆ Tongue feels clean rather than coated ◆ Profuse saliva ◆ Lack of thirst ◆ Possible fainting
LABOR PAINS Pain is experienced in childbirth as as result of contractions of the uterus that move the baby down the birth canal during labor. For most women labor is a painful business; for some it is excruciating. This may be because they have great sensitivity to pain or because the fetus is positioned in such a way that the uterus has to work harder than usual in order to push the baby out. Labor pains may be exacerbated by exhaustion, fear, anxiety, and sometimes anger. Homeopathic treatment aims to calm the emotions as well as to relieve pain and exhaustion. **SELF-HELP** Learn psychoprophylactic techniques (preventive measures that combine positive thinking and constructive breathing) at prenatal classes. These may help you restore a feeling of control in what can be a frightening situation. If you are extremely sensitive to pain, learn other relaxation techniques and consider acupuncture or hypnotherapy.	LABOR PAINS WITH GREAT SENSITIVITY TO PAIN	◆ Contractions that seem so painful they cause involuntary screaming and crying
	LABOR PAINS WITH GREAT IRRITABILITY	◆ Ineffectual contractions ◆ Pain extending into the rectum with a frequent urge to pass wind, urine, or stools ◆ Pain that causes spasms of the cervix, which does not dilate properly
	LABOR PAINS WITH A CONSTANT NEED FOR COMFORT AND SYMPATHY	◆ Labor progresses slowly ◆ Chilliness
BREAST-FEEDING PROBLEMS Several problems may arise during breast-feeding. The breasts may be too full for the baby to be able to latch onto a nipple properly. Expressing milk before nursing may solve the problem. The milk may be too watery or have a taste that the baby does not like arising from the mother's insubstantial diet, anxiety, exhaustion, or to strong-tasting foods that she has eaten. Pain as the baby suckles may be caused by inflammation of the breast tissue (see Mastitis, page 201), an abscess, or cracked nipples. **SELF-HELP** Bathe sore and cracked nipples after each feeding with a solution of calendula and hypericum (10 drops mother tinctures to 10 fl oz/300 ml boiled, cooled water). Do not use soap. Clean and dry the nipples thoroughly and apply hypericum or calendula ointment. Leave them exposed to the air regularly. Wear breast shields during pregnancy to draw out inverted nipples. **CAUTION** If there is engorgement or hardness, breast pain, fever, and tender glands under the arms, see a doctor within 12 hours.	THROBBING, INFLAMED BREASTS	◆ Engorgement or hardness of the breasts with red streaks on the skin ◆ Breasts feel heavy ◆ Hot, dry skin ◆ Possible mastitis or breast abscess
	PAIN WHEN THE BABY SUCKLES, CAUSING ANGER IN THE MOTHER	◆ Inflamed nipples that are very tender to the touch ◆ Great pain as the baby suckles
	ENGORGED BREASTS	◆ Milk is of poor quality ◆ Baby has difficulty latching onto a nipple ◆ Breasts are so full that they cause great discomfort ◆ Possible chilliness or perspiration, especially if the mother is overweight

PSYCHOLOGICAL SYMPTOMS	SYMPTOMS BETTER	SYMPTOMS WORSE	REMEDY & DOSAGE
◆ Irritability that is worse in the morning ◆ Harsh criticism of others	◆ With warmth and sleep ◆ From applying firm pressure to the stomach ◆ From washing or applying wet compresses to the stomach ◆ In the evening	◆ In cold, windy weather ◆ From spicy foods ◆ From taking stimulants ◆ From stress ◆ Between 3 A.M. and 4 A.M.	**Nux vomica** (*see page 63*) 6c every 2 hours up to 3 days
◆ Tearfulness ◆ Great desire for support and reassurance ◆ Self-pity	◆ From cold drinks or applying cold compresses to the stomach ◆ From sympathy and crying ◆ With the hands above the head ◆ With gentle exercise ◆ In fresh air	◆ In hot, stuffy rooms ◆ In the evening ◆ From rich, fatty foods ◆ Lying on the left side	**Pulsatilla** (*see page 61*) 6c every 2 hours up to 3 days
◆ Irritability and contempt ◆ Great desire for something but it is not known exactly what	◆ In fresh air	◆ From bending forward ◆ With movement ◆ With warmth ◆ Lying down ◆ From stress caused by embarrassment	**Ipecac.** (*see page 45*) 6c every 2 hours up to 3 days
◆ Nervousness and restlessness between contractions ◆ Tearfulness and despair	◆ With warmth ◆ Lying down ◆ From sucking ice	◆ With emotional excitement ◆ From strong smells and noise ◆ In fresh air ◆ In cold ◆ At night	**Coffea** (*see page 50*) 30c every 5 minutes up to 10 doses
◆ Irritability ◆ Impatience ◆ Great criticism of others	◆ With warmth and sleep ◆ From applying firm pressure or wet compresses to the abdomen ◆ In the evening ◆ From being left alone	◆ In cold ◆ Near noise ◆ From taking stimulants ◆ From eating ◆ From stress	**Nux vomica** (*see page 63*) 30c every 5 minutes up to 10 doses
◆ Restlessness ◆ Tendency to cry at the least provocation ◆ Great need for comfort and reassurance	◆ From crying and sympathy ◆ With the hands above the head ◆ With gentle movement ◆ In fresh air ◆ From applying cold compresses to the abdomen	◆ With heat ◆ In extremes of temperature ◆ Lying on the painful side ◆ In the evening and at night	**Pulsatilla** (*see page 61*) 30c every 5 minutes up to 10 doses
◆ Possible delirium with wide, staring eyes if temperature is very high	◆ When standing or sitting upright ◆ In warm rooms ◆ From applying warm compresses to the breasts	◆ With jarring, near noise ◆ From applying pressure to the breasts ◆ Lying down, especially on the right side	**Belladonna** (*see page 39*) 30c hourly up to 10 doses
◆ Anger ◆ Spitefulness and rudeness ◆ Great tendency to complain	◆ From applying cold compresses to the breasts ◆ From perspiring	◆ With heat ◆ At night	**Chamomilla** (*see page 46*) 30c every 4 hours up to 6 doses
◆ Worry about new responsibilities ◆ Anxiety causing forgetfulness and apprehension ◆ Anxiety about symptoms having been observed	◆ Lying down ◆ From massaging the breasts ◆ After breakfast	◆ From drinking milk ◆ From physical or mental exertion ◆ From climbing stairs ◆ In cold rooms ◆ From bathing	**Calc. carb.** (*see page 77*) 30c 4 times daily up to 3 days

MEN'S HEALTH

MEDICALLY SPEAKING, men are less complicated than women. The most troublesome of their problems that are suitable for self-help are usually the result of infections. The urethra in the male is much longer than that in the female and therefore tends to be less susceptible to invasion by germs. Men thus experience fewer problems with urinary control and infection than women. However, because the urethra

DISORDER	SPECIFIC AILMENT	PHYSICAL SYMPTOMS
ERECTILE DYSFUNCTION Problems with erection may result from physical causes, for example, injury or surgery to the genitals or spine; from chronic illnesses such as diabetes; from nervous disorders; or from taking drugs, either medically prescribed or recreational, or alcohol. Erectile dysfunction may also occur because of tiredness, or a lack of appropriate stimulation. Most physical problems occur because there is an insufficient supply of blood to the penis. The stresses of modern life or anxiety about sexual intercourse may further inhibit the ability to initiate or sustain an erection. SELF-HELP To reduce the psychological problems that may accompany erectile dysfunction, try to maintain a relaxed state of mind when making love. Forget about penetrative sexual intercourse for a while and concentrate on giving and receiving pleasure in areas of the body other than the genitals. CAUTION If symptoms persist, see a doctor.	ERECTILE DYSFUNCTION IN ANTICIPATION OF FAILURE	◆ Penis remains cold and small ◆ Possible premature ejaculation if erection does occur ◆ Great desire for sweet foods
	ERECTILE DYSFUNCTION CAUSED BY BRUISING	◆ Penis is bruised as a result of injury ◆ Penis feels sore and tender to the touch ◆ Possible premature ejaculation if erection does occur
	ERECTILE DYSFUNCTION CAUSED BY SEXUAL EXCESS	◆ Erection is not firm enough for penetration ◆ General weakness and nervous exhaustion ◆ Penis remains cold and small ◆ Possible premature ejaculation if erection does occur
HYDROCELE A soft, painless swelling of the scrotum, hydrocele is due to a buildup of excess fluid in the sheath surrounding the testes. It may be precipitated by injury and is common in older men, although in most cases the cause is unknown. The condition may be congenital. The swelling may be caused by inflammation, infection, or, very occasionally, a tumor. Usually hydrocele is just monitored, but fluid may need to be drained off should the swelling become too great. CAUTION If symptoms persist beyond a month, see a doctor.	HYDROCELE FOLLOWING INJURY	◆ Bruising with painful swelling of the scrotum and testicle ◆ Swelling may be filled with blood
	HYDROCELE WITH AN ACHING TESTICLE	◆ Testicle aches during thundery weather ◆ Association with orchitis (inflammation of a testicle) ◆ Right testicle is the one usually affected
BALANITIS This swelling and soreness of the foreskin may result from the friction of underwear, or from irritation caused by condoms or contraceptive creams. It may be associated with herpes or diabetes. SELF-HELP Bathe the foreskin and head of the penis (glans) in a solution of hypericum and calendula (see page 271) every four hours, then apply calendula ointment. CAUTION If symptoms persist for five days, see a doctor.	BALANITIS WITH INFLAMMATION OF THE FORESKIN AND GLANS	◆ Inner surface of the foreskin is irritated and inflamed ◆ Possible itching ◆ Possible discharge of offensive-smelling pus ◆ Possible ulceration
YEAST INFECTION Often transmitted from an infected partner, this fungal infection albicans yeast grows under the foreskin, causing inflammation. SELF-HELP Bathe the penis in a solution of hypericum and calendula (see page 271) four times daily. Apply calendula ointment. CAUTION If symptoms persist beyond 14 days, see a doctor. Make sure that your partner also goes for treatment.	YEAST INFECTION WITH INFLAMMATION AND DISCHARGE	◆ Inner surface of the foreskin is inflamed and itchy ◆ Head of the penis is red, with a raised rash that is itchy ◆ Possible itchy, smelly discharge from the penis

is connected to the testes, epididymis, and prostate gland any kidney, bladder, or urethral infection can spread easily to the reproductive system (*see page 198*). Disorders of that system are the subject of this section. Men's sexual activity can be extended into later life by following a lifestyle that promotes general good health, including a balanced diet, sufficient exercise, and effective stress control. Men may be reluctant to seek medical help for their ailments, especially those concerning the reproductive system. Many conditions are, however, easily treated if diagnosed early, and respond well to homeopathy. Neglect, on the other hand, can lead to complications that threaten fertility, sexual function, or even life.

PSYCHOLOGICAL SYMPTOMS	SYMPTOMS BETTER	SYMPTOMS WORSE	REMEDY & DOSAGE
◆ High sex drive but lack of self-confidence and expectation of failure to achieve or sustain an erection	◆ From loosening clothing ◆ From warm drinks ◆ From urinating	◆ From wearing tight clothing ◆ In very hot rooms ◆ From overeating	**Lycopodium** (*see page 59*) 30c twice daily up to 5 days
◆ Desire to be left alone ◆ Denial that there is a problem ◆ Refusal to get medical help ◆ Fear of being touched	◆ From bathing in cold water ◆ From adopting a sexual position that avoids putting pressure on the bruised area	◆ If touched ◆ From further injury or bruising ◆ From sexual excesses	**Arnica** (*see page 37*) 30c twice daily up to 5 days
◆ Anxiety about health ◆ Fear of death ◆ Increase in sexual thoughts despite decline in sexual function	◆ From applying firm pressure to the penis ◆ With rest ◆ From ejaculating	◆ If touched ◆ From a sprain or injury ◆ From sexual excesses	**Agnus castus** (*see page 173*) 30c twice daily up to 5 days
◆ Desire to be left alone ◆ Denial that there is a problem ◆ Refusal to get medical help	◆ From bathing in cold water ◆ From adopting a sexual position that avoids putting pressure on the bruised area	◆ If touched ◆ With movement ◆ Lying for too long on one side	**Arnica** (*see page 37*) 30c 3 times daily up to 3 weeks
◆ Nervousness ◆ Fear of thunderstorms and great sensitivity to approaching storms	◆ With heat ◆ With continuous movement ◆ Lying in bed with the legs pulled up to the chest	◆ Before thunderstorms ◆ In windy weather ◆ With rest, from standing, and on starting to move	**Rhododendron** (*see page 162*) 6c 3 times daily up to 3 weeks
◆ Restlessness at night ◆ Loss of willpower ◆ Indifference ◆ Suspicion	◆ In moderate temperatures ◆ With rest ◆ From scratching the affected area ◆ In the morning	◆ At night ◆ From perspiring ◆ From getting overheated ◆ In cold air and drafts	**Merc. sol.** (*see page 85*) 6c every 4 hours up to 5 days
◆ Restlessness at night ◆ Loss of willpower ◆ Indifference ◆ Suspicion	◆ In moderate temperatures ◆ With rest ◆ From scratching the affected area ◆ In the morning	◆ At night ◆ From perspiring ◆ From getting overheated or too cold ◆ From urinating	**Merc. sol.** (*see page 85*) 6c 4 times daily up to 14 days

HEALTH IN LATER LIFE

AS PEOPLE GET OLDER, they appreciate that health is something more than just the good fortune to have a body in proper working order. Maintaining health in later life has to do with genetic makeup, past and current lifestyles, and relationships with family, friends, and with the community, on whom a person may increasingly depend if health deteriorates and energy levels fall. Health and well-being in later life

DISORDER	SPECIFIC AILMENT	PHYSICAL SYMPTOMS
DIZZINESS In later life dizziness is commonly due to postural hypotension (low blood pressure on standing or sitting) or drugs. It may be exacerbated by osteoarthritis (*see page 196*). More seriously, dizziness may be indicative of Parkinson's disease (degeneration of nerve centers coordinating movement), cervical spondylosis (bony outgrowths on neck vertebrae restricting blood supply to the brain), or arteriosclerosis (hardening and narrowing of arteries, especially those supplying the brain). These conditions affect balance. Mild, early symptoms may respond to self-help remedies. **SELF-HELP** Keep physically active and maintain a good diet. Minimize the risk of falls in the home by, for example, securing floor coverings and attaching handrails along staircases. **CAUTION** If there is no improvement within two weeks, see a doctor. If dizziness increases rapidly, see a doctor within 24 hours. If dizziness causes a fall, see a doctor within two hours.	DIZZINESS AFTER A FALL OR INJURY	◆ Dizziness on standing up from a sitting or lying position ◆ Dizziness decreases after lying down ◆ Head movement creates a sensation of everything turning with it
	DIZZINESS WITH NAUSEA	◆ Dizziness is worse with movement and is associated with nausea ◆ Extreme sensitivity to noise that makes the dizziness worse ◆ Chilliness
	DIZZINESS THAT IS WORSE IN COLD WEATHER	◆ Dizziness with a tendency to fall forward and sideways ◆ Sensation of the head being compressed
CONFUSION Confusion is characterized by an inability to organize thoughts coherently and poor short-term memory. Elderly people are prone to confusion resulting from infection, alcohol, or drugs. Chronic confusion may be due to dementia (*see below*). Sudden onset may indicate a serious condition, such as hypothermia (fall in body temperature to less than 95°F/35°C), a stroke (*see page 187*), a brain tumor, or hypoglycemia (abnormally low blood-sugar levels). **SELF-HELP** Make sure that the diet is balanced. Try the breathing techniques used in yoga to reduce stress. **CAUTION** If there is no improvement within three weeks, see a doctor. If there is acute confusion, see a doctor within 12 hours.	CONFUSION WITH SUSPICION	◆ General slowing down of physical activity so that tasks take a long time to complete ◆ Weakness after eating ◆ Tendency to lose weight even when eating well
	CONFUSION WITH DELUSIONS	◆ Weakness when walking ◆ Noises in the head that resemble explosions ◆ Spasms in the neck or the bladder when urinating ◆ Sensation of the head being separated from the body
SENILE DEMENTIA A general decline in mental ability is caused by the progressive loss of function of brain cells. This occurs if arteries supplying blood to the brain become blocked, or as a result of a number of conditions, including Alzheimer's disease and stroke (*see page 187*). One of the first symptoms is a deterioration in short-term memory so that it becomes increasingly difficult to follow conversations or to read. As the condition progresses, there is a gradual loss of interest in previously enjoyed pursuits, as well as mood swings. There may be a loss of social or sexual inhibitions. Diagnosis needs care, since a deteriorating mental state may be caused by a variety of medical conditions, dietary deficiencies, the use of alcohol or drugs, or depression. **SELF-HELP** The diet should be balanced between proteins and carbohydrates, and include plenty of fresh fruits and vegetables. **CAUTION** If symptoms persist beyond a month, see a doctor.	SENILE DEMENTIA IN PEOPLE WHO WERE ONCE INTELLECTUALLY SHARP	◆ Craving for sweet foods ◆ Susceptibility to digestive problems such as bloating, excessive flatulence, and constipation ◆ Fullness after eating only small amounts of food ◆ Generally thin and withered appearance
	SENILE DEMENTIA WITH SUSPICION	◆ Weakness and fatigue ◆ Possible early stages of an enlarged prostate gland in men ◆ Slowing down of all movements
	SENILE DEMENTIA IN HIGH-STRUNG PEOPLE	◆ Numbness and tingling sensation in the fingers and toes ◆ Burning pains all over the body, but especially in the stomach ◆ Desire for salt and ice-cold drinks

can be planned for, as with any foreseeable situation, and the better the plan, the easier life will be. Bodily systems may ultimately fail because of inherited weaknesses, but to what extent they fail and how quickly they do so will also depend on nutrition, level of exercise, lifestyle, and attitudes toward life. Constitutional homeopathic treatment (*see page 176*) aims to establish a holistic approach to correcting imbalances in body systems, and maintaining a sense of vitality and well-being in a person as he or she gets older. Homeopathic remedies are particularly well suited to aging bodies that may be less able than young ones to metabolize conventional drugs with speed and efficiency.

PSYCHOLOGICAL SYMPTOMS	SYMPTOMS BETTER	SYMPTOMS WORSE	REMEDY & DOSAGE
• Denial that there is a problem • Desire to be left alone • Refusal to get medical help	• Lying down, especially with the head lower than the body • In the open air • From bathing in cold water • From sitting up straight	• From injury • If touched • With sleep • From getting up	**Arnica** (*see page 37*) 6c every 8 hours up to 14 days
• Nervousness • Concern that time is passing too quickly • Association with nervous exhaustion after long suffering	• With rest • From drinking warm water	• Near noise • If touched • With the eyes closed • With the slightest movement	**Theridion** (*see page 169*) 6c every 8 hours up to 14 days
• Association with a deep sense of grief • Failing memory necessitating double-checking everything	• From cold drinks • With gentle movement • With warmth	• In dry, cold wind • From stooping	**Causticum** (*see page 79*) 6c every 8 hours up to 14 days
• Tasks are carried out without adequate thought • Lack of confidence and a concern about being mocked • Suspicion of strangers and unfamiliar places	• From walking in the open air • From being alone	• From being in company • In cold • After meals	**Baryta carb.** (*see page 76*) 6c twice daily up to 3 weeks
• Great excitement and heightened awareness of sensations • Possible out-of-body experiences • Fear of the dark and of demons • Laughter at anything • Forgetfulness	• In the open air • From bathing in cold water • With rest	• In the dark • From physical or mental exertion • From coffee	**Cannabis ind.** (*see page 43*) 6c twice daily up to 3 weeks
• Lack of confidence as memory and concentration begin to fail • Fear of being alone	• From warm drinks • From loosening clothing • In the open air	• From the pressure of clothing • With warmth • Between 4 P.M. and 8 P.M. • From overeating	**Lycopodium** (*see page 59*) 30c twice daily up to 14 days
• Failing memory leading to odd actions, thoughts, and perceptions • Suspicion that everyone is mocking, leading to a lack of self-confidence and desire to be alone	• From walking in the open air • From being alone • From wrapping up warmly	• From being in company • In cold • From stress	**Baryta carb.** (*see page 76*) 30c twice daily up to 14 days
• Agitation and apprehension • Great fear of the dark and of being alone • Failing memory leading to constant worry about others	• With sleep, even catnaps • From a massage • From eating	• Lying down • From emotional stress • From warm foods • From mental exertion	**Phosphorous** (*see page 94*) 30c twice daily up to 14 days

DISORDER	SPECIFIC AILMENT	PHYSICAL SYMPTOMS
NEURALGIA Nerve pain may occur anywhere in the body but is most commonly associated with nerves providing sensation to the face, mouth, nose, upper eyelids, sinuses, and scalp. Neuralgia consists of a severe, shooting pain on one side of the face that lasts for seconds or minutes. The pain may be linked to infection of the sinuses, ears, or teeth, but often the cause is unknown. It may be referred pain, which is felt in a different area from the location of infection, for example, but in an area that is served by a different branch of the same nerve. Nerves are very sensitive, and neuralgia can be triggered by touch, pressure, chewing, or drafts. It is common in people over 70, in whom it may result from nerve damage. **SELF-HELP** Hold a covered hot-water bottle against the affected area. Try breathing techniques (*see page 217*) to relax the muscles and hence relieve pressure on the nerves. **CAUTION** If there is no improvement within two weeks, consult a doctor.	NEURALGIA IN THE EAR	◆ Intense, shooting pains ◆ Tearing pain above the left ear, then the right ◆ Numbness of outer ear and reduced hearing first on the left side, then on the right ◆ Sensation of pressure on the top of the head ◆ Possible shivers up the back and left side
	NEURALGIA WITH BURNING PAINS	◆ Burning pains in the head ◆ Restlessness ◆ Exhaustion
	NEURALGIA ON THE LEFT SIDE OF THE FACE	◆ Violent, tearing pain on the left side ◆ Twitching facial muscles on the left side ◆ Dark red cheek ◆ Possible redness and watering of the left eye ◆ Painfully stiff shoulders and neck
SKIN PROBLEMS With age, the skin loses elasticity and plumpness. It becomes thin, and tiny blood vessels that are nearer the surface as a result are easily damaged. This causes bruising and discoloration, which commonly occur on the backs of the hands, forearms, and lower legs. The discoloration fades but never disappears. The skin may develop pigmented patches, possibly due to faulty fat metabolism. Itchy skin is common with age, and is often caused by dryness, eczema (*see page 240*), or dermatitis (inflammation of the skin). **SELF-HELP** Extra vitamin C and the application of arnica ointment may lessen bruising, while extra vitamin E may help to reduce the impact of pigmented patches. **CAUTION** If a pigmented patch that is more than ⅜ in (1 cm) in diameter becomes larger, inflamed, or encrusted, develops an irregular, notched outline or a dark area within it, or itches, oozes, or bleeds, consult a doctor.	ITCHY SKIN THAT IS WORSE FROM WASHING	◆ Dry, scaly, itchy skin ◆ Burning pains after scratching and washing the affected areas ◆ Diarrhea in the morning
	DIRTY-LOOKING SKIN	◆ Skin eruption with great itching that induces scratching until the skin is raw ◆ Oily, dirty-looking skin ◆ Possible distinctive, unpleasant body odor
	OILY SKIN WITH EXCESSIVE PERSPIRATION	◆ Profuse, offensive-smelling perspiration ◆ Skin is oily and constantly moist ◆ Intolerable itching
INCONTINENCE & FREQUENT URINATION Incontinence is not an inevitable feature of aging, and is often secondary to a urinary infection such as cystitis, constipation, an enlarged prostate or irritation of the vulva, or the use of drugs. It can also occur after a stroke or problems with the spinal cord. Stress incontinence – a leakage of urine when laughing, coughing, or sneezing as a result of weak pelvic floor muscles – is chiefly a women's complaint. Associated with advanced senile dementia (*see page 266*), incontinence may be more a question of attitude than physical disability. It is often worse in cold, from extreme excitement, or from anxiety. The most common causes of frequent urination are diuretic drugs prescribed for high blood pressure, and drinking tea, coffee, or alcohol. **SELF-HELP** Avoid drinking large amounts, and urinate regularly. Yoga or osteopathy may help relax or reposition muscles in the lower spinal area. Exercises for the pelvic floor muscles will strengthen them. **CAUTION** If symptoms persist for more than three days, or if frequent urination is associated with great thirst, see a doctor.	FREQUENT URINATION DAY AND NIGHT	◆ Stress incontinence ◆ Frequent urination during first stage of sleep ◆ Frequent urination due to overdistention of the bladder following urine retention ◆ Only small amounts of urine are passed, due to paralysis of muscles in the neck of the bladder
	FREQUENT URINATION THAT IS WORSE AT 4 A.M.	◆ Strongest urge to urinate is at around 4 A.M. ◆ Possible difficulty in starting a stream of urine ◆ Possible pain in the small of the back
	FREQUENT URINATION WITH CONSTIPATION	◆ Frequent urge to urinate or to pass stools if constipated ◆ Possible ineffectual urge to urinate ◆ Sensation of there being more urine to pass even immediately after urination ◆ Possible cramps in the bladder ◆ Chilliness

PSYCHOLOGICAL SYMPTOMS	SYMPTOMS BETTER	SYMPTOMS WORSE	REMEDY & DOSAGE
• Irritability • Despondency	• From taking deep breaths • On rising from a sitting position • With movement	• In drafts • With changes in temperature • Twice a day at the same times • If touched, from talking, sneezing, or biting hard • With stooping or walking	**Verbascum** (*see page 171*) 6c 4 times daily up to 14 days
• Great anxiety • Fear that recovery is unlikely and that death is a possibility • Fear of cancer	• From applying cold compresses to the affected area • In cold air • Lying in a semireclined position • With heat	• Between midnight and 2 A.M. • With physical or mental exertion • From cold drinks	**Arsen. alb.** (*see page 68*) 6c 4 times daily up to 14 days
• Fear of pointed objects • Possible association with long-term grief	• From applying cold compresses to the affected area • With rest • From applying pressure to the affected area	• If touched or from jarring • On stooping or turning the eyes • With movement • On exposure to tobacco smoke • From sexual intercourse	**Spigelia** (*see page 167*) 6c 4 times daily up to 14 days
• Impatience • Bad temper • Lack of interest in personal appearance	• In cold • From applying cold compresses to the affected area	• From washing • When warm in bed • From wearing woolen clothing	**Sulfur** (*see page 99*) 6c 4 times daily up to 14 days
• Fear that recovery is unlikely • Feeling of having been forsaken • Possible suicidal tendency	• Lying down • From eating • From profuse perspiration	• In cold • From coffee • From washing	**Psorinum** (*see page 111*) 6c 4 times daily up to 14 days
• Loss of memory and willpower • Nervous confusion and a tendency to stammer	• From being neither too hot nor too cold • With rest • From scratching the affected area	• At night • From perspiring • On becoming overheated • In drafts or cold conditions	**Merc. sol.** (*see page 85*) 6c 4 times daily up to 14 days
• Possible association with long-term grief • Failing memory necessitates double-checking everything • Sympathy for others' suffering	• From cold drinks • From washing • From being warm in bed	• In dry, cold, raw winds and drafts • At 3 A.M., 4 A.M., or in the evening	**Causticum** (*see page 79*) 6c every 4 hours up to 3 days
• Irritability • Anxiety and fear when left alone • Great sensitivity to noise	• With warmth • With movement • When sitting with the elbows on the knees	• In cold air and drafts • In winter • From coffee	**Kali. carb.** (*see page 88*) 6c every 4 hours up to 3 days
• Irritability • Tendency to be argumentative, find fault with others, and blame others • Great sensitivity to noise and light	• With rest • From passing stools or gas • With warmth	• In the early morning • From stress and overindulgence • From being angry • Near noise, in light, if touched	**Nux vomica** (*see page 63*) 6c every 4 hours up to 3 days

FIRST AID

THE AIMS OF FIRST AID are to save life, limit injury, ease pain and anxiety, and summon the most appropriate help available. All first-aid methods, whether they are associated with conventional medicine or complementary therapies, are based on a common-sense approach to dealing with a serious accident or a minor scrape. Homeopathic remedies can help relieve pain, allay anxiety and shock, and facilitate healing. They can be used in conjunction with any other medication.

IDENTIFYING PRIORITIES IN AN EMERGENCY

The most important things to do in an emergency are to keep a clear head and not to panic, to determine what the priorities are, and to act decisively and promptly. Ideally, at least one person in every household should be trained in first-aid procedures. Homeopathic remedies should be given only after the priorities listed below have been identified.

ASSESSING SERIOUS CONDITIONS

Make sure that you, the injured person, and your surroundings are safe. Gently shake him or her by both shoulders – without moving the neck in case of head or neck injuries – and ask a question or give a command. If there is no response, proceed with the ABC of resuscitation.
A–airway Make sure that his or her airway is open by gently tilting the head back (*see right*).
B–breathing See if the chest is rising and falling, and listen and feel for breathing against your ear. If the person is not breathing, call an ambulance immediately. Begin mouth-to-mouth resuscitation if you have been trained to do it.
C–circulation Feel the person's neck at the side of the windpipe to see if there is a pulse. Check whether there is any movement or noise, and if the skin is pale and clammy. If there is neither pulse nor breathing, administer cardiopulmonary resuscitation (CPR), but only if you have been trained in the correct first-aid methods.

OPENING THE AIRWAY
Lay the injured person on her back on a firm surface. Gently tilt back the forehead and lift the jaw. Make sure that there are no foreign objects inside the mouth.

UNCONSCIOUSNESS
If an injured person is unconscious, and you have already checked the airway, breathing, and life signs (*see* Assessing serious conditions, *left*) and you do not suspect serious head, spinal, or internal injuries or fractured limbs, carefully maneuver her into a safe position (*see right*) and call an ambulance. Do not leave an unconscious person unattended. Check the airway, breathing, and pulse every five minutes. Make sure that she is kept warm but does not become overheated.

Bach Rescue Remedy. Drip 2 drops into the injured person's mouth every 10 minutes until help arrives.

A SAFE POSITION
Carefully place an unconscious person in the position below. This will ensure that the body will be propped in a stable and comfortable position. The head is slightly lower than the body, reducing the risks of vomit being inhaled (since liquids can drain from the mouth) or the tongue being swallowed.

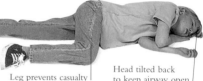

Leg prevents casualty from rolling onto front, inhibiting breathing

Head tilted back to keep airway open

BLEEDING
Check any open wounds to see if there is bleeding. If there is, apply a sterile pad and, if possible, a bandage. If there is a profuse flow of blood from the wound, call an ambulance. Place a sterile pad over the wound and apply firm pressure to the area until the bleeding stops or medical help arrives.

Arnica 30c every 10 minutes until the shock of the injury wears off or until medical help arrives, then every 8 hours for up to 4 days.

BURNS
If burns extend over an area larger than the palm of a hand, call an ambulance and carefully cover the affected parts with plastic wrap. Immerse a small burn in cold water for up to 10 minutes, then cover it with plastic wrap or a burn dressing. If neither is available, use a nonfluffy, clean dressing. Do not attempt to remove any pieces of clothing that may have adhered to the burned skin. Do not burst blisters or apply lotion, cream, or gel to the wounds. If the injured person is conscious, administer sips of water to minimize fluid loss.

Arnica 30c 3 doses only, then *Cantharis 30c* up to 6 doses or, if the burn continues to sting, *Urtica urens 6c* up to 6 doses.

FRACTURES

Evidence of a fracture includes pain, an inability to move the affected part, visible deformity, swelling, bruising, and shock. Try to immobilize the affected part to prevent further damage and blood loss. Bandage an arm against the chest or one leg to the other, for example. Pad out the bandages above and below the fracture so that clothes and blankets do not exert pressure on it. If the fracture is open, apply padding to each side of the bone, then cover the whole area with a sterile dressing. Apply pressure to the padding to help slow down the bleeding. Call an ambulance or, if the injury affects only a hand, take the injured person to a hospital.

Arnica 30c every 10 minutes until the shock of injury wears off, then every 8 hours up to 4 days. *Symphytum 6c* taken subsequently every 8 hours for up to 3 weeks will promote bone healing.

CHOKING

The airway may be obstructed by food, the tongue, vomit, or a foreign body, causing coughing, crying, and breathing difficulties. Check the mouth and remove any obvious obstructions. If the airway is totally obstructed and the person stops breathing, bend him forward if he is standing, or lay him on his side, and slap him sharply on the back between the shoulder blades three or four times with the heel of the hand. Check the mouth. In the case of a small child, lay the victim over your knee and use less force when slapping the back.

Aconite 30c every 10 minutes until the shock of this traumatic event wears off.

DROWNING

The priorities for a victim of drowning are to call an ambulance immediately and then start basic life support (*see* Assessing serious conditions, *opposite*).

ELECTROCUTION

If someone has been electrocuted, turn off the current at the outlet or circuit breaker. Keep the person away from water, which conducts electricity. Call an ambulance and start basic life support (*see* Assessing serious conditions, *opposite*). Look for any wounds. Lay a conscious person on the back, raise the legs slightly, and tilt the head to one side with the chin up. Place an unconscious victim in a safe position (*see opposite*) and cover her.

Aconite 30c every minute up to 10 doses if the victim is fearful or restless. If she is yawning, desperate for air, or turning blue, *Carbo veg. 30c* every minute up to 10 doses.

ASSEMBLING A FIRST-AID KIT

Many homeopathic pharmacies sell basic homeopathic first-aid kits containing between 12 and 18 remedies. These represent a good start, but check the contents before buying one to ensure that it includes the remedies that you need (*see below*). You may be able to exchange some remedies for others. For acute first-aid complaints, you will need remedies with a 30c potency; for less acute ailments, 6c potency. (Pregnant women should not take *Apis* of lower potency than 30c.)

STORING A FIRST-AID KIT All first-aid items should be kept together, preferably in a sturdy box, and stored in a cool, dry, and dark place. Kept like this, homeopathic remedies will retain their strength for years. Every adult member of a household should know where the first-aid kit is kept and have easy access to it, and it should always be placed well beyond the reach of young children.

ADMINISTERING REMEDIES Homeopathic remedies can be given in the same way to babies, children, and adults. Placed under the tongue, tablets or pilules dissolve quickly. For babies and small children, however, remedies made up of granules or powder may be preferable. These dissolve almost instantly and cannot be spat out. Alternatively, pilules can be crushed between two spoons.

The basic homeopathic remedies are easy and safe to take if a person is incapacitated by shock, anxiety, fear, or restlessness; creams, ointments, and solutions are both soothing and non-abrasive when applied to open wounds.

Homeopathic products can be used in conjunction with those of other medicinal therapies, such as herbal tinctures and creams. Aloe vera, for example, is very good for sunburns, while Bach Flower Remedies can be used to treat shock.

BASIC REMEDIES

These remedies for common minor injuries and emergencies make a good basic selection, which can be built up gradually. Dosages are suitable for adults, children, and babies.

- *Aconite 30c*
- *Apis 30c*
- *Arnica 6c, 30c*
- *Bryonia 30c*
- *Cantharis 6c, 30c*
- *Carbo veg. 30c*
- *Euphrasia 6c*
- *Hypericum 30c*
- *Ledum 6c*
- *Nux vomica 6c*
- *Phosphorus 6c*
- *Rhus tox. 6c*
- *Ruta 6c*
- *Silica 6c*
- *Symphytum 6c*
- *Urtica urens 6c*

MOTHER TINCTURES

Tinctures are used in solution for cleaning wounds – usually 10 drops of tincture to 5 cups (1.25 liters) cooled, boiled water. Euphrasia in a saline solution – 1 tsp (5 ml) salt to ¾ cup (150 ml) cooled, boiled water – is used for bathing eyes.

- Arnica
- Calendula
- Euphrasia
- Hypericum

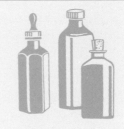

CREAMS & OINTMENTS

Homeopathic creams and ointments protect against infection, soothe pain, and promote healing. Creams are absorbed more quickly and are less greasy than ointments. (Arnica should not be applied to broken skin.)

- Arnica cream
- Calendula cream
- Calendula ointment
- Hypericum ointment
- Urtica ointment

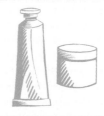

BASIC EQUIPMENT

A first-aid kit should include a variety of sizes and shapes of bandage and adhesive dressing, dressings such as sterile pads and gauze, sterile eye pads, scissors, tweezers, and safety pins.

- Sterile gauze and pads
- Crepe roller bandage
- Butterfly strips
- Triangular bandage
- Adhesive dressings
- Scissors and tweezers
- Safety pins

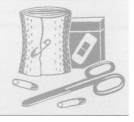

AILMENT	PHYSICAL SYMPTOMS	REMEDY & DOSAGE

MINOR CUTS & SCRAPES

Cuts and scrapes break the skin, allowing blood to get out and infection to get in. Surrounding and underlying tissue may also be torn and bruised.

ESSENTIAL TREATMENT Clean the wound very thoroughly using a sterile pad soaked in a solution of calendula and hypericum (*see page 271*). Apply calendula cream and cover with a sterile dressing. Leave the wound covered for up to three days.

CAUTION If the wound becomes more painful or develops pus, see a doctor.

◆ Cuts and scrapes surrounded by moderate to severe bruising	**Arnica** (*see page 37*) 30c every 2 hours for 6 doses, then 3 times daily up to 3 days
◆ Cuts and scrapes that feel numb and cold but are better from applying cold compresses	**Ledum** (*see page 152*) 6c every 2 hours for 6 doses, then 3 times daily up to 3 days
◆ Damage to the nerve, with shooting pains	**Hypericum** (*see page 148*) 30c every 2 hours up to 3 days

ANIMAL BITES

A bite can result in a puncture wound that produces little blood to wash away foreign bodies or bacteria. If the wound is deep, the tissue beneath may be damaged. Snakebites may have two puncture holes, with inflammation and localized pain. If the snake is poisonous, other parts of the body may be affected. Damage to the nervous system may cause a headache, vomiting, faintness, and breathing difficulties.

ESSENTIAL TREATMENT With all bites except venomous snakebites, hold the wound under running water for at least five minutes. Bathe with a solution of calendula and hypericum (*see page 271*). Pat dry with a sterile pad, cover with a dressing, and go to a hospital. With a venomous snakebite, immobilize the victim immediately and completely, and call an ambulance. Apply a bandage firmly over the bite to compress the site, then bandage the entire limb upward to deter the spread of venom in the body. If the head of a tick is buried in the skin, make sure that its whole body is removed using sterilized tweezers.

CAUTION All bites should be checked by a doctor.

◆ Bite associated with swelling, bruising, or pain	**Arnica** (*see page 37*) 30c every 5 minutes up to 10 doses
◆ Area surrounding the site of a bite has bluish purple appearance	**Lachesis** (*see page 152*) 6c every 8 hours up to 3 days
◆ Site of a bite is hot, red, and swollen	**Crotalus** (*see page 104*) 30c every 15 minutes up to 6 doses

STINGS

Many insect stings cause little more than local problems unless the victim has a severe allergic reaction (anaphylactic shock: *see page 206*). There may be swelling, pain, and – because the skin is broken – infection. In some regions of the world, however, the stings of certain insects, fish, and jellyfish may induce breathing difficulties or a loss of consciousness (*see page 270*), or may even be fatal.

ESSENTIAL TREATMENT Remove a stinger by brushing it off, and bathe the area with calendula solution (*see page 271*) to prevent infection. Do not suck out the poison. If a stinger cannot be removed, apply a paste of baking soda and water to the wound to alkalinize it. If a spine from a marine creature has entered the foot, immerse in water as hot as is bearable for at least 30 minutes to inactivate the venom.

CAUTION If a sting is in the mouth or throat, rinse with ice-cold water to prevent swelling and possible breathing difficulties, and go to a hospital immediately. If a sting produces a severe reaction, call an ambulance immediately.

◆ Sting associated with swelling, bruising, or pain	**Arnica** (*see page 37*) 30c every 5 minutes up to 10 doses
◆ Site of a sting feels cold and numb and is better from cold compresses	**Ledum** (*see page 152*) 6c every 8 hours up to 3 days
◆ Site of a sting is hot, red, and swollen	**Apis** (*see page 104*) 30c every 15 minutes up to 6 doses

AILMENT	PHYSICAL SYMPTOMS	REMEDY & DOSAGE
MINOR BURNS & SCALDS Burns are caused by heat, friction, or chemicals. Scalds are caused by hot liquids. **ESSENTIAL TREATMENT** Avoid touching the wound. For small burns and scalds, hold the affected area under cold, running water for up to ten minutes to reduce pain and swelling, and then leave exposed to the air. For larger burned or scalded areas, cover with plastic wrap or a sterile burn dressing if available (*see page 270*). **CAUTION** If the burned area is larger than the palm of a hand, see a doctor immediately.	◆ Immediate shock of injury	**Arnica** (*see page 37*) 30c every 15 minutes up to 3 doses
	◆ Blistering and searing or stinging pain that is better from the application of cold compresses to the wound	**Cantharis** (*see page 105*) 30c every 15 minutes up to 6 doses
	◆ Burn or scald that continues to sting	**Urtica urens** (*see page 170*) 6c every 15 minutes up to 10 doses
BLISTERS These are bubbles containing the serum from blood. They form beneath the surface of the skin in response to friction, burns, or scalds. **ESSENTIAL TREATMENT** Bathe with a solution of calendula and hypericum (*see page 271*), and then leave exposed to the air. **CAUTION** Never burst a blister. If a blister is larger than 1 in (2.5 cm), consult a doctor.	◆ Blister burns and itches, and is better from applying cold compresses	**Cantharis** (*see page 105*) 6c 4 times daily until pain wears off
	◆ Blister is red, swollen, and extremely itchy	**Rhus tox.** (*see page 162*) 6c 4 times daily until pain wears off
SPRAINS & STRAINS Sprains affect ligaments at a joint, and strains affect muscles. Both are caused by overstretching, which leads to swelling, stiffness, and pain when the joint is used. **ESSENTIAL TREATMENT** Support the injury in the most comfortable, raised position. Apply arnica cream and, if physically possible, bandage the affected part of the body firmly. Keep the injury raised and at rest. If there is swelling, apply cold compresses soaked in arnica solution (*see page 271*) or apply a covered ice pack. **CAUTION** If pain and swelling persist for more than a few hours, see a doctor.	◆ Pain, swelling, and stiffness immediately after the injury	**Arnica** (*see page 37*) 30c half-hourly up to 10 doses
	◆ Pain and stiffness continues	**Ruta** (*see page 163*) 6c 4 times daily until pain and stiffness wear off
BRUISING A bruise is created when the smallest blood vessels – the capillaries – are broken. Blood seeps into the surrounding tissue, but it soon clots and seals the damaged area, thus preventing further leakage. **ESSENTIAL TREATMENT** If the skin is unbroken, apply arnica cream. If the bruise is very painful and swollen, apply a covered ice pack or a cloth soaked in ice-cold water for ten minutes. Never apply an uncovered ice pack directly onto the skin. **CAUTION** If a bruise has not faded after one week, or the amount of bruising is disproportionately large for the injury, or bruising appears for no reason, consult a doctor.	◆ Bruising after damage to surface tissue	**Arnica** (*see page 37*) 30c every 10–15 minutes up to 10 doses
	◆ Bruising deep in a muscle, such as the quadriceps or hamstring, as a result of a sports injury	**Bellis** (*see page 129*) 30c every 10–15 minutes up to 10 doses

AILMENT	PHYSICAL SYMPTOMS	REMEDY & DOSAGE
SPLINTERS Splinters are small pieces of wood or metal that puncture the skin. The main risk is from infection, including tetanus. **ESSENTIAL TREATMENT** If the splinter is protruding, remove it carefully with tweezers. If it is just beneath the skin, sterilize the tip of a needle in a flame, let it cool, then gently lift the skin above the end of the splinter so that you can grasp the end with sterilized tweezers. Apply calendula cream. **CAUTION** If the wound develops pus, see a doctor.	◆ Pain and tenderness remaining after a splinter has been removed, or because tiny fragments of the splinter remain under the skin	**Silica** (*see page 97*) 6c 4 times daily up to 14 days
NOSEBLEEDS A nosebleed is the loss of blood from the membrane lining the inside of the nose, usually occurring only on one side. Nosebleeds are common in childhood, and are usually minor and easily stopped. They may be caused by trauma to the nose or by the weakening of blood vessels as a result of blowing the nose too hard. **ESSENTIAL TREATMENT** Lean over a bowl and pinch the lower part of the nose for at least ten minutes, then gradually release. If the bleeding has not stopped, repeat. **CAUTION** If bleeding has not responded to self-help measures within 20 minutes, or nosebleeds keep recurring, consult a doctor. If the nose bleeds following a head injury, call an ambulance immediately.	◆ Nosebleed following injury	**Arnica** (*see page 37*) 6c every 2 minutes up to 10 doses
	◆ Nosebleed following violent nose blowing	**Phosphorus** (*see page 94*) 6c every 2 minutes up to 10 doses
	◆ Blood is very bright red and nosebleed is accompanied by nausea	**Ipecac.** (*see page 45*) 6c every 2 minutes up to 10 doses
MINOR EYE & EAR INJURIES Both the surface of the eye and the outer ear canal are very delicate and can easily be damaged by injury or the entry of a foreign body. **ESSENTIAL TREATMENT** Gently wash away any dust or grit from an injured eye with cold water. Bathe the eye with a solution of calendula and hypericum (*see page 271*). If there is pain after the removal of a foreign body, bathe the eye with euphrasia solution (*see page 271*) every four hours. If there is a foreign body in the ear, such as a bee or other insect, wash out the ear with a tepid solution of calendula and hypericum. **CAUTION** All eye injuries must be examined by a doctor as soon as possible. If a chemical has entered an eye or there has been a penetrating wound, call an ambulance. If an object is stuck in the ear and does not float out easily when the ear is washed out, see a doctor as soon as possible. Do not insert anything into the ear.	◆ Black eye or bruising around an eye immediately after an injury	**Arnica** (*see page 37*) 6c every 2 hours up to 4 doses
	◆ Black eye with persistent pain that is better from applying cold compresses or an ice pack	**Ledum** (*see page 152*) 6c every 2 hours up to 10 doses
	◆ Persistent pain after removing a foreign body from an eye	**Euphrasia** (*see page 142*) 6c every 2 hours up to 3 doses
	◆ Persistent pain after removing a foreign body from an ear	**Hypericum** (*see page 148*) 30c half-hourly up to 10 doses
	◆ Postoperative pain when a foreign body has been surgically removed from an ear	**Arnica** (*see page 37*) 30c every 4 hours up to 6 doses

AILMENT	PHYSICAL SYMPTOMS	REMEDY & DOSAGE

FAINTING

Fainting is due to the temporary disruption of blood flow to the brain. It may be brought on by pain, hunger, or emotional stress. It should be differentiated from shock, which, particularly if it is caused by internal bleeding, may resemble a faint, especially if there is no obvious loss of blood.

ESSENTIAL TREATMENT A person who has fainted but is breathing normally should be placed in a safe position (*see page 270*) to keep the airway open. To prevent fainting – if there is nausea and unsteadiness, and the complexion is unusually pale – lie down and take deep breaths. Raise the feet to increase blood flow to the brain. Loosen tight clothing, and increase ventilation in the room.

CAUTION If a faint lasts for more than a few minutes, consider the possibility that the fainting might be caused by shock and, if necessary, call an ambulance.

* Fainting due to intense emotion

Ignatia (*see page 57*) 6c every 5 minutes up to 10 doses

* Fainting due to a scare or shock, particularly after witnessing an accident

Aconite (*see page 32*) 30c every 5 minutes up to 10 doses

* Fainting due to overexcitement

Coffea (*see page 50*) 6c every 5 minutes up to 10 doses

* Fainting in hot, stuffy surroundings

Pulsatilla (*see page 61*) 6c every 5 minutes up to 10 doses

* Fainting at the sight of blood

Nux vomica (*see page 63*) 6c every 5 minutes up to 10 doses

MOTION SICKNESS

This ailment occurs when the balance mechanism in the inner ear is upset by motion, especially while reading or focusing on stationary objects. Motion sickness is most common among children.

ESSENTIAL TREATMENT Avoid eating greasy foods and overeating before traveling. To prevent motion sickness, begin taking the appropriate remedy one hour before starting a journey. If there is vomiting, sip water frequently to avoid dehydration. If possible, increase ventilation in the vehicle in which you are traveling.

CAUTION People with insulin-dependent diabetes should be observed for hypoglycemia (*see page 191*) and given glucose or a sugary drink if necessary.

* Nausea and chilliness
* Giddiness and fainting
* Sensation as though there is a tight band around the head
* Worse from tobacco smoke

Tabacum (*see page 158*) 6c every 15 minutes up to 10 doses

* Giddiness and exhaustion with desire to lie down
* Sight of food induces nausea and increased salivation

Cocculus (*see page 124*) 6c every 15 minutes up to 10 doses

* Headache at the back of the eyes or over one eye
* Chilliness and constipation
* Worse from tobacco smoke, eating, and coffee

Nux vomica (*see page 63*) 6c every 15 minutes up to 10 doses

HEAT EXHAUSTION

This occurs in hot and humid climatic conditions and is caused by excessive fluid loss from the body.

ESSENTIAL TREATMENT Lie down in a cool place. If possible, direct the flow of air from an electric fan onto your body or lie beneath a wet sheet to cool down. Sip water or other clear liquids frequently to prevent dehydration.

CAUTION If the body temperature continues to rise, call an ambulance.

* Heat exhaustion accompanied by nausea and a severe headache that is worse with the slightest movement

Bryonia (*see page 42*) 30c every 5 minutes up to 10 doses

* Heat exhaustion accompanied by a throbbing, bursting headache, sweaty skin, and a hot face

Glonoinum (*see page 170*) 30c every 5 minutes up to 10 doses

A–Z QUICK REFERENCE

This quick-reference guide to the 322 remedies described in this book summarizes the possible key benefits of each remedy. It refers you to the appropriate page in the Materia Medica for more detailed information, as well as to other parts of the book where this remedy is recommended. Unlike in the rest of the book, in this guide the entries are arranged in alphabetical order by the commonly used, homeopathic names of the remedies. This will enable you quickly to locate details of the remedies you will find, for example, in a supermarket, pharmacy, or other store.

ABIES CAN.
Abies canadensis

KEY USES
- Digestive disorders associated with inflamed mucous membranes in the stomach and poor absorption of food
- Palpitations caused by nausea, bloating, and severe burning pains in the abdomen

See Materia Medica, *page 118*

ABIES NIG.
Resina piceae

KEY USES
- Indigestion, with a knotted sensation and stomach pains after eating

ABROTANUM
Artemisia abrotanum

KEY USES
- Chest symptoms that develop after skin eruptions have failed to come out
- Emaciation and debilitation of the lower limbs, possibly in children who fail to thrive, or have had polio
- Heart disease following the suppression of rheumatic symptoms
- Mumps that is transferred from the parotid glands to the testes

See Materia Medica, *page 126*

ABSINTHIUM
Artemisia absinthium

KEY USES
- Fits, seizures, and epilepsy in children
- Nervousness in children
- Terrible dreams and insomnia in children
- Trembling, grimacing, and unsteadiness, possibly linked to alcoholism
- Vertigo in children

See Materia Medica, *pages 126–27*

ACETIC AC.
Acidum aceticum

KEY USES
- Breathlessness
- Diabetes
- Fainting
- Hemorrhaging
- Postoperative exhaustion
- Severe burning pains and tenderness in the stomach
- Water retention

See Materia Medica, *pages 118–19*

ACONITE
Aconitum napellus

KEY USES
- Acute respiratory infections
- Eye and ear infections
- Fear, shock, and anxiety
- Problems in labor

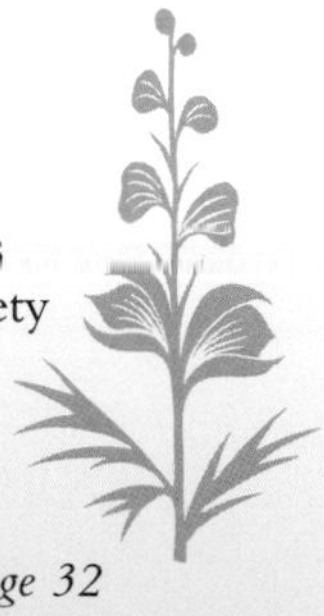

See Materia Medica, *page 32*
See also *pages 183, 186, 187, 196, 211, 212, 213, 218–19, 226–27, 228–29, 238–39, 244–45, 248–49, 250–51, 256–57, 275*

ACTAEA SPIC.
Actaea spicata

KEY USES
- Rheumatoid arthritis with pain that may be severe enough to make the limbs feel paralyzed

See Materia Medica, *page 120*

ADONIS
Adonis vernalis

KEY USES
◆ Asthma
◆ Edema
◆ Headaches
◆ Heart degeneration, perhaps following a severe bout of the flu or rheumatic fever

See Materia Medica, *page 121*

AESCULUS
Aesculus hippocastanum

KEY USES
◆ Dry, rough, burning throat
◆ Hemorrhoids
◆ Varicose veins

See Materia Medica, *page 121*
See also *pages 238–39*

AETHUSA
Aethusa cynapium

KEY USES
◆ Anxiety with associated diarrhea
◆ Confused state of mind with scattered thoughts
◆ Marked dullness and sluggish mental state
◆ Milk intolerance in children

See Materia Medica, *page 121*

AGARICUS
Agaricus muscarius

KEY USES
◆ Alcoholism
◆ Chilblains (cold sensitivity)
◆ Chorea
◆ Nervous system disorders
◆ Parkinson's disease

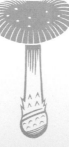

See Materia Medica, *page 33*
See also *pages 179, 186, 220–21, 230–31*

AGNUS CASTUS
Vitex agnus-castus

KEY USES
◆ Fatigue
◆ Impotence
◆ Loss of libido
◆ Postnatal depression
◆ Premature ejaculation

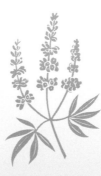

See Materia Medica, *page 173*
See also *pages 203, 264–65*

AGRAPHIS
Agraphis nutans

KEY USES
◆ Ear, nose, and throat infections linked to phlegm and deafness, chills that develop after exposure to cold winds, and swelling of the adenoids and tonsils

See Materia Medica, *page 122*

AILANTHUS
Ailanthus altissima

KEY USES
◆ Fevers with great weakness and congestion of the blood
◆ Infectious mononucleosis, with swollen tonsils and neck glands

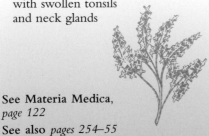

See Materia Medica, *page 122*
See also *pages 254–55*

ALFALFA
Medicago sativa

KEY USES
◆ Anorexia
◆ Cancer
◆ Chronic fatigue syndrome
◆ Insomnia
◆ Malnutrition and weight loss
◆ Nervous indigestion

See Materia Medica, *page 154*

ALLIUM CEPA
Allium cepa

KEY USES
◆ Allergies
◆ Eye irritation
◆ Hay fever and allergic rhinitis
◆ Neuralgic pains
◆ Phlegm
◆ Throat and chest infections

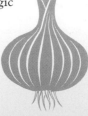

See Materia Medica, *page 34*
See also *pages 207, 224–25*

ALLIUM SAT.
Allium sativum

KEY USES
- Indigestion caused by a rich diet or by dietary change
- Tearing pains in the hip area and abdomen

See Materia Medica, *page 122*

ALOE
Aloe ferox 'Miller'

KEY USES
- Diarrhea
- Headaches
- Hemorrhoids
- Hepatitis

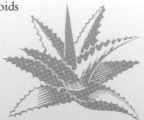

See Materia Medica, *page 35*
See also *pages 238–39*

ALUMEN
Aluminum potassium sulfuricum

KEY USES
- Bleeding hemorrhoids
- Bowel problems, especially in the elderly
- Deep anal aches
- Dysentery and bloody diarrhea
- Painful ulceration in the rectum
- Paralytic, sluggish muscle weakness
- Severe constipation, possibly due to uterine or rectal cancer

See Materia Medica, *page 123*

ALUMINA
Aluminum oxydatum

KEY USES
- Appetite disorders
- Constipation
- Dementia
- Fatigue
- Nervous disorders

See Materia Medica, *page 72*
See also *pages 238–39*

AMBROSIA
Ambrosia artemisiaefolia

KEY USES
- Hay fever, possibly involving eyes that water, smart, burn, and itch, a congested nose and head, watery phlegm, sneezing, nosebleeds, wheezy coughs, asthmatic irritations, or whooping cough, with diarrhea

See Materia Medica, *page 123*

AMMONIUM BROM.
Ammonium bromatum

KEY USES
- Coughs
- Epilepsy
- Neuralgic headaches
- Ovarian problems
- Sore eyes

See Materia Medica, *page 123*

AMMONIUM CARB.
Ammonium carbonicum

KEY USES
- Fatigue
- Poor circulation
- Respiratory illnesses
- Scarlet fever
- Skin conditions

See Materia Medica, *page 73*

AMMONIUM MUR.
Ammonium chloratum

KEY USES
- Enlarged glands
- Inflammatory eye conditions
- Liver complaints
- Menstrual disorders
- Respiratory disorders, such as a congested nose, sneezing, reduced sense of smell, sore throat, hoarseness, and thick, slimy mucus
- Sciatica and joint pains

See Materia Medica, *page 123*
See also pages 218–19

AMYL NIT.
Amylium nitrosum

KEY USES
- Heart symptoms, such as chest pains and feelings of oppression
- Hot flushes in conjunction with sunstroke, heart problems, or menopause

See Materia Medica, *page 124*

ANACARDIUM OCC.
Anacardium occidentale

KEY USES
- Exam nerves and phobias
- Leprosy
- Muscle complaints
- Skin eruptions
- Warts

See Materia Medica, *page 124*
See also *pages 254–55*

ANACARDIUM OR.
Anacardium orientale

KEY USES
- Chest pains
- Digestive disorders
- Low self-esteem
- Psychological problems
- Skin conditions

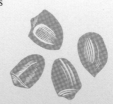

See Materia Medica, *page 36*

ANANTHERUM
Vetiveria zizianoides

KEY USES
- Hard, glandular swellings, especially in the neck
- Itchy skin eruptions, notably on the scalp and eyebrows
- Neuralgic headaches
- Skin disorders

See Materia Medica, *page 172*

ANGUSTURA
Galipea officinalis

KEY USES
- Nervous system disorders
- Rheumatic conditions

See Materia Medica, *page 144*

ANHALONIUM
Anhalonium lewinii

KEY USES
- Hallucinations with blurred or multi-colored vision disturbances
- Lack of coordination, possibly with muscle tremors, nausea, faintness, giddiness, and neuralgic pains and facial paralysis
- Mental exhaustion
- Migraines and other headaches

See Materia Medica, *page 124*

ANTIMONIUM CRUD.
Stibium sulfuratum nigrum

KEY USES
- Digestive disorders
- Gout
- Skin and nail conditions
- Skin infections with a rash
- Toothaches

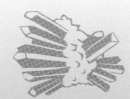

See Materia Medica, *page 98*

ANTIMONIUM TART.
Tartarus stibiatus

KEY USES
- Chicken pox
- Headaches
- Nausea
- Respiratory illnesses
- Skin conditions
- Whooping cough

See Materia Medica, *page 100*
See also *page 181*

APIS
Apis mellifica

KEY USES
- Bites and stings
- Cystitis
- Edema
- Fever
- Inflammation of the eyes, lips, mouth, or throat
- Urticaria

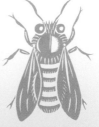

See Materia Medica, *page 104*
See also *pages 185, 186, 196, 202, 207, 242–43*

APOCYNUM
Apocynum cannabinum

KEY USES
- Edema associated with diseased organs, and possibly linked with Hodgkin's lymphoma or Bright's disease

See Materia Medica, *page 124*

ARANEA DIADEMA
Araneus diadematus

KEY USES
- Nervous system disorders accompanied by coldness, susceptibility to damp, and numbness

See Materia Medica, *page 125*

ARGENTUM MET.
Argentum metallicum

KEY USES
- Arthritis
- Bleeding between menstrual periods or heavy menopausal hemorrhaging
- Joint and bone disorders associated with the connective tissues, especially the cartilage
- Men's reproductive system disorders
- Ovarian pain, possibly due to cysts or tumors

See Materia Medica, *pages 125–26*

ARGENTUM NIT.
Argentum nitricum

KEY USES
- Anxiety and phobias
- Digestive problems
- Irritable bowel syndrome
- Multiple sclerosis
- Nervous disorders

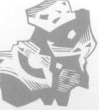

See Materia Medica, *page 74*
See also *pages 179, 185, 186, 189, 191, 202, 211, 238–39, 254–55*

ARNICA
Arnica montana

KEY USES
- Fever
- Joint and muscle pains
- Postpartum pain
- Shock, injury, and postoperative care
- Skin conditions
- Tooth and gum pains

See Materia Medica, *page 37*
See also *pages 185, 187, 201, 213, 230–31, 264–65, 266–67, 271*

ARSEN. ALB.
Acidum arsenicosum

KEY USES
- Digestive disorders
- Eye inflammation
- Food poisoning
- Headaches
- Respiratory illnesses

See Materia Medica, *page 68*
See also *pages 181, 182, 183, 185, 189, 190, 193, 194, 195, 200, 205, 207, 209, 212, 232–33, 236–37, 238–39, 240–41, 242–43, 244–45, 248–49, 268–69*

ARSEN. IOD.
Arsenicum iodatum

KEY USES
- Asthma
- Flu
- Hay fever

See Materia Medica, *page 126*
See also *pages 224–25*

ARTEMISIA
Artemisia vulgaris

KEY USES
- Chorea
- Convulsions and seizures, including petit mal in children
- Epilepsy
- Nervous disorders triggered by bad news, grief, or a blow to the head
- Sleepwalking

See Materia Medica, *page 127*

ARUM MAC.
Arum maculatum

KEY USES
- Asthma
- Respiratory tract problems, such as asthma, profuse phlegm, violent cough, and nasal polyps

See Materia Medica, *page 127*

ARUM TRIPH.
Arisaema triphyllum

KEY USES
- Allergic skin reactions
- Eczema
- Hay fever
- Scarlet fever

See Materia Medica, *page 126*
See also *page 207*

ARUNDO
Arundo mauritanica

KEY USES
- Allergies, especially hay fever, phlegmy inflammation, and extreme itching inside the nose
- Blepharitis
- Wet coughs with breathlessness

See Materia Medica, *page 127*
See also *page 207*

ASAFETIDA
Ferula assa-foetida

KEY USES
- Digestive disorders
- Nervous twitching

See Materia Medica, *page 143*

ASARUM
Asarum europaeum

KEY USES
- Alcoholism
- Aversion to sexual intercourse
- Digestive problems, possibly associated with anorexia
- Nervous hypersensitivity and edgy, hysterical behavior
- Severe insomnia

See Materia Medica, *page 127*

ASCLEPIAS TUB.
Asclepias tuberosa

KEY USES
- Phlegm
- Respiratory inflammation, such as bronchitis, the flu, pleurisy, or other feverish conditions with a painful, dry, hacking cough
- Rheumatic pains in the muscles and joints

See Materia Medica, *page 128*

ASTACUS
Astacus fluviatilis

KEY USES
- Enlarged and inflamed glands, especially in children and the elderly
- Inflammation in the liver area
- Urticaria, particularly if the rash is accompanied by cramps and pain

See Materia Medica, *page 128*

ASTERIAS
Asterias rubens

KEY USES
- Circulatory disorders, such as strokes
- Hard, swollen glands in the armpits
- High libido in women, causing restless sleep, erotic dreams, bad temper, and weepiness
- Left-sided symptoms, especially in women
- Obstinate constipation, especially during menopause
- Sharp breast pains at night

See Materia Medica, *page 128*

AURUM MET.
Aurum metallicum

KEY USES
- Angina
- Bone pains
- Depression
- Headaches
- Reproductive system problems

See Materia Medica, *page 75*
See also *pages 185, 186 187, 197, 203, 211, 212, 213*

AURUM MUR.
Aurum chloratum

KEY USES
- Cancer
- Edema, with a feeling of congestion in the liver, kidneys, and genitals
- Fibroids
- Heart conditions, such as palpitations and a sense of constriction in the chest

See Materia Medica, *page 128*
See also *pages 199, 209*

AVENA
Avena sativa

KEY USES
- Chronic insomnia
- Great weakness
- Low libido
- Male impotence, possibly linked with excessive sexual activity
- Nervous exhaustion

See Materia Medica, *page 129*

BACILLINUM
Bacillinum pulmo

KEY USES
- Respiratory problems, such as weak lungs, involving shortness of breath, hacking coughs, purulent mucus, asthma, and sharp pains in the heart area
- Skin conditions, such as eczema, pimples, ringworm, alopecia areata, and a susceptibility to fungal skin infections
- Tuberculosis and pneumonia

See Materia Medica, *page 129*
See also *pages 182, 183*

BADIAGA
Spongilla fluviatilis

KEY USES
- Hard, swollen glands in the neck and breasts
- Profuse mucus in the respiratory system, with copious phlegm, possibly due to the flu or hay fever
- Sneezing brought on by coughing

See Materia Medica, *page 167*

BAPTISIA
Baptisia tinctoria

KEY USES
- Acute fever
- Intestinal infections
- Septic conditions
- Throat infections

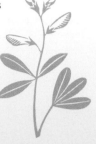

See Materia Medica, *page 40*

BARYTA CARB.
Barium carbonicum

KEY USES
- Anxiety and phobias
- Growth disorders in children
- Impotence
- Problems of the elderly
- Respiratory illnesses
- Swollen tonsils

See Materia Medica, *page 76*
See also *pages 187, 202, 266–67*

BARYTA MUR.
Barium chloratum

KEY USES
- Acutely swollen glands
- Mental disability in children with delayed development
- Nervous system disorders, such as seizures
- Retardation in elderly people
- Severe eczema
- Strokes

See Materia Medica, *page 129*
See also *page 194*

BELLADONNA
Atropa belladonna

KEY USES
- Acute fever and pain
- Headaches and migraines
- Menstrual pain
- Sore throat and dry cough

See Materia Medica, *page 39*
See also *pages 193, 196, 201, 205, 222–23, 224–25, 232–33, 240–41, 246–47, 248–49, 250–51, 252–53, 262–63*

BELLIS
Bellis perennis

KEY USES
- Muscle strain, sprains, and bruises
- Pain during pregnancy or after miscarriage or surgery
- Prolonged pain after injury
- Tumors on the sites of old injuries
- Varicose veins and congestion of the veins

See Materia Medica, *page 129*
See also *page 273*

BENZOIC AC.
Acidum benzoicum

KEY USES
- Cracking or swollen joints, possibly linked to gout
- Frothy, white stools
- Strong-smelling urine and incontinence at night
- Wandering pains

See Materia Medica, *page 119*

BERBERIS
Berberis vulgaris

KEY USES
- Cystitis
- Gallbladder problems
- Joint pains
- Kidney disorders
- Lower-back pains

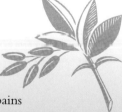

See Materia Medica, *page 41*

BISMUTH MET.
Bismuthum metallicum

KEY USES
◆ Violent abdominal pains, possibly with burning and ulceration in the stomach, bowels, and throat, accompanied by burping and flatulence

See Materia Medica, *page 130*

BORAX
Natrum tetraboracicum

KEY USES
◆ Cold sores on the lips
◆ Painful ulcers in the mouth or on the tongue
◆ Ulceration in the gastrointestinal tract

See Materia Medica, *page 157*
See also *page 211*

BORIC AC.
Acidum boricum

KEY USES
◆ Dizziness
◆ Eyes that are prone to swelling and conjunctivitis
◆ Headaches accompanied by nausea
◆ Heavy, nauseous feeling in the stomach
◆ Putrefying wounds
◆ Skin eruptions

See Materia Medica, *page 119*

BOTHROPS
Bothrops lanceolatus

KEY USES
◆ Bruising
◆ Hemorrhaging of thin blood that will not clot
◆ Severe premenstrual syndrome

See Materia Medica, *page 130*

BROMUM
Bromum

KEY USES
◆ Disorders of the thyroid, ovaries, or left testicle
◆ Respiratory problems such as colds

See Materia Medica, *page 130*
See also *page 209*

BRYONIA
Bryonia alba

KEY USES
◆ Breast problems
◆ Colds and flu
◆ Constipation
◆ Dry cough
◆ Headaches
◆ Joint pains

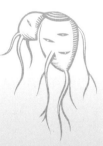

See Materia Medica, *page 42*
See also *pages 183, 196, 197, 201, 228–29, 238–39, 252–53, 258–59, 275*

BUFO
Bufo bufo

KEY USES
◆ Extremely high sex drive, with frequent masturbation, poorly developed sexual relationships, and sexual depravity
◆ Seizures
◆ Skin problems, such as blisters and itching, burning pustules

See Materia Medica, *pages 130–31*

CACTUS GRAND.
Selenicereus grandiflorus

KEY USES
◆ Constriction of the muscle fibers
◆ Heart conditions, especially pain triggered by angina
◆ Painful feeling of the body being caged and twisted

See Materia Medica, *page 165*
See also *page 185*

CADMIUM MET.
Cadmium metallicum

KEY USES
◆ Colitis
◆ Constipation
◆ Great fatigue
◆ Hemorrhoids
◆ Hernias in the diaphragm
◆ Painful abdominal bloating

See Materia Medica, *page 131*

CADMIUM SULF.
Cadmium sulfuricum

KEY USES
- Stomach problems accompanied by sharp, cutting abdominal pains, severe nausea, and vomiting

See Materia Medica, *page 131*
See also *page 212*

CALADIUM
Caladium seguinum

KEY USES
- Debilitation, forgetfulness, nervousness, and restlessness, perhaps following a feverish illness

See Materia Medica, *page 131*

CALC. CARB.
Calcium carbonicum Hahnemanni

KEY USES
- Anxiety and phobias
- Bone, joint, and dental problems
- Digestive disorders
- Headaches
- Women's health

See Materia Medica, *page 77*
See also *pages 181, 182, 183, 186, 194, 196, 199, 201, 202, 205, 207, 211, 212, 250–51, 254–55, 256–57, 258–59, 260–61, 262–63*

CALC. FLUOR.
Calcium fluoratum

KEY USES
- Bone malnutrition and deformity
- Brittle teeth
- Enlarged or varicose veins
- Hard lumps that develop on the skull and jaw
- Swollen, inflamed joints
- Tumors and growths

See Materia Medica, *pages 131–32*
See also *page 209*

CALC. IOD.
Calcium iodatum

KEY USES
- Adenoid complaints
- Enlarged tonsils
- Fibroids
- Thyroid enlargement during puberty

See Materia Medica, *page 132*
See also *page 199*

CALC. PHOS.
Calcium phosphoricum

KEY USES
- Bone and joint conditions
- Digestive disorders
- Fatigue
- Growth disorders
- Head pains
- Teething

See Materia Medica, *page 78*
See also *pages 193, 197, 201, 211*

CALC. SIL.
Calcium silicatum

KEY USES
- Boils, warts, or abscesses
- Lack of confidence
- Severe acne or acne rosacea

See Materia Medica, *page 132*

CALC. SULF.
Calcium sulfuricum

KEY USES
- Mucous membrane discharges, especially thick, yellow-colored phlegm or lumpy mucus with a cough
- Suppurating, yellow discharges of pus affecting wounds and other skin conditions, such as eczema, as well as the glands and bones

See Materia Medica, *page 132*

CALENDULA
Calendula officinalis

KEY USES
- Bleeding in the gums after a tooth extraction
- Cuts and broken skin
- Eczema
- Leg and varicose ulcers
- Postoperative wounds
- Ruptured muscles or tendons
- Torn perineal tissues following childbirth

See Materia Medica, *page 132*

CAMPHORA
Cinnamomum camphora

KEY USES
- Cholera
- Colds with chills and sneezing

See Materia Medica, *pages 136–37*

CANNABIS IND.
Cannabis sativa 'Indica'

KEY USES
- Disordered mental state
- Headaches
- Pain or paralysis in the legs
- Urinary tract infections

See Materia Medica, *page 43*
See also *pages 266–67*

CANNABIS SAT.
Cannabis sativa

KEY USES
- Reproductive system disorders, such as discharges from or narrowing of the urethra, inflammation of the penis, or acute gonorrhea
- Urinary tract disorders, such as infections and cystitis

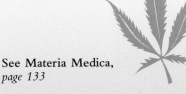

See Materia Medica, *page 133*

CANTHARIS
Cantharis vesicatoria

KEY USES
- Blisters
- Burns and scalds
- Excessive libido
- Gastritis, diarrhea, and dysentery
- Insect bites and stings
- Irritable bowel syndrome
- Severe cystitis
- Ulcerative colitis

See Materia Medica, *page 105*
See also *pages 189, 190, 260–61, 273*

CAPSICUM
Capsicum annuum var. *annuum*

KEY USES
- Infections that tend to suppurate
- Low vitality, perhaps in the elderly or those debilitated by alcoholism or prostate conditions
- Raw, burning throat

See Materia Medica, *page 133*
See also *page 202*

CARBO AN.
Carbo animalis

KEY USES
- Cancer
- Great fatigue
- Poor circulation with blue extremities
- Swollen, painful veins

See Materia Medica, *page 133*
See also *page 209*

CARBO VEG.
Carbo vegetabilis

KEY USES
- Breathing problems
- Chronic fatigue syndrome
- Fatigue
- Indigestion and flatulence
- Poor circulation

See Materia Medica, *page 44*
See also *pages 189, 193, 200, 205, 234–35, 236–37*

CARBOLIC AC.
Acidum carbolicum

KEY USES
- Constipation with foul breath
- Diarrhea, dysentery, or cholera
- Increased urine production
- Malignant or septic wounds
- Sudden burning, prickling, stinging pains and collapse, for example due to anaphylactic shock after a bee sting
- Vomiting due to sea sickness, pregnancy, or cancer

See Materia Medica, *page 119*

CARBON SULF.
Carbonium sulfuratum

KEY USES
- Chronic sciatic pain and twitching
- Digestive upsets
- Loss of sensation
- Progressive loss of vision
- Recurrent breathing difficulties
- Skin irritation
- Tinnitus

See Materia Medica, *page 134*
See also *pages 222–23*

CARCINOSIN
Carcinosinum

KEY USES
- Abdominal pains
- Chronic fatigue syndrome
- Insomnia
- Respiratory illnesses
- Skin growths and blemishes

See Materia Medica, *page 106*
See also *page 207*

CARDUUS
Silybum marianum

KEY USES
- Acute or chronic liver problems
- Gallbladder pains
- Gallstone colic
- Lung conditions, such as asthma
- Severe abdominal and liver pains

See Materia Medica, *page 166*

CASTOREUM
Castoreum

KEY USES
- Chronic fatigue syndrome in women
- Nervousness in conjunction with profuse sweating
- Sudden spasms of abdominal pain

See Materia Medica, *page 134*

CAULOPHYLLUM
Caulophyllum thalictroides

KEY USES
- Rheumatic pains affecting the small joints, particularly in conjunction with menstruation or uterine problems
- Uterine disorders, such as excessive bleeding and lack of uterine muscle tone

See Materia Medica, *page 134*

CAUSTICUM
Causticum Hahnemanni

KEY USES
- Cough
- Multiple sclerosis
- Skin conditions
- Sore throat and laryngitis
- Tremors and paralysis
- Urinary disorders

See Materia Medica, *page 79*
See also *pages 179, 196, 197, 201, 203, 205, 212, 213, 228–29, 242–43, 248–49, 266–67, 268–69*

CEANOTHUS
Ceanothus americanus

KEY USES
- Lethargy with swelling, tenderness, and pain in the spleen
- Nervous excitement with chilliness
- Serious blood or lymph disorders, such as leukemia or Hodgkin's disease

See Materia Medica, *page 134*

CEDRON
Simarouba cedron

KEY USES
- Neuralgic pains and other nervous system conditions, such as spasms or tics
- Recurrent fevers, such as those associated with malaria
- Severe headaches or migraines

See Materia Medica, *page 166*

CENCHRIS
Agkistrodon contortrix

KEY USES
- Breathlessness
- Congestion in the blood vessels
- Fear of rape, pins and pointed objects, going to sleep, and sudden death
- Mental and physical restlessness

See Materia Medica, *page 122*

CHAMOMILLA
Chamomilla recutita

KEY USES
- Colic and diarrhea
- Fever
- Irritability
- Menstrual and labor pains
- Toothaches, teething, and earaches

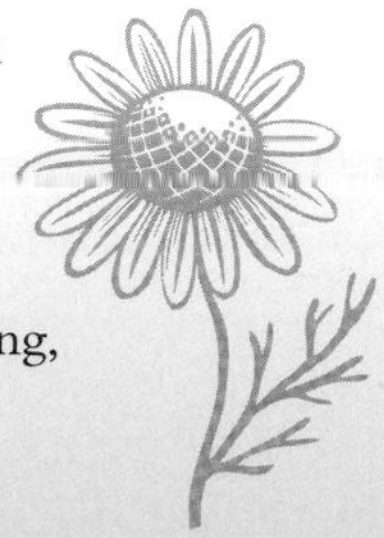

See Materia Medica, *page 46*
See also *pages 232–33, 246–47, 248–49, 262–63*

CHELIDONIUM
Chelidonium majus

KEY USES
- Gallstones
- Headaches
- Hepatitis
- Pneumonia
- Shoulder pains

See Materia Medica, *page 47*

CHENOPODIUM
Chenopodium ambrosioides var. anthelminticum

KEY USES
- Effects of strokes, particularly those involving right-sided paralysis
- Right-sided migraines

See Materia Medica, *page 135*

CHIMAPHILA
Chimaphila umbellata

KEY USES
- Men's complaints, such as enlarged prostate, urine retention, and a feeling that there is a ball in the pelvis
- Urinary tract disorders, such as painful urination, obstructed urine flow, and cystitis with blood in the urine

See Materia Medica, *page 135*
See also *page 202*

CHINA
Cinchona officinalis

KEY USES
- Digestive disorders
- Exhaustion caused by illness
- Fever and headaches
- Insomnia

See Materia Medica, *page 49*
See also *pages 186, 189, 205, 212, 258–59*

CHINA ARS.
Chininum arsenicosum

KEY USES
- Asthma, with a sensation of suffocation, oppressed breathing, or anxiety
- Great fatigue, perhaps following chronic fatigue syndrome, or a serious illness, such as malaria, or a debilitating epileptic attack

See Materia Medica, *page 135*

CHINA SULF.
Chininum sulfuricum

KEY USES
- Heavy, aching limbs
- Joint pains
- Recurrent fever, possibly due to malaria
- Severe head pain
- Sinking sensations when lying down
- Tender, sensitive spine
- Tinnitus

See Materia Medica, *page 136*
See also *pages 222–23*

CHIONANTHUS
Chionanthus virginicus

KEY USES
- Biliary colic
- Gallstones
- Headaches, especially those associated with nervous tension or menstruation, or accompanied by digestive upsets
- Jaundice
- Liver pains accompanied by colic, cramps, vomiting, and intestinal discomfort

See Materia Medica, *page 136*

CHOCOLATE
Chocolatum

KEY USES
- Fear of cars, accidents, illness, dogs, or being attacked
- Feelings of estrangement
- Great clumsiness and heaviness in the limbs, and constriction in the chest or head associated with nervous disorders
- Withdrawal and antisocial behavior

See Materia Medica, *page 136*

CICUTA
Cicuta virosa

KEY USES
- Nervous system problems, such as stammering, hiccups, sudden strong jerks or spasms
- Petit mal fits, epilepsy, or violent convulsions
- Skin disorders, often involving pustules that leave yellowish scabs, such as impetigo or eczema

See Materia Medica, *page 136*
See also *page 194*

CIMEX
Acanthia lectularia

KEY USES
- Anxiety, especially after a chill or drinking alcohol, and possibly followed by a fever
- Joint or muscle aches

See Materia Medica, *page 118*

CIMICIFUGA
Cimicifuga racemosa

KEY USES
- Depression
- Head and neck pains
- Menopause
- Menstrual problems
- Pregnancy

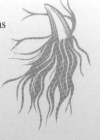

See Materia Medica, *page 48*

CINA
Artemisia cina

KEY USES
- Coughs and colds
- Intestinal worms
- Sleep problems
- Temper tantrums
- Twitching muscles

See Materia Medica, *page 38*
See also *pages 246–47*

CINNABARIS
Hydrargyrum sulfuratum rubrum

KEY USES
- Genital and rectal ulceration and warts
- Headaches, inflamed eyes, phlegm, and sore throat
- Painful menstruation, pregnancy, or labor
- Pimples, pustules, and skin eruptions
- Women's problems

See Materia Medica, *page 147*

CISTUS
Cistus canadensis

KEY USES
- Allergic rhinitis
- Chronic or recurrent sinusitis
- Frequent colds
- Glandular swelling and hardening, especially in the neck
- Tonsillitis
- Upper respiratory tract infections

See Materia Medica, *page 137*

CLEMATIS
Clematis recta

KEY USES
- Abnormal urine flow
- Moist, itchy pustules on the back of the head or skull
- Skin complaints
- Swollen glands, especially of prostate, testes, ovaries, or breasts
- Urethral inflammation

See Materia Medica, *page 137*

COCA
Erythroxylum coca

KEY USES
- Altitude sickness
- Breathlessness or asthma

See Materia Medica, *page 142*

COCCULUS
Anamirta cocculus

KEY USES
- Agitation
- Hypersensitivity to touch
- Muscle weakness, spasms in the legs, and gradual paralysis
- Sea and motion sickness, nausea, and vomiting
- Vertigo and dizziness

See Materia Medica, *page 124*
See also *page 275*

COCCUS CACTI
Dactylopius coccus

KEY USES
- Asthma
- Spasmodic coughing, especially whooping cough
- Urinary problems with pains in the kidneys

See Materia Medica, *page 140*

COFFEA
Coffea cruda

KEY USES
- Headaches
- Hot flushes during menopause
- Insomnia
- Overexcitement
- Palpitations
- Toothaches

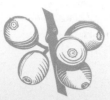

See Materia Medica, *page 50*
See also *pages 232–33, 244–45, 248–49, 262–63, 275*

COLCHICUM
Colchicum autumnale

KEY USES
- Illness accompanied by icy cold feeling in the stomach
- Muscle tissue disorders
- Nausea with colicky pains and painful distension of the abdomen
- Oversensitivity to external stimuli
- Problems with joint membranes, especially in the small joints
- Rheumatoid arthritis
- Ulcerative colitis

See Materia Medica, *page 137*
See also *pages 190, 197*

COLLINSONIA
Collinsonia canadensis

KEY USES
- Hemorrhoids
- Labor or pregnancy problems, such as itchy vulva during pregnancy, or diarrhea after labor
- Menstrual pain
- Pelvic aches

See Materia Medica, *page 137*

COLOCYNTHIS
Cucumis colocynthis

KEY USES
- Colic
- Diarrhea
- Facial neuralgia
- Menstrual problems
- Neuralgic pains

See Materia Medica, *page 52*
See also *pages 189, 190, 218–19, 236–37, 246–47*

COMOCLADIA
Comocladia dentata

KEY USES
- Nerve sensitivity
- Skin problems, such as extreme itching, burning, inflammation, and blistering

See Materia Medica, *page 138*

CONIUM
Conium maculatum

KEY USES
- Cysts, tumors, and cancer
- Enlarged prostate
- Nervous disorders
- Sexual problems
- Swollen breasts

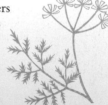

See Materia Medica, *page 51*
See also *pages 186, 201, 202, 203, 209, 258–59*

CONVALLARIA
Convallaria majalis

KEY USES
- Heart disorders with symptoms that include fluttery or noisy heartbeat, palpitations, poor circulation, and water retention
- Soreness of the uterus in conjunction with heart palpitations

See Materia Medica, *page 138*

COPAIVA
Copaifera officinalis

KEY USES
- Chronic bronchitis
- Colds
- Gonorrhea
- Leucorrhea
- Urethritis

See Materia Medica, *page 138*

CORALLIUM
Corallium rubrum

KEY USES
- Whooping and spasmodic coughs, accompanied by violent paroxysms, exhaustion, a smothering sensation, and the bringing up of blood

See Materia Medica, *pages 138–39*

CRATAEGUS
Crataegus laevigata

KEY USES
- Fast, feeble, and intermittent pulse
- Palpitations, possibly accompanied by fainting and collapse
- Rapid heartbeat
- Weak heart

See Materia Medica, *page 139*

CROCUS
Crocus sativus

KEY USES
- Hemorrhaging, such as nosebleeds or uterine bleeding
- Nervous excitement, with rapidly alternating moods and hysterical behavior

See Materia Medica, *page 139*

CROTALUS
Crotalus horridus horridus

KEY USES
- Bleeding
- Cancer
- Delirium
- Heart disorders
- Strokes
- Throat infections

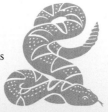

See Materia Medica, *page 107*
See also *page 209*

CROTALUS CASC.
Crotalus durissus terrificus

KEY USES
- Sensations of constriction, which is sometimes felt as a band around the throat or abdomen

See Materia Medica, *page 139*

CROTON
Croton tiglium

KEY USES
- Allergic skin conditions with extreme itching, such as eczema on the scrotum, or blistering rashes on the scrotum and penis
- Digestive problems, such as nausea and urgent diarrhea immediately after eating or drinking
- Headaches

See Materia Medica, *page 139*

CUBEBA
Piper cubeba

KEY USES
- Cystitis
- Gonorrhea
- Mucous membrane inflammation, particularly in the urinary tract
- Prostatitis

See Materia Medica, *page 160*

CUPRUM ARS.
Cuprum arsenicosum

KEY USES
- Irregular or weak heart function
- Poor kidney function
- Prolonged fluid loss, for example after injury or an operation

See Materia Medica, *page 140*

CUPRUM MET.
Cuprum metallicum

KEY USES
- Abdominal cramps
- Asthma
- Convulsions and epilepsy
- Coughs
- Exhaustion

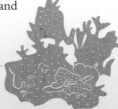

See Materia Medica, *page 80*
See also *pages 230–31*

CURARE
Strychnos toxifera

KEY USES
- Heaviness
- Numbness
- Physical weakness
- Piercing pains
- Progressive muscular paralysis and impaired reflex action

See Materia Medica, *page 168*

CYCLAMEN
Cyclamen europaeum

KEY USES
- Extreme indigestion that is aggravated by eating fats
- Menstrual problems

See Materia Medica, *page 140*

DIGITALIS
Digitalis purpurea

KEY USES
- Heart and circulatory disorders
- Liver problems, particularly in conjunction with heart problems

See Materia Medica, *pages 140–41*
See also *page 186*

DIOSCOREA
Dioscorea villosa

KEY USES
- Neuralgic and colicky pains, especially in the gastrointestinal system
- Renal colic, in men, associated with kidney stones, sharp pains radiating down the testicles and legs, and cold, clammy perspiration

See Materia Medica, *page 141*

DROSERA
Drosera rotundifolia

KEY USES
- Behavioral problems, especially in children
- Deep, violent, spasmodic coughs, especially whooping cough
- Growing pains in children, such as stiff ankles and pains in the joints and bones

See Materia Medica, *page 141*
See also *pages 250–51*

DULCAMARA
Solanum dulcamara

KEY USES
- Colds and coughs
- Diarrhea
- Hay fever and asthma
- Head and facial pains
- Joint pains
- Skin conditions

See Materia Medica, *page 62*
See also *pages 194, 226–27*

ECHINACEA
Echinacea angustifolia

KEY USES
- Abscesses, boils, and carbuncles
- Animal and insect bites and stings
- Cancer
- Diphtheria
- Fatigue
- Septicemia
- Swollen glands

See Materia Medica, *page 141*

ELAPS
Micrurus corallinus

KEY USES
- Hemorrhaging or other discharges characterized by black blood
- Right-sided paralysis after a stroke

See Materia Medica, *page 155*

EQUISETUM
Equisetum hyemale

KEY USES
- Bed-wetting in children during nightmares or other dreams
- Painful irritation of the bladder

See Materia Medica, *page 142*
See also *pages 248–49*

EUPATORIUM PER.
Eupatorium perfoliatum

KEY USES
- Flu or malarial fever accompanied by pains in the limbs

See Materia Medica, *page 142*

EUPHORBIUM
Euphorbia resinifera 'Berger'

KEY USES
◆ Burning pains in the bones, with a weak and dislocated feeling in the limbs, and sharp, cramping pains and weakness in the joints
◆ Itching, burning skin, possibly with warts, slow-healing ulcers, or yellow blistering as a result of erysipelas

See Materia Medica, *page 142*

EUPHRASIA
Euphrasia officinalis

KEY USES
◆ Colds
◆ Conjunctivitis
◆ Eye problems after an injury
◆ Hay fever
◆ Irritation in the eyes, with a heightened sensitivity to light

See Materia Medica, *pages 142–43*
See also *pages 220–21, 224–25*

FAGOPYRUM
Fagopyrum esculentum

KEY USES
◆ Eczema and itching skin
◆ Heart complaints associated with visibly pulsing arteries

See Materia Medica, *page 143*

FERRUM MET.
Ferrum metallicum

KEY USES
◆ Anemia
◆ Back and joint pains
◆ Circulatory problems
◆ Digestive disorders
◆ Headaches
◆ Severe fatigue

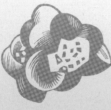

See Materia Medica, *page 81*

FERRUM PHOS.
Ferrum phosphoricum

KEY USES
◆ Colds
◆ Digestive disorders
◆ Earaches
◆ Fever
◆ Poor circulation
◆ Raynaud's disease
◆ Respiratory illnesses
◆ Urogenital problems

See Materia Medica, *page 82*
See also *pages 224–25*

FLUORIC AC.
Acidum hydrofluoricum

KEY USES
◆ Alopecia
◆ Bone conditions
◆ Discharges from the ears and nose
◆ Nail conditions
◆ Sexual problems
◆ Tooth decay
◆ Varicose veins

See Materia Medica, *page 69*
See also *page 209*

FRAXINUS
Fraxinus americana

KEY USES
◆ Fibroids and other tumors
◆ Heavy, painful menstruation
◆ Uterine problems, such as a uterus that is relaxed in tone or prolapsed

See Materia Medica, *page 143*
See also *page 199*

GELSEMIUM
Gelsemium sempervirens

KEY USES
◆ Acute bouts of flu or sore throat
◆ Hay fever
◆ Mental and physical paralysis linked with phobias, exam nerves, stage fright, and other anticipatory terrors

See Materia Medica, *page 144*
See also *pages 211, 224–25, 226–27, 254–55*

GLONOINUM
Trinitrum

KEY USES
◆ Heat exhaustion
◆ High blood pressure, especially in the elderly
◆ Hot flushes during menopause
◆ Severe headaches, accompanied by great confusion and a compulsion to hold the head and squeeze it

See Materia Medica, *page 170*
See also *page 275*

GNAPHALIUM
Gnaphalium polycephalum

KEY USES
- Foul-smelling diarrhea with colic
- Intense sciatic pains alternating with or followed by numbness
- Joint pains and rheumatic complaints
- Lumbago with numbness and heaviness in the affected area
- Scanty menstrual periods

See Materia Medica, *page 144*

GRANATUM
Punica granatum

KEY USE
- Expulsion of tapeworms

See Materia Medica, *pages 160–61*

GRAPHITES
Graphites

KEY USES
- Anxiety and shyness
- Digestive disorders
- Erectile problems
- Eye, ear, and nose conditions
- Menstrual problems
- Skin and nail conditions

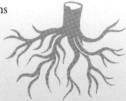

See Materia Medica, *page 83*
See also *pages 194, 195, 200, 201, 211, 212, 226–27, 240–41*

GRATIOLA
Gratiola officinalis

KEY USES
- Gastrointestinal problems, such as cramps in the pit of the stomach
- High sex drive, frequent masturbation, and nymphomania
- Migraines
- Sciatica

See Materia Medica, *pages 144–45*

GUAIACUM
Guaiacum officinale

KEY USES
- Arthritic or rheumatic joint pains, especially in the wrists
- Arthritic pains associated with swelling, tension, and tautness in the muscles
- Growing pains

See Materia Medica, *page 145*

HAMAMELIS
Hamamelis virginiana

KEY USES
- Hemorrhaging, such as heavy menstrual periods or nosebleeds
- Hemorrhoids
- Varicose veins

See Materia Medica, *page 145*
See also *pages 230–31, 238–39*

HECLA
Hecla lava

KEY USES
- Bone disorders, such as exostosis and osteitis
- Glandular swellings, especially in the neck
- Osteosarcoma and sarcoma, especially in the jaw, head, or legs
- Toothaches

See Materia Medica, *page 145*
See also *page 209*

HELLEBORUS
Helleborus niger

KEY USES
- Brain inflammation
- Depression
- Digestive disorders
- Headaches
- Nervous system disorders

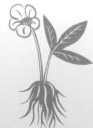

See Materia Medica, *page 55*

HELONIAS
Chamaelirium luteum

KEY USES
- Edema following uterine prolapse
- Suppressed menstruation
- Women's problems accompanied by severe fatigue

See Materia Medica, *page 135*

293

HEPAR SULF.
Hepar sulfuris calcareum

KEY USES
- Colds and phlegm
- Coughs and croup
- Digestive disorders
- Skin conditions
- Sore throat

See Materia Medica, *page 84*
See also *pages 194, 222–23, 226–27, 240–41, 250–51*

HYDRASTIS
Hydrastis canadensis

KEY USES
- Abnormal taste in the mouth
- Cancers of the liver, colon, or breast
- Phlegm
- Sinusitis
- Sore throat
- Stomach problems

See Materia Medica,
pages 147–48
See also *pages 226–27*

HYDROCOTYLE
Centella asiatica

KEY USES
- Excessive skin thickening, swelling, and distortion, like that occurring in elephantiasis
- Leprosy with no ulceration
- Lupus
- Psoriasis, with thickening and hardening of the affected area

See Materia Medica, *pages 134–35*

HYOSCYAMUS
Hyoscyamus niger

KEY USES
- Behavioral problems
- Coughs
- Delirium
- Paranoia

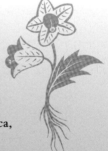

See Materia Medica,
page 56
See also *page 187*

HYPERICUM
Hypericum perforatum

KEY USES
- Injuries or wounds that feel more painful than they appear
- Nervous pains in phantom limbs after amputation
- Pain relief following operations, accidents, puncture wounds, and animal bites
- Tetanus prevention
- Toothaches or discomfort after dental treatment

See Materia Medica, *page 148*

IGNATIA
Ignatia amara

KEY USES
- Absent periods
- Digestive disorders
- Grief and distress
- Headaches
- Insomnia
- Phobias and fainting
- Sore throat

See Materia Medica, *page 57*
See also *pages 211, 212, 213, 234–35, 244–45, 256–57, 260–61, 275*

IODUM
Iodum

KEY USES
- Blockages in the eustachian tube
- Coughs
- Eating disorders
- Heat intolerance
- Overactive metabolism
- Prostate problems
- Respiratory illnesses
- Rheumatoid arthritis

See Materia Medica, *page 86*
See also *pages 197, 202, 222–23*

IPECAC.
Cephaelis ipecacuanha

KEY USES
- Asthma
- Coughs and wheezing
- Gynecological problems
- Migraines
- Morning sickness
- Nausea and vomiting

See Materia Medica, *page 45*
See also *pages 181, 236–37, 262–63*

IRIDIUM MET.
Iridium metallicum

KEY USES
- Exhaustion and anemia following a bout of illness
- Lameness or partial paralysis, particularly in the elderly
- Muscle pain and stiffness, with tender, swollen joints
- Neuralgic and sciatic nerve pains
- Suppurating abscesses in the armpits

See Materia Medica, *page 148*

IRIS

Iris versicolor

KEY USES
- Digestive disorders, such as nausea, severe diarrhea, and cholera
- Headaches and migraines

See Materia Medica, *page 148*

JUNIPER

Juniperus communis

KEY USES
- Menstrual pain
- Uterine muscle stimulant
- Water retention, possibly with advanced kidney disease

See Materia Medica, *pages 148–49*

KALI ARS.

Kalium arsenicosum

KEY USES
- Asthma
- Chronic skin conditions, such as eczema, psoriasis, acne, or ulcers
- Skin cancer
- Ulcerous varicose veins on the legs

See Materia Medica, *page 149*

KALI BICH.

Kalium bichromicum

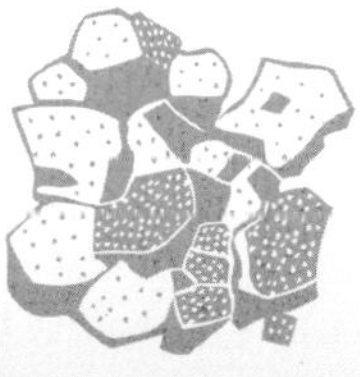

KEY USES
- Glue ear
- Headaches
- Indigestion
- Joint pains
- Phlegm and sinusitis
- Rheumatoid arthritis
- Skin conditions
- Sore throat, coughs, and croup

See Materia Medica, *page 87*
See also *pages 197, 226–27, 250–51*

KALI BROM.

Kalium bromatum

KEY USES
- Excessive sexual needs or impotence in men
- Ovarian cysts, tumors, or fibroids
- Psychosis, mania, paranoia, autism, or retardation
- Skin complaints, such as rosacea
- Stroke, epilepsy, or other seizures

See Materia Medica, *page 149*
See also *pages 193, 240–41*

KALI CARB.

Kalium carbonicum

KEY USES
- Asthma
- Coughs, whooping cough, and colds
- Incontinence
- Insomnia
- Joint or back pains, or osteoarthritis
- Kidney disorders
- Palpitations

See Materia Medica, *page 88*
See also *pages 181, 186, 196, 205, 250–51, 268–69*

KALI IOD.

Kalium iodatum

KEY USES
- Chronic phlegm or recurring sinusitis
- Copious and watery discharges, possibly with chronic allergic rhinitis
- Swellings, abscesses, or atrophy of the glands

See Materia Medica, *page 150*

KALI MUR.

Kalium chloratum

KEY USES
- Blockages of the eustachian tube
- Cancer
- Chronic mucus, nasal congestion, and nosebleeds
- Earaches or pains behind the ears
- Inflamed membranes or joints
- Sore throat
- Tonsillitis or swollen throat glands

See Materia Medica, *page 150*
See also *pages 209, 222–23, 226–27*

KALI NIT.

Kalium nitricum

KEY USES
- Asthma, croup, or bronchitis
- Nasal polyps, chronic irritation, phlegm, and sinusitis

See Materia Medica, *page 150*

KALI PHOS.
Kalium phosphoricum

KEY USES
- Abnormal discharges
- Back pains
- Chronic fatigue syndrome
- Excessive perspiration
- Hunger pains
- Insomnia

See Materia Medica, *page 89*

KALI SULF.
Kalium sulfuricum

KEY USES
- Asthma
- Chronic phlegm, or mucus in the nose, larynx, bronchi, or ears
- Glue ear
- Skin conditions such as eczema, psoriasis, ringworm, polyps, oily skin problems, and skin cancer

See Materia Medica, *pages 150–51*

KALMIA
Kalmia latifolia

KEY USES
- General muscle pains
- Heart disease
- Severe, sharp neuralgic pains in the muscles and joints

See Materia Medica, *page 151*

KREOSOTUM
Kreosotum

KEY USES
- Bleeding between menstrual cycles
- Candidiasis
- Disorders of the mucous membranes, especially in the vagina, cervix, and uterus
- Offensive-smelling menstrual flow

See Materia Medica, *page 151*
See also *pages 200, 248–49*

LAC CAN.
Lac caninum

KEY USES
- Breast problems
- Hypersensitivity
- Phobias
- Throat infections
- Vaginal bleeding and discharge

See Materia Medica, *page 108*

LAC DEFL.
Lac vaccinum defloratum

KEY USES
- Anemia and weakness following chronic disease
- Chronic liver disease
- Diabetes
- Headaches, especially those associated with menstruation
- Water retention related to heart disease

See Materia Medica, *page 151*

LACHESIS
Lachesis muta

KEY USES
- Heart disorders
- Poor circulation and varicose veins
- Sore throat
- Spasms and tremors
- Women's health

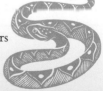

See Materia Medica, *page 109*
See also *pages 179, 186, 193, 199, 201, 212, 213, 258–59*

LACHNANTHES
Lachnanthes tinctoria

KEY USES
- Circulatory system disorders related to the head and chest
- Right-sided headaches, accompanied by great chilliness
- Tuberculosis

See Materia Medica, *page 151*

LATHYRUS
Lathyrus sativus

KEY USES
- Multiple sclerosis
- Pain in the lower back
- Total loss of sexual function
- Tremors
- Urinary incontinence
- Weakness and heaviness in the aftermath of the flu and other viral illnesses

See Materia Medica, *page 151*

LATRODECTUS MAC.
Latrodectus mactans

KEY USES
- Heart problems, especially angina
- Restlessness, particularly associated with acute angina attacks

See Materia Medica, *page 152*
See also *page 185*

LEDUM
Ledum palustre

KEY USES
- Black eyes and other eye injuries
- Bleeding into the eye chamber after an iridectomy
- Cuts and grazes
- Insect stings
- Open wounds, especially severe ones with bruising, puffy, purplish skin
- Rheumatic pains

See Materia Medica, *page 152*
See also *page 196*

LILIUM
Lilium lancifolium

KEY USES
- Depression
- Heart problems, such as angina
- Urinary disorders
- Women's health

See Materia Medica, *page 58*
See also *page 185*

LITHIUM CARB.
Lithium carbonicum

KEY USES
- Arthritic conditions
- Bones and muscles that are sore
- Distorted, swollen, tender, sore, and red joints
- Gout
- Hip pains
- Stiff limbs

See Materia Medica, *page 152*

LOBELIA
Lobelia inflata

KEY USES
- Breathlessness and asthma accompanied by great anxiety
- Nausea with giddiness
- Vomiting with profuse perspiration

See Materia Medica, *page 152*

LUPULUS
Humulus lupulus

KEY USES
- Burning in the urethra
- Delirium associated with drunkenness
- Greasy, clammy, profuse perspiration
- Hangovers with nausea, dizziness, and headaches
- Overexcitability
- Rheumatic pains
- Twitching, nervous tremors

See Materia Medica, *page 146*

LYCOPODIUM
Lycopodium clavatum

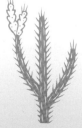

KEY USES
- Anxiety
- Chest infections
- Digestive disorders
- Urogenital problems

See Materia Medica, *page 59*
See also *pages 182, 191, 195, 196, 197, 200, 202, 203, 209, 211, 212, 218–19, 236–37, 242–43, 244–45, 264–65, 266–67*

LYCOPUS
Lycopus virginicus

KEY USES
- Overactivity of the thyroid gland, particularly during menopause
- Respiratory complaints in conjunction with heart problems
- Weak heart, erratic pulse, or heart disease

See Materia Medica, *page 153*

LYSSIN
Lyssin hydrophobinum

KEY USES
- Choking sensation when swallowing, with profuse saliva
- Excessive sexual energy
- Fear, irritability, and a desire to pass stools or urinate, triggered by sight or sound of running water
- Nervous system, throat, and sexual organ disorders, such as uterine prolapse
- Pain during sexual intercourse

See Materia Medica, *page 153*

MAG. CARB.
Magnesium carbonicum

KEY USES
- Acidity in the digestive system
- Constipation
- Diarrhea
- Exhaustion or chronic fatigue syndrome with swollen glands, lax muscles, and susceptibility to hernias

See Materia Medica, *page 153*

MAG. MUR.
Magnesium chloratum

KEY USES
- Children who are prone to digestive problems and whose parents regularly argue
- Chronic fatigue syndrome
- Digestive complaints, such as nausea, indigestion, and constipation
- Restlessness in bed
- Swollen glands

See Materia Medica, *page 153*

MAG. PHOS.
Magnesium phosphoricum

KEY USES
- Abdominal, menstrual, and other cramps
- Colic
- Earaches
- Headaches
- Neuralgia
- Toothaches

See Materia Medica, *page 90*
See also *pages 246–47, 256–57*

MAG. SULF.
Magnesium sulfuricum

KEY USES
- Dry skin
- Exhaustion or chronic fatigue
- Nausea
- Sleep problems
- Urinary disorders, possibly with digestive, skin, or menstrual problems and awkward limb movements

See Materia Medica, *page 154*

MALANDRINUM
Malandrinum

KEY USES
- Antidote to any adverse effects of a smallpox vaccination
- Dry, scaly, itchy skin with cracks or fissures
- Greasy, pustular skin eruptions
- Rough, unhealthy-looking skin

See Materia Medica, *page 154*

MANCINELLA
Hippomane mancinella

KEY USES
- Confused feelings about sexuality connected with fear of being possessed by evil spirits
- Fear of insanity and loss of mind control
- Obsessive behavior, even leading to a psychological breakdown
- Skin problems, such as dermatitis

See Materia Medica, *page 145*

MANDRAGORA
Mandragora officinarum

KEY USES
- Abdominal pains
- Congestive headaches
- Limbs that feel heavy, bruised, or sore
- Sciatica

See Materia Medica, *page 154*

MANGANUM MET.
Manganum metallicum

KEY USES
- Earaches
- Extremely sensitive bones, especially in children
- Great sensitivity to noise and wind
- Temporary reduction in hearing
- Tinnitus

See Materia Medica, *page 154*

MEDORRHINUM
Medorrhinum

KEY USES
- Genital warts and herpes
- Rhinitis, sinusitis, and asthma
- Testicular pains
- Urinary tract infections
- Women's health

See Materia Medica, *page 110*
See also *pages 197, 200*

MELILOTUS
Melilotus officinalis

KEY USES
- Circulatory problems
- Throbbing headaches

See Materia Medica, *pages 154–55*

MERC. CORR.
Hydrargyrum bichloratum

KEY USES
- Anxiety and restlessness
- Colitis
- Delirium and stupor during illness
- Dysentery
- Swollen glands
- Throat complaints, such as ulcerated tonsils

See Materia Medica, *page 146*
See also *page 190*

MERC. CYAN.
Hydrargyrum cyanatum

KEY USES
- Acute infectious diseases with rapidly sinking strength and a tendency to hemorrhage
- Throat and mouth conditions, such as diphtheria and tonsillitis

See Materia Medica, *pages 146–47*

MERC. DULC.
Hydrargyrum chloratum

KEY USES
- Agitation
- Apprehension
- Congested inflammation in the ears and eustachian tubes, leading to deafness and chronic fluid in the ear
- Restlessness

See Materia Medica, *page 146*

MERC. IOD. FLAV.
Hydrargyrum iodatum flavatum

KEY USES
- Ear infections affecting the right side
- Right-sided complaints, particularly throat infections, such as pharyngitis and tonsillitis

See Materia Medica, *page 147*

MERC. IOD. RUBER.
Hydrargyrum biiodatum

KEY USES
- Ulcerated sore throat with swollen glands and stiff muscles in the neck and throat

See Materia Medica, *page 146*

MERC. SOL.
Hydrargyrum metallicum

KEY USES
- Eye and ear infections
- Fever
- Mouth and throat conditions
- Osteoarthritis
- Phlegm and colds
- Thrush

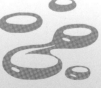

See Materia Medica, *page 85*
See also *pages 196, 200, 232–33, 250–51, 252–53, 254–55, 264–65, 268–69*

MERC. SULF.
Hydrargyrum sulfas

KEY USES
- Digestive disorders, sometimes combined with respiratory complaints
- Respiratory difficulties, such as pains in the chest and rapid breathing

See Materia Medica, *page 147*

MEZEREUM
Daphne mezereum

KEY USES
- Anxiety-related digestive system disorders
- Neuralgic pains around the teeth or face, and pains in the long bones
- Shingles affecting the chest
- Suppurating skin complaints, such as eczema and psoriasis

See Materia Medica, *page 140*
See also *page 194*

MILLEFOLIUM
Achillea millefolium

KEY USES
- Bleeding from injuries, internal bleeding, or menstrual irregularities
- Congestion in the ears, eyes, nose, and chest
- Profuse, painful uterine bleeding following childbirth or an abortion
- Severe colicky pain, diarrhea, or painful varicose veins, during pregnancy
- Sore nipples and suppressed breast milk after childbirth

See Materia Medica, *page 118*

MOSCHUS
Moschus moschiferus

KEY USES
- Fainting triggered by the slightest excitement, or by eating, menstruation, or heart disease
- General coldness or a chill in a specific area of the body
- Heightened physical and mental tension, which may cause spasms, twitches, and seizures in the muscles
- Hiccups

See Materia Medica, *page 155*

MUREX
Murex purpurea

KEY USES
- Digestive problems in women
- Intense premenstrual and menstrual pain
- Painful breasts, perhaps developing benign tumors

See Materia Medica, *page 155*

MURIATIC AC.
Acidum hydrochloricum

KEY USES
- Chronic fatigue syndrome
- Weakness or physical collapse after feverish illness, such as infectious mononucleosis or typhoid

See Materia Medica, *page 119*

MYGALE LAS.
Mygale lasiodora

KEY USES
- Chorea
- Twitching, convulsive movements, possibly accompanied by nausea, dimmed vision, and heart palpitations

See Materia Medica, *page 156*

NAJA
Naja naja

KEY USES
- Angina
- Erratic pulse
- Heart valve abnormalities
- Violent palpitations

See Materia Medica, *page 156*

NAT. ARS.
Natrum arsenicum

KEY USES
- Complaints associated with the chest, involving breathlessness, a dry, hacking cough, great sensitivity to smoke or dust, and restlessness

See Materia Medica, *page 156*

NAT. CARB.
Natrum carbonicum

KEY USES
- Colds, phlegm, and headaches
- Depression
- Digestive disorders
- Exhaustion
- Infertility
- Phobias
- Skin conditions and allergies

See Materia Medica, *page 91*
See also *pages 203, 207, 211, 212*

NAT. FLUOR.
Natrum fluoricum

KEY USES
- Aversion to sour-tasting things
- Cold sweats in the armpits
- Desire for alcohol
- Right-sided complaints

See Materia Medica, *page 156*

NAT. MUR.
Natrum chloratum

KEY USES
- Colds and mucus
- Digestive disorders
- Headaches and migraines
- Mouth and throat conditions
- Skin conditions
- Women's health

See Materia Medica, *page 92*

See also *pages 179, 186, 196, 205, 207, 212, 213, 218–19, 220–21, 224–25, 226–27, 232–33, 242–43*

NAT. PHOS.
Natrum phosphoricum

KEY USES
- Digestive disorders characterized by excess acidity and sour discharges
- Failure to thrive, in bottle-fed babies

See Materia Medica, *pages 156–57*

NAT. SULF.
Natrum sulfuricum

KEY USES
- Asthma
- Headaches caused by injury or those accompanied by increased salivation or strong intolerance to light
- Liver conditions, such as hepatitis and gallstones, colicky abdominal pains, and jaundice
- Severe or suicidal depression

See Materia Medica, *page 157*

NITRIC AC.
Acidum nitricum

KEY USES
- Anal fissures
- Cancer
- Candidiasis
- Hemorrhoids
- Mouth ulcers
- Phlegm
- Skin conditions
- Warts

See Materia Medica, *page 70*

See also *pages 200, 209*

NUX MOSCH.
Myristica fragrans

KEY USES
- Chronic constipation with fullness and bloating in the abdomen
- Confusion, dizziness, and fainting
- Dry tongue that sticks to the roof of the mouth
- Great drowsiness
- Loss of coordination
- Unquenchable thirst

See Materia Medica, *page 156*

NUX VOMICA
Strychnos nux-vomica

KEY USES
- Asthma
- Colds and the flu
- Cystitis
- Digestive disorders
- Headaches
- Irritability and insomnia
- Menstrual or pregnancy problems

See Materia Medica, *page 63*

See also *pages 186, 187, 189, 190, 200, 202, 207, 212, 213, 218–19, 224–25, 234–35, 236–37, 238–39, 244–45, 260–61, 262–63, 268–69, 275*

OLEANDER
Nerium oleander

KEY USES
- Cradle cap
- Dandruff
- Eczema
- Psoriasis

See Materia Medica, *page 157*

See also *page 194*

ONOSMODIUM
Onosmodium virginianum

KEY USES
- Exhaustion, characterized by trembling, a sensation of heaviness, and lack of coordination, possibly combined with diminished or absent sexual desire
- Eyestrain

See Materia Medica, *page 158*

OPIUM
Papaver somniferum

KEY USES
- Constipation
- Delirium tremens
- Grief
- Insomnia and narcolepsy
- Poststroke paralysis
- Shock and injury

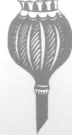

See Materia Medica, *page 60*

See also *pages 187, 213*

ORIGANUM
Origanum majorana

KEY USES
- Women's sexual problems involving obsession with sexual thoughts, restlessness, and swollen, itchy, and painful breasts

See Materia Medica, *page 158*

OXALIC AC.
Acidum oxalicum

KEY USES
- Angina with palpitations that are worse when lying down
- Pain in the spermatic cord
- Throbbing, crushing pain in the testes

See Materia Medica, *page 120*

PAEONIA
Paeonia officinalis

KEY USES
- Nightmares, especially those involving ghosts
- Rectal and anal problems, such as fissures and hemorrhoids

See Materia Medica, *page 158*

PALLADIUM MET.
Palladium metallicum

KEY USES
- Abdominal infections
- Head and limb pains, accompanied by irritability and impatience
- Ovarian pains and cysts, especially in the right side of the body
- Prolapsed or displaced uterus
- Sprained limbs
- Tired, cold, or tense limbs

See Materia Medica, *page 158*

PANAX GINSENG
Panax pseudoginseng

KEY USES
- Fatigue as a result of excessive sexual intercourse
- Paralytic weakness
- Rheumatic pain
- Sciatica

See Materia Medica, *page 159*

PAREIRA
Pareira brava

KEY USES
- Kidney colic
- Prostate disorders, such as an enlarged prostate gland
- Urinary disorders, involving painful urination, and severe pains on the left side of the lower back, and in the penis

See Materia Medica, *page 159*

PASSIFLORA
Passiflora incarnata

KEY USES
- Alcoholism
- Insomnia accompanied by hemorrhoids, pain in the coccyx, or discomfort during or just before menstruation
- Screaming children
- Whooping cough

See Materia Medica, *page 159*

PETROLEUM
Petroleum rectificatum

KEY USES
- Chilblains (cold sensitivity)
- Diarrhea and nausea
- Eczema and psoriasis
- Migraines
- Motion sickness

See Materia Medica, *page 93*
See also *page 195*

PHOSPHORIC AC.
Acidum phosphoricum

KEY USES
- Chronic fatigue syndrome
- Diabetes
- Diarrhea
- Exam nerves
- Exhaustion
- Grief or shock
- Growing pains
- Headaches

See Materia Medica, *page 71*
See also *pages 191, 205, 213*

PHOSPHORUS
Phosphorus

KEY USES
- Bleeding
- Burning pains
- Digestive disorders
- Palpitations
- Poor circulation
- Respiratory illnesses

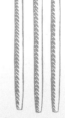

See Materia Medica, *page 94*

See also *pages 179, 181, 182, 183, 186, 190, 191, 199, 209, 211, 213, 228–29, 234–35, 236–37, 244–45, 266–67*

PHYTOLACCA
Phytolacca americana

KEY USES
- Breast problems
- Infectious mononucleosis
- Inflamed neck glands and tonsils
- Mumps
- Psoriasis

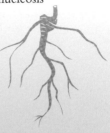

See Materia Medica, *page 159*

See also *pages 195, 201, 252–53, 254–55*

PICRIC AC.
Acidum picrinicum

KEY USES
- Indifference with mental and physical fatigue, which may develop into actual paralysis

See Materia Medica, *page 120*

PLANTAGO
Plantago major

KEY USES
- Bed-wetting problems
- Earaches
- Toothaches

See Materia Medica, *page 160*

PLATINA
Platinum metallicum

KEY USES
- Depression
- Head and facial pains
- Menstrual problems
- Numbness and cramps
- Oversensitivity of the female genitalia

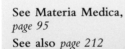

See Materia Medica, *page 95*

See also *page 212*

PLUMBUM MET.
Plumbum metallicum

KEY USES
- Constipation
- Diabetes
- Dupuytren's contracture
- Multiple sclerosis
- Muscle weakness
- Neurological conditions
- Vaginismus

See Materia Medica, *page 96*

See also *pages 179, 191, 260–61*

PODOPHYLLUM
Podophyllum peltatum

KEY USES
- Abdominal cramps
- Diarrhea
- Gastroenteritis
- Liver problems

See Materia Medica, *page 160*

PSORINUM
Psorinum

KEY USES
- Depression
- Diarrhea
- Ear and eye infections
- Phobias
- Respiratory illnesses
- Skin problems, such as rosacea and severe eczema

See Materia Medica, *page 111*

See also *pages 193, 194, 211, 268–69*

PULSATILLA
Pulsatilla pratensis subsp. *nigricans*

KEY USES
- Colds and coughs
- Digestive disorders
- Eye infections
- Sinusitis
- Women's health

See Materia Medica, *page 61*

See also *pages 183, 189, 196, 201, 202, 207, 212, 213, 218–19, 220–21, 222–23, 226–27, 228–29, 230–31, 234–35, 236–37, 240–41, 252–53, 256–57, 262–63, 275*

PYROGEN.
Pyrogenium

KEY USES
- Fevers, for example during menstruation
- Flu
- Genital tract infections following childbirth or an abortion
- Infections
- Pelvic infections in women
- Red-streaked skin
- Septic states, such as abscesses that never fully heal

See Materia Medica, *page 161*

QUERCUS
Quercus robur

KEY USES
- Acute alcohol poisoning
- Chronic spleen disorders, such as an enlarged spleen caused by recurrent malaria or alcoholism
- Recurrent gout
- Reduction in desire for alcohol

See Materia Medica, *page 161*

RADIUM BROM.
Radium bromatum

KEY USES
- Acute rheumatic pains
- Conditions arising from radiation poisoning or treatment, such as ulcers from X-ray burns
- Neuralgic pains
- Psoriasis, eczema, dermatitis, acne rosacea, skin blemishes, or moles
- Skin cancer

See Materia Medica, *page 161*

RANUNCULUS BULB.
Ranunculus bulbosus

KEY USES
- Muscle, joint, and skin problems, possibly occurring simultaneously

See Materia Medica, *page 161*

RAPHANUS
Raphanus sativus var. niger

KEY USES
- Extreme abdominal distension
- Postoperative pain

See Materia Medica, *page 162*

RHEUM
Rheum officinale

KEY USES
- Chronic diarrhea, with yellow or green, frothy or fermented stools that are sour-smelling
- Colicky pain, often accompanied by shivering and an urge to pass stools
- Nausea

See Materia Medica, *page 162*

RHODODENDRON
Rhododendron chrysanthum

KEY USES
- Hydrocele
- Joint problems, such as gout, arthritis, or rheumatic pain

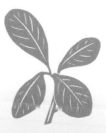

See Materia Medica, *page 162*
See also *pages 264–65*

RHUS TOX.
Rhus toxicodendron

KEY USES
- Musculoskeletal problems, such as cramps, sprains, strains, restless legs, rheumatic or arthritic pains, and sciatica
- Skin conditions, such as chicken pox, shingles, herpes, rosacea, eczema, or diaper rash
- Skin eruptions with blisters

See Materia Medica, *pages 162–63*
See also *pages 187, 193, 194, 197, 218–19, 230–31, 246–47, 252–53, 273*

RHUS VEN.
Rhus venenata

KEY USES
- Flaking, itching skin, possibly with patches of thickening or hardening, and a tendency for the skin to crack

See Materia Medica, *page 163*

RICINUS
Ricinus communis

KEY USES
◆ Diarrhea, especially in children
◆ Nausea and profuse vomiting

See Materia Medica, *page 163*

RUMEX CRISPUS
Rumex crispus

KEY USES
◆ Asthma
◆ Whooping cough, dry, tickling coughs, croup, or other hard, hacking coughs

See Materia Medica, *page 163*

RUTA
Ruta graveolens

KEY USES
◆ Chronic arthritis
◆ Eyestrain
◆ Sprains and strains, especially repetitive strain injuries
◆ Stiff, sore lower back or sciatica

See Materia Medica, *pages 163–64*
See also *pages 220–21, 273*

SABADILLA
Schoenocaulon officinale

KEY USES
◆ Inflammation of the respiratory mucous membranes, possibly due to hay fever, asthma, tonsillitis, or a cold

See Materia Medica, *page 164*

SABAL
Serenoa repens

KEY USES
◆ Genitourinary disorders, such as frequent urination, urine retention as a result of prostate enlargement, gonorrhea, or inflammation of the seminal tubes
◆ Sexual and general fatigue

See Materia Medica, *page 166*
See also *page 202*

SABINA
Juniperus sabina

KEY USES
◆ Genital warts
◆ Infertility
◆ Itching, burning external genitalia
◆ Phimosis, swelling of the upper penis, and gonorrhea
◆ Uterine problems, such as pale red, clotting hemorrhages

See Materia Medica, *page 149*
See also *page 203*

SALICYLIC AC.
Acidum salicylicum

KEY USES
◆ Ear problems, especially tinnitus, vertigo, and progressive deafness
◆ Physical weakness
◆ Severe headaches
◆ Ulceration of the mucous membranes, such as mouth ulcers

See Materia Medica, *page 120*
See also *pages 222–23*

SAMBUCUS
Sambucus nigra

KEY USES
◆ Asthma
◆ Bronchitis
◆ Croup
◆ Whooping cough

See Materia Medica, *page 164*

SANGUINARIA
Sanguinaria canadensis

KEY USES
◆ Asthma
◆ Hay fever

See Materia Medica, *page 164*

SANICULA
Aqua sanicula

KEY USES
- Digestive symptoms, involving bloating, sour burps, and an urge to pass stools after eating
- Low vitality due to slow digestion and undernourishment
- Menstrual disorders

See Materia Medica, *page 125*

SARSAPARILLA
Smilax officinalis

KEY USES
- Urinary tract problems, such as cystitis, characterized by a constant urge to urinate, pain as urination ends, and possibly blood in the urine

See Materia Medica, *page 166*

SCORPION
Scorpio europaeus

KEY USES
- Great fears, especially those of driving and of accidents, rooted in the abdomen, and possibly with sharp cramps below the ribs

See Materia Medica, *page 164*

SCUTELLARIA
Scutellaria laterifolia

KEY USES
- Chronic fatigue syndrome
- Headaches with possible dizziness, twitching muscles, and sensitivity to light
- Nervous exhaustion, possibly as a result of illness, continuous, tiring work, or overstudying

See Materia Medica, *page 165*

SECALE
Secale cornutum

KEY USES
- Flows of watery blood between menstrual periods
- Hypercontraction of the muscles in the uterus
- Menstrual cramps
- Puerperal sepsis
- Uterine bleeding
- Weak contractions during labor

See Materia Medica, *page 165*

SELENIUM MET.
Selenium metallicum

KEY USES
- Chronic fatigue syndrome
- Great weakness, especially if the body temperature increases
- Multiple sclerosis

See Materia Medica, *page 165*
See also *page 202*

SENECIO
Senecio aureus

KEY USES
- Appetite loss
- Bleeding in congested and inflamed kidneys
- Bleeding in the lungs or the throat
- Excitability
- Insomnia
- Menstrual problems
- Nosebleeds

See Materia Medica, *page 165*

SENEGA
Polygala senega

KEY USES
- Chest and phlegmy conditions, such as bronchitis, tuberculosis (especially in the elderly), and coughs

See Materia Medica, *page 160*

SEPIA
Sepia officinalis

KEY USES
- Digestive disorders
- Fatigue
- Headaches
- Phlegm
- Poor circulation
- Skin conditions
- Women's health

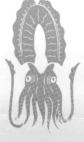

See Materia Medica, *page 112*
See also *pages 186, 195, 196, 199, 203, 211, 212, 242–43, 256–57, 258–59, 260–61*

SILICA

Silicea terra

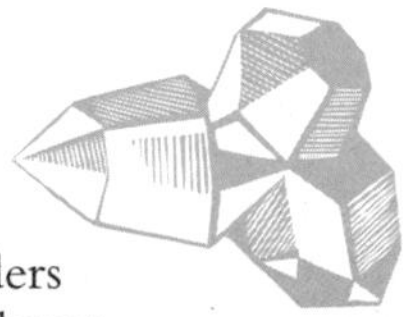

KEY USES
- Coughs
- Diabetes
- Digestive disorders
- Ear, nose, and throat problems
- Headaches
- Skin, teeth, nail, and bone conditions

See Materia Medica, *page 97*
See also *pages 191, 193, 196, 199, 201, 209, 220–21*

SINAPSIS

Brassica nigra

KEY USES
- Colds
- Hay fever
- Intense sneezing
- Pharyngitis
- Phlegm
- Sweating

See Materia Medica, *page 130*

SOLIDAGO

Solidago virgaurea

KEY USES
- Fibroids
- Kidneys that feel distended, sore, aching, and tender

See Materia Medica, *pages 166–67*

SPIGELIA

Spigelia anthelmia

KEY USES
- Headaches or migraines
- Heart murmurs or valve disorders
- Neuralgic or rheumatic pains
- Palpitations
- Rheumatic heart disease or angina
- Sinus infections

See Materia Medica, *page 167*
See also *pages 185, 197, 268–69*

SPONGIA

Euspongia officinalis

KEY USES
- Heart complaints, involving palpitations and great exhaustion
- Upper respiratory tract infections

See Materia Medica, *page 143*

SQUILLA

Urginea maritima var. *rubra*

KEY USES
- Chronic respiratory conditions, such as bronchitis (in the elderly), pleurisy, coughs, and asthma
- Measles in children

See Materia Medica, *page 170*

STANNUM MET.

Stannum metallicum

KEY USES
- Exhaustion after chronic respiratory problems
- Nervous system disorders
- Serious respiratory infections, such as bronchitis or pneumonia

See Materia Medica, *page 167*

STAPHYSAGRIA

Delphinium staphisagria

KEY USES
- Grief
- Headaches and toothaches
- Insomnia
- Joint pains
- Skin conditions, such as psoriasis
- Styes
- Urogenital problems, such as cystitis

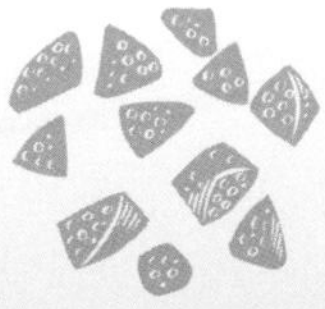

See Materia Medica, *page 54*
See also *pages 195, 213, 220–21, 260–61*

STICTA

Lobaria pulmonaria

KEY USES
- Chronic phlegm that is difficult to expel and causes stuffiness, a dull, heavy feeling in the head, and a dry, tickly throat
- Pneumonia
- Respiratory problems asssociated with hay fever or other allergic reactions, the flu, or bronchitis

See Materia Medica, *page 152*

STRAMONIUM
Datura stramonium

KEY USES
- Asthma
- Bronchitis
- Chorea
- Fever
- Phobias
- Violence and mania

See Materia Medica, *page 53*
See also *page 211*

STRONTIUM CARB.
Strontium carbonicum

KEY USES
- Acute conditions following an operation or injury, such as fainting, exhaustion, chills, violent palpitations, and collapse
- Heart conditions, including angina, phlebitis, and terrible pains in the muscles and bones

See Materia Medica, *page 167*

SULFUR
Sulfur

KEY USES
- Digestive disorders
- Men's health
- Respiratory illnesses
- Skin conditions
- Women's health

See Materia Medica, *page 99*
See also *pages 186, 190, 194, 195, 196, 201, 202, 207, 211, 212, 234–35, 240–41, 242–43, 246–47, 252–53, 258–59, 260–61, 268–69*

SULFUR IOD.
Sulfur iodatum

KEY USES
- Chronic, itchy skin complaints, such as weeping eczema, acne, boils, pustules, hives, and lichen planus

See Materia Medica, *page 168*

SULFURIC AC.
Acidum sulfuricum

KEY USES
- Diabetes
- Extreme fatigue following an injury, concussion, or operation, especially if healing is slow

See Materia Medica, *page 120*

SYMPHYTUM
Symphytum officinale

KEY USES
- Abscesses in the psoas muscle
- Eye injuries
- Malignant bone tumors on the face
- Sprains and fractured or badly set bones
- Tingling pain from old injuries to the bone, cartilage, and periosteum

See Materia Medica, *page 168*

SYPHILINUM
Syphilinum

KEY USES
- Asthma
- Constipation
- Eye inflammation
- Headaches
- Menstrual problems and miscarriages
- Obsessive-compulsive behavior
- Ulcers

See Materia Medica, *page 113*

TABACUM
Nicotiana tabacum

KEY USES
- Acute digestive upsets, especially during pregnancy or chemotherapy
- Diarrhea or habitual constipation with rectal paralysis or spasms
- Motion sickness
- Severe nausea

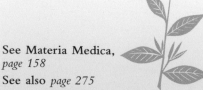

See Materia Medica, *page 158*
See also *page 275*

TARAXACUM
Taraxacum officinale

KEY USES
- Digestive disorders
- Gallbladder inflammation
- Gallstones
- Headaches associated with gastric problems
- Urinary problems

See Materia Medica, *page 168*

TARENTULA
Tarentula hispanica

KEY USES
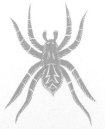
- Angina and heart disorders
- Cystitis
- Diabetes
- Mood swings
- Multiple sclerosis
- Restless limbs and chorea
- Women's health

See Materia Medica, *page 114*
See also *pages 179, 191*

TARENTULA CUB.
Tarentula cubensis

KEY USES
- Acute infections such as diphtheria
- Pain relief during a slow death
- Septic conditions, such as carbuncles, septicemia, painful abscesses, ulcers, and gangrene
- Severe coughs, such as whooping cough, if there is great prostration
- Slow-developing fever

See Materia Medica, *pages 168–69*

TELLURIUM MET.
Tellurium metallicum

KEY USES
- Back pains
- Eye and ear infections
- Skin conditions, such as psoriasis, ringworm, herpes, and eczema on the eyelids and behind the ears

See Materia Medica, *page 169*

TEREBINTHUM
Terebinthina laricina

KEY USES
- Burning pain and bleeding of the mucous membranes
- Inflammation of the urinary tract or kidneys, accompanied by hemorrhaging, water retention, and edema in the hands and feet

See Materia Medica, *page 169*

TEUCRIUM MARUM
Teucrium marum

KEY USES
- Fibroids in the uterus
- Fibrous tumors on the eyelids
- Gonorrhea
- Intestinal worms
- Polyps of the nose, ears, vagina, and rectum

See Materia Medica, *page 169*

THEA
Camellia sinensis

KEY USES
- Extreme forms of behavior in children and adults, including irritability, mental restlessness, violent impulses, and psychiatric problems
- Indigestion
- Insomnia
- Overactive nervous system
- Palpitations or other heart problems

See Materia Medica, *page 133*

THERIDION
Theridion curassavicum

KEY USES
- Acute sensitivity of the bones, nerves, and spine
- Diabetes

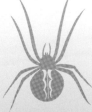

See Materia Medica, *page 169*
See also *pages 191, 266–67*

THLASPI
Capsella bursa-pastoris

KEY USES
- Fibroids
- Hemorrhaging, especially during pregnancy, causing great pain
- Nosebleeds during pregnancy
- Violent cramping in the uterus, associated with hemorrhaging, between menstrual periods, during pregnancy, following labor, or after a miscarriage or abortion

See Materia Medica, *page 133*

THUJA
Thuja occidentalis

KEY USES
- Catarrh (phlegm) and sinusitis
- Headaches
- Menstrual problems
- Skin conditions
- Urogenital problems

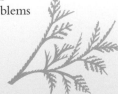

See Materia Medica, *page 64*
See also *pages 202, 212, 242–43*

TUBERCULINUM
Tuberculinum Koch

KEY USES
- Allergies
- Arthritic pains
- Colds
- Coughs and acute bronchitis
- Hay fever
- Neurotic behavior

See Materia Medica, *page 115*
See also *page 207*

URANIUM NIT.
Uranium nitricum

KEY USES
- Diabetes with water retention and increased urination
- Digestive disorders, such as indigestion, bloating, and abdominal gas
- High blood pressure
- Kidney inflammation
- Liver problems

See Materia Medica, *page 170*
See also *page 191*

URTICA URENS
Urtica urens

KEY USES
- Blistering, burning, stinging, red rashes caused by insect bites, stings, shellfish, and plants
- Burnt, blistered skin
- Swollen or itchy skin eruptions
- Urticaria

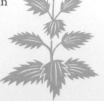

See Materia Medica, *page 170*
See also *pages 242–43, 273*

USTILAGO
Ustilago zeae

KEY USES
- Slow, congestive bleeding following miscarriage or labor
- Women's problems, such as uterine fibroids

See Materia Medica, *page 171*

UVA URSI
Arctostaphylos uva-ursi

KEY USES
- Chronic bladder irritation
- Digestive, respiratory, or childbirth symptoms accompanying a urinary disorder
- Enlarged prostate gland
- Inflammation and stones in the kidneys

See Materia Medica, *page 125*

VALERIANA
Valeriana officinalis

KEY USES
- Neuralgic pains, rapid pulse, and blood congestion in the head

See Materia Medica, *page 171*

VERATRUM ALB.
Veratrum album

KEY USES
- Collapse
- Diarrhea
- Emotional problems
- Vomiting and nausea
- Weakness and fainting

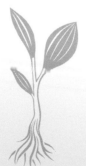

See Materia Medica, *page 65*

VERATRUM VIR.
Veratrum viride

KEY USES
- Asthma
- Intense fever
- Manic behavior
- Pleurisy
- Pneumonia
- Puerperal fever

See Materia Medica, *page 171*

VERBASCUM
Verbascum thapsiforme

KEY USES
- Coughs
- Irritation and inflammation of the bladder, ears, or respiratory tract
- Neuralgic pains in the face and teeth
- Painful colds

See Materia Medica, *page 171*
See also *pages 268–69*

VESPA
Vespa crabro

KEY USES
- Constipation
- Disorders of the female reproductive organs
- Mucous membrane problems
- Premenstrual depression
- Red, swollen skin complaints, such as boils, itchy bumps, weals, and lentil-shaped spots
- Stinging, burning pains

See Materia Medica, *page 171*

VIBURNUM
Viburnum opulus

KEY USES
- False labor
- Painful menstruation
- Pains following labor
- Recurrent miscarriage
- Threatened abortion

See Materia Medica, *page 172*

VINCA
Vinca minor

KEY USES
- Burning leg ulcers
- Cradle cap
- Excessive menstrual flow
- Itchy, burning skin
- Warm scalp with foul-smelling eruptions and corrosive itching
- Weeping eczema

See Materia Medica, *page 172*

VIOLA TRI.
Viola tricolor

KEY USES
- Obstinate skin problems, such as impetigo, rashes, eczema, rosacea, and pustular eruptions
- Urinary problems, such as sharp pains in the urethra and bed-wetting at night

See Materia Medica, *page 172*
See also *page 193*

VIPERA
Vipera berus

KEY USES
- Phlebitis
- Recurrent nosebleeds
- Varicose veins

See Materia Medica, *page 172*

VISCUM ALB.
Viscum album

KEY USES
- Generalized tremors and uncontrollable jerking after a fright
- Neuralgic pains, especially headaches
- Seizures including petit mal and epilepsy that may be accompanied by breathing problems
- Tearing joint pains

See Materia Medica, *pages 172–73*

WYETHIA
Wyethia helenoides

KEY USES
- Hay fever with itching in the ears, palate, and the back of the nose, a scalding sensation in the mouth, and violent sneezing

See Materia Medica, *page 173*
See also *page 207*

ZINC. MET.
Zincum metallicum

KEY USES
- Eczema and viral skin infections
- Headaches
- Nervous exhaustion
- Twitching limbs, such as restless legs
- Urogenital problems

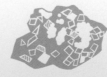

See Materia Medica, *page 101*
See also *pages 230-31*

ZINGIBER
Zingiber officinale

KEY USES
- Asthma
- Digestive disorders, including nausea, vomiting, and colicky pain in the abdomen, with chronic excess mucus production in the intestine

See Materia Medica, *page 173*

HOW TO FIND A PRACTITIONER

THERE ARE TWO KINDS of homeopathic practitioners in the US: medically and nonmedically qualified. The former are MDs who are also qualified homeopaths; they are sometimes registered with the American Institute of Homeopathy. Nonmedically qualified homeopaths are qualified as homeopaths but not as MDs. Training standards vary in this latter group, and the author recommends contacting one of the many organizations listed opposite to help ensure training standards have been met. Medically qualified homeopathic practitioners are subject to the rules of the American Medical Association (AMA), while nonmedically trained practitioners may register with one or more of the homeopathic organizations listed on the facing page and are subject to the society's code of ethics.

Personal recommendation can be an effective way of choosing a homeopath. It is often best to seek the advice of family members and friends who have visited a homeopath, or ask your physician to refer you. It may help if the homeopath then writes to your physician outlining the homeopathic treatment planned, and it is always recommended that you continue under the care of your physician. Homeopaths should freely provide information about their service and expected course of treatment. If you are not at ease with the philosophy and practice of a particular homeopath, feel free to find a different practitioner. A good homeopath should aim to establish a rapport based upon trust and empathy.

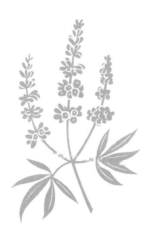

ORGANIZATIONS

The following organizations can help with finding a reputable homeopathic practitioner in a particular area:

American Association of Naturopathic Physicians
601 Valley Street, Suite 105, Seattle, WA 98109
Tel: (206) 298–0126/Fax: (206) 298–0129
E-mail: 74602.3715@compuserve.com
Online: www.naturopathic.com

American Institute of Homeopathy
801 North Fairfax Street, Suite 306, Alexandria, VA 22314
Tel: (703) 246–9501
Online: www.healthy.net/aih

Arizona Homeopathic Medical Association
Suite 300, 2525 West Greenway Road, Phoenix, AZ 85023
Tel: (602) 978–1722/Fax: (602) 942–3787

Hahnemann College of Homeopathy
80 Nicol Avenue, Point Richmond, CA 94801
Tel: (510) 412–9040/Fax: (510 412–9044

Hahnemann Medical Clinic
80 Nicol Avenue, Point Richmond, CA 94801
Tel: (510) 412–9040/Fax: (510 412–9044

Homeopathic Academy of Naturopathic Physicians
P.O. Box 12488, Portland, OR 97212
Online:www.healthy.net/pan/pa/homeopathic/hanp/index.html

Homeopathic Educational Services
2124 Kittredge Street, Berkeley, CA 94704
Tel: (510) 649–0294/Fax: (510) 649–1955
E-mail: mail@homeopathic.com
Online: www.homeopathic.com

National Center for Homeopathy
801 North Fairfax Street, Suite 306, Alexandria, VA 22314
Tel: (703) 548–7790/Fax: (703) 548–7792
E-mail: nchinfo@igc.org
Online: www.homeopathic.org

North American Society of Homeopaths
122 East Pike Street, Suite 1122, Seattle, WA 98122
Tel: (541) 345–9815
E-mail: nash@homeopathy.org
Online: www.homeopathy.org

SUPPLIERS OF HOMEOPATHIC REMEDIES

Arrowroot Standard Direct Ltd.
83 East Lancaster Avenue, Paoli, PA 19301
Tel: (800) 234–8879/Fax: (800) 296–8998
E-mail: customerservice@arrowroot.com
Online: www.arrowroot.com

Baileys
175 Harvard Avenue, Allston, MA 02134
Tel: (617) 782–7202/Fax: (617) 782–4328
E-mail: baileyspharm@juno.com
Online: www.baileyspharm.com

Biological Homeopathic Industries
11600 Cochiti SE, Albuquerque, NM 87123
Tel: (505) 293–3843/Fax: (505) 275–1672
E-mail: info@heelbhi.com
Online: www.heelbhi.com

Boericke and Tafel, Inc.
2381 Circadian Way, Santa Rosa, CA 95407
Tel: (707) 571–8202/Fax: (707) 571–8237
E-mail: bandt@sonic.net

Boiron-Bornemann Inc
Box 449, 6 Campus Avenue, Newtown Square, PA 19073
Tel: (800) BLU-TUBE/Fax: (800) 999–4373
E-mail: boiron@worldnet.att.net
Online: www.boiron.com

Dolisos America Inc.
3014 Rigel Avenue, Las Vegas, NV 89102
Tel: (800) DOLISOS/Fax: (702) 871–9670
E-mail: DolisosAm@aol.com
Online: www.plantes-et-medecines.com

Hahnemann Laboratories, Inc.
1940 Fourth Street, San Rafael, CA 94901
Tel: (800) 4 ARNICA/(415) 451–6978
Fax: (415) 451–6981
E-mail: mqremmaker@aol.com
Online: www.hahnemannlabs.com

HealthCo Northwest
170 West Ellendale, Dallas, OR 97338
Tel: (503) 831–0871/(888) 715–6398
Fax: (503) 831–0873
E-mail: dockperson@aol.com
Online: www.healthco-nw.com

King Bio Pharmaceuticals Inc.
1264 New Leicester Highway, Asheville, NC 28806
Tel: (800) 543–3245/Fax: (828) 683–2222
E-mail: orders@kingbio.com
Online: www.kingbio.com

Leicester Pharmacy
1060 Main Street, Leicester, MA 01524
Tel: (508) 892–8166/Fax: (508) 892–1896

Luyties Pharmacal Company
4200 Laclede Street, St. Louis, MO 63108
Tel: (314) 533–9600/Fax: (314) 535–9600
E-mail: luytiesstl@aol.com

Mediral International Inc.
5260 East 39th Avenue, Denver, CO 80207
Tel: (877) 633–4725/(303) 331–6161
Fax: (303) 355–4155
E-mail: info@mediral.com
Online: www.mediral.com

Newton Homeopathic Laboratories Inc.
2360 Rockaway Ind. Boulevard, Conyers, GA 30207
Tel: (800) 448–7256/(770) 922–2644
Info line: (800) NOSODE 3
Fax: (800) 760–5550/(770) 388–7768
E-mail: mailinfo@newtonlabs.net
Online: www.newtonlabs.net

Santa Monica Homeopathic Pharmacy
629 Broadway, Santa Monica, CA 90401
Tel: (310) 395–1131/Fax: (310) 395–7861
E-mail: smhomeopathic@hotmail.com
Online: www.healingedge.com/santa.html

Standard Homeopathic Company
PO Box 61067, 204–210 West 131st Street, Los Angeles, CA 90061
Tel: (800) 624–9659/Fax: (310) 516–8579
Online: www.hylands.com

BIBLIOGRAPHY

This selected listing of reference works is provided as a guide for those who are interested in learning more about the history, science, and present-day practice of homeopathy.

GENERAL

Blackie, M.
Classical Homoeopathy
(Beaconsfield Publishers, 1986)

Blackie, M.
The Challenge of Homoeopathy
(Unwin Hyman, 1985)

Boericke, W.
Materia Medica with Repertory
(Boericke & Tafel, 1927)

Castro, M.
The Complete Homeopathy Handbook: a Guide to Everyday Health Care
(Macmillan, 1995)

Clark, J. H.
Dictionary of Materia Medica
(Homoeopathic Publishing Company, 1925, 3 volumes)

Coulter, C. R.
Portraits of Homeopathic Medicines, Volume 2
(North Atlantic Books, 1988)

Coulter, C. R.
Portraits of Homeopathic Medicines, Volume 1
(North Atlantic Books, 1986)

Hahnemann, Samuel
(tr. L. H. Tafel from 2nd enlarged German edition of 1835)
The Chronic Diseases
(C. Ringer & Company, 1838, 2 volumes)

Jouanny, J.
Essentials of Homoeopathic Therapeutics
(Laboratoire Boiron, 1985)

Kent, J. T.
(eds. Chand, D. H. & Schmidt, P.)
Final General Repertory
(Natural Homoeopathic Pharmacy, 1980)

Kent, J. T.
Materia Medica
(Sinha Roy, 1970)

Lessell, C. B.
Homoeopathy for Physicians
(Thorsons, 1983)

Lockie, A.
The Family Guide to Homeopathy
(Hamish Hamilton, 1998)

Lockie, A. & Geddes, N.
The Complete Guide to Homeopathy
(Dorling Kindersley, 1995)

Morrison, R.
Desktop Guide to Keynotes and Confirmatory Symptoms
(Hahnemann Clinic Publishing, 1993)

Nash, E. D.
Leaders in Homoeopathic Therapeutics
(Boericke & Tafel, 1946)

Neatby, E. A. & Stoneham, T. G.
A Manual of Homoeopathic Therapeutics
(Staple Press, 1948)

Schroyens, F. (ed.)
Synthesis Repertorium Homoeopathicum
(Homoeopathic Book Publishers, 1995)

Shepherd, D.
A Physician's Posy
(C. W. Daniel Company, 1969)

Shepherd, D.
Magic of the Minimum Dose
(C. W. Daniel Company, 1964)

Tyler, M. L.
Homoeopathic Drug Pictures
(C. W. Daniel Company, 1942)

Vermeulen, F.
Concordant Materia Medica
(Emryss, 1977)

Vermeulen, F.
Synoptic Materia Medica
(Merlijn Publishers, 1992)

THEORY OF HOMEOPATHY

Bradford, D. L.
The Life and Letters of Samuel Hahnemann
(Royal Publishing House, 1970)

Campbell, A.
The Two Faces of Homoeopathy
(Robert Hale, 1984)

Gaier, H.
Thorsons Encyclopedic Dictionary of Homoeopathy
(Thorsons, 1991)

Hael, R.
Samuel Hahnemann: his Life and Works
(Homoeopathic Publishing Company, 1922, 2 volumes)

Hahnemann, Samuel
(tr. Künzli, J., Naude, A., & Pendleton, P.)
The Organon of Medicine
(Gollancz, 1986)

Hobhouse, R. W.
The Life of Samuel Hahnemann
(World Homoeopathic Links, 1984)

Kent, J. T.
Lectures on Homoeopathic Philosophy
(Erhart & Carl, 1937)

Livingstone, R.
Evergreen Medicine
(Asher Asher, 1991)

Pelikan, W.
The Secrets of Metals
(Anthroposophic Press, 1973)

Roberts, A. H.
The Principles and Art of Cure by Homoeopathy
(Homoeopathic Publishing Company, 1936)

Scholten, J.
Homoeopathy and Minerals
(Stichting Alonissos, 1996)

Ullman, D.
Homoeopathy: Medicine for the 21st Century
(Thorsons, 1989)

Vannier, L.
Typology in Homoeopathy
(Beaconsfield Publishers, 1992)

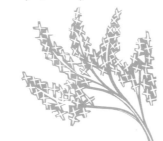

Vithoulkas, G.
Homoeopathy: Medicine of the New Man
(Thorsons, 1985)

Wheeler, C. E.
*The Principles and Practice
of Homoeopathy*
(Heinemann, 1940)

Whitmount, E. C.
The Alchemy of Healing
(North Atlantic Books, 1993)

Whitney, J.
*Vitalistic Medicine from Ancient Egypt
to the 21st Century*
(Open Doors Books, 1998)

HOMEOPATHY
& COMPLEMENTARY MEDICINE

Bach, Edward
Heal Thyself
(C. W. Daniel Company, 1978)

Bach, Edward
The Twelve Healers and Other Remedies
(C. W. Daniel Company, 1973)

Bown, D.
*The Royal Horticultural Society
Encyclopedia of Herbs*
(Dorling Kindersley, 1995)

Chevalier, A.
The Encyclopedia of Medicinal Plants
(Dorling Kindersley, 1996)

Day, C.
*The Homoeopathic Treatment of
Small Animals*
(C. W. Daniel Company, 1990)

**Foundation for Integrated
Medicine**
*Integrated Healthcare – A Way Forward
for the Next Five Years?*
(Foundation for Integrated
Medicine, 1998)

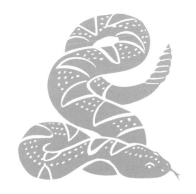

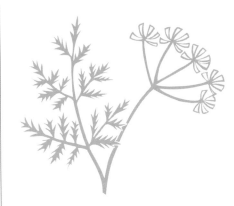

Gilbert, P.
*A Doctor's Guide to Helping Yourself
with Biochemic Tissue Salts*
(Thorsons, 1984)

Grossinger, R.
Plant Medicine
(North Atlantic Books, 1990)

Murray, M. & Pizzorno, J.
Encyclopedia of Natural Medicine
(Optima, 1990)

Newman-Turner, R.
Naturopathic Medicine
(Thorsons, 1984)

Ody, P.
*The Herb Society's Complete
Medicinal Herbal*
(Dorling Kindersley, 1993)

Polunin, M. & Robbins, C.
The Natural Pharmacy
(Dorling Kindersley, 1992)

Sharma, R.
*The Element Family Encyclopaedia
of Health*
(Element, 1998)

Tisserand, R.
The Art of Aromatherapy
(C. W. Daniel Company, 1977)

Vincent, C. & Furnham, A.
*Complementary Medicine: a Research
Perspective*
(Wiley, 1997)

SELF-HELP

Cummings, S. & Ullman, D.
*Everybody's Guide to Homoeopathic
Medicines: Taking Care of Yourself
and Your Family with Safe and
Effective Remedies*
(Tarcher, 1997)

Panos, M. B. & Heimlich, J.
Homoeopathic Medicine at Home
(Corgi, 1980)

Pratt, N.
Homoeopathic Prescribing
(Beaconsfield Publishers, 1980)

Sharma, C.
*A Manual of Homoeopathy and
Natural Medicine*
(Turnstone Press, 1975)

Stevenson, J. H.
*Helping Yourself with Homoeopathic
Remedies*
(Thorsons, 1976)

HOMEOPATHY FOR WOMEN

Jahr, G. H. G.
Diseases of Females
(Bhatta-Charrya & Company, 1939)

Lockie, A. & Geddes, N.
The Women's Guide to Homoeopathy
(Hamish Hamilton, 1992)

Yingling, W. A.
The Accoucher's Emergency Manual
(Set, Dey & Company, 1936)

HOMEOPATHY FOR CHILDREN

Herscu, P.
The Homeopathic Treatment of Children
(North Atlantic Books, 1991)

HOMEOPATHY & FIRST AID

Gibson, D. H.
*First Aid Homeopathy in Accidents
and Ailments*
(British Homoeopathic Association,
1982)

Tyler, M. L. & Weir, J.
Acute Conditions, Injuries, etc.
(British Homoeopathic Association,
1932)

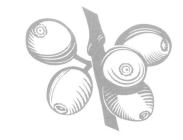

INDEX

Page numbers in **bold** type indicate the main entries for remedies and ailments. Names in *italic* denote Latin names of homeopathic remedies. **Bold** names identify the main alphabetic entries for remedies by their common remedy names, with cross-references from those names to the Latin remedy names as necessary.

A

S

ACKNOWLEDGMENTS

AUTHOR'S ACKNOWLEDGMENTS

First and foremost I am deeply indebted to Serena Scrine R. S. Hom. for all her help in writing this book. She has gone far beyond her original role as researcher, helping to shape the book from the outset. Without her energy, encouragement, and vision, I am sure this book would not have turned out so well.

I am most grateful to John Morgan of Helios Pharmacy and to the British Homeopathic Association, particularly Enid Segall, who so kindly helped me through the nomenclature crisis.

I would also like to thank Barbara Lockie for her understanding, support, and research, as well as David, Kirsty, Alistair, and Sandy for their research and encouragement.

Thanks also go to Dennis and Mary Thompson for their extensive research on herbal medicine and aromatherapy oils; David Warkentin and his team for MacRepertory and Reference Works, which have proved invaluable in the writing of this book; Minerva Books for reference works; and Dragon's Health Club in Guildford for advice on physical fitness and exercise.

In addition, I would like to thank the practice staff for all their help and support, including Pat Web, Chris Donne, Claire Lindsay, Lesley Holloway, Marjorie Edmonds, and Kate Sarama who kept everything ticking over and helped with the odd bit of typing. Thanks also to Gail Hart for her magnificent slaving over a hot word processor.

Finally, thanks to my agents Lutyens and Rubinstein and everyone at Dorling Kindersley, especially Stephanie Farrow and Jude Garlick.

Dr. Lockie can be reached at www.drlockie.com

PUBLISHERS' ACKNOWLEDGMENTS

Dorling Kindersley is very grateful to Dr. David Riley for his expert advice as consultant on the American edition of this book and would also like to thank Constance Novis, Jill Hamilton, Constance M. Robinson, Judit Bodnar, and Mary Sutherland for their editorial work on this edition.

Thanks go to Janice Anderson, Salima Hirani, Lucy Hurst, and Christa Weil for editorial help; Penelope Cream for proofreading the manuscript; and Sue Bosanko for the index. Many thanks to John Dinsdale, Phil Gilderdale, Laura Jackson, Anne Renel, Marga Ruiz, and Rachana Shah for design assistance; Nicola Cox and Conrad Van Dyk for DTP assistance; and Sarah Young for the remedy illustrations. Thanks to Anna Grapes and Jamie Robinson for picture research and all at the DK picture library, particularly Neale Chamberlaine.

Thanks to Peter Anderson, Andy Crawford, Steve Gorton, and Ian O'Leary for photography.

Special thanks to Olivia Forsey, Salima Hirani, Andrew Krag, and Bridget Roseberry for modelling.

Dorling Kindersley is particularly grateful to the following for their expert help, advice, and knowledge: Michael Bate (Weleda (UK) Ltd., Derby); Eamonn Byrne (School of Horticulture, Kew); Dr. Sue Davidson; Maurice and Janet Elliott (Old Hall Plants, Suffolk); Kate Haywood (Royal Horticultural Society, Wisley); and Tony Pinkus (Ainsworths Pharmacy, London).

Many thanks also to the following for their kind help in supplying or obtaining equipment, plants, or materials for photography: Barwinnock Herbs (Ayrshire); Bob and Liz Farrow; John Hamer; Jeff Hope (Torz & Macatonia, London); Christopher Jackson; Anthony Lymon Dixon (Arne Herbs, Bristol); Tim Pitt; Jane Seppings (Winter Flora Ltd., Suffolk); and Richard Tayler.

PICTURE CREDITS

The publisher would like to thank the following for their kind permission to reproduce their photographs:

a = above; c = centre; b = below/bottom; l = left; r = right; t = top.

AKG London: 12 bl, 13 cr, 14 t, 15 tr, 16 tl, Erich Lessing 12 tr, 18 bl; **Bridgeman Art Library, London/New York**: Phillips, The International Fine Art Auctioneers 72 bl; **Bruce Coleman Ltd**: Alain Compost 50 bl; **Colorific!**: Anthony Joyce 60 bl; **Mary Evans Picture Library**: 23 tr, 51 bl, 92 bl, 105 bl, 114 bl; **Geoscience Features**: Dr B. Booth 44 tr; **Katz Pictures**: The Mansell Collection 57 bl; **Magnum**: Hiroji Kubota 217 bl; **Mark T. O'Shea**: 107 tr, 109 tr; **Royal London Homeopathic Hospital**: 17 tr; **Science Photo Library**: Jean-Loup Charmet 22 b, CNRI 115 tr, 177 cl, Custom Medical Stock Photo 113 tr, Vaughan Fleming 87 tr, NIH, Custom Medical Stock Photo 106 tr, Alfred Pasieka 110 tr, J. C. Revy 111 tr; **Seven Seas Ltd**: 90 bl; **SuperStock Ltd**: 217 br; **Telegraph Colour Library**: Adamsmith Productions 177 bl, Ancil Nance 217 tr, Paul Aresu 177 br, Stephen Simpson 177 tr; **Dana Ullman, M.P. H., Homeopathic Educational Services, US**: 17 bl, 19 tr, 20